Autonomic Nervous System and Sleep

Sudhansu Chokroverty
Pietro Cortelli
Editors

Autonomic Nervous System and Sleep

Order and Disorder

Springer

Editors
Sudhansu Chokroverty
School of Graduate Medical Education
Seton Hall University
South Orange, NJ
USA

Pietro Cortelli
IRCCS-ISNB, PADG1, Osp Bellaria - Pad G1
DIBINEM University of Bologna
Bologna
Italy

ISBN 978-3-030-62262-6 ISBN 978-3-030-62263-3 (eBook)
https://doi.org/10.1007/978-3-030-62263-3

This Springer imprint is published by the registered company Springer Nature Switzerland AG
The registered company address is: Gewerbestrasse 11, 6330 Cham, Switzerland

Foreword

In the past several decades, a great deal has been learned about sleep, the state in which human beings spend about one third of their lives. It has become evident that sleep is crucial to the normal consolidation of memories, a function so vital that perhaps it is the long-sought reason that the phenomenon of sleep has weathered the challenges of evolution. Disordered breathing during sleep is now one of the most common medical problems diagnosed in people of all ages. Abnormal sleep is a major symptom of psychiatric disorders and may contribute to the cause of exacerbations of depression and anxiety. It is also related to weight control and various endocrine functions. Unproductive sleep is a risk factor for an array of cardiac disorders, and it is a widely held hope that one might die peacefully in one's sleep. If so, we would have the connection between sleep and the heart to thank. It is becoming clear that there is virtually no system that is not impacted by sleep.

What is the interface between the protean functions of the nervous system and sleep? Clearly, this is mainly the autonomic nervous system. The autonomic nervous system has also undergone intense study since its discovery just over 100 years ago. Yet, there has never been a single volume dedicated to the relationship of the autonomic nervous system and sleep, until now. In ***Autonomic Nervous System and Sleep: Order and Disorder,*** two distinguished experts, one in sleep and the other in the autonomic nervous system, collaborated to produce and edit an authoritative tome addressing virtually every important facet of the interface between these two interlocking, largely unconscious aspects of the function of the human nervous system.

For the benefit of the newcomer, the book begins with the basics of the anatomy and physiology of the autonomic nervous system, the sleep-wakefulness network, and the control over the cardiovascular system. Part II is a review of the most important laboratory testing procedures used in the evaluation of patients suspected of harboring a disorder of sleep and/or the autonomic nervous system. The bulk of the book is in Part III, in which virtually every important clinical syndrome is reviewed in an authoritative manner. The volume editors have chosen a cast of superstars, each with deep expertise in the various disorders of the sleep–autonomic interface. The chapters are both scientifically rigorous and clinically useful, such that the book can be used either as a reference volume or a handbook, rigorously edited by Professors Chokroverty and Cortelli, such that it will be a classic that will be procured and valued by students, residents, faculty, and experts.

Martin A. Samuels, MD

Founding Chair Emeritus, Department of Neurology,
Brigham and Women's Hospital, Miriam Sydney
Joseph Distinguished Professor of Neurology,
Harvard Medical School,
Boston, MA, USA

Preface

Since its early discovery in the late nineteenth century, the autonomic nervous system (ANS), subserving a very important function of the human body along with its significance, remained largely neglected or poorly recognized by the clinicians for the next 75 years or so. It is now recognized that there is a dynamic coupling among the ANS, particularly the central autonomic network (CAN), somatic central (CNS), peripheral nervous system, and sleep-wake neurons in the CNS. Traditional thinking has been centered on the role of ANS in wakefulness, but there are profound changes in the ANS during sleep (normal sleep is now considered a vital function of human health). There is not a single textbook available describing this significant interaction between the ANS and sleep, although there are journal articles and a few scattered chapters in textbooks. It is therefore now an opportune moment to bring out this dynamic bidirectional relationship (anatomically and functionally), discussing its significance and clinical implications in a comprehensive (yet not encyclopedic) textbook. This close coupling between the ANS, sleep, and the CNS reflects a mind–body interaction during human sleep-wake states.

We, the editors, have succeeded in attracting some of the world's leading experts in the fields of autonomic and sleep medicine to contribute to this volume, which bodes well and will enhance the stature of this textbook.

The volume is divided into three broad parts: I. Basics, II. Laboratory Evaluation, and III. Clinical Aspects, addressing the order and disorder of the interaction between the ANS and sleep and capturing many of the recent advances in 30 chapters. It should be useful not only to sleep specialists and senior trainees but also to general internists, pulmonary physicians, pediatricians, family physicians, otolaryngologists, dentists , neurosurgeons, and neuroscientists interested in patients suffering from sleep and autonomic dysfunction as well as those paramedical and ancillary staff with an interest in sleep and autonomic medicine (e.g., nurses, technologists, and other healthcare workers). Finally, this book should be useful to both the beginners and those advanced in the field.

Edison, NJ, USA — Sudhansu Chokroverty, MD
Bologna, Italy — Pietro Cortelli, MD, PhD

Acknowledgments

First, we like to thank all the contributors for their scholarly and insightful writings and their patience and dedication to see the volume in production. Additionally, we wish to thank all those (authors, editors, and publishers) responsible for granting permission to reproduce illustrations, tables, and boxes that have been published previously in other books and journals. We owe a great deal to Gregory Sutorius, senior editor of clinical medicine at Springer Nature, New York, NY, for his professionalism, dedication, and commitment to see the book in print as quickly as possible. We must thank Katherine Kreilkamp at Springer whose functions included formatting, preparation of proofs, and pushing through production. We also like to thank the other dedicated staff at Springer, New York, who played a significant role in producing the book in its final format.

The senior editor (SC) wishes to thank Chelsea Reimer, editorial assistant to the *Sleep Medicine* journal, for her valiant support and dedication for organizing the table of contents, keeping an eye on the contributors for prompt revision, making corrections, editing, and typing, in addition to her major function as editorial assistant to the journal. Last but not least, the senior editor must acknowledge his wife, Manisha Chokroverty, MD, for her usual and unfailing and continued support, love, patience, and tolerance throughout the long period of writing, editing, and proof reading during the production and publication of the book.

We would like to acknowledge with gratitude Professor Martin A. Samuels, Professor of Neurology at Harvard Medical School and Emeritus Chairman of Neurology at Brigham and Women's Hospital, Boston, MA, for his thoughtful "FOREWORD" written for this book.

Contents

Contributors

Editors

Sudhansu Chokroverty, MD, FRCP Hackensack Meridian Health, Neuroscience Institute at JFK, JFK University Medical Center, Edison, NJ, USA

Seton Hall University & Hackensack Meridian School of Medicine at Seton Hall, South Orange, NJ, USA

Rutgers Robert Wood Johnson Medical School, New Brunswick, NJ, USA

Pietro Cortelli, MD, PhD IRCCS Istituto di Scienze Neurologiche, Bologna, Italy

Department of Biomedical and NeuroMotor Sciences (DIBINEM), University of Bologna, Bologna, Italy

Contributors

Elio Clemente Agostoni, MD Sleep Medicine Center, Department of Neuroscience, Grande Ospedale Metropolitano Niguarda, Milan, Italy

Roberto Amici, MD Department of Biomedical and NeuroMotor Sciences (DIBINEM), University of Bologna, Bologna, Italy

Fiona C. Baker, PhD SRI International, Menlo Park, CA, USA

Jacquie Baker, PhD University Hospital, London Health Sciences Centre, London, ON, Canada

Luca Baldelli, MBBS Department of Biomedical and NeuroMotor Sciences (DIBINEM), University of Bologna, Bologna, Italy

Lucie Barateau, MD Sleep-Wake Disorders Center, Department of Neurology, National Reference Network for Narcolepsy, Gui-de-Chauliac Hospital, CHU Montpellier, Montpellier, France

PSNREC, University Montpellier, INSERM 1061, Montpellier, France

Francesca Baschieri, MD Department of Biomedical and NeuroMotor Sciences (DIBINEM), University of Bologna, Bologna, Italy

Eduardo E. Benarroch, MD Division of Autonomic Disorders, Department of Neurology, Mayo Clinic, Rochester, MN, USA

Sushanth Bhat, MD Neuroscience Institute, Hackensack Meridian Health, JFK Medical Center, Seton Hall University, Edison, NJ, USA

Rebecca Burdayron, BSc Department of Educational and Counselling Psychology, McGill University, Montréal, QC, Canada

Hôpital en Santé Mentale Rivière-des-Prairies, CIUSSS du Nord-de-l'Ile-de-Montréal, Montréal, QC, Canada

Giovanna Calandra-Buonaura, MBBS IRCCS Istituto di Scienze Neurologiche, Bologna, Italy

Department of Biomedical and NeuroMotor Sciences (DIBINEM), University of Bologna, Bologna, Italy

Yves Dauvilliers, MD, PhD Sleep-Wake Disorders Center, Department of Neurology, National Reference Network for Narcolepsy, Gui-de-Chauliac Hospital, CHU Montpellier, Montpellier, France

PSNREC, University Montpellier, INSERM 1061, Montpellier, France

Massimiliano de Zambotti, PhD SRI International, Menlo Park, CA, USA

Alex Desautels, MD, PhD Department of Neurology, University of Montréal, Montréal, QC, Canada

Center for Advanced Research in Sleep Medicine, Sacré-Coeur Hospital, Montréal, QC, Canada

Luigi Ferini-Strambi, MD UO Neurology – Sleep Disorder Center, Department of Clinical Neurosciences, IRCCS San Raffaele Hospital, "Vita-Salute" San Raffaele University, Milan, Italy

Thea Giacomini, MD Child Neuropsychiatry Unit, IRCCS Giannina Gaslini Institute, Genoa, Italy

Department of Neuroscience, Rehabilitation, Ophthalmology, Genetics and Maternal and Child Sciences (DINOGMI), University of Genoa, Genoa, Italy

Kevin S. Gipson, MD, MS Division of Pediatric Pulmonology and Sleep Medicine, Department of Pediatrics, Massachusetts General Hospital, Harvard Medical School, Boston, MA, USA

Christian Guilleminault, MD, DM, DBiol Stanford Sleep Medicine Center, Psychiatry and Behavioral Sciences, Stanford University, Stanford, CA, USA

Pietro Guaraldi, MD PhD IRCCS Istituto di Scienze Neurologiche, Bologna, Italy

Valeria Iodice, MD, PhD Queen Square Institute of Neurology, University College London, London, UK

Autonomic & Neurovascular Medicine Centre, Hospital of St John & St Elizabeth, London, UK

Autonomic Unit, National Hospital for Neurology & Neurosurgery, Queen Square, London, UK

Horacio Kaufmann, MD Dysautonomia Center, Department of Neurology, New York University School of Medicine, New York, NY, USA

Ramesh K. Khurana, MD Neurology Division, Department of Medicine, MedStar Union Memorial Hospital, Baltimore, MD, USA

Kurt Kimpinski, MD, PhD, FRCPC School of Kinesiology, Western University, London, ON, Canada

Department of Clinical Neurological Sciences, University Hospital, London Health Sciences Centre, London, ON, Canada

Schulich School of Medicine & Dentistry, Western University, London, ON, Canada

Suresh Kotagal, MBBS Center for Sleep Medicine and Department of Neurology, Mayo Clinic, Rochester, Minnesota, USA

Daniela Lucini, MD, PhD Department of Medical Biotechnology and Translational Medicine (BIOMETRA), Istituto Clinico Humanitas, University of Milan, Milan, Italy

Sara Marelli, PhD UO Neurology – Sleep Disorder Center, Department of Clinical Neurosciences, IRCCS San Raffaele Hospital, "Vita-Salute" San Raffaele University, Milan, Italy

Christopher J. Mathias, DPhil, DSc, FRCP Queen Square Institute of Neurology, University College London, London, UK

Autonomic & Neurovascular Medicine, Lindo Wing, St Mary's Hospital, Imperial College Healthcare Trust, London, UK

Autonomic & Neurovascular Medicine Centre, Hospital of St John & St Elizabeth, London, UK

Mitchell G. Miglis, MD Autonomic Division, Department of Neurology and Neurological Sciences; Sleep Medicine Division, Department of Psychiatry and Behavioral Sciences, Stanford University, Palo Alto, CA, USA

Lino Nobili, MD, PhD Child Neuropsychiatry Unit, IRCCS Giannina Gaslini Institute, Genoa, Italy

Department of Neuroscience, Rehabilitation, Ophthalmology, Genetics and Maternal and Child Sciences (DINOGMI), University of Genoa, Genoa, Italy

William C. Orr, PhD University of Oklahoma Health Sciences Center, Oklahoma City, OK, USA

OU Medical Center, Gastroenterology, Oklahoma City, OK, USA

Andrew P. Owens, BA Hons, PGDip, MSc, PhD Department of Old Age Psychiatry, Institute of Psychiatry, Psychology & Neuroscience, Kings College, London, UK

Massimo Pagani, MD Department of Medical Biotechnology and Translational Medicine (BIOMETRA), University of Milan, Milan, Italy

Jose-Alberto Palma, MD, PhD Dysautonomia Center, Department of Neurology, New York University School of Medicine, New York, NY, USA

Liborio Parrino, MD, PhD Sleep Disorders Center, Department of Medicine and Surgery, University Hospital Parma, Parma, Italy

Marie-Hélène Pennestri, PhD Department of Educational and Counselling Psychology, McGill University, Montreal, QC, Canada

Hôpital en Santé Mentale Rivière-des-Prairies, CIUSSS du Nord-de-l'Ile-de-Montréal, Montreal, QC, Canada

Giuseppe Plazzi, MD, PhD IRCCS Istituto di Scienze Neurologiche, Bologna, Italy

Department of Biomedical and NeuroMotor Sciences (DIBINEM), University of Bologna, Bologna, Italy

Paola Proserpio, MD Sleep Medicine Center, Department of Neuroscience, Grande Ospedale Metropolitano Niguarda, Milan, Italy

Federica Provini, MD, PhD IRCCS Istituto di Scienze Neurologiche, Bologna, Italy

Department of Biomedical and NeuroMotor Sciences (DIBINEM), University of Bologna, Bologna, Italy

Samih Raad, MD Department of Pulmonary, Critical Care & Sleep Medicine, University of Oklahoma Health Sciences Center, Oklahoma City, OK, USA

Maria Salsone, MD UO Neurology – Sleep Disorder Center, Department of Clinical Neurosciences, IRCCS San Raffaele Hospital, "Vita-Salute" San Raffaele University, Milan, Italy

Institute of Molecular Bioimaging and Physiology, National Research Council (IBFM-CNR), Cantazaro, Italy

Kamal Shouman, MD Division of Autonomic Disorders, Department of Neurology, Mayo Clinic, Rochester, MN, USA

Alessandro Silvani, MD, PhD Department of Biomedical and NeuroMotor Sciences (DIBINEM), University of Bologna, Bologna, Italy

Walter Struhal, MD Abteilung für Neurologie, Universitätsklinikum Tulln; and Karl Landsteiner Privatuniversität für Gesundheitswissenschaften, Tulln, Austria

Anastasios Tentolouris, MD, MSc First Department of Propaedeutic Internal Medicine, School of Medicine, Laiko General Hospital, National and Kapodistrian University of Athens, Athens, Greece

Nikolaos Tentolouris, MD, PhD First Department of Propaedeutic Internal Medicine, School of Medicine, Laiko General Hospital, National and Kapodistrian University of Athens, Athens, Greece

Roberto Vetrugno, MD, PhD Department of Neurology–Neurophysiology, Casa di Cura Madre Fortunata Toniolo, Bologna, Italy

Jennifer Zitser, MD Global Brain Health Institute, Department of Neurology & Neurological Sciences, University of California, San Francisco, San Francisco, CA, USA

Movement Disorders Unit, Department of Neurology, Tel-Aviv Sourasky Medical Center, Sackler Faculty of Medicine, Tel Aviv University, Tel Aviv, Israel

Giovanna Zoccoli, MD, PhD Department of Biomedical and NeuroMotor Sciences (DIBINEM) and Department of Physiology, University of Bologna, Bologna, Italy

Introduction

1

Sudhansu Chokroverty and Pietro Cortelli

The modern era of the autonomic nervous system (ANS) began with the demonstration by Gaskell of "craniosacral" and "thoracolumbar" outflows in 1886 [1], as well as introduction of the term "the autonomic nervous system" by Langley in 1898 [2]. Despite an early recognition of the ANS, the topic has remained largely neglected in the fields of basic science, clinical neurology, and clinical medicine in general. Modern scientists have shown a dynamic interaction between the central autonomic network (CAN) and sleep-wake generating neurons [3–9] in the central nervous system (CNS). In 1972, Lugaresi et al. [10] clearly demonstrated by polygraphic recording during sleep in humans dynamic and coordinated oscillations between cerebral activity (as documented by fluctuating and cyclic EEG changes, subsequently coined *cyclic alternating pattern* (CAP) by Terzano and co-investigators [11]) and many physiological characteristics, particularly cardiovascular and respiratory systems (as documented by periodic changes in blood pressure [BP]), heart rate (HR), and breathing. These oscillations reflect a compelling coupling between somatic and the autonomic nervous systems during sleep. This coupling results from an interaction between neuroanatomical substrates and neurophysiological changes during sleep and wakefulness. These changes reflect mind–body (brain–body) interplay during human sleep-wake states. Most of our thinking processes and intellectual efforts are directed at activities during wakefulness. However, there has been an increasing awareness about the importance of sleep and how its dysfunction impacts our life. Good sleep is now recognized as a vital sign of human health and increasing attention is being paid toward this topic which still remains a mystery to these scientists. Sleep has its own world with its own rhythms and rituals. Sleep commands all the vital functions of the human body (e.g., circulation, respiration, endocrine secretion, gastrointestinal, and genitourinary health) controlled by both the somatic and autonomic nervous systems working in unison to maintain not only our internal homeostasis but also how to respond to the external world [12]. The ANS through its anatomical and functional organization impacts every body system and organ and this fact is the key to maintaining internal homeostasis ("milieu") in the human body. The close interrelationship of the ANS in terms of neural circuits [13], functions, neurotransmitters, and neuromodulators with sleep-wake states makes it important to have a basic knowledge about the order and disorder of the ANS in sleep-wakefulness for understanding its impact on various diseases and for designing appropriate treatment. Our concept about the ANS has been evolving over the past half a century pointing to new directions in research in the field. In addition to nocturnal sleep, it is also important to consider napping (brief daytime sleep), as well as the relationship between nocturnal sleep and napping; the results, however, have been contradictory [14, 15]. The various studies [14, 16] only account for sleep duration but not sleep architecture (e.g., sleep stages). In addition, it is important to think about chronobiological, behavioral, and medical aspects of napping. Naps themselves, particularly short naps, may not have detrimental effects; on the other hand, naps may be consequences (adverse effects of comorbid health issues or may be secondary to age-related brain and body changes). Furthermore, sleep regulates immune process and indirectly inflammation. Sleep and inflammation have a bidirectional relationship. On the one hand, sleep disorders (e.g., insomnia and sleep apnea) promote inflammation in a nonspecific manner; on the other hand, the immune system modulates sleep

S. Chokroverty (✉)
Hackensack Meridian Health, Neuroscience Institute at JFK, JFK University Medical Center, Edison, NJ, USA

Seton Hall University & Hackensack Meridian School of Medicine at Seton Hall, South Orange, NJ, USA

Rutgers Robert Wood Johnson Medical School, New Brunswick, NJ, USA
e-mail: Sudhansu.chokroverty@hmhn.org

P. Cortelli
IRCCS Istituto di Scienze Neurologiche, Bologna, Italy

Department of Biomedical and NeuroMotor Sciences (DIBINEM), University of Bologna, Bologna, Italy

S. Chokroverty, P. Cortelli (eds.), *Autonomic Nervous System and Sleep*, https://doi.org/10.1007/978-3-030-62263-3_1

and inflammation causing daytime sleepiness. Of note, there are different types of naps, for example, recovery, prophylactic, appetitive, fulfillment, and essential naps [14]. For control of other body systems see Chaps. 2 and 3.

Before discussing the ANS changes in sleep including age-related changes it is essential to have a basic understanding of sleep which has fascinated and intrigued mankind for centuries. During sleep there is suspension of environmental awareness but the internal awareness is dominated by a dream-like state. Bremer's experimental sections in cats in 1935 producing *cerveau isolé* [17] (intercollicular section) and *encéphale isolé* (medullospinal transection) introduced the concept of passive theory of sleep (see also Chap. 4). This was supported initially by the discovery of ascending reticular activating system (ARAS) by Moruzzi and Magoun in 1949 (see Chap. 4) [18] introducing the concept of passive theory of sleep mechanism (deafferentation). However, this theory was challenged later by Batini et al.'s experiment [19] of midpontine trigeminal transection in cats in 1959 (see Chap. 4) that lies a few millimeters below the transection producing *cerveau isolé* preparation strengthening the active theory of mechanism of sleep. Contemporary theory of sleep recognizes both "active" (e.g., activation of the ARAS including aminergic, serotonergic, histaminergic, laterodorsal tegmental (LDT), and pedunculopontine tegmental (PPT) cholinergic nuclei, and glutamatergic neurons), and "passive" (e.g., withdrawal of afferent stimuli and deactivation of ARAs and other wake-promoting neurons) [20–22] mechanisms.

Non-traditionally, human existence may be divided into six states [12, 23; unpublished observation] (see also Chap. 4): (i) active wakefulness (AW), (ii) relaxed wakefulness (RW), (iii) pre-dormitum (a term used by McDonald Critchley [24] to a stage between relaxed wakefulness and stage 1 of non-rapid eye movement (NREM) sleep), (iv) NREM or quiet sleep, (v) REM or active sleep, and (vi) post-dormitum (sleep inertia or sleep drunkenness, a state between sleep and awakening first thing in the morning).

AW is characterized by EEG desynchronization, active waking eye movements (WEMs), prevalent skeletal muscle activity and dominance of sympathetic activity [23, 25]. During active W homeostatic mechanism is overshadowed by the catabolic state of intense muscle activity and is reflected in alterations of physiological variables (e.g., O_2, CO_2, H+) [12].

RW is characterized by a desynchronized EEG with well-organized and well-modulated posteriorly dominant alpha activity in the adults, persisting postural muscle tone and stable ANS with the slight sympathetic dominance [21, 23]. In contrast, synchronized EEG, slow eye movements (SEMs) mildly decreased postural muscle tone and parasympathetic dominance are the features of quiet or NREM sleep. Active or REM sleep, on the other hand, is characterized by (i) desynchronized EEG with sawtooth waves; (ii) postural muscle atonia or hypotonia (lowest muscle tone during sleep); (iii) variable sympathetic-parasympathetic activity (parasympathetic dominance with intermittent activation of sympathetic tone); (iv) rapid eye movements (REMs); and (v) myoclonic twitching and jerks (transient phasic muscle bursts) [25].

Thus, the two basic states (NREM and REM) differ considerably in terms of physiological variables [23]. NREM is dominated by homeostatic regulation (relatively stable). In contrast, during REM sleep homeostasis is suspended and poikilostasis is dominant (may be termed poikilstatic) [12]. Homeostasis refers to the integrated physiological functions, whereas poikilostasis signifies disintegrated physiological functions [12]. Physiological events in these two states should be described in terms of the somatic nervous system (i.e., somatic behavior) and the ANS (i.e., autonomic behavior) [12]. Proof of functional dichotomy between these two states of sleep may be exemplified by the effects of thermal load. Exposure to warm environment (37 °C) during NREM sleep will cause tachypnea but not in REM sleep. Exposure to cold environment (4 °C) is characterized by shivering as evidenced by increased neck muscle (EMG) activity in NREM sleep but there is absence of EMG activity in neck muscles during REM sleep [12].

To understand further the interaction between the ANS and sleep in terms of its impact on health and disease, it is essential to know the profound changes in the ANS during sleep [26]. Essentially there are two changes in the ANS during sleep: The parasympathetic tone increases in NREM sleep with further increase in REM sleep; the sympathetic tone decreases in both NREM and REM sleep with intermittent hyperactivation during REM, particularly in phasic REM sleep. Sleep onset (SO) is an unstable state, whereas the deepest stage of sleep (stage N3 or slow wave sleep [SWS]) is the most stable stage. Factors for stability in SWS include the following [12, 27]: (i) increased arousal threshold in N3 compared with N1 or N2, preventing arousal-related instability; (ii) increased genioglossus single motor unit activity during this stage (possibly related to higher upper airway resistance; (iii) higher $PaCO_2$ during N3; (iv) a theoretical possibility of increased central respiratory drive; (v) finally, stage N3 is seen mostly in non-CAP EEG stage (in terms of CAP- non-CAP EEG oscillations) instead of the unstable EEG CAP stage. Respiration is very unstable at SO and is most likely related to arousal fluctuations [26] and loss of wakefulness stimuli. At SO there are also changes in frequency, tidal volume, and changes in blood gas tension. There may be a few periods of apnea at SO.

In addition to significant sleep-related changes in the ANS and the CNS, it is also important to be aware of age-related changes in these systems [28] to assess autonomic and other functions in diseased and healthy individuals. Loss or functional alterations (decrease) of wake-active (wake-promoting) neurons (e.g., orexinergic, cholinergic, histaminergic, noradrenergic, dopaminergic, and serotonergic neurons) in the elderly seem to be due to age-related structural alterations in the brain. These changes may account for sleep disturbance in the aging and neurodegenerative diseases. This reduction of neurons and neuronal circuits including synapses (structural or functional loss) [28] may be responsible for daytime sleepiness (napping). Similarly, there are age-related changes in the ANS [28] which may be responsible for sleep and autonomic function alterations in the elderly. Therefore, it is important to have age-matched controls for evaluation of autonomic function laboratory tests. One must consider these age-related changes in order to address the interaction between the ANS and sleep, and their impact on physiological changes in normal sleep and diseased states. Another important recent discovery is the presence of the glymphatic system in rats, mice, and guinea pigs [29] with indirect indications (from sophisticated magnetic resonance imaging [MRI] studies of the brain) of its presence even in human beings [30]. The brain has no lymphatic system, and this drainage system (named glymphatic system because of its close association with astrocytes and oligodendroglia) located in the brain's perivascular spaces appears to expand during sleep for removing waste metabolic products of the brain (e.g., amyloid). Sleep deprivation is therefore thought to be an important factor in the pathogenesis of many neurodegenerative diseases (e.g., Alzheimer's disease [AD] and Parkinson's disease [PD]).

It is also important to understand significance of autonomic function (AF) tests and the autonomic clinician must have a basic knowledge about the type of AF tests to perform both during wakefulness and sleep (see Chaps. 9 and 12). Anatomical substrates for central autonomic control (see Chaps. 2 and 3) subserving a variety of integrative functions [6, 31] include the following structures: (i) spinal cord, (ii) brain stem, (iii) cerebellum; (iv) hypothalamus; (v) amygdala; and (vi) some parts of the cerebral cortex (see further on). The major control systems include cardiovascular, respiratory, gastrointestinal (including swallowing, gut motility, and secretions) and genitourinary systems (including micturition and sexual functions). Cardiovascular functions are controlled by both cortical and subcortical structures. Major cerebral cortical centers include insula, anterior cingulate gyrus, medial prefrontal cortex, and hypothalamus (see Chap. 2). Main supraspinal centers comprise (see Chap. 2) neurons located in the locus coeruleus, the rostral ventrolateral medulla (RVLM), nucleus tractus solitarius (NTS) and the brain stem parasympathetic premotor neurons in the dorsal motor nucleus (DMN) and the nucleus ambiguus (NAS) belonging to the vagus nerve. Sympathetic premotor neurons in the RVLM descend to the spinal sympathetic preganglionic motor neurons in the intermediolateral centers of T1–L2 spinal cord segments (see Chap. 3). BP, HR, cardiac contractility causing vasoconstriction or vasodilation are controlled by the two divisions (sympathetic and parasympathetic) of the ANS. For control of other body systems see Chaps. 2 and 3.

An important dysautonomic sign is orthostatic hypotension (OH, see Chap. 3 for understanding mechanism of OH). Orthostatic hypotension can be brought on by a decrease in baroreceptor sensitivity (age-related), volume depletion, autonomic failure, neurological diseases, medical disorders, and iatrogenic causes (medications and surgical sympathectomy) (see Chap. 12, Section "General and Specific Clinical Manifestations of Autonomic Dysfunction and Physiology of Orthostatic Blood Pressure Control").

Autonomic control shows a wide variation in all three major sleep-wake states (W, NREM, and REM), and most variations in ANS control occur during REM sleep [12, 26]. In REM sleep ANS control functions through an "open loop," that is, without any feedback between wakefulness and NREM sleep whereas the latter two states use a "closed loop" (i.e., receiving feedback). The specific neural factors responsible for autonomic control remain unknown. It is, however, important to know the factors controlling autonomic regulation in order to understand normal and abnormal human physiology in sleep and wakefulness. A number of sleep disorders (both primary and secondary) affect the ANS. A dynamic interaction among the sympathetic, parasympathetic, and enteric divisions of the ANS and the CNS confer profound hemodynamic and physiological changes in almost every system of the body causing significant clinical implications [3–5, 7].

Stage REM is a period of predominant vagal tone interspersed with bursts of sympathetic hyperactivity [26], changes in the rate and rhythm of the heart beat as well as appearance of ectopic beats are noted in the electrocardiogram (EKG) of normal sleeping individuals. In addition to relative bradycardia in NREM sleep, brady-tachyarrhythmias in REM sleep there may be other relatively benign cardiac arrhythmias noted in REM sleep which include sinus pauses, and partial heart block as a result of heightened parasympathetic tone [32–34]. Brodsky et al. [35] documented sinus pauses in young male medical students. Ventricular premature beats decrease during sleep as a result of reduced sympathetic activity [36–38]. Prolongation of QT interval may occur in normal man during sleep posing a risk factor for susceptible individuals with long QT syndrome [36–38].

The most susceptible time for myocardial infarction, stroke, and sudden cardiac death is in the morning between 6 am and 11 am [39, 40]. The reason is not definitely known but is multifactorial and may include increased platelet aggregability, sympathetic surge during REM sleep in the early morning hours just before final wake up from sleep, alteration of endothelial function leading to vascular disease as well as increased morning plasma catecholamines [26, 27,

41, 42]. These factors are particularly serious in those with existing coronary arterial or other cardiovascular diseases. There is an overall reduction of 10–20% of BP compared to daytime waking level [27, 41, 42]. This is known as normal dipping. A failure of dipping, reverse dipping (e.g., increased BP) or extreme dipping (more than 20% reduction in BP during sleep) are all risk factors for increased cardiovascular morbidity and mortality. There is also an increased coagulability during sleep as a result of increased tissue plasminogen activator (tPA) inhibitor 1 (PAI-I) and a decrease in tPA [43]. Thus, increased platelet aggregation and coagulability, and endothelial dysfunction in the early morning hours play a major role in early morning increased incidence of cardiovascular catastrophes or sudden cardiac death [27, 40, 41, 43].

In this single comprehensive text, we the editors and superb contributors (experts in the fields of the ANS and sleep) have been able to capture the interaction of the ANS with the CNS in almost all body systems and organs; this interaction is altered in sleep compared to wakefulness. In three broad sections (basic, laboratory, and clinical) the eminent scientists and contributors have made a valiant effort to discuss how the ANS changes in sleep may impact human health and diseases including primary sleep disorders. The ANS and sleep show a bidirectional relationship: autonomic dysfunction may affect sleep and, in turn, sleep and its disorders may affect ANS functions. In view of the fact that there is a forceful coupling among the CNS, the ANS, and various body systems and organs, it is understandable that the central autonomic network with its ascending and descending projections connecting the central and peripheral autonomic neurons and the somatic nervous system controls vital functions of the body maintaining internal homeostasis. The fact the ANS plays a central role directing essential and fundamental functions of the body, particularly its role during sleep has not been sufficiently emphasized in various textbooks, book chapters, or journal articles. In this comprehensive (but not encyclopedic) textbook we have addressed all the facts about the ANS and sleep interaction as well as the ANS alterations in sleep, and how these impact primary and comorbid (neurological and other medical-psychiatric disorders) sleep dysfunction. This new knowledge about the sleep–ANS interaction will enhance our understanding of the pathophysiology of various disorders and help to introduce new lines of therapy to improve morbidity, mortality, and prognosis of a variety of sleep and other medical-neurological diseases.

In conclusion, the ANS–CNS–sleep interaction explains mind–body (including brain–heart and other organs) interplay. This volume should be useful to sleep specialists, neurologists, and internists (especially those specializing in pulmonary, cardiovascular, and gastrointestinal medicine) dealing with sleep and autonomic failure or hyperactivity, family physicians, psychiatrists, psychologists, pediatricians, otolaryngologists, dentists, neurosurgeons, and neuroscientists interacting with patients suffering from sleep and autonomic dysfunction as well as those interested in understanding sleep and the ANS (e.g., technologists, nurses, and other healthcare professionals). This book should be useful to both beginners and those advanced in the field.

References

1. Gaskell WH. On the structure, distribution and function of the nerves which innervate the visceral and vascular systems. J Physiol. 1886;7(1):1–80.
2. Langley JN. The autonomic nervous system, part 1. Cambridge: W. Heffer and Sons; 1921.
3. de Zambotti M, Trinder J, Silvani A, Colrain IM, Baker FC. Dynamic coupling between the central and autonomic nervous systems during sleep: a review. Neurosci Biobehav Rev. 2018;90:84–103.
4. de Zambotti M, Willoughby AR, Franzen PL, Clark DB, Baker FC, Colrain IM. K-complexes: interaction between the central and autonomic nervous systems during sleep. Sleep. 2016;39(5):1129–37.
5. Silvani A, Calandra-Buonaura G, Dampney RA, Cortelli P. Brain-heart interactions: physiology and clinical implications. Philos Transact A Math Phys Eng Sci. 2016;374(2067):20150181.
6. Benarroch EE. Central autonomic network: functional organization and clinical correlations. Armonk: Futura Publishing Co., Inc.; 1997.
7. Quigley EMM, Conklin JL. The "big brain" and the "little brain". Interactions between the enteric and central nervous system in the gut functions. In: Quigley EM, Dfeiffer RF, editors. Neurogastroenterology. Philadelphia: Elsevier/Butterworth-Heinmann; 2004.
8. Samuels MA. Neurally induced cardiac damage. Definition of the problem. Neurol Clin. 1993;11(2):273–92.
9. Sforza FA, Arida RM, Cysneiros RM, Terra VC, Sonoda EY, de Albuquerque M, Cavalheiro EA. The brain-heart connection: implications for understanding sudden unexpected death in epilepsy. Cardiol J. 2009;16(5):394–9.
10. Lugaresi E, Coccagna G, Mantovani M, Lebrun R. Some periodic phenomena arising during drowsiness and sleep in man. Electroencephalogr Clin Neurophysiol. 1972;32(6):701–5.
11. Terzano MG, Parrino L, Sherieri A, et al. Atlas, rules and recording techniques for the scoring of cyclic alternating pattern (CAP) in human sleep. Sleep Med. 2001;2(6):537–53.
12. Parmeggiani PL. Systemic homeostasis and poikilostasis in sleep. London: Imperial College Press; 2011. p. 1–121.
13. Bartsch RP, Liu KK, Bashan A, Ivanov PC. Network physiology: how organ systems dynamically interact. PLoS One. 2015;10(11):e0142143.
14. Mantua J, Spencer RMC. Exploring the nap paradox: are mid-day sleep bouts a friend or foe? Sleep Med. 2017;37:88–97.
15. Mantau J, Spencer RMC. The interactive effects of nocturnal sleep and daytime naps in relation to serum C-reactive protein. Sleep Med. 2015;16:1213–6.
16. Chen G, Chen L, Wen J, Yao J, Li L, Lin L, et al. Associations between sleep duration, daytime nap duration, and osteoporosis vary by sex, menopause, and sleep quality. J Clin Endocrinol Metab. 2014;99(8):2869–77.
17. Bremer F. Cerveau isolé et physiologic du sommeil. CR Soc Biol (Paris). 1935;118:1235–44.

18. Moruzzi G, Magoun H. Brain stem reticular formation and activation of the EEG. Electroencephalogr Clin Neurophysiol. 1949;1:455–73.
19. Batini C, Moruzzi G, Palestini M, et al. Effects of complete pontine transections on sleep-wakefulness rhythm: the ucidpontine pre trigeminal preparation. Areh Ital Biol. 1959;97:1–12.
20. España RA, Scammell TE. Sleep neurobiology from a clinical perspective. Sleep. 2011;34(7):845–58.
21. Saper CB, Fuller PM, Pedersen NP, Lu J, Scammell TE. Sleep state switching. Neuron. 2010;68(6):1023–42.
22. Lu J, Sherman D, Devor M, Saper CB. A putative flip-flop switch for control of REM sleep. Nature. 2006;441(7093):589–94.
23. Lugaresi E, Provini F, Montaga P. The neuroanatomy of sleep. Considerations on the role of the thalamus in sleep and a proposal for caudorostral organization. Rev Eur J Anat. 2004;8(2):85–93.
24. McDonald C. The pre-dormitum. Rev Neurol (Paris). 1955;93:101–6.
25. American Academy of Sleep Medicine. International classification of sleep disorders. 3rd ed. Darien: American Academy of Sleep Medicine; 2014.
26. Parmeggiani PL. The autonomic nervous system in sleep. In: Kryger MH, Roth T, Dement WC, editors. Principles and practice of sleep medicine. Philadelphia: Saunders; 1994. p. 194–203.
27. Chokroverty S. Physiological changes in sleep. In: Chokroverty S, editor. Sleep disorders medicine: basic science, technical considerations and clinical aspects. 4th ed. New York: Springer Science & Business Media; 2017. p. 153–94.
28. Katzman R, Terry R. Normal aging of the nervous system. In: Katzman R, editor. The neurology of aging. Philadelphia: Davis; 1983.
29. Nedergaard M. Neuroscience. Garbage truck of the brain. Science. 2013;340(6140):1529–30.
30. Berezuk C, Ramirez J, Gao F, Scott CJ, Huroy M, Swartz RH, et al. Virchow-Robin spaces: correlations with polysomnography-derived sleep parameters. Sleep. 2015;38(6):853–8.
31. Benarroch EE. Baroreflex Failure. In: Benarroch EE, editor. Central autonomic network: functional organization and clinical correlations. Armonk: Futura Publishing Company, Inc; 1997. p. 482–4.
32. Parish JM, Shepard JW Jr. Cardiovascular effects of sleep disorders. Chest. 1990;97(5):1220–6.
33. Osuna E, Patino G. REM sleep-related complete heart block: is it a specific sleep-related disorder? Sleep Med. 2006;7(4):387–8.
34. Verrier RL, Kirby DA. Sleep and cardiac arrhythmias. Ann N Y Acad Sci. 1988;533:238–51.
35. Brodsky M, Wu D, Denes P, Kanakis C, Rosen KM. Arrhythmias documented by 24 hour continuous electrocardiographic monitoring in 50 male medical students without apparent heart disease. Am J Cardiol. 1977;39(3):390–5.
36. Vatta M, Dumaine R, Varghese G, Richard TA, Shimizu W, Aihara N, et al. Genetic and biophysical basis of sudden unexplained nocturnal death syndrome (SUNDS), a disease allelic to Brugada syndrome. Hum Mol Genet. 2002;11(3):337–45.
37. Samuels M. Introduction to neurocardiology. In: Mathias CJ, Bannister R, editors. Autonomic failure. 5th ed. Oxford: Oxford University Press; 2013. p. 669–76.
38. Muller JE, Stone PH, Turi ZG, Rutherford JD, Czeisler CA, Parker C, et al. Circadian variation in the frequency of onset of acute myocardial infarction. N Engl J Med. 1985;313(21):1315–22.
39. Cohen MC, Rohtla KM, Lavery CE, Muller JE, Mittleman MA. Meta-analysis of the morning excess of acute myocardial infarction and sudden cardiac death. Am J Cardiol. 1997;79(11):1512–6. Erratum in: Am J Cardiol 1998;81(2):260
40. Otto ME, Svatikova A, Barretto RB, Santos S, Hoffmann M, Khandheria B, Somers V. Early morning attenuation of endothelial function in healthy humans. Circulation. 2004;109(21):2507–10.
41. Fabbian F, Smolensky MH, Tiseo R, Pala M, Manfredini R, Portaluppi F. Dipper and non-dipper blood pressure 24-hour patterns: circadian rhythm-dependent physiologic and pathophysiologic mechanisms. Chronobiol Int. 2013;30(1–2):17–30.
42. Larochelle P. Circadian variation in blood pressure: dipper or non-dipper. J Clin Hypertens (Greenwich). 2002;4(Suppl 1):3–8.
43. Gram J, Kluft C, Jespersen J. Depression of tissue plasminogen activator (t-PA) activity and rise of t-PA inhibition and acute phase reactants in blood of patients with acute myocardial infarction (AMI). Thromb Haemost. 1987;58(3):817–21.

Part I

Basics

Central Autonomic Network

2

Kamal Shouman and Eduardo E. Benarroch

Overview

The central nervous system controls autonomic function via several interconnected areas distributed throughout the neuraxis. Whereas these areas have been referred to as central autonomic network (CAN), they control many other functions including arousal and respiration [1]. One major output of this integrated network is mediated by preganglionic sympathetic and parasympathetic neurons. Central autonomic control areas are hierarchically organized. Areas in the medulla and lower pons relay interoceptive information to the forebrain and mediate cardiovascular, respiratory, gastrointestinal, and micturition reflexes. They include the nucleus of the solitary tract (NTS), reticular formation of the rostral ventrolateral medulla (VLM), rostral ventromedial medulla (RVMM) including the caudal raphe nuclei, medullary respiratory groups, parabrachial nucleus (PB), and pelvic organ stimulating center (formerly known as pontine micturition center or Barrington nucleus). Areas in the upper pons and midbrain integrate autonomic control with pain modulation, responses to stress, behavioral arousal, and motor responses. They include the periaqueductal gray (PAG), the pedunculopontine tegmental nucleus (PPT/PPN), and locus coeruleus (LC). The hypothalamus functions as a pattern generator of integrated autonomic, endocrine and behavioral responses to ensure bodily homeostasis and adaptation to the environment. The hypothalamic autonomic output originates primarily from the paraventricular nucleus (PVH), dorsomedial nucleus (DMH), and lateral hypothalamic area, including the group of neurons that synthesize orexin (Orx, also known as hypocretin, Hcrt). The core telencephalon areas controlling autonomic function are the amygdala, insular cortex, and anterior and midcingulate cortex (Fig. 2.1). Many areas initially defined by their prominent role in controlling autonomic function, such as the C1 area of the RVLM, are now recognized to have a major role in mechanisms of arousal, respiratory activation, and immune modulation [2]. Although the functional anatomy of the central control of autonomic function has been best characterized in experimental animals [3–11], several functional neuroimaging studies show that many of the same areas are activated during autonomic responses in humans [12–20].

K. Shouman (✉) · E. E. Benarroch
Division of Autonomic Disorders, Department of Neurology, Mayo Clinic, Rochester, MN, USA
e-mail: shouman.kamal@mayo.edu

Neurotransmission and Effector Mechanisms of the Central Autonomic Control

Inputs and Signaling in the Central Autonomic Network

Brain areas controlling autonomic function receive and integrate inputs from four major sources: interoceptive, humoral, “limbic”, and circadian. Interoceptive inputs from visceral, pain, and thermal receptors are relayed by spinal afferents via ascending projections to lamina I of the dorsal horn or via cranial nerve afferents that relay in the NTS. Humoral signals from the blood (e.g., levels of glucose or cytokines) or cerebrospinal fluid (CSF, such as pH) can reach the central autonomic areas either directly or indirectly via sensory circumventricular organs [21]. These include the subfornical organ (SFO), organum vasculosum of the lamina terminalis (OVLT) and the area postrema. Forebrain “limbic” areas such as the amygdala and anterior cingulate cortex provide autonomic control signals in response to behaviorally relevant stimuli that trigger emotion, such as pain or social cues. Circadian signals are provided by the suprachiasmatic nucleus [22].

The primary neurotransmitter mediating excitatory interactions among the different components of the central autonomic control network is L-glutamate; the primary inhibitory transmitter is γ-aminobutyric acid (GABA). These are also the primary neurotransmitters (sometimes together with the

S. Chokroverty, P. Cortelli (eds.), *Autonomic Nervous System and Sleep*, https://doi.org/10.1007/978-3-030-62263-3_2

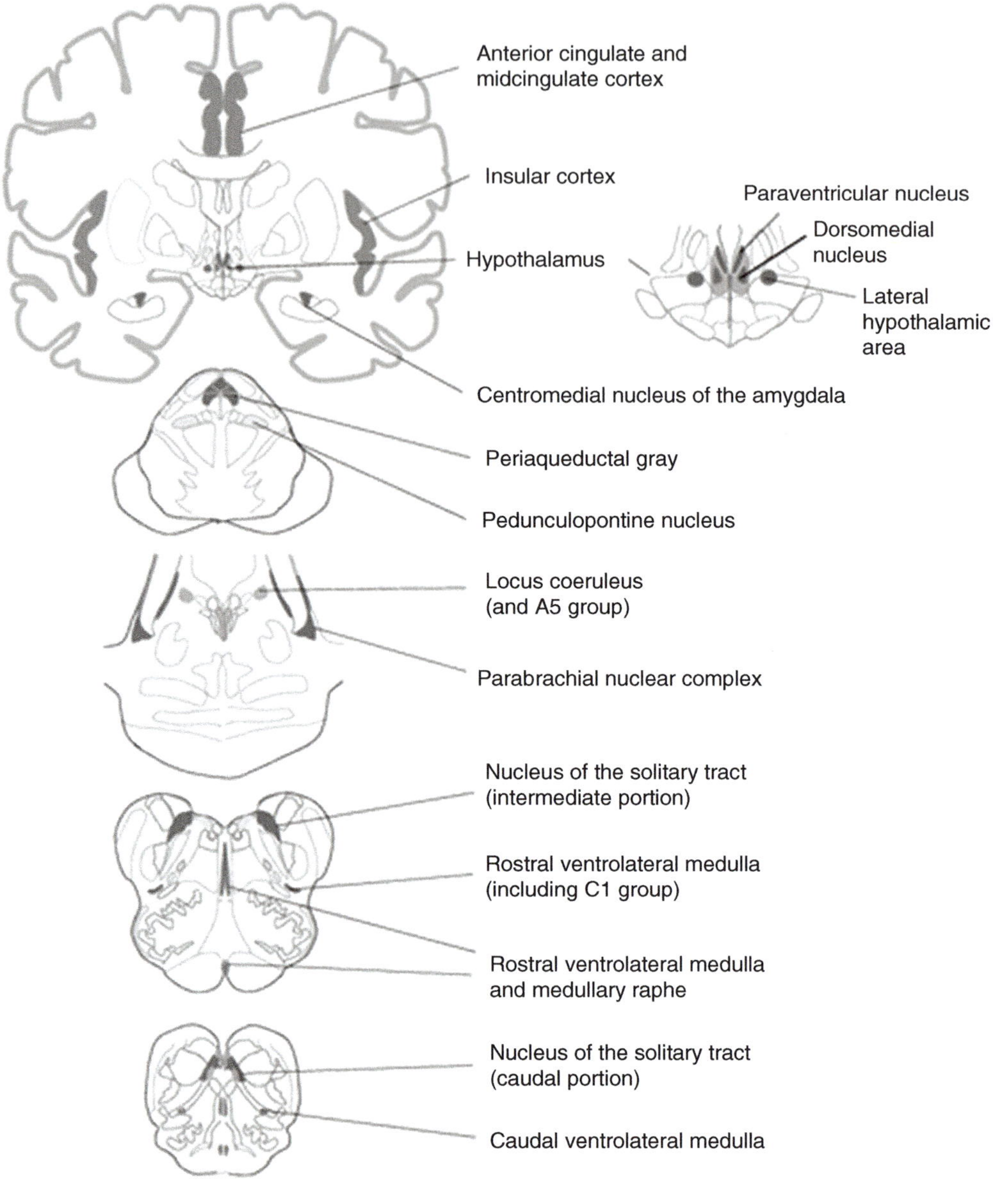

Fig. 2.1 *Main structures within the central autonomic network.* Telencephalic areas include the amygdala, insular cortex, and anterior and midcingulate cortex; these areas are involved in high level autonomic control in the setting of emotion and cognition. Hypothalamic areas include paraventricular nucleus, dorsomedial nucleus, and lateral hypothalamic area (including orexin neurons); these areas are involved in integrate control of autonomic, endocrine, and other response to internal stressors. Areas in the rostral brain stem include the periaqueductal gray, the pedunculopontine tegmental nucleus, and locus coeruleus; these areas participate in autonomic control in relation to arousal state and stress response. Areas in the lower brain stem include nucleus of the solitary tract, reticular formation of the rostral ventrolateral medulla including C1 area, and rostral ventromedial medulla including the caudal raphe nuclei; they participate in autonomic reflexes and are the final premotor autonomic regions innervating the preganglionic autonomic neurons

inhibitory amino acid glycine) of circuits controlling respiration and the sleep-wake cycle. Autonomic, respiratory, and arousal circuits are modulated in a state-dependent function by cholinergic, monoaminergic, and peptidergic influences from the brainstem, basal forebrain, and hypothalamus and by local interactions mediated by nitric oxide (NO), purines, endocannabinoids, and other signals. There is increasing evidence of a fundamental role of astrocytes in many of these interactions.

Outputs of the Central Autonomic Network

The final effectors of the central control of autonomic function are the preganglionic sympathetic and parasympathetic neurons. These neurons are cholinergic and elicit fast excitation of autonomic ganglia and enteric neurons via ganglion type nicotinic receptors.

The sympathetic preganglionic neurons are located in the thoracolumbar spinal cord at the T1 to L2 segments, primarily in lamina VII forming the intermediolateral column (IML). These neurons form separate functional units that are activated in a selective manner in response to different stimuli. In normal conditions, the preganglionic sympathetic subunits are differentially recruited to mediate distinct patterns of sympathetic responses coordinated by descending inputs form the medulla and hypothalamus [23]. The sympathetic output is critical for maintenance of blood pressure, local regulation of blood flow, thermoregulation, and responses to exercise and internal or external stressors. The preganglionic sympathetic axons terminate on paravertebral, prevertebral, and terminal ganglia, as well as the adrenal medulla. The primary neurotransmitter in sympathetic postganglionic neurons is norepinephrine; the exception is sympathetic postganglionic neurons innervating the sweat glands, which are cholinergic as well as vasodilator nerves in the muscles and coronary arteries.

The parasympathetic output can be subdivided from the functional standpoint into outputs to cranial effectors via cranial nerves III, VII, and IX; outputs to the thoracic and abdominal viscera mediated by the vagus nerve (cranial nerve X); and outputs from pelvic organs (bladder, rectum, and sexual organs) originating from sacral preganglionic neurons. Parasympathetic output mediates organ-specific reflexes. The primary neurotransmitter of most parasympathetic ganglion and enteric nervous system (ENS) neurons is acetylcholine; the parasympathetic output is also mediated by non-cholinergic neurons that release NO and vasoactive intestinal polypeptide (VIP).

Cranial parasympathetic reflexes mediate pupillary constriction and accommodation, lacrimal and salivary gland secretion, and cranial vasodilation. Vagal reflexes are critical for beat-to-beat control of the heart rate and activation of upper gastrointestinal motility. Vagal preganglionic neurons are located in the dorsal motor nucleus of the vagus (DMV) and ventrolateral portion of the nucleus ambiguus (NAmb) in the medulla [24]. The DMV mediates all vago-vagal reflexes controlling motility and secretion in the gastrointestinal and respiratory tracts [25]. The ventrolateral portion of the NAmb provides vagal output to cardiac ganglion neurons controlling the sinus node [11, 24]. Sacral preganglionic nucleus controls micturition, defecation, and sexual function [10, 26].

Segmental Control of Preganglionic Neurons

Preganglionic sympathetic and sacral parasympathetic neurons in the spinal cord mediate segmental reflexes triggered by activation of primary afferents and involving local excitatory or inhibitory interneurons [23]. Typical examples are somatosympathetic reflexes triggered by pain or other somatic stimuli and storage reflexes triggered by bladder afferents during urinary stage. In normal conditions, this segmental spinal preganglionic apparatus is incorporated into specific patterns of response under the influence of descending supraspinal pathways originating in the brainstem or spinal cord. Interruption of these supraspinal descending pathways above the spinal T5 level results in massive, unpatterned reflex activation of sympathetic preganglionic neurons in response to segmental inputs such as visceral distension or nociceptor stimulation. This constitutes autonomic dysreflexia, manifested primarily with severe hypertension [27].

Lower Brainstem Areas Controlling Cardiovascular, Respiratory, and Gastrointestinal Functions

Nucleus of the Solitary Tract

The NTS is the first relay station of visceral afferents that initiate medullary reflexes and relay visceral and taste information to rostral brain areas [28, 29]. The rostral portion of the NTS receives input from taste receptors via facial, glossopharyngeal, and vagus nerve afferents; the intermediate portion receives gastrointestinal afferent input via the vagus nerve; and the caudal portion receives inputs from carotid baroreceptors and chemoreceptors via the glossopharyngeal afferents and inputs from cardiac, pulmonary, and upper airway receptors via vagal afferents. The topographic organization of afferent inputs to the NTS has been confirmed with functional neuroimaging in humans [30]. In addition to cranial nerve afferents, the NTS receives a projection from spinal neurons of lamina I conveying inputs from nociceptors, muscle receptors, thermoreceptors, and visceral receptors. The NTS also receives inputs from the area postrema, which lacks a blood–brain barrier and serves as a sensor of signal from the blood and CSF [31]. Virtually all afferents to the NTS are glutamatergic; some primary afferents also release substance P, adenosine triphosphate (ATP), and NO. Many of these cotransmitters presynaptically regulate glutamate release from primary afferents [28].

The NTS is the first relay station for gastrointestinal, cardiovascular, and respiratory reflexes. NTS projections to the DMV mediate vago-vagal gastrointestinal reflexes [25]; projections to the nucleus ambiguus mediate baroreflex-triggered decrease in the heart rate [11]; projections to the caudal VLM mediate baroreflex-triggered indirect inhibition of sympathoexcitatory neurons of the rostral ventrolateral medulla (RVLM) [5, 32]; and direct projections from the NTS to the RVLM mediated chemoreflex-triggered sympathoexcitation [33]. Inputs from the NTS to medullar and pontine respiratory groups mediate reflexes that control ventilation [34]. The NTS contains a complex network of inhibitory GABAergic neurons that receive descending inputs from several sources and participate in modulation of cardiovascular, respiratory, and gastrointestinal reflexes in response to emotion, stress, and other behavioral states. Astrocytes may have an important role in regulation of transmission in the NTS [35]. The second major function of the NTS is to provide ascending viscerosensory information to rostral areas, including the periaqueductal gray (PAG), hypothalamus, thalamus, and amygdala. These ascending inputs reach these areas either directly or via a relay in the parabrachial (PB) nuclear complex [36].

Rostral Ventrolateral Medulla

The RVLM contains premotor sympathetic excitatory neurons that project to the intermediolateral cell column [5]. These RVLM neurons are glutamatergic and include a subset that also synthesizes epinephrine (C1 group). Glutamatergic inputs from the RVLM activate preganglionic neurons that increase blood pressure and heart rate via input to noradrenergic sympathetic ganglion cells innervating muscle, splanchnic and renal vessels, and heart. The pathway from the RVLM to the preganglionic neurons is critical for tonic, reflex, and adaptive control of blood pressure [3]. The sympathoexcitatory RVLM neurons are inhibited by inputs from NTS neurons activated by baroreceptor afferents; this effect is mediated by GABAergic neurons of the caudal VLM projecting to the RVLM [5, 32]. C1 neurons also innervate the hypothalamus and other brainstem areas involved in control of respiration, arousal, and stress. Studies in rodents using selective optogenetic activation or inactivation of C1 neurons showed that these cells mediate the sympathoexcitatory effects of internal stressors such as hypoxia [2, 8]. Stimulation of C1 neurons not only results in sympathoexcitation but also causes arousal from NREM sleep and increase in ventilation. All the effects of C1 neuron stimulation are profoundly reduced during REM compared to NREM sleep and wakefulness [37]. Selective C1 neuron silencing resulted in only a small reduction of blood pressure in conscious animals under normoxic conditions but reduced sympathetic nerve activity and arterial blood pressure during anesthesia, prevented the sympathoexcitatory response to hypoxia, and abolished the increase in sympathetic activity resulting from baroreceptor denervation [38].

Rostral Ventromedial Medulla and Medullary Raphe

The rostral ventromedial medulla (RVMM) and medullary raphe, including the serotonergic neurons of nucleus raphe pallidus (RPa), contain premotor sympathoexcitatory neurons that are critical for thermoregulatory responses to cold [39]. These neurons receive inputs from thermosensitive neurons in the hypothalamus and project to preganglionic sympathetic neurons that activate noradrenergic output that elicit skin vasoconstriction and lipolysis in the brown fat. Whereas RVMM are not primarily involved in control of blood pressure and are not controlled by the baroreflex, they elicit tachycardia in response to external stressors [40]. Some neurons of the RPa and raphe obscurus are chemosensitive and respond to hypercapnia [41]. They innervate several components of the medullary respiratory network to promote ventilation [41].

Medullary Respiratory Circuits

The respiratory central pattern generator is located in the lower brainstem and includes several rhythm-generating components that drive downstream premotor neurons innervating spinal respiratory and cranial motoneurons [42]. These pattern generators respond to stimuli from central and peripheral chemoreceptors that interact to regulate the pattern of respiration and trigger sympathoexcitatory and cardiovagal responses to maintain optimal tissue oxygenation. The preBötzinger complex (preBötC) located in the ventrolateral medulla is the critical pattern generator of inspiration. It contains glutamatergic excitatory neurons that project to all medullary and pontine premotor respiratory regions [43].

Studies in rodents indicate that the primary central chemosensitive zone is the retrotrapezoid nucleus (RTN) located in ventral medullary surface [44]. The RTN contains glutamatergic neurons and are activated by increased PCO_2, both via intrinsic acid sensitive channels and by paracrine signals released from neighboring astrocytes. These neurons also receive input from peripheral chemoreceptors activated by hypoxia via a relay in the NTS and thus integrate central and peripheral chemosensitive signals. The RTN stimulates respiration via glutamatergic inputs to the preBötC and other brainstem respiratory groups. Respiratory chemosensitivity also involves serotonergic neurons of the medullary raphe, including the RPa and nucleus raphe obscurus [41]. The control of phrenic, intercostal, and abdominal motoneurons innervating inspiratory and expiratory muscles depends on descending inputs from premotor respiratory neurons located in a continuous column along the ventrolateral medullary reticular formation and referred to as the ventral respiratory column. These neurons of the ventral respiratory column receive input from the medullary and pontine respiratory pattern generators, central chemoreceptive areas, and NTS and send direct projections to respiratory motoneurons of the spinal cord. The respiratory network also controls the phasic activity of muscles that the control upper airway via inputs to the nucleus ambiguus, hypoglossal, trigeminal, and facial nuclei.

Parabrachial Nuclear Complex

The parabrachial (PB) nuclear complex consists of three major subdivisions: lateral PB (LPB), medial PB, and the Kölliker–Fuse nucleus (KF) [36] and provides an interface between medullary reflexes and forebrain mechanisms regulating cardiovascular, respiratory, and other homeostatic functions. The PB subnuclei also relay interoceptive inputs (pain, visceral, and temperature sensation) from lamina I of the dorsal horn and NTS to the thalamus, hypothalamus, and amygdala. The PB nuclear complex receives topographically and functionally organized descending projections from the forebrain, including the anterior cingulate, prefrontal, and insular cortices; several areas of the hypothalamus; and central nucleus of the amygdala [45].

The outputs from the PB complex subnuclei are mediated by glutamate and several neuropeptides. These outputs participate in control of arousal, respiration, cardiovascular function, thermoregulation, and control of food and salt intake. For example, the medial PB contains glutamatergic neurons that are critical for cortical arousal via projections to the basal forebrain [46]. The LPB contains glutamatergic neurons that mediate arousal in response to hypercapnia; these neurons also express calcitonin-gene-related peptide (CGRP) [47]. Components of the PB nuclear complex, including the external LBP, lateral crescent, and KF, constitute the so-called pontine respiratory group, which has a major role in phase-switching of respiratory activity [43, 48]. Glutamatergic neurons in this complex are activated by hypercapnia and project to the ventrolateral medullary premotor respiratory column, the cranial nerve nuclei controlling the upper airway, and the phrenic nucleus in the spinal cord [49]. The LPB also participates in control of arterial blood pressure, as well as sodium and fluid homoeostasis [50]. It receives inputs from arterial baroreceptors and cardiac receptors via the NTS and projects back to the NTS and to the RVLM, including the C1 group; via these projections, different portions of the lateral PB may exert either excitatory or inhibitory influences on baroreflex responses and sympathetic output [51, 52]. Neurons of the LPB receive inputs from lamina I neurons receiving inputs from skin thermoreceptors and convey these inputs to the hypothalamus [39]. LPB neurons expressing CGRP also relay satiety signals from the gut and nociceptive signals from lamina I to the amygdala and thalamus [53].

Pelvic Organ Stimulating Center

The pelvic organ stimulating center is a recent term for a nucleus located in the dorsal pontine tegmental field and previously known as the Barrington nucleus or pontine micturition center [10]. This nucleus sends direct excitatory projections to all parasympathetic motoneurons in the sacral cord innervating the pelvic organs, including not only the bladder but also the distal colon, rectum, and internal genital organs. Collaterals of the pelvic organ stimulating center fibers have access to the inhibitory premotor interneurons in the sacral cord, innervating the nucleus of Onuf, so that contraction of the bladder, rectum, and uterus occurs together with relaxation of the pelvic floor striated muscles, which is important for micturition, defecation, and parturition [26]. A group of neurons in the pontine lateral tegmental field just caudal and ventrolateral to the pelvic organ stimulating center and referred to as pelvic floor stimulating center projects directly to the somatic motoneurons in the nucleus of Onuf in the upper sacral cord innervating the striated muscles of the pelvic floor [10].

Upper Brainstem and Behavioral State-Dependent Regulation of Autonomic Output

Periaqueductal Gray

The periaqueductal gray (PAG) provides an anatomical and functional interface between the forebrain areas involved in cognitive and emotional processing and lower brainstem circuits mediating autonomic reflexes, pain modulation, and motor responses. The PAG has been subdivided into four columns: dorsomedial, dorsolateral, lateral, and ventrolateral; each is characterized by specific inputs, outputs, and functions [9]. The PAG receives afferents from the forebrain (predominantly orbitomedial prefrontal, anterior cingulate, and anterior insular cortex, amygdala, and hypothalamus), brainstem (including the NTS, PB complex, and monoaminergic groups), and sensory neurons of the dorsal horn and trigeminal nucleus. The different columns of the PAG provide efferents to the thalamus, hypothalamus, and brainstem. Via its descending projections, the PAG coordinates specific patterns of cardiovascular, respiratory, motor and pain modulatory responses associated with stress and emotional arousal [9]. The dorsolateral PAG receives inputs from the amygdala and its stimulation generates increases in sympathetic activity and respiratory rate that resemble responses naturally evoked by psychological stressors. The lateral PAG receives inputs from somatic pain receptors and generates increases in sympathetic activity via direct descending projections to the RVLM, as well as analgesia and motor activation as part of a fight-or-flight response. The ventrolateral PAG contains different groups of neurons involved in several functions. Neurons that receive nociceptive inputs from visceral and deep receptors trigger sympathoinhibition, cardiovagal activation, opioid-mediated analgesia, and inhibition of motor activity as a part of the "playing death" response [9]. Other neurons receive inputs from bladder afferents and control the micturition reflex via projections to the pelvic organ stimulating center [10]. The ventrolateral PAG also contains REM-off neurons that participate in reciprocal inhibitory interactions with pontine REM-on neurons in the subcoeruleus/sublaterodorsal nucleus of the pons [54]. The presence of dopaminergic neurons in this area participates in arousal maintenance [55].

Locus Coeruleus

The locus coeruleus (LC) contains norepinephrine-synthesizing neurons that send diffuse projections throughout the central nervous system and have a major role in arousal, attention, and stress response [56]. In humans, the most extensive innervation targets somatosensory, motor, prefrontal, and parietal cortices. The LC also sends ascending projections to the amygdala, entorhinal cortex, hippocampal formation, thalamus, basal forebrain, and hypothalamus. Descending projections of the LC innervate autonomic areas such as the DMV, sacral preganglionic neurons, and central gray as well as dorsal horn of the spinal cord. The LC receives a wide variety of afferent inputs from several sources, including the prefrontal and anterior cingulate cortices, central nucleus of the amygdala, posterior lateral hypothalamus, PPN, and C1 neurons of the RVLM. The LC has a major role in attention, emotional memory, and response to stress. Noradrenergic neurons of the LC, like serotonergic neurons in the rostral raphe nuclei and histaminergic neurons of the tuberomammillary nucleus of the hypothalamus, have high firing rates during wakefulness, reduced firing during NREM sleep, and virtual cessation of firing during REM sleep. The LC, together with other catecholaminergic cells groups, including area A7 and nucleus subcoeruleus region, provides polysynaptic collateral projections to both the IML and the ventral horn. These catecholaminergic presympathetic-premotor neurons send polysynaptic collaterals to skeletal muscle and the adrenal gland, and have an important role in somatomotor–sympathetic integration [57].

Pedunculopontine Tegmental Nucleus

The pedunculopontine tegmental nucleus (PPT/PPN) contains intermingled populations, of cholinergic, glutamatergic, and GABAergic neurons that differentially influence cortical activity and sleep-wake states via projections to the thalamus, hypothalamus, and brainstem. Cholinergic (as well as glutamatergic) PPN/PPT neurons promote arousal and REM sleep, reduce muscle tone necessary for locomotion, and increase dopamine release from midbrain neurons in response to reward [58]. The PPT/PPN contains functionally distinct areas affecting respiration, cardiovascular function, and activity of upper airway muscles. The PPT/PPN sends excitatory cholinergic projections to the RVLM, including the C1 area [59]. Putative command neurons in the PPT/PPN are connected to both motor and autonomic areas and may integrate the somatomotor and sympathetic functions during different behaviors, including arousal and locomotion [60].

Hypothalamus: Pattern Generator for Basic Survival Functions

Functional Organization

The hypothalamus functions as a pattern generator of responses mediated by neural circuits critical for basic vital functions, including energy metabolism, fluid and electrolyte balance, thermoregulation, wake-sleep cycle, responses to internal or environmental stressors, and reproduction [7]. The preoptic hypothalamus contains neuronal circuitry critical for circadian rhythms, thermoregulation, electrolyte-balance, wake-sleep regulation, and reproduction. The tuberal hypothalamus includes nuclei that participate in control of feeding, autonomic, and endocrine responses to stress, aggression, and sexual behavior. The posterior hypothalamus provides output to the arousal system. The hypothalamus incorporates information from sensory afferents, humoral signals, and emotional circuits, and compares these inputs to basic set-points for parameters such as blood temperature, sodium, glucose, and hormone levels. The hypothalamus then activates autonomic, endocrine, and behavioral responses to maintain homeostasis or overcome stressors.

Autonomic Output

The autonomic output of the hypothalamus originates primarily from the paraventricular nucleus (PVN), dorsomedial nucleus (DMH), and adjacent lateral hypothalamic area, including the orexin/hypocretin (Orx/Hcrt) group, with a small contribution from the arcuate (infundibular) nucleus. These nuclei contain neurons that project to preganglionic sympathetic or parasympathetic neurons either directly or, more commonly, via brainstem areas.

The PVN is critical for integrated responses to internal stressors, including hypoglycemia, hypovolemia, and circulating cytokines in the setting of inflammation. Preautonomic autonomic neurons send direct projections to the IML, NTS, and RVLM, including the C1 group [61, 62]. There is topographic organization of PVN neurons controlling sympathetic outflow to different target organs, such as the heart and the kidney. These receive information from visceral receptors, including low pressure cardiac receptors relayed by the NTS and the A1 and A2 noradrenergic neurons in the medulla; signals such as plasma osmolarity and angiotensin II via the median preoptic nucleus, SFO, and OVLT; and signals such as levels of insulin and leptin controlling food intake via inputs from the arcuate nucleus. In general, PVN presympathetic neurons do not appear to have a major role in regulating sympathetic responses to short-term homeostatic changes but have a major role in responses to longer-term challenges, such as sustained water deprivation or chronic intermittent hypoxia [62]. Whereas presympathetic PVN neurons are not primarily affected by the baroreflex, they can modify baroreflex gain during exercise or in response to psychiatrical stressors via projections to the NTS [63].

The DMH has a major role in sympathoexcitatory and respiratory response to psychological stressors [40, 64] and also has a key role in sympathoexcitatory responses to exposure to cold [65]. These responses are largely mediated by DMH projections to the RVMM, including the RPa. The RPa contains premotor sympathoexcitatory neurons that trigger stress-induced tachycardia and cold-induced skin vasoconstriction and thermogenesis by the brown adipose tissue via direct projections to the IML [39]. The DMH also projects very heavily to other hypothalamic regions, the amygdala, medial prefrontal cortex, and PB complex.

The perifornical region is a major source of sympathetic vasomotor and respiratory drive during arousal or psychological stress via its direct projection to the RVMM and IML, dorsomedial medulla, and Kölliker–Fuse nucleus (reviewed by Dampney [40]). The Orx/Hcrt neurons located in the lateral hypothalamus, DMH and perifornical region have a major role in maintenance of wake state and trigger autonomic and respiratory responses associated to stress and reward. These neurons project to arousal-mediating cholinergic and monoaminergic cell groups, PAG, RVLM, RVMM, PB/Kölliker–Fuse nuclei, and preBötC [66]. Orexin increases blood pressure, heart rate, sympathetic nerve activity, and respiration; these are components of arousal and are necessary to allow the expression of motivated behaviors [67]. The firing rate of orexin neurons is altered greatly during a variety of behaviors, including the different phases of sleep, exercise, and psychological stress.

Limbic Areas Involved in Emotion, Cognition, and Autonomic Control

The core telencephalic areas controlling autonomic outputs are the amygdala, insular and anterior cingulate cortex areas. These areas are consistently activated in humans during tasks associated with sympathetic or parasympathetic responses [12–20]. They are interconnected with each other and control autonomic outputs via projections to the hypothalamus and brainstem and are core components of the emotion or "anterior limbic" system, which also includes the orbitofrontal cortex; nucleus accumbens and hypothalamus [68, 69]. Central autonomic commands to preganglionic neurons may be sent as predictive signals about the expected sensory consequences resulting from activation of the target organs; these commands are also sent as a feedforward efference copy to viscerosensory areas that receive feedback information resulting from the actual response of the target organ. The mismatch between feedforward commands and feedback signals generates an error prediction signal that is utilized in the CNS to modify the autonomic commands and/or the sensory predictions [70].

Amygdala

The amygdala provides automatic tagging of the valence (positive or negative) and intensity of innate or conditioned environmental stimuli and thereby their behavioral relevance [68]. The outputs of the amygdala to the hypothalamus and brainstem trigger automatic survival responses. Its outputs to the orbitofrontal cortex, hippocampus, and nucleus accumbens contribute to representation of value for reward (incentive)-based behavior, modulate episodic memory, and contribute to social cognition [71]. The amygdala is a nuclear complex subdivided into lateral, basal, and central nuclei; these nuclei participate in intrinsic circuits for encoding, retrieval, and extinction of emotional memories. Neurons in the lateral nucleus respond to concurrent neutral (conditioned) inputs from cortical sensory association areas and emotionally relevant (positive or negative) unconditioned stimuli directly from the thalamus or PB nuclei; the lateral amygdala is thus the primary site for associative (Pavlovian) learning. Information from the lateral nucleus is then channeled and processed via the basal nucleus to the central nucleus, which also receives direct input via the PB. The medial portion of the central nucleus (CeM) and neighboring bed nucleus of the stria terminalis form a tightly interconnected unit involved in organizing defensive responses to a wide range of threats [72]. The CeM projects to the hypothalamus, PAG, PB complex, and medullary autonomic and motor areas. These outputs trigger sympathetic or parasympathetic activation, adrenocortical hormone secretions, and motor responses such as vocalization, freezing, and startle [73].

Insular Cortex

The insular cortex is involved in a wide range of sensory, cognitive, affective, and motor functions and receives inputs from multiple sources [74, 75]. The dorsal posterior insula is the primary interoceptive cortex and integrates visceral, pain, and temperature sensations conveyed to subnuclei in the ventromedial portion of the thalamus that receive inputs pathways from lamina I, NTS, and PB nuclear complex. The anterior insula, via its interconnections with the amygdala, anterior cingulate, and orbitofrontal cortex, integrates these interoceptive signals with emotional and cognitive processing to contribute to the conscious awareness of bodily sensation [74]. For example, functional magnetic resonance (fMRI) studies showed increased activity of the anterior insula during tasks in which subjects attend to the timing of their heartbeats [76]. The insula is also a visceromotor area controlling both the sympathetic and parasympathetic outputs, primarily via a relay in the lateral hypothalamus [77]. Studies in rodents and effect of lesions in humans suggest that there may be a lateralization of insular control of cardiovascular function [77]. Consistent with this possibility, fMRI studies showed greater activation of the right than the left insular cortex in association with increase in heart rate in response to mental stress [77] or during baroreflex-mediated sympathoexcitation elicited by the Valsalva maneuver [78]. Normal subjects, who reacted with an increase in heart rate during mental stress, had larger activation of the right insular cortex and anterior shift in activity compared to subjects that did not react. This putative lateralization of autonomic control, with predominance of sympathetic activation from the right insula, has been linked to susceptibility to cardiac arrhythmias and other cardiovascular changes after stroke [79]. Functional imaging studies also showed that in response to emotional stressors associated with increased sympathetic activity, there is also asymmetric activation of the amygdala, PAG, and DMH [80]. As the DMH triggers sympathetically mediated increase in heart rate in response to emotional stressors via input to the RPa, this could predispose to stress-induced cardiac arrhythmias [80].

Anterior and Midcingulate Cortices

The cingulate cortex is a complex structure that is subdivided into four main sectors, anterior cingulate (ACC), midcingulate (MCC), posterior cingulate, and retrosplenial cortex [81], that are involved in different aspects of emotional processing. The ACC includes a subgenual and pregenual regions that are strongly interconnected with the orbitofrontal cortex and the amygdala and send strong projections to the lateral hypothalamus, PAG, PB, and medullary autonomic areas. Stimulation of the pregenual ACC during presurgical brain mapping in patients with epilepsy elicited emotional face expression, interoceptive sensations, and autonomic responses that included hot flushes in the face, cold sweats, and tachycardia; many patients explicitly interpreted these symptoms in terms of fear and anxiety [82]. In contrast, stimulation of the anterior MCC elicited goal-oriented behaviors but no autonomic responses. Together with the insular cortex, the pregenual ACC and anterior MCC are central nodes of the so-called salience network. Functional neuroimaging showed that the intrinsic connectivity within this network correlates positively with resting muscle sympathetic nerve activity [83]. Previous studies also showed that measures of sympathetic activity, such as sympathetic skin response, were coupled to enhanced activity in the anterior midcingulate (referred to as dorsal ACC in these studies) and insular cortices [84]. In contrast, sympathetic indices were negatively correlated with activity of the subgenual cingulate and adjacent ventromedial prefrontal cortex, which are components of "default mode network" [84]. Activation of the subgenual ACC strongly correlates with indices of cardiovagal activity, such as heart rate variability [85].

Summary

The CNS areas controlling autonomic functions are closely interconnected; integrate autonomic with respiratory, arousal, and other homeostatic responses. These areas participate in state-dependent control of these functions not only during wakefulness but also across sleep states [86, 87], in response to emotion, and during attentional and other behavioral tasks [40]. Optogenetic studies in rodents and fMRI studies in humans have provided insight into the functional organizations of these areas. Integration of the information from animal and human studies will help in elucidating the mechanisms of abnormal autonomic control in CNS disorders, which are also typically associated with abnormalities in sleep.

References

1. Benarroch EE. Brainstem integration of arousal, sleep, cardiovascular, and respiratory control. Neurology. 2018;91(21):958–66.
2. Stornetta RL, Guyenet PG. C1 neurons: a nodal point for stress? Exp Physiol. 2018;103(3):332–6.
3. Dampney RA. Central neural control of the cardiovascular system: current perspectives. Adv Physiol Educ. 2016;40(3):283–96.
4. Saper CB. The central autonomic nervous system: conscious visceral perception and autonomic pattern generation. Annu Rev Neurosci. 2002;25:433–69.
5. Guyenet PG. The sympathetic control of blood pressure. Nat Rev Neurosci. 2006;7(5):335–46. Review
6. McAllen RM, Spyer KM. The location of cardiac vagal preganglionic motoneurones in the medulla of the cat. J Physiol. 1976;258(1):187–204.
7. Saper CB, Lowell BB. The hypothalamus. Curr Biol. 2014;24(23):R1111–6.
8. Guyenet PG, Stornetta RL, Bochorishvili G, Depuy SD, Burke PG, Abbott SB. C1 neurons: the body's EMTs. Am J Physiol Regul Integr Comp Physiol. 2013;305(3):R187–204.
9. Bandler R, Keay KA, Floyd N, Price J. Central circuits mediating patterned autonomic activity during active vs. passive emotional coping. Brain Res Bull. 2000;53(1):95–104.
10. Holstege G. How the emotional motor system controls the pelvic organs. Sex Med Rev. 2016;4(4):303–28.
11. Gourine AV, Machhada A, Trapp S, Spyer KM. Cardiac vagal preganglionic neurones: an update. Auton Neurosci. 2016;199:24–8.
12. Critchley HD. Neural mechanisms of autonomic, affective, and cognitive integration. J Comp Neurol. 2005;493(1):154–66.
13. Cechetto DF, Shoemaker JK. Functional neuroanatomy of autonomic regulation. NeuroImage. 2009;47(3):795–803.

14. Kreibig SD. Autonomic nervous system activity in emotion: a review. Biol Psychol. 2010;84(3):394–421.
15. Beissner F, Meissner K, Bar KJ, Napadow V. The autonomic brain: an activation likelihood estimation meta-analysis for central processing of autonomic function. J Neurosci. 2013;33(25):10503–11.
16. Shoemaker JK, Norton KN, Baker J, Luchyshyn T. Forebrain organization for autonomic cardiovascular control. Auton Neurosci. 2015;188:5–9.
17. Macefield VG, Henderson LA. “Real-time” imaging of cortical and subcortical sites of cardiovascular control: concurrent recordings of sympathetic nerve activity and fMRI in awake subjects. J Neurophysiol. 2016;116(3):1199–207.
18. Macey PM, Ogren JA, Kumar R, Harper RM. Functional imaging of autonomic regulation: methods and key findings. Front Neurosci. 2015;9:513.
19. Sklerov M, Dayan E, Browner N. Functional neuroimaging of the central autonomic network: recent developments and clinical implications. Clin Auton Res. 2019;29(6):555–66.
20. Kimmerly DS. A review of human neuroimaging investigations involved with central autonomic regulation of baroreflex-mediated cardiovascular control. Auton Neurosci. 2017;207:10–21.
21. Sisó S, Jeffrey M, González L. Sensory circumventricular organs in health and disease. Acta Neuropathol. 2010;120(6):689–705.
22. Albrecht U. Timing to perfection: the biology of central and peripheral circadian clocks. Neuron. 2012;74(2):246–60.
23. Deuchars SA, Lall VK. Sympathetic preganglionic neurons: properties and inputs. Compr Physiol. 2015;5(2):829–69.
24. Hopkins DA, Bieger D, deVente J, Steinbusch WM. Vagal efferent projections: viscerotopy, neurochemistry and effects of vagotomy. Prog Brain Res. 1996;107:79–96.
25. Travagli RA, Anselmi L. Vagal neurocircuitry and its influence on gastric motility. Nat Rev Gastroenterol Hepatol. 2016;13(7):389–401.
26. Fowler CJ, Griffiths D, de Groat WC. The neural control of micturition. Nat Rev Neurosci. 2008;9(6):453–66.
27. Eldahan KC, Rabchevsky AG. Autonomic dysreflexia after spinal cord injury: systemic pathophysiology and methods of management. Auton Neurosci. 2018;209:59–70.
28. Cutsforth-Gregory JK, Benarroch EE. Nucleus of the solitary tract, medullary reflexes, and clinical implications. Neurology. 2017;88(12):1187–96.
29. McRitchie DA, Tork I. The internal organization of the human solitary nucleus. Brain Res Bull. 1993;31(1–2):171–93.
30. Topolovec JC, Gati JS, Menon RS, Shoemaker JK, Cechetto DF. Human cardiovascular and gustatory brainstem sites observed by functional magnetic resonance imaging. J Comp Neurol. 2004;471(4):446–61.
31. Price CJ, Hoyda TD, Ferguson AV. The area postrema: a brain monitor and integrator of systemic autonomic state. Neuroscientist. 2008;14(2):182–94.
32. Dampney RA, Polson JW, Potts PD, Hirooka Y, Horiuchi J. Functional organization of brain pathways subserving the baroreceptor reflex: studies in conscious animals using immediate early gene expression. Cell Mol Neurobiol. 2003;23(4–5):597–616.
33. Guyenet PG. Regulation of breathing and autonomic outflows by chemoreceptors. Compr Physiol. 2014;4(4):1511–62.
34. Zoccal DB, Furuya WI, Bassi M, Colombari DS, Colombari E. The nucleus of the solitary tract and the coordination of respiratory and sympathetic activities. Front Physiol. 2014;5:238.
35. Lin LH, Moore SA, Jones SY, McGlashon J, Talman WT. Astrocytes in the rat nucleus tractus solitarii are critical for cardiovascular reflex control. J Neurosci. 2013;33(47):18608–17.
36. Fulwiler CE, Saper CB. Subnuclear organization of the efferent connections of the parabrachial nucleus in the rat. Brain Res. 1984;319(3):229–59.
37. Abbott SB, Coates MB, Stornetta RL, Guyenet PG. Optogenetic stimulation of c1 and retrotrapezoid nucleus neurons causes sleep state-dependent cardiorespiratory stimulation and arousal in rats. Hypertension. 2013;61(4):835–41.
38. Wenker IC, Abe C, Viar KE, Stornetta DS, Stornetta RL, Guyenet PG. Blood pressure regulation by the rostral ventrolateral medulla in conscious rats: effects of hypoxia, hypercapnia, baroreceptor denervation, and anesthesia. J Neurosci. 2017;37(17):4565–83.
39. Morrison SF, Nakamura K, Madden CJ. Central control of thermogenesis in mammals. Exp Physiol. 2008;93(7):773–97.
40. Dampney RA. Central mechanisms regulating coordinated cardiovascular and respiratory function during stress and arousal. Am J Physiol Regul Integr Comp Physiol. 2015;309(5):R429–43.
41. Teran FA, Massey CA, Richerson GB. Serotonin neurons and central respiratory chemoreception: where are we now? Prog Brain Res. 2014;209:207–33.
42. Del Negro CA, Funk GD, Feldman JL. Breathing matters. Nat Rev Neurosci. 2018;19(6):351–67.
43. Feldman JL, Del Negro CA, Gray PA. Understanding the rhythm of breathing: so near, yet so far. Annu Rev Physiol. 2013;75:423–52.
44. Guyenet PG, Bayliss DA. Neural control of breathing and CO2 homeostasis. Neuron. 2015;87(5):946–61.
45. Moga MM, Herbert H, Hurley KM, Yasui Y, Gray TS, Saper CB. Organization of cortical, basal forebrain, and hypothalamic afferents to the parabrachial nucleus in the rat. J Comp Neurol. 1990;295(4):624–61.
46. Kaur S, Pedersen NP, Yokota S, Hur EE, Fuller PM, Lazarus M, et al. Glutamatergic signaling from the parabrachial nucleus plays a critical role in hypercapnic arousal. J Neurosci. 2013;33(18):7627–40.
47. Kaur S, Wang JL, Ferrari L, Thankachan S, Kroeger D, Venner A, et al. A genetically defined circuit for arousal from sleep during hypercapnia. Neuron. 2017;96(5):1153–67. e1155
48. Chamberlin NL, Saper CB. Topographic organization of respiratory responses to glutamate microstimulation of the parabrachial nucleus in the rat. J Neurosci. 1994;14(11 Pt 1):6500–10.
49. Yokota S, Kaur S, VanderHorst VG, Saper CB, Chamberlin NL. Respiratory-related outputs of glutamatergic, hypercapnia-responsive parabrachial neurons in mice. J Comp Neurol. 2015;523(6):907–20.
50. Davern PJ. A role for the lateral parabrachial nucleus in cardiovascular function and fluid homeostasis. Front Physiol. 2014;5:436.
51. Chamberlin NL, Saper CB. Topographic organization of cardiovascular responses to electrical and glutamate microstimulation of the parabrachial nucleus in the rat. J Comp Neurol. 1992;326(2):245–62.
52. Hayward LF, Felder RB. Lateral parabrachial nucleus modulates baroreflex regulation of sympathetic nerve activity. Am J Phys. 1998;274(5):R1274–82.
53. de Lacalle S, Saper CB. Calcitonin gene-related peptide-like immunoreactivity marks putative visceral sensory pathways in human brain. Neuroscience. 2000;100(1):115–30.
54. Fuller PM, Saper CB, Lu J. The pontine REM switch: past and present. J Physiol. 2007;584(Pt 3):735–41.
55. Lu J, Jhou TC, Saper CB. Identification of wake-active dopaminergic neurons in the ventral periaqueductal gray matter. J Neurosci. 2006;26(1):193–202.
56. Benarroch EE. Locus coeruleus. Cell Tissue Res. 2018;373(1):221–32.
57. Nam H, Kerman IA. Distribution of catecholaminergic presympathetic-premotor neurons in the rat lower brainstem. Neuroscience. 2016;324:430–45.
58. Mena-Segovia J, Bolam JP. Rethinking the pedunculopontine nucleus: from cellular organization to function. Neuron. 2017;94(1):7–18.
59. Padley JR, Kumar NN, Li Q, Nguyen TB, Pilowsky PM, Goodchild AK. Central command regulation of circulatory function mediated

by descending pontine cholinergic inputs to sympathoexcitatory rostral ventrolateral medulla neurons. Circ Res. 2007;100(2):284–91.
60. Krout KE, Mettenleiter TC, Loewy AD. Single CNS neurons link both central motor and cardiosympathetic systems: a double-virus tracing study. Neuroscience. 2003;118(3):853–66.
61. Saper CB, Loewy AD, Swanson LW, Cowan WM. Direct hypothalamo-autonomic connections. Brain Res. 1976;117(2):305–12.
62. Dampney RA, Michelini LC, Li DP, Pan HL. Regulation of sympathetic vasomotor activity by the hypothalamic paraventricular nucleus in normotensive and hypertensive states. Am J Physiol Heart Circ Physiol. 2018;315(5):H1200–14.
63. Michelini LC. Differential effects of vasopressinergic and oxytocinergic pre-autonomic neurons on circulatory control: reflex mechanisms and changes during exercise. Clin Exp Pharmacol Physiol. 2007;34(4):369–76.
64. Fontes MA, Xavier CH, de Menezes RC, Dimicco JA. The dorsomedial hypothalamus and the central pathways involved in the cardiovascular response to emotional stress. Neuroscience. 2011;184:64–74.
65. Dimicco JA, Zaretsky DV. The dorsomedial hypothalamus: a new player in thermoregulation. Am J Physiol Regul Integr Comp Physiol. 2007;292(1):R47–63.
66. Nattie E, Li A. Respiration and autonomic regulation and orexin. Prog Brain Res. 2012;198:25–46.
67. Kuwaki T, Zhang W. Orexin neurons as arousal-associated modulators of central cardiorespiratory regulation. Respir Physiol Neurobiol. 2010;174(1–2):43–54.
68. LeDoux J. The amygdala. Curr Biol. 2007;17(20):R868–74. Review
69. Rolls ET. Limbic systems for emotion and for memory, but no single limbic system. Cortex. 2015;62:119–57.
70. Barrett LF, Simmons WK. Interoceptive predictions in the brain. Nat Rev Neurosci. 2015;16(7):419–29.
71. LeDoux J. Rethinking the emotional brain. Neuron. 2012;73(4):653–76.
72. Fox AS, Shackman AJ. The central extended amygdala in fear and anxiety: closing the gap between mechanistic and neuroimaging research. Neurosci Lett. 2019;693:58–67.
73. Venkatraman A, Edlow BL, Immordino-Yang MH. The brainstem in emotion: a review. Front Neuroanat. 2017;11:15.
74. Craig AD. Significance of the insula for the evolution of human awareness of feelings from the body. Ann N Y Acad Sci. 2011;1225:72–82.
75. Nieuwenhuys R. The insular cortex: a review. Prog Brain Res. 2012;195:123–63.
76. Schulz SM. Neural correlates of heart-focused interoception: a functional magnetic resonance imaging meta-analysis. Philos Trans R Soc Lond Ser B Biol Sci. 2016;371(1708):20160018.
77. Cechetto DF. Cortical control of the autonomic nervous system. Exp Physiol. 2014;99(2):326–31.
78. Macey PM, Rieken NS, Kumar R, Ogren JA, Middlekauff HR, Wu P, et al. Sex differences in insular cortex gyri responses to the valsalva maneuver. Front Neurol. 2016;7:87.
79. Oppenheimer S, Cechetto D. The insular cortex and the regulation of cardiac function. Compr Physiol. 2016;692:1081–133.
80. Fontes MAP, Filho ML, Santos Machado NL, de Paula CA, Souza Cordeiro LM, Xavier CH, et al. Asymmetric sympathetic output: the dorsomedial hypothalamus as a potential link between emotional stress and cardiac arrhythmias. Auton Neurosci. 2017;207:22–7.
81. Vogt BA. Submodalities of emotion in the context of cingulate subregions. Cortex. 2014;59:197–202.
82. Caruana F, Gerbella M, Avanzini P, Gozzo F, Pelliccia V, Mai R, et al. Motor and emotional behaviours elicited by electrical stimulation of the human cingulate cortex. Brain. 2018;141(10):3035–51.
83. Taylor KS, Kucyi A, Millar PJ, Murai H, Kimmerly DS, Morris BL, et al. Association between resting-state brain functional connectivity and muscle sympathetic burst incidence. J Neurophysiol. 2016;115(2):662–73.
84. Critchley HD, Nagai Y, Gray MA, Mathias CJ. Dissecting axes of autonomic control in humans: insights from neuroimaging. Auton Neurosci. 2011;161(1–2):34–42.
85. Lane RD, Weidenbacher H, Smith R, Fort C, Thayer JF, Allen JJ. Subgenual anterior cingulate cortex activity covariation with cardiac vagal control is altered in depression. J Affect Disord. 2013;150(2):565–70.
86. Benarroch EE. Control of the cardiovascular and respiratory systems during sleep. Auton Neurosci. 2019;218:54–63.
87. Silvani A, Dampney RA. Central control of cardiovascular function during sleep. Am J Physiol Heart Circ Physiol. 2013;305(12):H1683–92.

Functional Neuroanatomy of the Peripheral Autonomic Nervous System

3

Sudhansu Chokroverty and Sushanth Bhat

Introduction

John Newport Langley, a Cambridge (England) physiologist, coined the term "autonomic nervous system (ANS)" in 1898, a term that included the thoracolumbar sympathetic and craniosacral (later termed parasympathetic) outflows as well as the local nervous system of the gut (came to be known later as the enteric nervous system (ENS) [1–5]). It is notable that he also introduced the terms "pre-and postganglionic" fibers in 1895. Following the demonstration by W. H. Gaskell of the craniosacral and thoracolumbar outflows toward the end of the nineteenth century [6], Langley proposed the term parasympathetic for the craniosacral outflow in 1905 and sympathetic for the thoracolumbar outflow [1, 2]. For some incomprehensible reason, the ENS was only recognized decades later in 1970 [3] (see below). Despite this early recognition of the ANS, which permeates throughout entire body systems and organs subserving vital functions for living beings, this important component of the nervous system has been a long neglected topic in the field until Shy and Drager [7] in 1960 directed our attention to a relentlessly progressive neurodegenerative disease initially involving the central autonomic neurons and later somatic nervous system (cerebellar-parkinsonian or parkinsonian-cerebellar syndrome). Since then there has been a surge of interest, particularly among academic neurologists. (Many physicians, however, remain uncertain even now about how to deal with disorders of the ANS).

The ANS basically controls the body's internal environment, maintaining the internal homeostasis (steady state) without conscious perception (involuntary) of almost all organs and systems in the body (e.g., cardiovascular, respiratory, gastrointestinal, and genitourinary systems, and endocrine functions as well as the Harvard physiologist Walter B. Cannon's "fight-or-flight" response under stressful situations (1915)) [8]. In contrast, the somatic (voluntary) nervous system is responsive to the external environment with conscious perception [8]. These two systems work in unison to control the body's homeostasis, constantly adapting to in order to keep the vital functions stable. It is astonishing to think how the ANS has been neglected by clinicians for nearly a century after the introduction of the topic by Langley.

Traditionally, the ANS has been divided into two divisions (the third division was reintroduced later): sympathetic and parasympathetic, and each division has central and peripheral components [9–15]. These are predominantly efferent fibers, but autonomic afferent fibers also exist, participating in vital reflex and other functions (see below). The internal homeostasis is maintained by three divisions of the ANS (sympathetic nervous system [SNS], the parasympathetic nervous system [PNS], and the enteric nervous system; see below), which are closely integrated and influenced by the central autonomic network [3, 15–17]) (see also Chap. 2). For a detailed description, readers are referred to some excellent texts [4, 5, 15]. Figures 3.1, 3.2, and 3.3 schematically outline the traditional two extrinsic divisions of the ANS and their connections.

The Sympathetic Efferent Organization

Anatomically the SNS is located at a central (spinal) level from C8-T1 to L1–L2 segments of the spinal cord and a peripheral level. The intermediolateral neurons in the

S. Chokroverty (✉)
Hackensack Meridian Health, Neuroscience Institute at JFK, JFK University Medical Center, Edison, NJ, USA

Seton Hall University & Hackensack Meridian School of Medicine at Seton Hall, South Orange, NJ, USA

Rutgers Robert Wood Johnson Medical School, New Brunswick, NJ, USA
e-mail: Sudhansu.Chokroverty@hackensackmeridian.org

S. Bhat
Neuroscience Institute, Hackensack Meridian Health, JFK Medical Center, Seton Hall University, Edison, NJ, USA

S. Chokroverty, P. Cortelli (eds.), *Autonomic Nervous System and Sleep*, https://doi.org/10.1007/978-3-030-62263-3_3

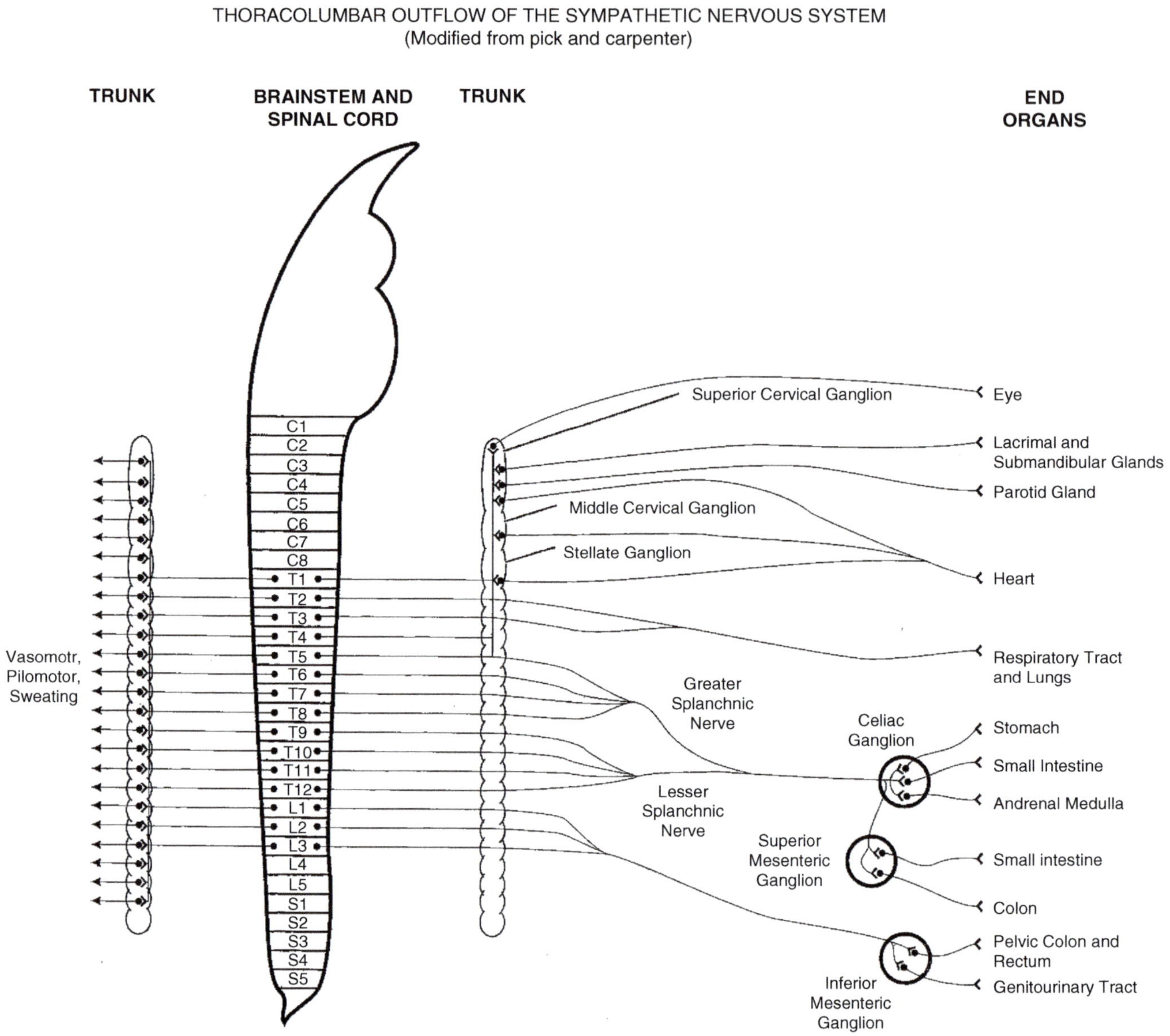

Fig. 3.1 Thoracolumbar outflow of the sympathetic nervous system shown schematically. (Modified from Pick [4] and Carpenter [11])

thoracolumbar spinal segments provide preganglionic nerve fibers, which are thinly myelinated fibers (white rami communicantes) measuring 2–3 μm in diameter and leave the intermediolateral column neurons along the ventral roots from C8 or T1 to L2 segments of the spinal cord (see Fig. 3.3). These preganglionic fibers then leave the ventral roots and pass to the nearest paravertebral sympathetic chain (trunk) located bilaterally on two sides of the vertebral column consisting of a series of ganglia connected with intervening nerves (see Figs. 3.1 and 3.2). The sympathetic chain extends from the base of the skull to the coccyx where the two trunks join in front of the coccyx to form a terminal ganglion called coccygeal or ganglion impar. There are three cervical ganglia (superior, middle, and inferior or stellate ganglia), 10–12 thoracic, four lumbar and four sacral ganglia, for a total of 22–23 ganglia (see Fig. 3.1). The preganglionic sympathetic fibers passing to the sympathetic chain may pursue one or more of the following three routes [16]: 1. Immediately synapse at the same level with a ganglion to leave the trunk as postganglionic fibers; 2. Ascend or descend in the sympathetic chain and leave the chain (trunk) as postganglionic fibers after synapsing with the paravertebral ganglia; 3. Leave the thoracic paravertebral trunk as splanchnic nerves (the greater, lesser, and least splanchnic nerves) to synapse with the nearby prevertebral ganglia (e.g., celiac, aorticorenal, superior, and inferior mesenteric ganglia, including previsceral and terminal ganglia). The postganglionic nerve fibers emerge to innervate the abdominal and pelvic viscera [4, 5, 15]. Some preganglionic fibers will pass through the chain to directly innervate the adrenal medulla. The preganglionic sympathetic fibers destined to innervate pupils of the eye and skin of the head and neck pass through the stellate and middle cervical ganglia without synapsing to the superior cervical ganglia where fibers synapse and postganglionic unmyelinated fibers (Gray

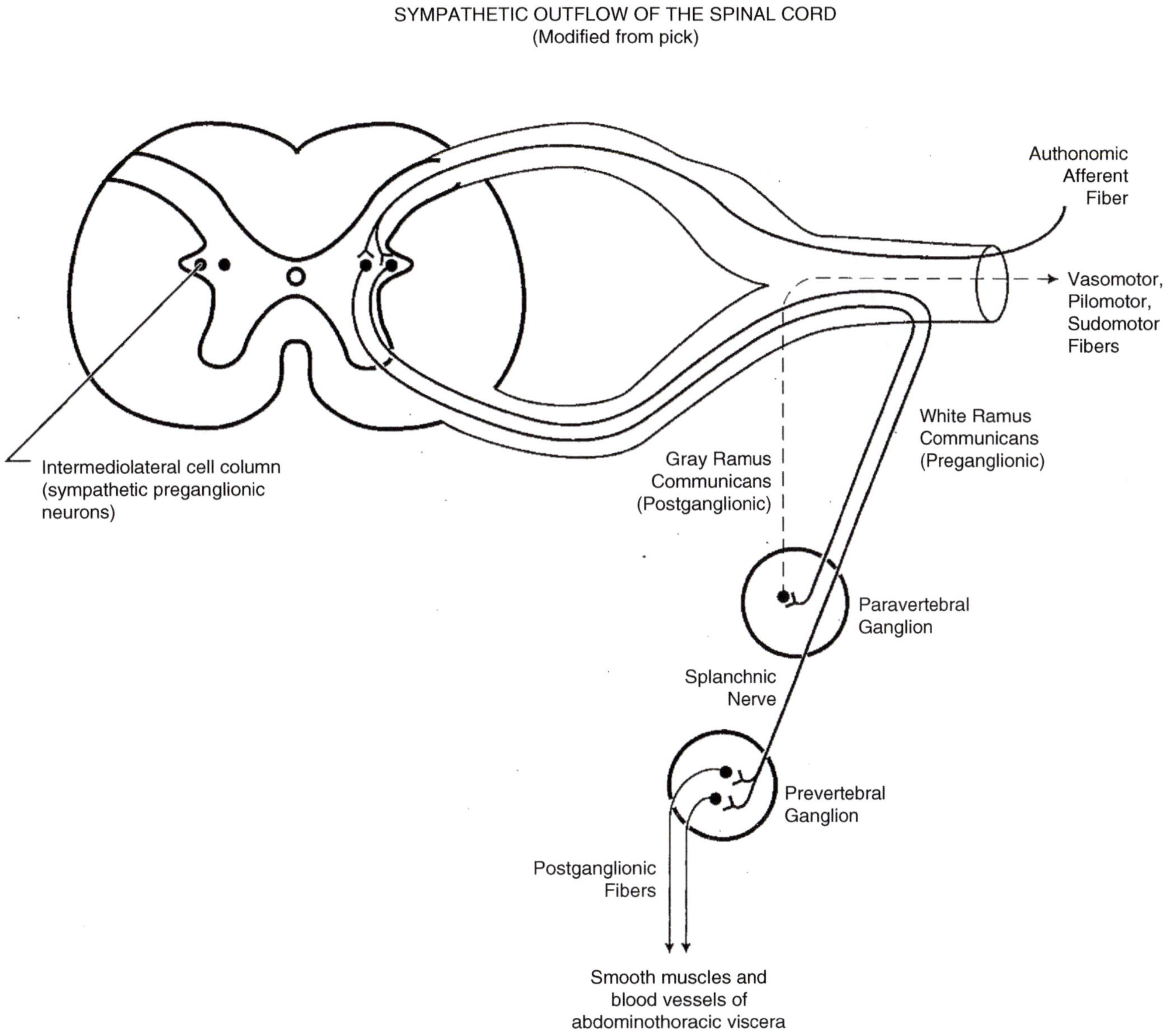

Fig. 3.2 Schematic diagram to show sympathetic outflow of the spinal cord

rami communicantes) innervate pupils and other structures in the head and neck. Prevertebral ganglia are located in the midline, anterior to the vertebral column. Previsceral or terminal ganglia are located close to the peripheral target structures. In the SNS, the preganglionic fibers are short but the postganglionic fibers are long. This lengthwise arrangement is reversed in the PNS, that is, the preganglionic fibers are long, whereas the postganglionic fibers are short. The postganglionic sympathetic fibers, which are unmyelinated, travel as gray rami communicantes along the spinal and peripheral nerves to the blood vessels to control limb circulation (vasomotor), sweat glands (sudomotor), and arrectores pilorum muscles of the skin (pilomotor), as well as the blood vessels of the voluntary muscles and the bones of all four limbs.

The sympathetic fibers from T1-T4 spinal segments and the cervical ganglia form the cardiac plexus to control the rhythm and contraction of the heart. The respiratory system is innervated by T2-T7 segments through stellate ganglion and upper five thoracic ganglia forming the pulmonary plexus. The esophageal plexus is formed by the postganglionic fibers from T2-T7 spinal cord segments with synapses at stellate and T2-T4 thoracic ganglia. Stomach, duodenum, and pancreas are controlled by T6-T10 segments through celiac ganglia. Celiac, aorticorenal, superior, and inferior mesenteric ganglia receiving innervation from T6-L2 segments control the rest of the small intestine and colon, including the rectum and anus. The genitourinary system is controlled by the hypogastric plexus receiving innervation from T10-L2 spinal cord segments. L1 and L2 spinal cord segments (through hypogastric plexus) control ejaculation in men. The T4-T9 segments control the upper trunk, whereas T10-L2 segments control the lower trunk below the umbili-

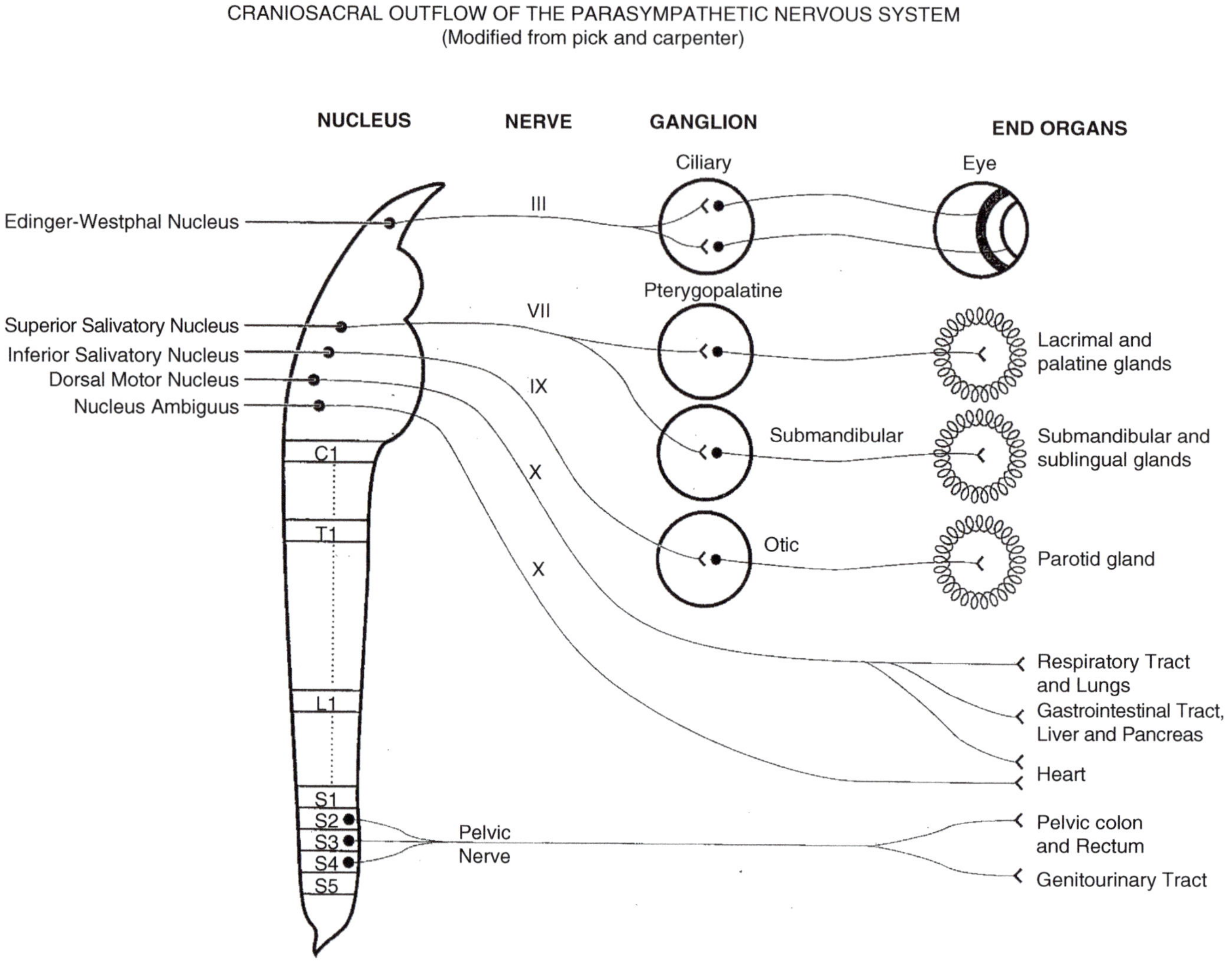

Fig. 3.3 Craniosacral outflow of the parasympathetic nervous system shown schematically. (Modified from Pick [4] and Carpenter [11])

cus. The rostral four thoracic segments innervate the upper limbs, while T12-L2 segments innervate the lower limbs. The ciliospinal center (of Budge) for pupillary dilatation is located in the C8-T1 segments. The splanchnic neurons from T4-L2 segments send impulses to the abdominal viscera.

The Parasympathetic Efferent Organization

The efferent parasympathetic nervous system (PNS) consists of the cranial and sacral subdivisions. The parasympathetic preganglionic neurons are located within the nuclei of the third, seventh, ninth, and tenth cranial nerves. The tectal outflow arises from the Edinger–Westphal nucleus in the midbrain, which sends preganglionic fibers to the ciliary ganglion from which the postganglionic fibers innervate the ciliary muscle of accommodation and sphincter pupillae muscle for pupilloconstriction.

The salivatory nuclei are located in the reticular formation at the pontomedullary junction. The superior salivatory nucleus sends efferent secretomotor and vasodilator fibers through the chorda tympani branch of the seventh nerve to innervate the lacrimal, sublingual, submandibular, and mucosal glands in the nasal cavity and palate.

The inferior salivatory nucleus sends efferent preganglionic fibers through the ninth cranial nerve to the otic ganglion, and via the auriculotemporal nerve, a branch of the mandibular division of the trigeminal nerve, innervates the parotid gland.

The preganglionic fibers from the dorsal motor nucleus of the vagus and the nucleus ambiguus in the medulla travel to innervate the heart and the smooth muscles of the thoracoabdominal viscera.

The preganglionic neurons of the sacral division of the parasympathetic system are located in the gray matter lateral to the central canal of the second, third and fourth sacral divisions of the spinal cord, and travel in the ventral spinal roots. These fibers form the nervi erigentes or the pelvic nerves and terminate in the postganglionic cell bodies located in the pelvic plexus. The postganglionic fibers originating from the pelvic plexus terminate at the distal segment of the sigmoid colon, the rectum, the urinary bladder, and the reproductive system.

The urinary bladder, including the lower urinary tract, is controlled by three groups of neurons (the pelvic, hypogastric, and pudendal nerves):

- The sacral parasympathetic (S2-S4 segments) forming the pelvic nerves
- The thoracolumbar SNS (T10-L2 segments of the spinal cord) fibers forming the hypogastric nerves
- The sacral somatic segments (S2-S4) forming the pudendal nerve

The Enteric Nervous System

Although Langley in 1898 [2] alluded to the local nervous system of the gut, the enteric nervous system (ENS) has not been known to the medical community until recognized in 1970 [3]. The ENS, derived from the word enteron (gut), also known as the "little brain" of the gut, plays an important role in the functional relationship with the "big brain" (brain–gut axis [17]). The ENS can function to an extent autonomously and semi-independently, but input from the traditional ANS and CNS ("big brain") influences gastro-intestinal (G-I) function through modulation of the ENS [17–22]. The ENS contains three groups of neurons [19–22]: the intrinsic primary afferent neurons, interneurons, and enteric motor neurons (efferent), forming networks to control alimentary behavior. The ENS subserves its functions by using two distinct intestinal plexuses: the myenteric plexus of Auerbach located between outer longitudinal and inner circular smooth muscles (involuntary) of the gut and the submucosal plexus of Meissner. The ENS, using several neuronal circuits, is involved in sensory-motor integration controlling intestinal motility, secretion, local blood flow, absorption, and to an extent these ENS circuits also modulate endocrine and immune functions [17–22]. The intestinal motility (motor pattern) basically consists of two types [20]: the propulsive stereotyped movements of peristalsis and spontaneous cyclical migrating motor complex (MMC). The ENS system involved in these movements consists of the intrinsic afferent neurons, interneurons, and efferent motor neurons forming neural circuits. Both the inner circular and the outer longitudinal smooth muscles of the gut are driven by the enteric neuronal circuits to initiate and propel these movements. The propulsive peristaltic movements are initiated by the sequential contractions of the circular smooth muscles beginning orally and propagating aborally. The enteric neuronal circuits also initiate the spontaneous cyclical MMC, propagating slowly aborally every 90 minutes, which has a circadian rhythm [23] with the lowest velocity during sleep without consistent relationship to the non-rapid eye movement (NREM) / REM sleep cycle [24]. The intrinsic ENS neurons directly control the gut motility and secretion, whereas the extrinsic parasympathetic and sympathetic divisions of the ANS originating from the CNS modulate the ENS neurons at the circuits. The central parasympathetic premotor neurons located in the dorsal motor nucleus (DMN) of the vagus nerve control (excitatory) most of the gut except the distal sigmoid colon and rectum, which are controlled by the parasympathetic outflow of the sacral (S2-S4) segments of the spinal cord. The premotor sympathetic neurons of the thoracolumbar outflow provide inhibitory control of the gut smooth muscles but exert excitatory control over the internal anal and vesical sphincters. In addition to these enteric motor neurons, there are primary enteric afferent neurons responding to both mechanical and chemical stimuli, and these afferent projections from the gut integrate with the central autonomic network for appropriate motor response (see also Chap. 2). These intrinsic primary afferents from the enteric neurons transmit impulses to the CNS via nodose ganglion of the vagus nerve (tenth cranial) and terminate onto the NTS, which provides CNS stimuli for sending efferent message mainly from the DMN of the vagus nerve to the effector organs. These are also somatic afferents projecting to the CNS via dorsal root ganglia. The ENS thus works in concert with the ANS and CNS to maintain the internal homeostasis and stability of the gastrointestinal tract. In addition, the interaction between the "little brain" and "big brain" maintains an awareness of what has been happening in the gut throughout 24 hours (brain–gut axis) [17].

Autonomic Afferent Fibers

In contrast to the general misperception, the ANS contains not only motor or efferent neurons (consisting of two neuron chains: preganglionic and postganglionic motor neurons) but also afferent fibers [3–5, 9, 15, 16, 25] (sensory neurons) transmitting signals to the CAN with its ascending and descending projections to other central ANS structures in the CNS to maintain stability of the internal environment (see also Chap. 2) . The role of the intrinsic primary afferent originating from neurons of the ENS through brain–gut interaction is to maintain the stability of the internal milieu ("*milieu intérieur*," the term coined by Claude Bernard in 1854) of the alimentary tract (see description above).

An example of an important parasympathetic afferent includes the baroreceptor and chemoreceptor afferents arising from presso- and chemo-receptors located in the carotid sinus and aortic arch [9, 10, 13, 18]. The afferent fibers for these reflexes are mediated by the sinus nerve of Hering, a branch of the glossopharyngeal (ninth cranial) nerve and the aortic nerve of Cyon and Ludwig, a branch of the vagus (tenth cranial) nerve. These fibers send afferent impulses from the mechanoreceptors and chemoreceptors in the walls of the carotid artery, heart, and aorta to the CNS structures controlling circulation and respiration. The baroreceptor afferents terminate on the nucleus tractus solitarius (NTS) [9, 10, 18], an important relay station in the medulla receiving visceral afferents from the cardiovascular, respiratory, and gastrointestinal tracts, as well as taste fibers, and afferents from the baroreceptors and chemoreceptors (see also Chap. 2) (Fig. 3.4). The NTS sends impulses to the medullary reticular formation (ventrolateral medulla), which in turn sends descending bulbospinal projections for vasomotor mediation to the intermediolateral column cells of the spinal cord. The latter through the thoracolumbar sympathetic outflow exerts specific influences on the sympathetic nerves supplying the heart, blood vessels, and adrenal medulla but has no effect on non-cardiorespiratory sympathetic nerves, for example, pupils, sweating, and piloerection. Sympathetic afferent fibers from the viscera traveling with the splanchnic nerves have been described, and other afferents join the somatic nerves on their way to the dorsal root ganglia. The afferents from the respiratory tract and pulmonary receptors terminate also on the NTS via the vagus (tenth cranial) nerve. Finally, general visceral afferents from the gastrointestinal tract also project to the NTS. The efferents arising from the adjacent DMN influence gastrointestinal tract motility and secretion via the vagus nerve and the ENS. The autonomic afferent fibers consist of viscerosensory (e.g., the enteric afferent fibers from cell bodies in the ENS, baroreceptors, and chemoreceptors), somatosensory (e.g., thermoreceptors and noci-

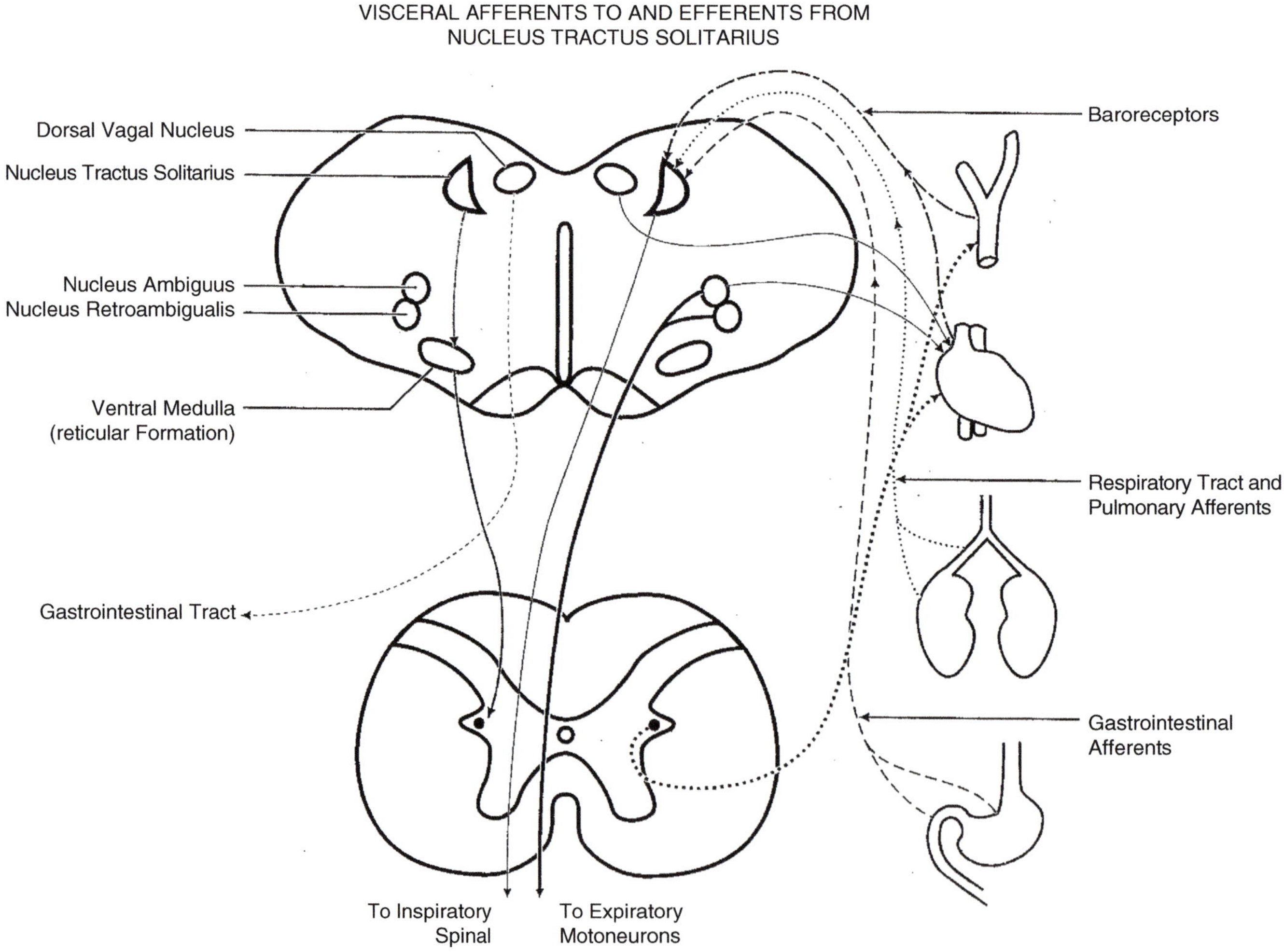

Fig. 3.4 Visceral afferents to and efferents from nucleus tractus solitarius

ceptors), and special sensory fibers (e.g., taste, salivation, and balance receptors in the inner ear) [15, 16, 25]. The afferent ANS fibers most likely participate in visceral sensation and autonomic reflexes, such as respiratory, viscerosomatic, baroreceptor, and vasomotor reflexes.

Pharmacology and Physiology of the ANS (See Also Chap. 5)

Two physiologists, Henry Dale (1914) [26] from London, England, and Otto Loewi (1921) [27] from Frankfurt, Germany, are responsible for discovering acetylcholine as the principal neurotransmitter for the ANS, for which they shared the 1936 Nobel Prize for Medicine [25].

Two chemical transmitters, acetylcholine and norepinephrine, help mediate autonomic functions [14, 25]. Acetylcholine is the neurotransmitter for the preganglionic neurons of both sympathetic and parasympathetic systems, while it is the neurotransmitter for all parasympathetic postganglionic and sympathetic postganglionic fibers innervating sweat glands. For central autonomic regulation, cholinergic neurons play a significant role. There are two receptors for acetylcholine: muscarinic and nicotinic receptors.

Norepinephrine is the neurotransmitter for the sympathetic nervous system. It is released at the postganglionic sympathetic nerve terminals. Two adrenergic receptors, α (alpha) receptors (α1 and α2) and β (beta) receptors (β1 and β2), are responsible for binding of norepinephrine released from the sympathetic nerve endings. The effects of alpha receptors in general are excitatory and those of beta receptors are inhibitory except for the receptors in the heart where they are excitatory. The sympathetic vasodilator fibers to the skeletal muscles and coronary blood vessels may contain cholinergic or beta receptors.

The adrenal medulla, part of the adrenal gland, receives sympathetic preganglionic neurons, but in response to the neurotransmitter acetylcholine it secretes largely adrenaline (epinephrine) with a small amount of noradrenaline (norepinephrine) [22, 25] and a very small amount of dopamine.

The principal neurotransmitter in the ENS, as in other parts of the ANS, is acetylcholine, which is excitatory. There are also inhibiting neurotransmitters like nitric oxide (NO) and vasoactive intestinal polypeptide (VIP). At least 30 neurotransmitters have been identified [17–22] in the ENS, including serotonin, substance P, neuropeptide Y, GABA, and dopamine.

Physiology

The Sherringtonian concept of "*final common motor pathway*" can also be applied (as suggested by Janig in 1986) [25, 28] to the peripheral autonomic nervous system calling it a "*final common autonomic pathway*" as the most important component of the ANS for ultimate control to maintain a stable internal milieu (homeostasis).

There is a general misconception of a functional universal antagonism between the SNS and the PNS. In fact, the two systems act synergistically to get the best possible autonomic function (e.g., the SNS governs ejaculation, and PNS erection in men to get an effective reproductive function, which does not imply opposite effect), although many appear to have reciprocal and opposing effects [9, 14, 25]. Physiological changes following stimulation of the sympathetic nervous system consist of the following responses: increase in heart rate and blood pressure, piloerection, sweating, pupillary dilation, bronchodilation, vasoconstriction, hyperglycemia, inhibition of the gastrointestinal motility, contraction of the internal anal and urinary bladder sphincters, release of renin and norepinephrine, and secretion of epinephrine (adrenaline) from the adrenal medulla, ejaculation in men, glycogenolysis, and neoglucogenesis.

Parasympathetic responses following activation of the system include the following: bradycardia, vasodilation, pupillary constriction, bronchoconstriction, increased gut motility and peristalsis, increased glandular secretions, contraction of the detrusor muscles in the urinary bladder, and penile erection in men.

There are striking physiological changes in the ANS during sleep (see Chap. 5) [29, 30]. The fundamental changes are two: (1) there is an increased parasympathetic tone during REM sleep and NREM sleep and (2) the sympathetic tone decreases in both stages with intermittent hyperactivation in REM sleep, particularly during phasic eye movements. Because of these sleep-related physiological changes there is pupillary constriction during sleep as well as bradycardia and slight fall of blood pressure (BP); BP fall in sleep is known as "dipping." Respiration is highly vulnerable during sleep because of absence of participation of the voluntary breathing system (only the autonomic or metabolic system remains active), decreased firing rates with reduced participation of the central respiratory neurons in the medulla and pons, as well as impaired hypoxic and hypercapnic ventilatory responses, resulting in mild sleep-related hypoventilation.

Clinico-Anatomical Correlation

From an account of the functional neuroanatomy of the autonomic nervous system as described above, it will now be easy to understand the various clinical manifestations resulting from the autonomic deficits [9].

Pathogenesis of Orthostatic Hypotension An important feature of autonomic failure is orthostatic hypotension in the erect posture manifested clinically by orthostatic intolerance symptoms (e.g., dizziness, syncope or presyncope, blurring of vision, nausea, and light headedness) resulting from cerebral hypoperfusion. To understand the mechanism of orthostatic hypotension following lesions of the ANS (central or peripheral), it is important to understand the mechanism of maintenance of circulation and BP in the upright posture in a healthy individual [9, 13, 14]. On assuming an upright position there is an intense gravitational stress on the circulation with a shift of blood from the upper to the lower body (about 500–700 mL) and a decrease in central blood volume. This causes diminished venous return to the heart with diminished stroke volume and cardiac output, resulting in a transient postural hypotension with a decrease in blood flow through various organs, including the brain and the splanchnic region. Because of this transient postural fall of BP, immediate compensatory measures are initiated using the neural mechanism through the baroreceptor reflex pathway. This is followed by delayed compensation of humoral and physical (see below) mechanisms.

The baroreceptors in the carotid sinus and aortic arch are immediately stimulated as a result of hypotension as part of body's defense mechanism with transmission of afferent impulses to the nucleus tractus solitarius, an important structure for the baroreflex mechanism in the brainstem. This is followed by sympathetic stimulation from ventral medulla and vagal inhibition. As a result, within 30–45 seconds of assuming the upright position, peripheral resistance, venous return, and cardiac output are all increased, resulting in the restoration of BP to its baseline level in the supine position. The primary baroreceptor mechanism is helped by the humoral mechanism of release of plasma catecholamines, renin and aldosterone, and the physical factors of accumulation of excess tissue fluid in the legs, "muscle pump," and respiratory actions. The neural compensatory mechanism may fail as a result of lesion of the afferent arc, the medullary center, or the efferent arc of the baroreflex mechanism [9, 13, 14]. The lesions in the central nervous system could be in the medulla, the supramedullary regions controlling the nucleus tractus solitaries, or in the pathways from the nucleus tractus solitarius to the ventral medulla, and from there to the intermediolateral neurons of the spinal cord. Hence, diversely located lesions involving the brainstem, hypothalamus, other forebrain and limbic regions, as well as intermediolateral neurons of the spinal cord, sympathetic ganglia, and postganglionic sympathetic fibers, and afferent fibers to NTS may cause orthostatic hypotension.

Extensive lesions of the lumbosacral spinal cord may involve the parasympathetic and sympathetic innervation of the urinary bladder, causing symptoms of urgency, hesitation, and frequency of micturition, dribbling, incontinence, and retention of urine.

Lesions of the sacral parasympathetic neurons in the second, third, and fourth sacral regions may cause erectile dysfunction in men; this is often an early manifestation of autonomic neuropathy. Sympathetic neuropathy affecting the urogenital system may cause retrograde ejaculation of semen into the urinary bladder or failure of ejaculation in men.

The sweat glands are innervated by the postganglionic sympathetic fibers, which receive innervation from the intermediolateral neurons in the spinal cord. Involvement of these sympathetic fibers as well as those in the brainstem or the hypothalamus will cause impairment of sweating in the face, trunk, or the limbs, depending on the site of the lesions.

A perusal of the functional neuroanatomy would make it easily understandable why a lesion of the cervical sympathetic fibers may cause. Horner syndrome or a lesion of the Edinger–Westphal nucleus, or its efferent parasympathetic outflow will cause impairment of pupillary response to light and accommodation. Similarly, lesions of the superior and inferior salivatory nuclei or their efferents will cause diminished lacrimation (dryness of the eyes) and dryness of the mouth.

The heart and circulation are under the control of the sympathetic and parasympathetic nervous systems, and a lesion of the central autonomic network or involvement of its afferent and efferent connections will cause cardiac autonomic denervation, resulting in either persistent tachycardia or other cardiac arrhythmias.

A consideration of the central respiratory mechanism and the close interrelationship among autonomic, respiratory, and hypnogenic neurons makes it plausible to think that lesions in the central brainstem or adjacent structures may cause a variety of respiratory changes in cases of autonomic failure. These changes are particularly notable during sleep in the most well-recognized central degenerative autonomic neuropathy, namely, the Shy–Drager syndrome [3, 14, 31] or multiple system atrophy with progressive autonomic failure. A variety of respiratory changes are noted in this condition [31] (see also Chap. 12).

Lesions of the dorsal vagal motor nucleus of the medulla and its efferent connections will cause difficulty in swallowing and vomiting due to gastroesophageal atony. Other examples of intestinal motility disorders include achalasia, intestinal pseudo-obstruction, irritable bowel syndrome causing constipation or intermittent diarrhea (IBS-C or IBS-D), and urinary or fecal incontinence [22]. These gastrointestinal motility disorders may be caused by an enteric neuropathy due to dysfunction of the myenteric plexus neurons or secondary to an effect on the extrinsic ANS modulating the intrinsic ENS.

The following case example (adapted from Wilson-Pauwels et al., case study 1, [15]) illustrates the role of the

ANS in understanding the concept of "fright-fight-or-flight," the phrase introduced by Cannon [8].

During a short vacation in Maui, an island located in Hawaii, a 20-year-old woman decided to take a swim in the ocean. Suddenly she noticed that the tide was going out and she had difficulty in maintaining her orientation and began to drift farther and farther from the shore. She got frightened and started swimming back to the shore. Her breathing was becoming faster and faster, and she noticed that her heart had begun to pound. She was not particularly a good swimmer but realized that she was having superhuman strength, which enabled her muscles to act vigorously so that she was able to swim against the tide to the shore. On reaching the shore and arriving at the beach she noticed her breathing was rapid, her heart was racing, she was pale, and was having cold sweat in her extremities. She was resting flat, and in course of the next several minutes she began to feel normal; her respiration and heart rate returned to her normal baseline state.

Questions:	1. What is "fright- fight-or-flight" reaction?
	2. How do you explain her vigorous increase of strength?
	3. What are the mechanisms for her respiratory and heart rate changes?
	4. How do you explain her pallor and cold clammy sweaty limbs?

Comments (Based on Clinico-Anatomo-Physiological Correlation)

Answer to Questions 1–3 As discussed previously, the phrase "fright-fight-or-flight" was coined by Cannon [8] to describe a physiologic response to a threat ("fright"), real or perceived, in order to defend from the threat ("fight"), to escape from it ("flight"), or both. These efforts require vigorous energetic action and heavy use of the muscles. The chain of events occurs as follows (steps 1 to 4):

- **Step 1:** In response to a perceived threat the body through the senses (e.g., the eyes [vision] or ears [auditory perception]) sends signals to the amygdala, a part of the limbic system located in the medial temporal lobe bilaterally and responsible for emotional processing. The amygdala immediately sends distressed signals to the hypothalamus, the main ganglion of the autonomic nervous system (ANS), a sort of command center communicating with the rest of the body through the ANS, controlling all the vital organs (e.g., the heart, the lungs, gastrointestinal, genitourinary, and endocrine systems).
- **Step 2:** In this situation of "fright- fight-or-flight" reaction the hypothalamus sends bursts of sympathetic activity (the sympathetic system is predominately located in the posterior hypothalamus). As a result of sympathetic hyperactivity, a cascade of events occur supporting "fight-or-flight" response in the body with a characteristic physiological manifestation as described in step 3.
- **Step 3:** Adrenaline is released from adrenal glands (through activation of hypothalamo–pituitary–adrenal [HPA] axis) [32], and adrenaline is secreted from the adrenal glands. Noradrenaline (norepinephrine) is released from the postganglionic sympathetic nerves, causing vasomotor changes with vasodilatation and increased blood flow to the muscles and coronary arteries, encouraging muscle activation, cardioexcitation, as well as vasoconstriction in the skin and splanchnic regions, and bronchiodilatation with increased oxygen inhalation. In addition, there is increased glycogenolysis (in the liver and muscles), making excess glucose available for extra energy as well as increased cortisol secretion through activation of the HPA axis.
- **Step 4:** The above changes provide excessive energy throughout the body. These physiological changes cause a characteristic clinical presentation that can be summarized as follows: The subject manifests increased BP and heart rate (heart racing with palpitation), hyperventilation, panting, cold, clammy (sweaty) extremities, pallor of the skin of the face and the limbs, piloerection ("goose bumps"), and pupillary dilatation. The sympathetic nervous system uses two types of receptors to bring on the above physiological changes: α receptors (α1 and α2) and β receptors (β1 and β2)—α receptor activation causes vasoconstriction, relaxation of the gut muscles and pupillary dilatation, whereas β receptor activation causes vasodilatation of muscle vessels and coronary arteries, increased heart rate and cardiac contraction (increasing cardiac output), and bronchodilation (allowing increased airflow in and out of the lungs).

Answer to Question 4 How do you explain her cold clammy (sweaty) limbs with pallor of the skin?

Vasoconstriction in the cutaneous vessels caused pallor. Vasoconstriction in the splanchnic region made blood available to muscles and other regions, including the brain, and is responsible for increased peripheral resistance and BP.

Sweating was caused by intense sympathetic stimulation of the sweat glands, which helped dissipate heat generated by intense muscle activation.

It is notable that this description of "fight-or-flight" reaction in the above subject supports the concept of an "autonomic storm" ("autonomic dysreflexia and hyperactivity").

References

1. Langley JN. On the union of cranial autonomic (visceral) fibres with the nerve cells of the superior cervical ganglion. J Physiol. 1989;23(2):240–70.
2. Langley JN. The autonomic nervous system, part 1. Cambridge: W. Heffer and Sons; 1921.
3. Furness JB, Costa M. The enteric nervous system. Edinburgh: Churchill Livingstone; 1987.
4. Pick J. The autonomic nervous system. Philadelphia: JB Lippincott; 1970.
5. Kuntz A. The autonomic nervous system. Philadelphia: Lea & Febiger; 1953.
6. Gaskell WH. On the structure, distribution and function of the nerves which innervate the visceral and vascular systems. J Physiol. 1886;7(1):1–80.
7. Shy GM, Drager GA. A neurological syndrome associated with orthostatic hypotension: a clinical-pathologic study. AMA Arch Neurol. 1960;2(5):511–27.
8. Cannon WB. Bodily changes in pain, hunger, fear and rage: an account of recent researches into the function of emotional excitement. New York/London: D. Appleton & Co; 1915.
9. Chokroverty S. Functional anatomy of the autonomic nervous system: autonomic dysfunction and disorders in the CNS. In: Correlative neuroanatomy and neuropathology for the clinical neurologists. American Academy of Neurology Course No. 144. Minneapolis: American Academy of Neurology; 1991. p. 77–103.
10. Lowey AD. Anatomy of the autonomic nervous system: an overview. In: Lowey AD, Spyer KM, editors. Central regulation of autonomic functions. New York: Oxford University Press; 1990. p. 3–16.
11. Carpenter MB. Human neuroanatomy. 7th ed. Baltimore: Williams & Wilkins; 1976.
12. Lutherer LO, Williams JL, Everse SJ. Neurons of the rostral fastigial nucleus are responsive to cardiovascular and respiratory challenges. J Auton Nerv Syst. 1989;27(2):101–12.
13. Spyer KM. The central nervous organization of reflex circulatory control. In: Lowey AD, Spyer KM, editors. Central regulation of autonomic functions. New York: Oxford University Press; 1990. p. 168–88.
14. Chokroverty S. Autonomic dysfunction in olivopontocerebellar atrophy. In: Duvoisin RC, Plaitakis A, editors. Advances in neurology: Olivopontocerebellar atrophies. New York: Raven Press; 1984. p. 105–41.
15. Wilson-Pauwells L, Stewart PA, Akesson EJ. Autonomic nerves: basic science, clinical aspects, case studies. Hamilton: BC Dekker; 1997.
16. Johnson RH, Lambie DG, Spalding JMK. The Autonomic nervous system. In: Joynt RJ, editor. Clinical neurology, vol. 4. Philadelphia: Lippincott-Raven; 1986. p. 1–94.
17. Quigley EMM, Conklin JK. The "big brain" and the "little brain": central nervous systems in the regulation of gut function. In: Quigley EMM, Pfeiffer RF, editors. Neurogastroenterology. Philadelphia: Butterworth-Heinemann; 2004. p. 3–14.
18. Benarroch EE. Enteric nervous system: functional organization and neurologic implications. Neurology. 2007;69(20):1953–7.
19. Goyal RK, Hirano I. The enteric nervous system. N Engl J Med. 1996;334(17):1106–15.
20. Costa M, Brooks SJK, Henning GW. Anatomy and physiology of the enteric nervous system. Gut. 2000;47(Suppl 4):iv15-9; discussion iv26
21. Wood JD. Enteric neurobiology: discoveries and directions. Adv Exp Med Biol. 2016;891:175–91.
22. Albanese A, Brisinda G, Mathias CJ. The autonomic nervous system and gastrointestinal disorders. In: Appenzeller O, editor. The autonomic nervous system. Part II, dysfunctions, Handbook of clinical neurology, vol 75. Amsterdam/New York: Elsevier; 2000. p. 613–63.
23. Kumar D, Wingate DL, Rukebsuch Y. Circadian variation in the propagation velocity of the migrating motor complex. Gastroenterology. 1986;91(4):926–30.
24. Kumar D, Idzikowski C, Wingate DL, Soffer EE, Thompson P, Siderfin C. Relationship between enteric migrating motor complex and the sleep cycle. Am J Phys. 1990;259(6 Pt 1):G983–90.
25. Janig W, Habler JJ. Organization of the autonomic nervous system: structure and function. In: Appenzeller O, editor. The autonomic nervous system. Part II, dysfunctions, Handbook of clinical neurology, vol 75. Amsterdam/New York: Elsevier; 2000. p. 1–52.
26. Dale HH. The action of certain esters and ethers of choline, and their relation to muscarine. J Pharmacol Exp Ther. 1914;6(2):147–90.
27. Loewi O. Über humorale Übertragbarkeit der Herznervenwirkung. IMitteilung Pflügers Arch Ges Physiol. 1921;189(1):239–24.
28. Jänig W. Spinal cord integration of visceral sensory systems and sympathetic nervous system reflexes. Prog Brain Res. 1986;67:255–77.
29. Parmeggiani PL, Morrison AR. Alterations of autonomic functions during sleep. In: Lowey AD, Spyer KM, editors. Central regulation of autonomic functions. New York: Oxford University Press; 1990.
30. Chokroverty BS. Physiological changes in sleep. In: Chokroverty S, Ferini-Strambi L, editors. Oxford textbook of sleep disorders. Oxford: Oxford University Press; 2017. p. 43–52.
31. Chokroverty S. Assessment of sleep disturbances in autonomic failure. In: Mathias CJ, Bannister R, editors. Autonomic failure: a textbook of clinical disorders of the autonomic nervous system. 5th ed. Oxford: Oxford University Press; 2001. p. 410–23.
32. Spiga F, Walker JJ, Terry JR, Lightman SL. HPA axis rhythms. Compr Physiol. 2014;4(3):1273–98.

4 Functional Neuroanatomy and Mechanism of Sleep

Sudhansu Chokroverty

Introduction and Historical Note

Before discussing functional neuroanatomy and mechanism of sleep, a brief historical note with some general comments is included in order to place the topic in proper perspective.

General Comments

Traditionally, our existence on this planet is divided into three neurobehavioral states: wakefulness (W), non-rapid eye movement (NREM) and rapid eye movement (REM) sleep [1]. I should like to add three more making a total of six distinct behavioral and electrophysiological States (stages) with their own controls, functions, rhythms and rituals [2–4] (S. Chokroverty, unpublished observations):

1. Active Wakefulness (AW)
2. Relaxed Wakefulness (RW)
3. Predormitum (a term introduced by McDonald Critchley [4]) to denote a stage between RW and stage 1 of NREM sleep

4a. Stage 1 NREM sleep signifying pre-sleep behavior with generators in the brainstem separate from those for other stages of NREM and REM sleep [2]

4b. Stage N2 (lighter stage of NREM sleep) with appearance of characteristic sleep spindles and K complexes accompanied by delta waves (0.5–2 Hz) occupying less than 20% of each epoch

4c. Slow wave sleep (SWS) or deeper stage of NREM sleep) with delta waves occupying 20% or more in each epoch

5. REM sleep with its distinctive signatures of rapid eye movements (REMs), muscle atonia and low amplitude mixed frequency electroencephalogram (EEG) waves as well as sawtooth waves (STW)
6. Post-dormitum (also known as sleep inertia or sleep drunkenness [5], a stage between the end of night's sleep and full wakefulness in the morning). This is a transient physiological state characterized by hypovigilance, grogginess, confusion, and impaired cognitive and behavioral performance.

Historical Note

It is notable that the great cataclysmic influenza pandemic (also known as the Spanish flu) in the early twentieth century (probably from 1915–1927) caused by an unknown influenza virus (this was identified later in 1933 after analyzing viral RNA sequences in the preserved postmortem tissues from the victims [6]) that killed 50–100 million people. This pandemic in many patients caused a dreadful neurologic illness termed "encephalitis lethargica." The influenza pandemic devastated Northern Europe (probably beginning in Romania first), spreading later to the rest of the globe killing 50–100 million individuals [6]. This pandemic of the past causing brain disease taught us a great deal about sleep-wakefulness. An insightful young Austrian neurologist, Constantin von Economo, made careful observations of these patients during their illness and then participated in postmortem pathological study of those unfortunate victims who later died. He made the following astute clinicopathological observations: Those who had extensive lesions in the posterior hypothalamus had suffered from excessive and irresistible sleepiness, and an inability to maintain wakefulness (comprising about 50–60% of the patients) whereas those whose lesions were in the anterior hypothalamus complained of severe insomnia when they

S. Chokroverty (✉)
Hackensack Meridian Health, Neuroscience Institute at JFK, JFK University Medical Center, Edison, NJ, USA

Seton Hall University & Hackensack Meridian School of Medicine at Seton Hall, South Orange, NJ, USA

Rutgers Robert Wood Johnson Medical School, New Brunswick, NJ, USA
e-mail: Sudhansu.Chokroverty@hackensackmeridian.org

S. Chokroverty, P. Cortelli (eds.), *Autonomic Nervous System and Sleep*, https://doi.org/10.1007/978-3-030-62263-3_4

were alive (about 10% of von Economo's encephalitis). Based on these observations he made two memorable predictions:

1. Sleep-wake-generating neurons are located in the hypothalamus; its anterior region is responsible for regulating sleep and posterior region for wakefulness
2. His second prediction was even more profound and prophetic: The cause of this disease (narcolepsy) named after Gélineau (1880) and earlier (1877) alluded to by Westphal is located in the lateral-posterior hypothalamus. These observations were published between 1917 and 1931 [7–9]

The sleep community had to wait for about 70 years to scientifically prove von Economo's two predictions (see further on).

von Economo's concept about localization of sleep-wake-generating neurons in the diencephalon was overshadowed by two experimental preparations in the cats by the Belgian physiologist, Frederick Bremer, in 1935 producing *cerveau isolé* after intercollicular transection in the midbrain causing sleepiness, and *encéphale isolé* after transection at the junction of medulla and spinal cord in cats resulting in wakefulness [10]. Bremer thus postulated a passive theory of sleep as a result of withdrawal of all environmental afferent stimuli. This experiment and subsequent discovery of the brainstem reticular activating system in 1949 (see below) also shifted the focus of the research from diencephalon to the brainstem region [2]. An ascending reticular activating system (ARAS) was identified by Moruzzi and Magoun in 1949 in the central part of the brainstem stimulation of which caused arousal and wakefulness, whereas lesion caused stupor, and disfacilitation with withdrawal of afferent stimuli at sleep onset [11]. The passive theory of Bremer was forcefully challenged by a group of Italian physiologists led by Battini in 1959 [12] by producing (pretrigeminal midpontine transaction) in the cats which is located a few millimeters below 'Cerveau isolé' preparation causing wakefulness which implied that between these two sections (intercollicular in the mesencephalon and pretrigeminal pontine cats) there are wake-promoting neurons. We know that laterodorsal tegmental (LDT) and pedunculopontine tegmental (PPT) cholinergic neurons are located in the pontomesencephalic junction which are active during wakefulness and REM sleep but inactive during NREM sleep [13].

The role of the thalamus in sleep-wake generation remained neglected for a long time until the discovery of "Fatal Familial Insomnia (FFI)" in 1986 by Lugaresi and coworkers from Bologna, Italy [14]. Although Hess, a Swiss physiologist, using electrical stimulation in cats initially thought that the anterior hypothalamus contained deactivating structures thus confirming von Economo's observation, he subsequently concluded that true sleep occurred only on stimulating the thalamus [15]. This observation, however, did not get a strong support from the world sleep research community, particularly after strong criticism about the technical procedure by Bremer [16, 17]. It is notable that as early as 1923 Tromner [18] provided reason for localization of the sleep center in the thalamus and later [19] suggested in disagreement with von Economo's prediction [7] that the anterior hypothalamic sleep center simply exerted pressure on the thalamus for generating sleep. Lugaresi and collaborators [14], however, clearly documented the important role played by the thalamus in sleep regulation after clinicopathological observation in FFI of degeneration of mediodorsal and anteroventral nuclei of the thalamus associated with severe insomnia. This observation was subsequently strengthened by electrophysiological documentation by Steriade and collaborators [20] of a significant role played by the thalamus in NREM sleep generation. Their study demonstrated that the thalamus is the first relay station at which reduction of afferent signals takes place at sleep onset. Their research also showed that sleep spindles are generated in the thalamic reticular nucleus, and delta oscillation of NREM sleep has two generators: one in the thalamus and the other in the cerebral cortex.

It is notable that von Economo's first prediction was proven correct by the scientific community about 70 years after von Economo's remarkable prediction about the existence of sleep-wake neurons in hypothalamus. We have now clear evidence about the role of ventrolateral preoptic (VLPO) and median preoptic (MnPO) neurons in the control of onset and maintenance of NREM sleep (mainly) and posterior hypothalamic tuberomammillary histaminergic (TMH) neurons in promoting wakefulness. The contemporary theory for sleep-wake regulation [21] lends strong support to what von Economo postulated in the beginning of the last century.

Following this brief historical note and some general comments about sleep-wakefulness I shall now summarize the contemporary concept and mechanism of wake-sleep states. But before I begin my discussion in the next section, I must mention why I am devoting this much space to functional neuroanatomy and mechanism of sleep-wake states in a book on sleep and the autonomic nervous system (ANS). This is because there is a dynamic interaction between the ANS, particularly the central autonomic network (CAN) with its reciprocal ascending and descending projections, and sleep-wake-generating neurons located in the brainstem, the diencephalon, and the cerebral cortex including the limbic system [22] (see also Chap. 2). Besides this close interrelationship (anatomically and physiologically) between the CAN and sleep-wake neurons and circuits, it is important to understand the significance of this dynamic coupling with profound bidirectional changes among these neurons which has implications in various somatic and autonomic disorders including primary and secondary (comorbid) sleep disorders. There has been a remarkable progress in the last century in uncovering our understanding of the molecular mechanism and functional neuroanatomy of sleep-wakefulness.

In the literature there has been an undue emphasis on the mechanism of NREM and REM sleep but we should really focus on the question of "How do we remain awake" (as suggested by Kleitman in the 1930s [23]). Kleitman in his book mentioned "without wakefulness sleep cannot be said to exist" [23]. Human beings remain asleep during developmental stage inside the mother's womb and wake up for the first time when born [23]. Even in the newborn, sleep occupies 16 hours a day. I shall first outline the functional neuroanatomy and mechanism of wakefulness, NREM and REM sleep. The concluding paragraphs will summarize some conceptual mechanism of sleep-wake states as well as cycling of NREM-REM throughout the night.

Neuroanatomical Substrates and Control of Wake-Sleep States

There is not a single wake or sleep center but the neurons responsible for these states are located in separate parts of the CNS as interconnecting circuits and systems rather than as discrete centers. These conclusions are based on the following experimental methods to characterize wake-sleep neuroanatomical substrates or generators (Box 4.1): i. Discrete lesions; ii. Stimulation including optogenetic stimulation; iii. Transection; iv. Ablation; v. Chemical injections into discrete neuronal substrates; vi. Intracellular recordings; vii. c-fos (immediate early genes immunoreactivity [c-fos, a protein released in response to activation of certain neuronal structures]); and vii. Neuroimaging including positron emission tomographic (PET) and single photon emission tomographic (SPECT) scans as well as brain functional magnetic resonance imaging (fMRI) for mapping the brain networks.

Box 4.1 Methods to Characterize Anatomical Substrates and Generators for Sleep-Wakefulness

Discrete lesions
Stimulation including optogenetic stimulation
Transection
Ablation
Chemical injections into discrete substrates
Intracellular recordings
c-fos (immediate early genes) immunoreactivity (c-fos, a protein released in response to activation of certain neuronal structures)
Neuroimaging including positron emission tomographic (PET) and single photon emission tomographic (SPECT) scans as well as brain functional magnetic resonance imaging (fMRI) for mapping brain networks

Neuroanatomical Substrates and Control of Wakefulness

Box 4.2 lists the neuroanatomical substrates of wakefulness. The most important structure is the ascending reticular activating system (ARAS), a part of the reticular formation (RF) of the brainstem [24]. The existence of RF has been known since the late nineteenth century as a group of loosely scattered neurons with interconnecting fibers in the center of the brainstem but its function has not been definitely known. There were scant reports dealing with wakefulness and arousal until the serendipitous discovery by Moruzzi and Magoun in 1949 of the ascending reticular activating system (ARAS) in the central core of the upper pons and mesencephalon receiving collaterals from the specific afferent sensory systems in the lateral part of the brainstem transmitting environmental stimuli to the thalamus and sensory cerebral cortex. The RF has an ascending projection (two branches) to the thalamus, the forebrain, and the cerebral cortex and a descending projection to the lower brainstem and spinal cord utilizing tegmentoreticular (TRT) and spinoreticular (SRT) tracts. The ventral branch arises from the cholinergic laterodorsal tegmental (LDT) and pedunculopontine tegmental (PPT) nuclei and activates the cerebral cortex through its projection to the intralaminar, relay and reticular nuclei of the thalamus and diffuse thalamocortical projections (prominent in the frontal cortex). There is also a

Box 4.2 Neuroanatomical Substrates of Wakefulness

Reticular formation (RF), particularly the ascending reticular activating system (ARAS)
Diffuse thalamocortical projections (DTCP)
Cholinergic projections to the thalamus from the laterodorsal tegmental (LDT) and pedunculopontine (PPT) nuclei
Ascending arousal system originating from locus ceruleus (LC) noradrenergic and dorsal raphe (DR) serotonergic neurons through the basal forebrain
Lateral hypothalamic orexin/hypocretin neurons with their diffuse ascending and descending projections covering the entire central nervous system (CNS) and the autonomic nervous system (ANS)
Posterior hypothalamic tuberomammillary histaminergic projection through the forebrain
Cholinergic projections from the basal forebrain nucleus basalis of Meynert diffusely to the cerebral cortex
Glutamatergic projection from *preceruleus*—from dorsal part of sublaterodorsal (SLD) tegmental nuclei through parabrachial area (PBA) and through the basal forebrain diffusely to the cerebral cortex
Dopaminergic neurons from ventrolateral periaqueductal gray (VLPAG), ventral tegmental area (VTA) and substantia nigra (SN) pars compacta projecting widely
Parts of prosencephalon (forebrain), particularly frontal, temporal, parietal and limbic cortices

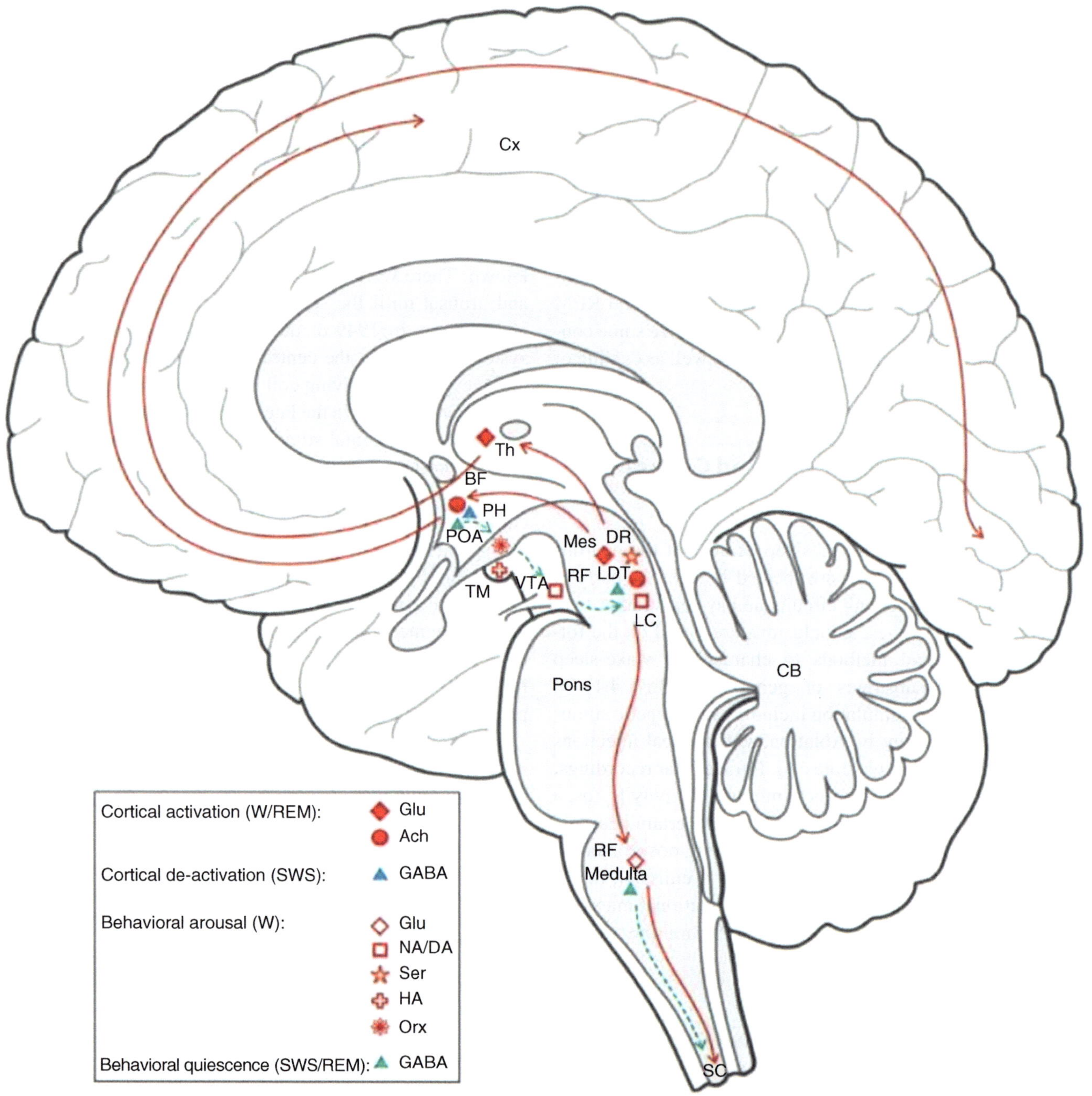

Fig. 4.1 Ascending arousal projections (two branches) form reticular formation (RF), including the ascending reticular activating system, to activate the cerebral cortex (CX) and maintain vigilance, awareness and wakefulness. Th Thalamus, BF Basal forebrain, PH Posterior hypothalamus, POA Preoptic area, TM Tuberomammillary nucleus, DR Dorsal raphe, LDT Laterodorsal tegmental nucleus, MES Mesencephalon, CB Cerebellum (From Saper et al. [27] © 2005, with permission Springer Nature)

glutamatergic projection from the parabrachial nucleus through basal forebrain (BF) taking part in this activation [25]. The dorsal projection (second branch of ARAS) uses an extrathalamic route through the lateral and posterior hypothalamus to the basal forebrain and cerebral hemispheres. This projection arises from the noradrenergic locus ceruleus (LC), serotonergic dorsal raphe (DR), dopaminergic (DA), ventrolateral periaqueductal gray (VLPAG), ventral tegmental area (VTA), substantia nigra (SN), and histaminergic tuberomammillary nucleus (TMN) in the posterior hypothalamus as well as the orexin/hypocretin neurons in the lateral hypothalamus/perifornical region and cholinergic neurons in the nucleus basalis Meynert of the basal forebrain. This second branch through the extrathalamic route projects diffusely to the cerebral cortex including the limbic system. The ascending arousal system

(ARAS) has two branches (Fig. 4.1): ventral and dorsal [26, 27]. The Orexin/Hypocretin system consisting of only about 70,000 neurons has widespread ascending and descending connections to the entire CNS and ANS (Fig. 4.2) [28]. Thus, the ARAS through its diffuse projections to the thalamus and the cortex activates the cerebral cortex and is responsible for maintaining wakefulness, arousal and awareness. The descending projection of RF is responsible for motor control and maintenance of muscle tone. Therefore, the principal neuroanatomical substrate responsible for wakefulness, arousal and vigilance is the ARAS (see Box 4.2 for all neuroanatomical substrates for wakefulness) transmitting environmental stimuli to the cerebral cortex including the limbic system to control awareness, con-

Box 4.3 Neurotransmitters and Neuromodulators Involved in Arousal and Wakefulness

Acetylcholine	
Noradrenaline	
Orexin/hypocretin	
Serotonin (5-hydroxytryptamine)	
Histamine	
Dopamine	
Glutamate	Intermingled within the ARAS and are released maximally during wakefulness
Aspartate	

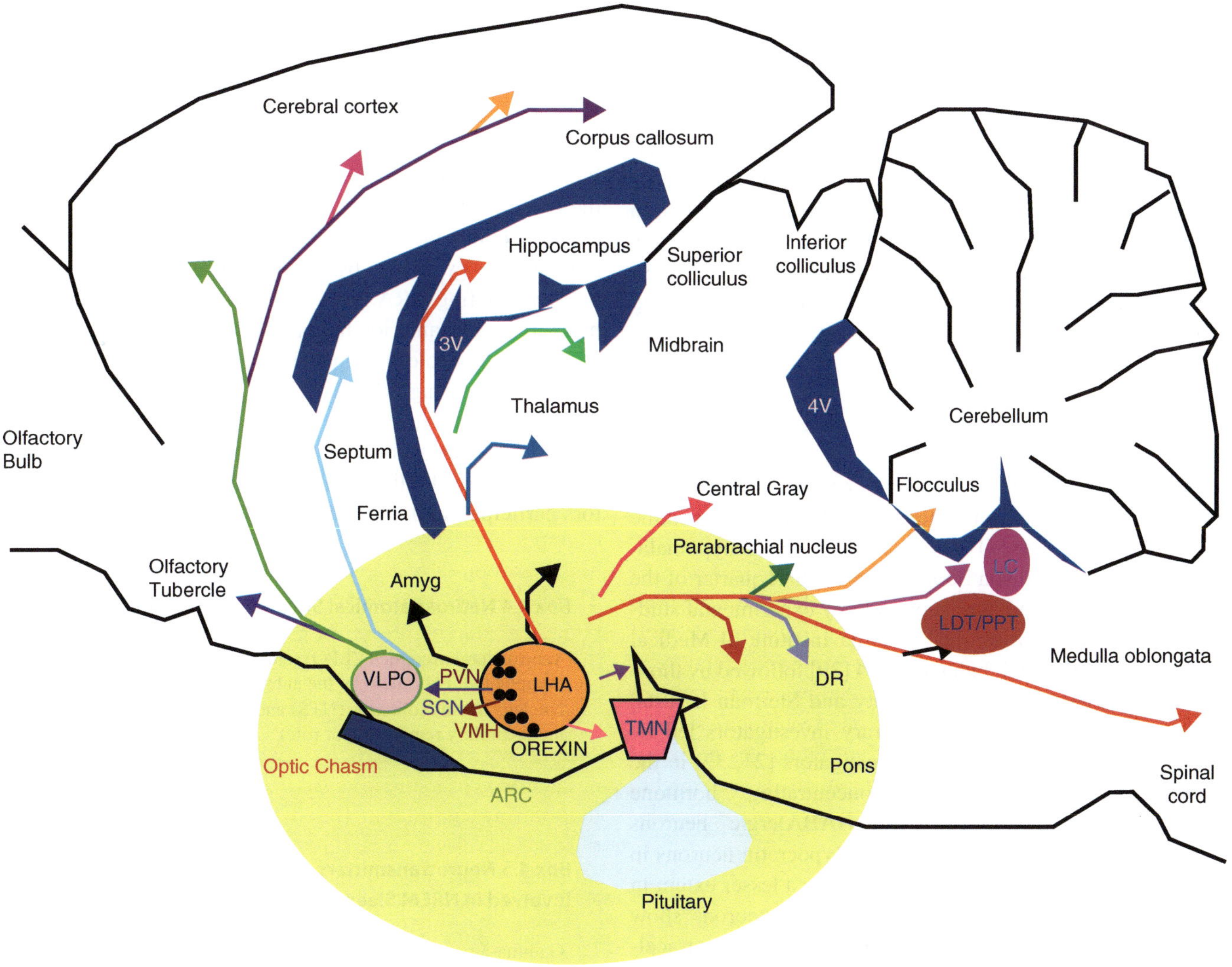

Fig. 4.2 Diffuse ascending and descending projections from lateral hypothalamic area (LHA) of the orexin/hypocretin throughout the central nervous system and the autonomic nervous system. DR Dorsal raphe, VLPO Ventrolateral preoptic nucleus, TMN Tuberomammillary nuclei, PVN Paraventricular nucleus, VMH Ventromedial hypothalamic nucleus, SCN Suprachiasmatic nucleus, Amyg Amygdala, (*red arrow* just before DR: Dorsal raphe: Locus ceruleus), ARC Arcuate nucleus. (From Chokroverty and Provini [28], © 2017, with permission Springer Science+Business Media)

sciousness and emotion assisted by neurostimulators and neuromodulators (Box 4.3). In addition, corticofugal projection to the ARAS creates cortical-subcortical as well as subcortical-cortical control system to maintain a balance in preventing hyperactivation. A breakdown in this intricate balance will result in sleep-wake disturbance causing either insomnia (hyperarousal) or excessive daytime sleepiness (EDS) as a result of disruption of wake-promoting neurons.

Other neuroanatomical structures besides the ARAS participating in maintaining wakefulness include the suprachiasmatic nucleus (SCM) of the hypothalamus through its anatomical connection to the wake-sleep-promoting neurons besides its principal function of regulating circadian rhythm. Animal experiments by Moruzzi, Magoun and others have clearly shown that stimulation of ARAS will activate the cerebral cortex producing desynchronized EEG and wakeful behavior, whereas lesion in the ARAS, particularly the portion in the midbrain, will result in sleep, stupor or coma depending on the extent and severity of the lesion. The wake-promoting neurons including LDT, PPT, LC, DR, TM or DA and orexin fire maximally during wakefulness and are disfacilitated during sleep. The LDT and PPT also fire maximally during REM sleep, whereas LC, DR, TM or DA fall silent in REM sleep and show weak firing intensity in NREM sleep. Excitatory amino acids, glutamic and aspartic acids intermingle within the ARAS and are released maximally during wakefulness.

Neuroanatomical Substrates of NREM Sleep

i. Hypothalamus NREM sleep-generating neurons are mainly located in the ventrolateral preoptic (VLPO) and the median preoptic (MnPO) nuclei of the anterior hypothalamus as suggested by von Economo in the first quarter of the last century [7–9] and later supported by experimental studies first by Dikshit from the All India Institute of Medical Sciences in New Delhi, India, in 1934 [29] followed by those of Nauta in 1946 [30] and McGinty and Sterman in 1968 [31] and finally by the contemporary investigators led by Saper as well as Sherin and co-investigators [21, 32] in the 1990s. Additionally, melanin-concentrating hormone (MCH)/gamma-aminobutyric acid-(GABA)ergic neurons located near wake-promoting Orexin/Hypocretin neurons in the lateral hypothalamus also contribute to a lesser extent in the generation of SWS. These hypnogenic neurons show increased firing rates at sleep onset as evidenced by intracellular recordings and increased expression of c-fos immunoreactivity as well as by optogenetic stimulation of MCH neurons. The VLPO and MnPO neurons (both use the inhibitory neurotransmitter and neuromodulator GABA and galanin) actively participate in NREM sleep onset (MnPO) and maintenance as well as consolidation (VLPO).

ii. Brainstem Nucleus tractus solitarius (NTS) and parafacial zone (Pz), a node of sleep active rostral medullary neurons identified in rats, play a minor role in NREM sleep generation [26]. This node located in the upper medulla dorsal to the facial nerve projects to the wake-promoting parabrachial nucleus (PBN) in the pons [26]. The medial PBN expresses c-fos positive immunoreactivity (i.e., active neurons) after sleep but not after wakefulness, and hence these are sleep active neurons. Pz lesion causes increased wakefulness but reduced SWS. More than 50% of Pz sleep-active neurons use inhibitory transmitter/modulator GABA/glycine.

iii. Role of Thalamus The active role of the thalamus in NREM sleep function (sleep spindles and slow oscillations) has been revived by Lugaresi et al. (see Section I above) after discovery of FFI (originally suggested by Hess in 1944 [15] but remained neglected).

iv. Role of Suprachiasmatic Nucleus The SCM located in the anterior hypothalamic region primarily controls the circadian rhythm but also plays a minor role in sleep-wake regulation as evidenced by its anatomical connection to both wake-promoting ARAS and sleep-promoting VLPO-MnPO neurons of the anterior hypothalamus. Therefore, SCM in addition to its role in controlling sleep timing (circadian), particularly during REM sleep and NREM-REM cycling, also participates in the homeostatic regulation (minor role) of NREM sleep state. Box 4.4 lists neuroanatomical substrates and Box 4.5 lists neurotransmitters and neuromodulators participating in NREM sleep.

Box 4.4 Neuroanatomical Substrates of NREM Sleep

Ventrolateral preoptic (VLPO) (clustered) and median preoptic (MnPO) nuclei of the anterior hypothalamus
Nucleus tractus solitarius (NTS) and parafacial zone (Pz) in the medullary region (minor role)

Box 4.5 Neurotransmitters and Neuromodulators Involved in NREM Sleep Generation

Gamma-aminobutyric acid (GABA): inhibitory
Galanin: inhibitory
Melanin-concentrating hormone (MCH/GABA)
Adenosine

Neuroanatomical Substrates of REM Sleep

The neuroanatomical substrates for REM sleep are outlined in Box 4.6. Neurotransmitters and neuromodulators actively participating in REM sleep generation are listed in Box 4.7. The dorsal pons is the primary region for the control of REM sleep as clearly shown by Jouvet [33] in his transection of the brainstem of cats (Fig. 4.3) [28, 34, 35]. For instance, a transection at pontomesencephalic junction disclosed all the REM-generating neurons below the transection whereas section at pontomedullary junction revealed the REM-generating neurons above the cut. The crucial experiment was a transection at the pontomesencephalic and pontomedullary junctions leaving an isolated pons showing all the signs of REM sleep-generating neurons. The pons is thus shown to be necessary and sufficient for generating REM sleep. To understand REM sleep-generating mechanism we need to explain about the essential physiological components of REM sleep and then introduce three main animal models available trying to explain mechanism of REM sleep. The REM sleep's key components are listed in Box 4.8 and discussed further while outlining the three REM sleep animal models.

Box 4.6 Neuroanatomical Substrates of REM Sleep

Pontine sublaterodorsal (SLD) tegmental nucleus in rats (equivalent to *perilocus ceruleus alpha* in cats and subcoeruleus nucleus in humans): glutamatergic
Laterodorsal tegmental (LDT) and pedunculopontine tegmental (PPT) nuclei at pontomesencephalic junction: cholinergic
Lateral hypothalamic melanin-concentrating hormone (MCH) /GABAergic neurons next to orexin/hypocretin
Anterior hypothalamic extended (diffuse) ventrolateral preoptic (VLPO) neurons
Anterior hypothalamic suprachiasmatic nuclei
Part of limbic cortex including amygdala, hippocampus, anterior cingulate gyrus, bed nucleus of stria terminalis.

Box 4.7 Neurotransmitters and Neuromodulators Involved in REM Sleep

Acetylcholine (excitatory)
Gamma-aminobutyric acid (GABA) (inhibitory)
Glycine (inhibitory)
Melanin-concentrating hormone (MCH)/GABA
GABA/galanin—extended ventrolateral preoptic (VLPO) and median preoptic (MnPO)

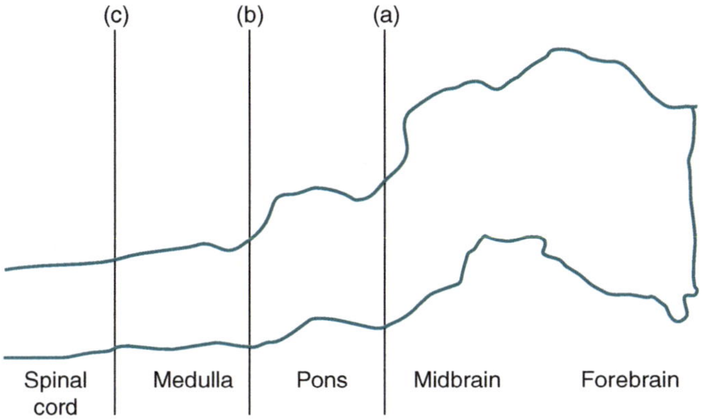

Fig. 4.3 Schematic sagittal section of the cat brain stem. (**a**) Pontomesencephalic junction; (**b**) Pontomedullary junction; (**c**) *Medullospinal* cord junction. (From Chokroverty and Provini [28], © 2017, with permission Springer Science+Business Media) (From Chokroverty and Provini [28], with permission Springer Nature)

Animal Models

i. McCarley–Hobson [13] reciprocal interaction (or activation synthesis) model based on reciprocal interaction of "REM-on" cholinergic LDT-PPT neurons at pontomesencephalic junction and "REM-off" LC noradrenergic and DR serotonergic neurons is the earliest and most well-known for REM generation and maintenance (Fig. 4.4) [28, 36]. This self-excitatory and negative self-inhibitory feedback model is analogous to the mathematical Lotka–Volterra predator–prey equations. The role of GABAergic neurons (both local and distal) in the REM sleep generation has been emphasized in the last modification of the reciprocal interaction model by McCarley [36].

ii. Lu and Co-workers from the Saper Group [37] introduced a "flip-flop" switch interaction model in rats to explain

Box 4.8 Essential Components of Physiological REM Sleep

Rapid eye movements (REMs): "phasic" REM
Desynchronized electroencephalogram (EEG) (tonic REMs) and sawtooth waves (phasic REM)
Electromyographic features:
Muscle atonia or marked hypotonia (tonic REM)
Transient myoclonic bursts or twitchings (phasic REM)
Others (partial list of phasic bursts during phasic REM):
Middle ear muscle activity (MEMA)
Periorbital integrated potentials (PIPS)
Phasic tongue movements
Hippocampal theta rhythm (animal EEG)
Up and down swings of blood pressure, heart rate and respiration
Ponto-geniculo-occipital (PGO) waves (mostly described during animal experiments, but also found in some human cases during depth recording

REM sleep mechanism (Fig. 4.5) [28] switching between GABAergic "REM-off" neurons in the deep mesencephalon, ventral periaqueductal gray (VLPAG) and lateral pontine tegmentum (LPT), and GABAergic "REM-on" neurons in the sublaterodorsal tegmental nucleus (SLD) in the dorsolateral pons (equivalent to peri-locus ceruleus alpha in the cat and subceruleus in humans). The ascending glutamatergic projections from the dorsal extension of SLD, named precoeruleus neurons to medial septum, are responsible for hippocampal theta and other EEG rhythms during REM sleep. REM muscle atonia is related to descending glutamatergic projections from ventral SLD directly to spinal interneurons without any apparent relay in the ventromedial medulla (VMM) inhibiting (hyperpolarizing) spinal ventral horn cells by both GABAergic and glycinergic mechanisms (inhibitory). Cholinergic and aminergic neurons do not form part of the "flip-flop" switch and play a modulatory role. Since the original description these workers made some modifications [38]. Based on recent studies [38], investigators concluded in agreement with Luppi's group (Fig. 4.6) [28, 39] that glutamatergic neurons play a significant role in REM sleep generation. Ventral SLD descending glutamatergic neurons may cause muscle atonia by activating GABA/glycinergic premotor neurons in the VMM (indirect projection) as well as to the spinal cord interneurons (direct projections). VLPAG and the adjacent LPT in the reticular formation containing GABA are the "REM-off" neurons which are silent during REM sleep and exert tonic inhibitory control over glutamatergic "REM-on" or REM executive neuron in SLD during NREM sleep and wakefulness. These "REM-off" neurons thus "gate" the appearance of REM sleep. The extended VLPO region (GABAergic) projections to VLPAG and LPT (REM-off) to cause increased firing of the cells thus indirectly supporting REM sleep generation. MCH neurons have projections to both SLD as well as VLPAG and LPT for controlling REM sleep. The latest suggestion from this group [38] regarding cortical activation during REM sleep is noteworthy: The SLD dorsal preceruleus glutamatergic neurons project to the basal forebrain through a relay in pontine para-

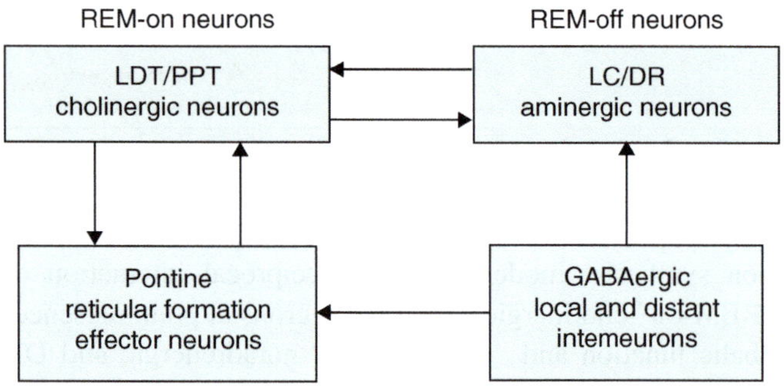

Fig. 4.4 McCarley–Hobson REM sleep model of reciprocal interaction between cholinergic REM-on and aminergic REM-off neurons. LDT Laterodorsal tegmental nucleus, PPT *Pedunculopontine tegmental nucleus*, LC Locus ceruleus, DR Dorsal raphe, GABA Gamma-aminobutyric acid. (From Chokroverty and Provini [28], © 2017, with permission Springer Science+Business Media)

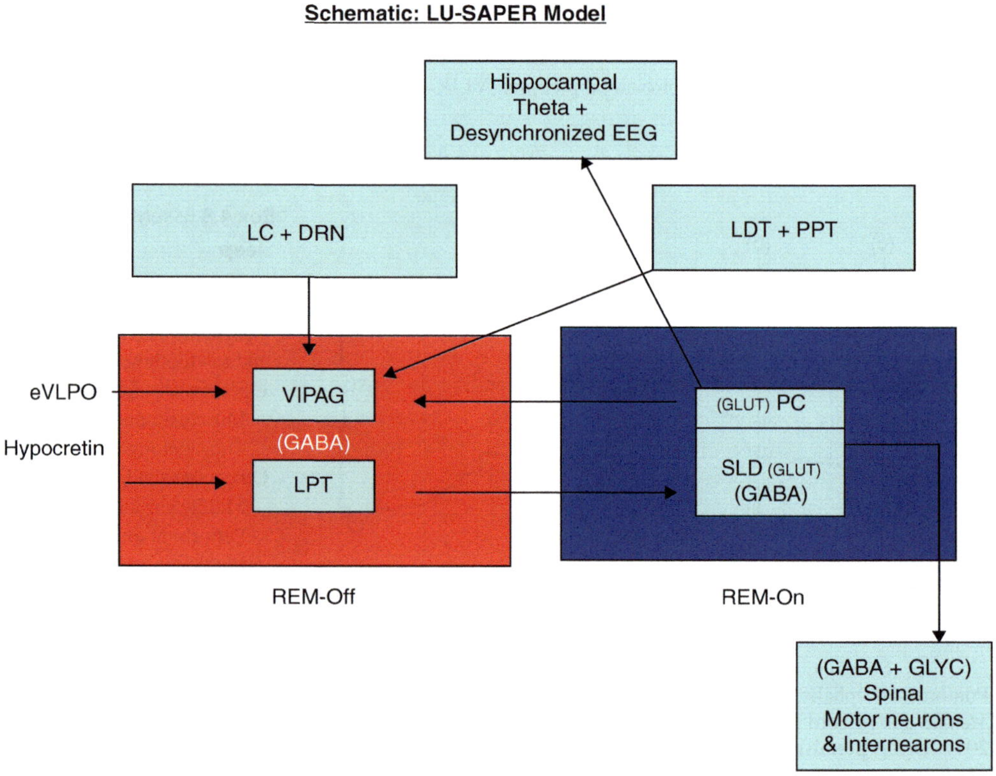

Fig. 4.5 "Flip-flop" switch original model of Saper's group schematically shown to explain REM sleep mechanism. SLD Sublaterodorsal nucleus, GABA Gamma-aminobutyric acid, GLUT Glutamatergic neurons, GLYC Glycinergic neurons, PC Preceruleus, LDT Laterodorsal tegmental nucleus, PPT *Pedunculopontine tegmental nucleus*, LC Locus ceruleus, DRN Dorsal raphe nucleus. (From Chokroverty and Provini [28], © 2017, with permission Springer Science+Business Media)

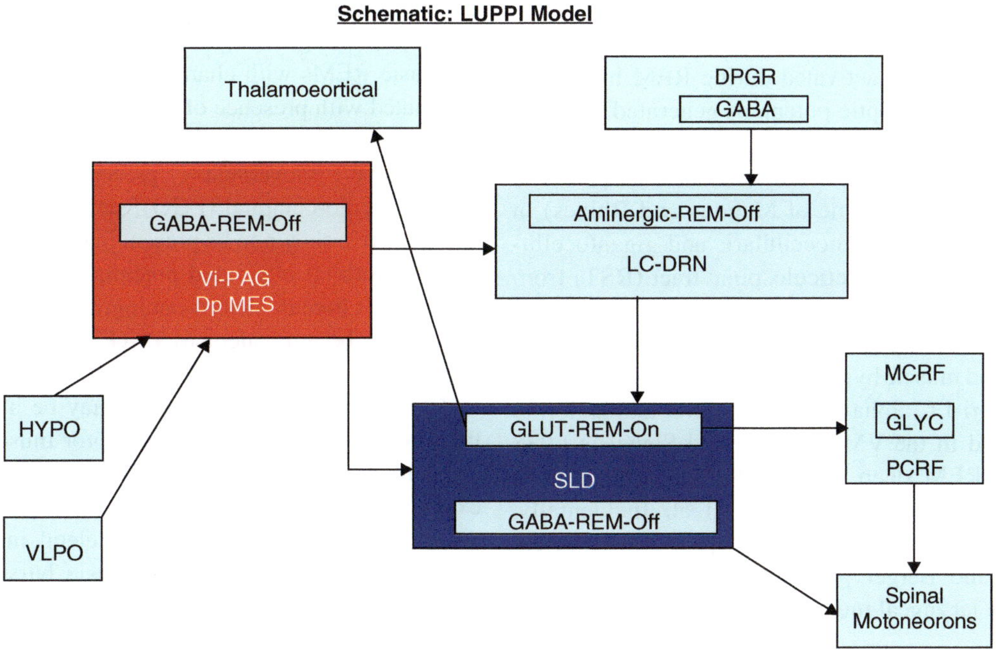

Fig. 4.6 Luppi's original model schematically shown to explain REM sleep mechanism in rats. GLUT Glutamatergic neurons, GABA Gamma-aminobutyric acid, LC Locus ceruleus, DRN Dorsal raphe nucleus, GLYC Glycinergic neurons, VLPO Ventrolateral preoptic nuclei of anterior hypothalamus, VLPAG Ventrolateral periaqueductal Grey region, DpMES Deep mesencephalic reticular neurons, MCRF-PCRF Magnocellular and parvocellular reticular formation, eVLPO Hypothalamic extended VLPO nuclei, HYPO Lateral hypothalamic orexin/hypocretin. (From Chokroverty and Provini [28], © 2017, with permission Springer Science+Business Media)

brachial nucleus; thus, this pathway (septo-hippocampal) may generate hippocampal theta and other REM EEG rhythms.

iii. The Model Proposed by Luppi's Group [40] stated that at REM sleep onset there is an activation of "REM-on" glutamatergic neurons in the SLD. These REM-generating neurons would be inhibited (hyperpolarized) during wakefulness and NREM sleep by tonic GABAergic input from REM-off neurons located in the deep mesencephalic, VLPAG and LPT regions and a few GABAergic neurons in the SLD as well as by active firing of monoaminergic "REM-off" neurons. Muscle atonia would be caused by both indirect and direct projections utilizing glycinergic and GABAergic premotor neurons in the magnocellular and parvocellular reticular nuclei in the VMM as well as in the interneurons in the spinal cord and causing hyperpolarization of the motor neurons. Ascending dorsal SLD glutamatergic neurons are responsible for cerebral cortical activation and REM EEG pattern through projections to the thalamus and thalamocortical pathways along with cholinergic neurons from LDT/PPT to the reticular thalamic nuclei and basal forebrain regions. In this model also cholinergic neurons do not play a significant role but a modulating and permissible influence. In their latest experiment Luppi et al. suggested that SLD neurons are mainly involved in REM muscle atonia only but not for other components of REM sleep, thus creating certain contradictions in hypothesis for REM sleep regulation [38]. It is important to note that the conclusion of Luppi and co-investigators regarding SLD glutamatergic neurons is based on solid experimental evidence. Following REM sleep deprivation studies in rats they noted that during REM recovery sleep, c-fos activated SLD neurons were not cholinergic (i.e., there was no increase of choline acetyltransferase, the enzyme synthesizing acetylcholine); also the enzyme synthesizing GABA, glutamic acid decarboxylase (GAD) did not increase in the majority of the SLD neurons, and hence most of them were not GABAergic. But most of the SLD neurons expressed vesicular glutamate transporter 2 (vGLUT2), a specific marker of glutamatergic neurons.

Essential Physiological Components of REM Sleep

Box 4.8 lists the core physiological components of REM sleep.

i. REM Motor Atonia Most of the muscles show atonia or marked hypotonia during REM sleep (lowest muscle tone compared with that in all other sleep stages and wake state except oculomotor muscles, middle ear and diaphragmatic muscles. What is the mechanism of REM muscle atonia?

This has been briefly mentioned above. In 1979 Sakai and co-investigators suggested an anatomical pathway (Fig. 4.7) [41], which is activated during REM hypotonia [42]: inhibitory post-synaptic potentials generated by interneurons in the region of peri-LC alpha ventral to LC are transmitted by the lateral tegmento reticular tract (TRT) to the VMM (the inhibitory zone of Magoun and Rhines) in and around the nucleus magnocellularis and gigantocellularis in the paramedianus. Reticulospinal tract (RST) from this region projects to the spinal cord ventral horn cells causing hyperpolarization (documented by Chase and Morales [43]) and muscle hypotonia or atonia. Experimental lesions in the peri-LC alpha region by Jouvet and Delorme in 1965 [44] and in the VMM by Lai and Siegel in 1988 [45] producing REM sleep without atonia can be cited in support of this hypothesis by Sakai et al. Incidentally, Jouvet's group first described in 1959 [46] REM muscle atonia in cats and Berger [47] described such atonia in human intrinsic laryngeal muscles in 1961.

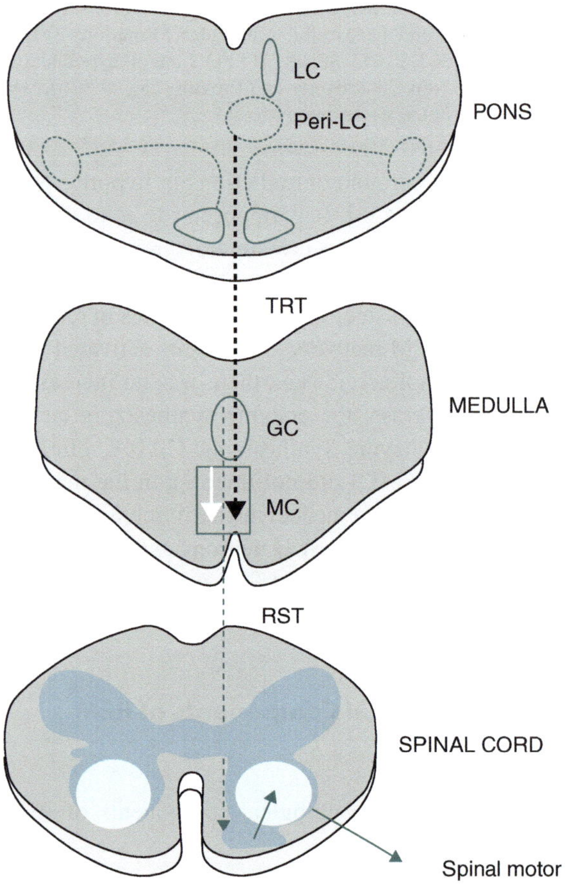

Fig. 4.7 REM muscle atonia pathway schematically shown. LC Locus ceruleus, Peri-LC Perilocus ceruleus alpha, TRT Tegmentoreticular tract, RST Reticulospinal tract, GC Gigantocellularis of medullary reticular formation, MC Magnocellularis of medullary reticular formation.(From Chokroverty and Provini [28], © 2017, with permission Springer Science+Business Media)

ii. Rapid Eye Movements (REMs) The second most characteristic finding during normal REM sleep is the presence of phasic REMs with characteristic morphological features associated with presence of muscle atonia except in the oculomotor and diaphragmatic muscles. These REMs are saccadic eye movements preceded immediately by pontogeniculo-occipital (PGO) waves in animal EEGs [48] and later also shown to be present in human depth recordings [49]. Periorbital integrated potentials (PIPs) (Fig. 4.8) [28] recorded in human electro-oculograms (EOGs) [50, 51] are thought to be equivalent to PGO waves. Why there is an absence of muscle atonia in the oculomotor muscles remains undetermined and conjectural. It may be hypothesized that the inhibitory drive to the oculomotor muscles is too weak (or remaining below threshold) and easily overcome by excitatory drive (it is notable that excitatory drive breaks through inhibitory drive in the skeletal muscles as manifested by transient myoclonic phasic bursts seen in these muscles during overnight polysomnography recording). The other suggestion is that the hypothetical atonia pathway (see above) does not project to connect with the oculomotor nuclei in the pontomesencephalic region.

iii. REM Sleep EEG This is manifested by desynchronized EEG with low amplitude mixed frequency waves (predominantly alpha and beta frequency with some theta rhythms) resembling waking EEG as well as sawtooth waves (2–7 Hz with characteristic morphological appearance seen best in frontocentral derivation) appearing just before phasic eye movements of REM sleep (see Fig. 4.8). The mechanism of generation of REM sleep EEG has been described above.

iv. Central Pattern Generators (CPGs) or the Mesencephalic and Spinal Locomotor Generators The existence of CPGs is well known in animals but scantily described in humans [52]. These are inhibited during normal REM sleep but postulated to be activated [52] during REM sleep behavior disorder (RBD), most likely in conjunction with activation of descending glutamatergic corticospinal and corticobulbar tracts to spinal ventral motor and cranial motor neurons, respectively, apparently bypassing the basal ganglia. These projections from activated CPGs and central motor cortex appear to be responsible for generating abnormal, mostly violent movements of RBD. The mechanism of inhibition and activation of CPGs remains to be documented.

Summary of Mechanisms of Sleep

In this last section, I will limit my discussion to some general comments and concentrate mostly on NREM sleep rather than REM sleep mechanism as the latter has been described under the heading of animal models.

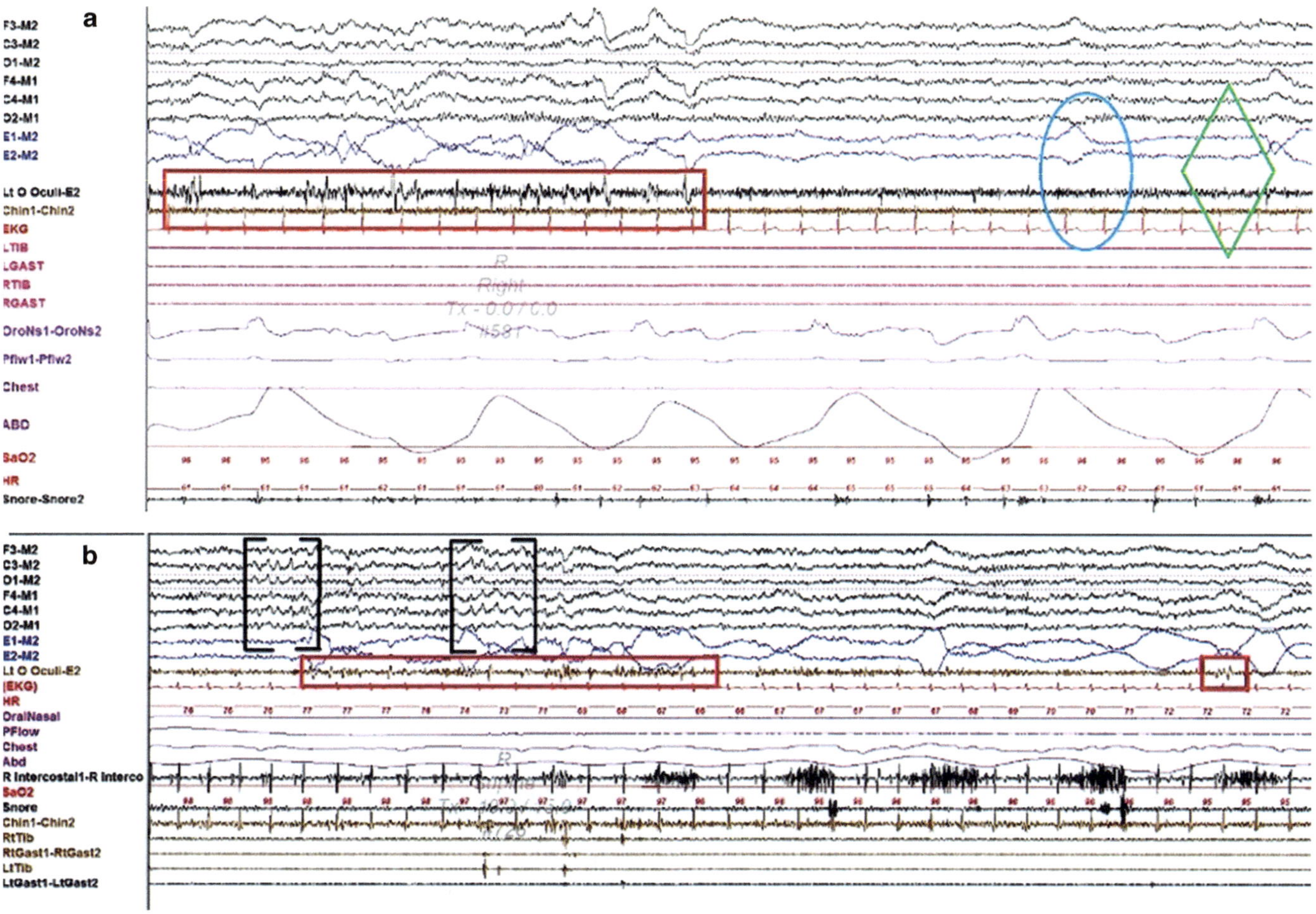

Fig. 4.8 A 60-second epoch of a polysomnography segment showing periorbital integrated potentials (PIPS, Horizontal rectangular bars in both a and b) (vertical boxes, sawtooth waves) The blue in 'a': REMs without PIPS. The green diamond in 'a': no REMs and no PIPS. In 'b' in the left hand column note: part of central apnea (no effort and no flow, and absence of Intercostal EMG bursts); in the right hand column: portion of obstructIve apnea (no flow but presence of effort along with Intercostal [inspiratory] EMG bursts). Chokroverty et al. [41], with permission Elsevier

Simply put spontaneous sleep results from a disruption of a dynamic equilibrium between the mutually antagonistic arousal and hypnogenic systems [16, 17]. Spontaneous sleep represents the final outcome of a chain of disinhibition and inhibition resulting in deactivation (i.e., inhibition) of the brainstem ARAS [16, 17, 26]. The main stimulus for this mechanism includes decrement of tonic activity in the ARAS resulting from various factors (e.g., blocking of environmental sensory afferent stimuli and a cascade of disfacilitation). Bremer [16, 17] suggested that a functional inhibition of the reticular formation would release suppression in many regions in the forebrain thus reinforcing disinhibition (i.e., excitation) of hypnogenic neurons. Of note, at sleep onset there is an increase of recurrent inhibition at the thalamocortical levels [53]. It is also known that relative immobility and closure of the eyelids block the activating sensory inflow [54]. It is important to remember that corticofugal projections provide excitation in the brainstem ARAS in case of functional or otherwise suppression of the ARAS tone [55, 56].

Both active and passive theories govern the generation of NREM sleep. The contemporary theory for the mechanism of sleep is cleverly explained by Saper's group [21, 37, 38] as a "flip-flop" switch (borrowing an engineering term as follows [of note, similar term applies to both NREM and REM sleep]): At sleep onset VLPO and MnPO ("Sleep-on" neurons) fire rapidly inhibiting brain stem waking and hypothalamic orexinergic and histaminergic waking neurons; at the same time there is reciprocal disinhibition of VLPO and MnPO neurons thus further exciting the "sleep-on" neurons. (Fig. 4.9) [21]. Orexin/hypocretin is thought to stabilize the switch. At wake onset wake active neurons fire rapidly and reciprocally inhibiting "sleep-on" neurons, and simultaneously reinforcing disinhibition of wave promoting neurons. Thus, interlinked excitation and inhibition [25] (reciprocal interaction) [16, 17, 21, 25, 38, 57] similar to that described above for REM sleep mechanism) results in mutually self-reinforcing or self-sustaining mechanism. There is acceleration of one group of neurons (e.g., "sleep-on") and

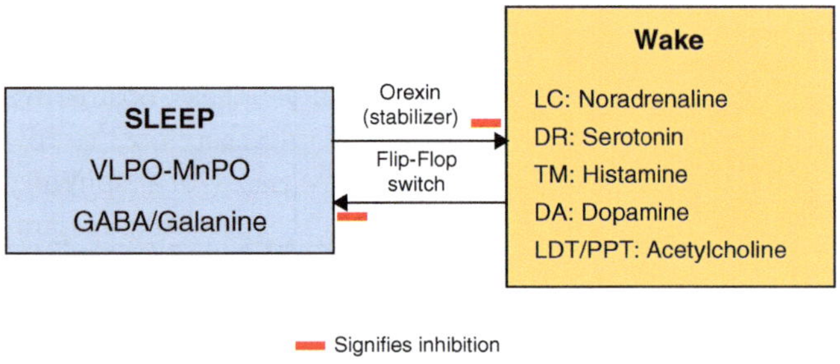

Fig. 4.9 Sleep switch (flip-flop switch) between the hypothalamus and the brainstem showing schematically mutual inhibition between sleep-promoting ventrolateral preoptic (VLPO), median preoptic (MnPO), and wake-promoting neurons [21]
During sleep VLPO-MnPO neurons fire rapidly inhibiting wake-promoting neurons thus causing disinhibition and reinforcement of their own firing. In contrast, during wakefulness there is rapid firing of wake-promoting neurons and inhibition of VLPO-MnPO neurons resulting in disinhibition of wake-on neurons. There is thus a reciprocal interaction like a "flip-flop" switch between two groups of antagonistic neurons. Orexin (hypocretin) is thought to stabilize the behavior of the switch; the switch will be destabilized if there is instability on either end
DR Dorsal raphe, TM Tuberomammillary, LC Locus ceruleus, DA Dopaminergic, LDT/PPT Laterodorsal tegmental/pedunculopontine tegmental

deceleration of the other contrasting group (e.g., "wake-on") and vice versa fulfilling the principle of reciprocal interaction [16, 17, 25]. Disruption of one end of the switch will destabilize the entire switch causing instability [21, 57]. Similar activation but to a smaller extent also occurs at sleep onset of the NTS and Pz in the lower brainstem with reciprocal interaction of the upper brainstem ARAS independent of the hypothalamic brainstem switch described above. MCH neurons in the lateral hypothalamus next to orexin neurons play a minor role in NREM sleep but play a major role (master generator) in REM sleep and REM-NREM cycling.

What causes firing of VLPO and MnPO neurons at sleep onset? This is somewhat controversial. It is thought to be due to a progressive accumulation of adenosine (assumed to be a physiological sleep factor) in the basal forebrain during prior wakefulness acting through adenosine A1 and A2A receptors [58]. The role of other sleep factors (e.g., prostaglandin D2, the cytokine interleukin- IB (IL-IB), growth hormone releasing factor (GHRF) and muramyl peptides) remains undetermined. It is noteworthy that as early as 1909 Ishimori [59] from Japan as well as Legendre and Pieron [60] from France in 1913 observed sleep-promoting substances in the cerebrospinal fluid of animals during prolonged wakefulness.

What causes the sleep-wake and NREM-REM cycles? These are controlled by a population of neurons that are dispersed and intermingled in an intricate and widespread network of neurons distributed throughout the reticular core extending from the caudal brainstem to the thalamus, the hypothalamus and the basal forebrain [2, 20, 21, 25, 37, 38, 56] (the network includes the brainstem, diencephalon, basal forebrain and cerebral hemispheres including limbic cortex). As stated above, acceleration in one group of cells can lead to deceleration in another group [16, 17, 26]. Thus, reciprocal oscillations of activity generate cyclic changes in cortical activity and behavior-promoting sleep-wake as well as NREM-REM cycling during sleep at night [16, 17, 26]. Both the homeostatic and circadian processes take part in these biological phenomena.

In conclusion, neurophysiological investigations in the last 80–90 years have shown that inhibition and disinhibition (i.e., facilitation) play the most significant role in sleep-wake generation illustrating (as so aptly expressed by Bremer [17]) the visionary concept of Sherrington.

References

1. Iber C, American Academy of Sleep Medicine, et al. The AASM manual for the scoring of sleep and associated events: rules, terminology and technical specifications. Westchester: American Academy of Sleep Medicine; 2007.
2. Lugaresi E, Provini F, Montagna P. The neuroanatomy of sleep. Considerations on the role of the thalamus in sleep and a proposal for a caudorostral organization. Eur J Anat. 2004;8(2):85–93.
3. Parmeggiani PL. Systemic homeostasis and poikilostasis in sleep. London: Imperial College Press; 2011.
4. Critchley M. The pre-dormitum. Rev Neurol (Paris). 1955;93:101–6.
5. Tassi P, Muzet A. Sleep inertia. Sleep Med Rev. 2000;4(4):341–53.
6. Morens DM, Taubenberger JK. Influenza cataclysm, 1918. N Engl J Med. 2018;379(24):2285–7.
7. von Economo C. Encephalitis lethargica. Wien Klin Weshr. 1917;30:581–3.
8. von Economo C. Sleep as a problem of localization. J Nerv Ment Dis. 1930;71:249–59.
9. von Economo C. Encephalitis lethargica, its sequalae and treatment. Newman KO, translator. London/Oxford: Oxford University Press; 1931.
10. Bremer F. Cerveau isolé et physiologic du sommeil. CR Soc Biol (Paris). 1935;118:1235–41.
11. Moruzzi G, Magoun HW. Brain stem reticular formation and activation of the EEG. Electroencephalogr Clin Neurophyisol. 1949;1(4):455–73.
12. Batini C, Moruzzi G, Palestini M, Rossi GF, Zanchetti A. Effects of complete pontine transections on the sleep-wakefulness rhythm: the midpontine pretrigeminal preparation. Arch Ital Biol. 1959;97:1–12.
13. Seriade M, McCarley RW. Brain control of wakefulness and sleep. 2nd ed. New York: Kluwer, Academic/Plenum; 2005.
14. Lugaresi E, Medori R, Montagna P, Baruzzi A, Cortelli P, Lugaresi A, et al. Fatal familial insomnia and dysautonomia with selective degeneration of thalamic nuclei. N Engl J Med. 1986;315(16):997–1003.
15. Hess WR. Das Schlafsyndrom als Folge dienzephaler Reizung. Helv Physiol Pharmacol Acta. 1944;2:30–344.
16. Bremer F. The neurophysiological problem of sleep. In: Adrian ED, Bremer F, Jasper HH, editors. Brain mechanisms and consciousness: a symposium organized by the council for international orga-

nizations of medical sciences, Quebec, 1953. Oxford: Blackwell Scientific Publications; 1954. p. 137–62.
17. Bremen F. Cerebral hypnogenic centers. Ann Neurol. 1977;2(1):1–6.
18. Tromner E. Schlaf und Lethargica. Zbl ges Neurol Psychiat. 1923;33:508.
19. Tromner E. Schlaf und Enzephalitis. Zbl ges Neurol Psychiat. 1926;101:786–97.
20. Steriade M. Neurophysiologic mechanisms of non-rapid eye movement (resting sleep). In: Chokroverty S, editor. Sleep disorders medicine. 2nd ed. Philadelphia: Elsevier/Butterworth; 1999. p. 51–62.
21. Saper CB, Chou T, Scammell TE. The sleep switch: hypothalamic control of sleep and wakefulness. Trends Neurosci. 2001;24(12):726–31.
22. Lowey AD. Anatomy of the autonomic nervous system: an overview. In: Lowey AD, Spyer KM, editors. Central regulation of autonomic functions. New York: Oxford University Press; 1990. p. 3–16.
23. Kleitman N. Sleep and wakefulness. Chicago: University of Chicago Press; 1939. Midway Reprint Edition; 1963. p. 3–7.
24. Brodal A. The reticular formation of the brain stem: anatomical and functional considerations. Edinburgh: Oliver and Boyd; 1957.
25. Anaclet C, Griffith K, Fuller PM. Activation of the GABAergic parafacial zone maintains sleep and counteracts the wake-promoting action of the psychostimulants armodafinil and caffeine. Neuropsychopharmacology. 2018;43(2):415–25.
26. Jones BE. Neuroanatomical, neurochemical, and neurophysical bases of waking and sleeping. In: Chokroverty S, Ferini-Strambi L, editors. Oxford textbook of sleep disorders. Oxford: Oxford University Press; 2017. p. 23–32.
27. Saper CB, Scammell TE, Lu J. Hypothalamic regulation of sleep and circadian rhythms. Nature. 2005;437(7063):1257–63. https://www.nature.com/articles/nature04284
28. Chokroverty S, Provini F. Sleep, breathing, and neurologic disorders. In: Chokroverty S, editor. Sleep disorders medicine. New York: Springer Science+Business Media; 2017. p. 787–890.
29. Dikshit VV. Action of acetylcholine on the "sleep center". J Physiol. 1934;83:42.
30. Nauta WJH. Hypothalamic regulation of sleep in rats: an experimental study. J Neurophysiol. 1946;9:285–316.
31. McGinty DJ, Sterman MB. Sleep suppression after basal forebrain lesions in the cat. Science. 1968;160(3833):1253–5.
32. Sherin JE, Shiromani PJ, McCarley RW, Saper CB. Activation of ventrolateral preoptic neurons during sleep. Science. 1996;271(5246):216–9.
33. Jouvet M. Paradoxical sleep—a study of its nature and mechanisms. Prog Brain Res. 1965;18:20–62.
34. Jouvet M. Recherches sur les structures nerveuses et les mécanismes responsible des différentes phases du sommeil physiologique. Arch Ital Biol. 1962;100:125-2-6. http://sommeil.univ-lyon1.fr/articles/jouvet/arch_ital_biol/sommaire.php. Accessed 16 Aug 2020. (*Article in French*).
35. Siegel JM. Mechanisms of sleep control. J Clin Neurophysiol. 1990;7(1):49–65.
36. McCarley RW. Neurobiology of REM and NREM sleep. Sleep Med. 2007;8(4):302–30.
37. Lu J, Sherman D, Devor M, Saper CB. A putative flip-flop switch for control of REM sleep. Nature. 2006;441(7093):589–94.
38. Vetrivelan R, Lu J. Neural circuitry regulating REM sleep and its implication in REM sleep behavior disorder. In: Schenck C, Hogl B, Videnovic A, editors. Rapid eye movement sleep behavior disorder. Cham: Springer Nature; 2019. p. 559–77.
39. Luppi PH, Fort P. Neurochemistry of sleep: an overview of animal experimental work. In: Aminoff MJ, Boller F, Swaab DF, series editors. Handbook of clinical neurology, Vol 98., 3rd series. Montagna P, Chokroverty, volume editors. Sleep disorders part I. Amsterdam: Elsevier; 2011. p. 173–190.
40. Luppi PH, Clement O, Peyton C, Fort P. Neurobiology of REM sleep. In: Chokroverty S, Ferini-Strambi L, editors. Oxford textbook of sleep disorders. Oxford: Oxford University Press; 2017. p. 15–22.
41. Chokroverty S, Bhat S, Rubinstein M. Periorbital integrated potentials: useful phasic REM sleep markers. Sleep Med. 2017;37:74–6. https://doi.org/10.1016/j.sleep.2017.06.016.
42. Sakai K, Sastre JP, Salvert D, Touret M. Tegmentoreticular projections with special reference to the muscular atonia during paradoxical sleep in the cat. Brain Res. 1979;176(2):233–54.
43. Chase M, Morales FR. Phasic changes in motoneuron membrane potential during REM periods of active sleep. Neurosci Lett. 1982;34(2):177–82.
44. Jouvet M, Delorme F. Locus coeruleus et sommeil paradoxical. CR Soc Biol (Paris). 1965;159:895–9.
45. Lai YY, Siegel JM. Medullary regions mediating atonia. J Neurosci. 1988;8:4790–6.
46. Jouvet M, Michel F. Corrélations électromyographiques du sommeil chez le chat décortiqué et mésencéphalique chronique. CR Soc Biol (Paris). 1959;153:422–5.
47. Berger RJ. Tonus of extrinsic laryngeal muscles during sleep and dreaming. Science. 1961;134(3482):840.
48. Datta S, Hobson A. Neuronal activity in the caudolateral peribrachial pons: relationship to PGO waves and rapid eye movements. J Neurophysiol. 1994;71(1):95–109.
49. Fernández-Mendoza J, Lozano B, Seijo F, Santamarta-Liébana E, Ramos-Platón MJ, Vela-Bueno A, Fernández-González F. Evidence of subthalamic PGO-like waves during REM sleep in humans: a deep brain polysomnographic study. Sleep. 2009;32(9):1117–26.
50. Benson K, Zarcone VP Jr. Phasic events of REM sleep: phenomenology of middle ear muscle activity and periorbital integrated potentials in the same normal population. Sleep. 1979;2(2):199–212.
51. Chokroverty S, Bhat S, Rubinstein M. Periorbital integrated potentials: useful phasic REM sleep markers. Sleep Med. 2017;37:74–6.
52. Tassinari CA, Rubboli G, Gardella E, Cantalupo G, Calandra-Buonaura G, Vedovello M, et al. Central pattern generators for a common semiology in fronto-limbic seizures and in parasomnias. A neuroethologic approach. Neurol Sci. 2005;26(Suppl 3):S225–32.
53. Steriade M, Apostol V, Oakson M. Control of unitary activation in the cerebello-thalamic pathway during wakefulness and synchronized sleep. J Neurophysiol. 1971;34(3):389–413.
54. Rougeul A. Concomitants électrographiques de l'assoupissement. Etude sur le chat et perspectives phylogénétiques fonctionnelles [Electrographic concomitants of sleep onset. Study in the cat and functional phylogenetic perspectives]. Rev Electroencephalogr Neurophysiol Clin. 1973;3(1):7–20. (*Article in French*)
55. Livingston RB, Hernandez-Peon R, French JD. Corticofugal projections to brain stem activating system. Fed Proc. 1953;12:89–90.
56. Bremer F, Terzuolo C. Rôle de l'écorce cérébrale dans le processus du réveil. Arch Internat Physiol. 1952;60(2):228–31.
57. Saper CB, Fuller PM. Wake-sleep circuitry: an overview. Curr Opin Neurol. 2017;44:186–92.
58. Porkka-Heiskanen T, Strecker RE, Thakkar M, Bjorkum AA, Greene RW, McCarley RW. Adenosine: a mediator of the sleep-inducing effects of prolonged wakefulness. Science. 1997;276(5316):1265–8.
59. Ishimori K. True causes of sleep—a hypnogenic substance as evidenced in the brain of sleep-deprived animals. Tokyo Igakkai Zasshi. 1909;23:429–57.
60. Legendre R, Pieron H. Recherches sur le besoin de sommeil consécutif à une veille prolongée. Z Allerg Physiol. 1913;14:235–62.

Physiological Changes in the Autonomic Nervous System During Sleep

5

Roberto Amici and Giovanna Zoccoli

Autonomic Function and Behavioral States

A behavioral state can be defined as the set of values that describe the level of activity of the physiological variables at a given point in time [1, 2]. Accordingly, each behavioral state is characterized by a specific pattern of autonomic nervous system (ANS) activity. The ANS, working together with the somatomotor and the neuroendocrine system, allows the body to maintain its internal homeostasis, as well as to optimize the interaction between the organism and the external environment. Since wakefulness and sleep are behaviors characterized by different levels of activity and interaction with the external environment, it is unsurprising that a consistent remodulation of ANS activity occurs during the transition from wakefulness to sleep [3]. Furthermore, sleep itself is a state showing an intrinsic heterogeneity. In fact, in non-rapid eye-movement sleep (NREMS), as well as during quiet wakefulness, physiological adjustments work effectively to maintain stable internal conditions (i.e., maintenance of body homeostasis); in contrast, during rapid eye-movement sleep (REMS) the regulatory control of physiological variables follows an apparently "non-homeostatic" modality that has been defined as "poikilostatic" [1, 2]. The ANS regulates the majority of the body's internal processes (e.g., blood pressure, cardiac activity, breathing, and body temperature) via afferent visceral and efferent sympathetic and parasympathetic pathways [4]. Given the functional dichotomy in terms of control theory between NREMS and REMS [5], the ANS activity changes dramatically even across sleep stages.

Sleep-dependent changes in autonomic control may be evaluated using different techniques: either indirectly, through photoplethysmographic-type methods; or invasively, through microneurographic recording of sympathetic nerve activity (SNA). Currently, the analysis of the spontaneous oscillations of heart period (HP, i.e. the reciprocal of heart rate, HR) and blood pressure (BP) provides information on sympathetic and parasympathetic activity to the heart and blood vessels and is more frequently utilized [6]. Altogether these different approaches indicate that, compared to previous wakefulness, during NREMS the contribution of the parasympathetic section increases, while that of the sympathetic section decreases, in accordance with the reduced metabolic and somatic activity of this sleep stage. During REMS, sympathetic activity shows great variability, and parasympathetic discharge displays phasic changes, reflecting the apparently non-homeostatic regulatory modality of this state. Moreover, both in humans and in laboratory animals, during REMS sympathetic vasomotor activity shows a heterogeneity of activation on a regional basis, with a decreased outflow in splanchnic and renal nerves, and an increased activity in muscle nerves.

The ANS and other regulatory systems that allow the body to cope with changes in the environment (external and internal) and to maintain homeostasis also operate in a predictive manner, allowing the organism to anticipate the occurrence of environmental stimuli that recur regularly, by promoting the appropriate corrective responses in advance [7]. This sophisticated predictive regulatory mechanism is controlled by circadian clocks, which are coordinated by the suprachiasmatic nucleus (SCN) in the anterior hypothalamus. The SCN acts as a pacemaker, generating and maintaining biological rhythms of around 24 hours in synchronization with the light-dark cycle. Neurons in the SCN project to the paraventricular nucleus (PVN) of the hypothalamus and other hypothalamic nuclei involved in the control of autonomic activity, as well as projecting to the hypothalamic neurons associated with the promotion of sleep (ventrolateral preoptic area, VLPO) (Fig. 5.1). Thus, wake-sleep changes that occur in autonomic activity based on changes in behavioral-dependent body's requirements are inscribed on

R. Amici (✉) · G. Zoccoli
Department of Biomedical and NeuroMotor Sciences (DIBINEM)-Physiology, Alma Mater Studiorum-University of Bologna, Bologna, Italy
e-mail: roberto.amici@unibo.it

S. Chokroverty, P. Cortelli (eds.), *Autonomic Nervous System and Sleep*, https://doi.org/10.1007/978-3-030-62263-3_5

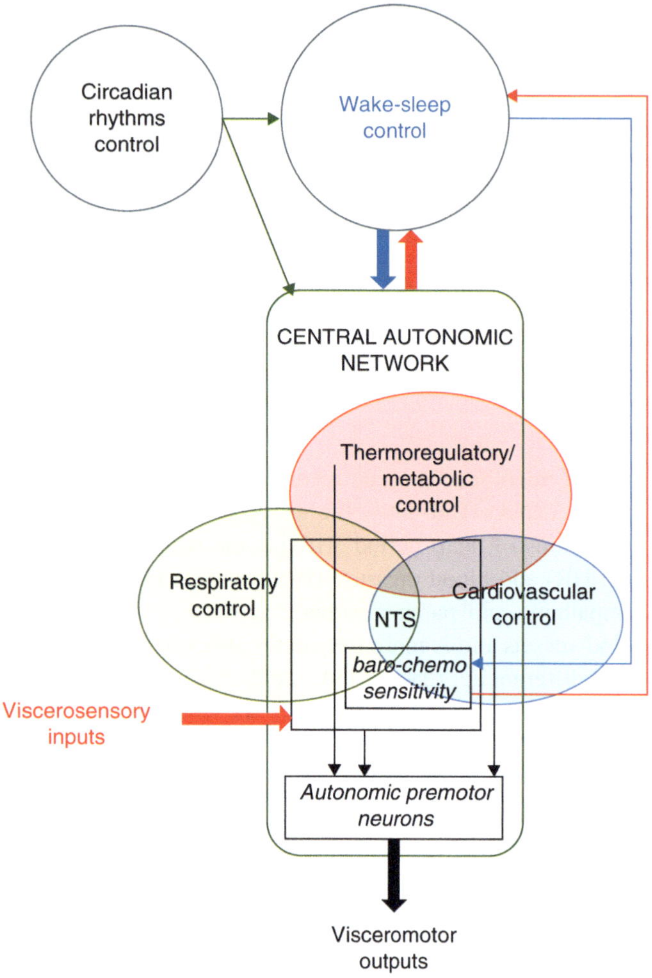

Fig. 5.1 The central autonomic network (CAN) is a neural system controlling autonomic activity, which in integration with neuroendocrine and behavioral responses operates for the maintenance of homeostasis and for the survival of the individual and of the species. It includes the limbic cortical and subcortical regions, as well as the hypothalamus and different brainstem nuclei; these are reciprocally interconnected and receive viscerosensory inputs, mainly through the nucleus of the tractus solitarius (NTS). In the CAN, nuclei involved in respiratory, cardiovascular, and thermoregulatory/metabolic regulation are largely overlapped. Their integrated activity generates specific patterns of visceromotor commands. CAN activity is regulated according to the behavioral states, including the wake-sleep cycle. Reciprocally, afferent visceral sensory information activating the CAN may produce a modulatory effect on the centers for wake-sleep state control. Moreover, wake-sleep dependent changes in autonomic activity are modulated by circadian clocks, which are coordinated by the suprachiasmatic nucleus in the anterior hypothalamus. This allows anticipating the occurrence of environmental stimuli that recur regularly, by promoting appropriate physiological responses in advance

the circadian modulation of physiological functions. Therefore, the hypothalamic integrative control allows the suitable autonomic (and endocrine) profile for wakefulness, NREMS and REMS to be anticipatorily established.

The aim of this chapter is to describe the functional changes in the ANS, which characterize the transitions from quiet wakefulness, through NREMS, to REMS. Emphasis will be placed on the autonomic regulation of respiratory and cardiovascular activity, and on the role of the ANS in the control of body temperature and energy expenditure.

Sleep, Autonomic Function, and Respiratory Regulation

Even if brainstem respiratory neurons make inspiratory skeletal muscles contract by activating somatic motor neurons, ventilation is strongly affected by ANS activity. Respiratory function is under the control of the same central autonomic network that controls other visceral functions [8], and the activity of the medullary respiratory neurons of the dorsal respiratory group (DRG, which includes the neurons of the solitary tract nucleus, NTS) is directly modulated by the vagal afferents coming from the lungs, and by the afferents coming from chemoreceptors and baroreceptors (see Fig. 5.1). Different hypothalamic regions, such as PVN, the perifornical area (PFA), the dorsomedial hypothalamus (DMH), the lateral hypothalamic area (LHA), and the posterior hypothalamus, were identified as the primary nuclei for respiratory control [9]. PVN neurons are connected with various brainstem and spinal cord regions involved in respiratory control [10], such as the parabrachial nucleus, retrotrapezoid nucleus, and NTS. Of note, vasopressin and oxytocin-containing PVN neurons project to the pre-Bötzinger complex (preBötC, the major putative respiratory pacemaker) and directly to the phrenic nucleus in the cervical spinal cord [11]. PVN plays a role in driving baseline respiration, but it is mainly involved in the mediation of the respiratory response to hypoxia. PFA is a region for mediation of respiration, arousal and other autonomic regulation as well. It is extensively interconnected with the DMH [12, 13], and DMH neurons likely regulate autonomic and respiratory activity via projections to the PFA. Finally, LHA, which represents a central chemoreception site [14] directly connected with preBötC neurons [15], plays a role in the maintenance of baseline respiration together with the posterior hypothalamus. PFA, DMH, and LHA all contain orexinergic neurons [16], projecting to the autonomic and respiratory centers in the brainstem, but their role in modulation of breathing is still unclear [9]. The central circuits that control respiratory activity are in close connection and in part overlap with those that control cardiocirculatory activity [8] (see Fig. 5.1); for example, medullary parasympathetic preganglionic neurons that control the cardiac sinoatrial node are subjected to a direct modulation by the central respiratory drive [18] besides integrating inputs from baroreceptors, chemoreceptors, and trigeminal receptors [17]. This represents the principal mechanism responsible for respiratory sinus arrhythmia [19].

It is worth noting that not only the control of breathing activity by the ANS in a sleep-dependent manner, but also changes in breathing such as those seen when transitioning from wakefulness to sleep [20], also modulate the ANS [4]; they can act both directly, through central circuits, and reflexively, since the reduction of the tidal volume during sleep produces a change in the response of the pulmonary afferents [21].

Several changes occur in respiratory function during sleep, due to the loss or the reduction of different control mechanisms working during wakefulness. During sleep, the main input controlling breathing is represented by chemical signals, coming from peripheral and central chemoreceptors. However, chemo-responsiveness is reduced during sleep: ventilatory responses to hypoxia are decreased in NREMS and REMS, and even if CO_2 remains the main regulator for breathing, ventilatory response to hypercapnia is also reduced, and tolerance to high levels of CO_2 increases. As a result, a reduction of minute ventilation is accompanied by an increase in arterial pCO_2 of 3–8 mmHg. During sleep, apnea threshold is reached (and breathing stops) when arterial pCO_2 falls 2–6 mm Hg below the normal stable value for sleep, a value that broadly corresponds to normal arterial pCO_2 in wakefulness [22]. While at sleep onset respiratory instability may appear, with increases and decreases in breathing amplitude, during stable NREMS ventilation is regular, the indices of its variability are very low and minute ventilation progressively drops. During REMS, minute ventilation decreases further, breathing becomes irregular, displaying phasic changes in respiratory amplitude and frequency that parallel the occurrence of REMS and may include central apneas [23]. REMS are also associated with inhibition of upper airway dilator muscles, favoring the occurrence of obstructive apneas [24]. The irregular respiratory pattern of REMS is a very robust phenomenon, and it is not affected by hypoxia, hypercapnia, chemodenervation, or vagotomy [24].

Sleep, Autonomic Function, and Cardiovascular Regulation

Autonomic regulation of cardiac and circulatory functions significantly differs across the wake-sleep cycle, to maintain peripheral blood supply matching the appropriate metabolic requirements of various organs. During NREMS, parasympathetic control of the heart increases, while cardiac and vascular sympathetic activity decreases compared to wakefulness. Accordingly, HR and BP decrease, as well as muscle sympathetic nerve activity (MSNA) (in addition to splanchnic and renal sympathetic nerve activity, as shown in laboratory animals); LF component of BP variability decreases, while HF component of RR variability increases, with a reduction of LF/HF ratio [6, 25]. The mechanisms underlying HR and BP changes in NREMS are not yet fully understood; in mice BP decrease during NREMS is mainly due to a decrease in sympathetic vasoconstriction, while HR reduction is obtained by balancing cardiac parasympathetic activation and sympathetic withdrawal [26]. Changes in sympathetic and parasympathetic activity on heart and vessels are a consequence of central command that both directly control autonomic premotor neurons and modulate baroreflexes [27] (see Fig. 5.1). While the effects of sleep on baroreflex sensitivity (BRS) are inconsistent and insubstantial [28], during NREMS a reset of the baroreflex toward lower values of BP and HR compared with wakefulness has been described [29]. The overall reduction of the sympathetic tone during NREMS may be interrupted by sympathetic neural surges generated by external or internal stimuli. Causing transit arousal, autonomic activation accompanies arousal from sleep, but it can also be generated in the absence of EEG modifications (autonomic activation) or with EEG modifications other than those characteristic of the arousal (subcortical arousal) [30]. During NREMS stage N2 EEG K-complex are associated with bursts of MSNA and phasic increases in BP [31]. Leg movements during sleep also entail substantial sympathetic activation [32]. Disturbances and frequent arousals during the night, as in the context of sleep-disordered breathing, may thus represent a stressful condition for the cardiovascular system [33]. In particular, while in normal subjects BP and SNA decline significantly during NREMS, they both reach very high levels during sleep in patients with obstructive sleep apnea, in which sympathetic nerve discharge remains very high even when they are awake [34].

REMS is characterized by phasic changes in sympathetic and parasympathetic activity, leading to accelerations and decelerations in heart rhythm, respectively, associated with bursts of phasic rapid eye movements, PGO waves, myoclonic twitches, and breathing irregularities, which produces large fluctuations of cardiovascular variables. In particular, due to increased sympathetic activity to the heart and blood vessels during REMS [26] mean values of BP and HR are higher than during NREMS, even if the values remain lower than those recorded during wakefulness [28]. Accordingly, during REMS, the LF component of the HR variability and LF/HF ratio increase compared to NREMS [3]. Different evidences suggest that the hemodynamic pattern of REMS is mainly produced by the activation of central commands controlling premotor autonomic neurons, and it is only modulated by sinoaortic reflexes [28]. The prevalence of central commands on baroreflex regulation of cardiac function during REMS is confirmed by studies assessing the spontaneous fluctuations in heart period (HP, that is, the reciprocal of HR) and BP in the time domain during the different wake-sleep states [35]. In particular, cross-correlation analysis of HP and BP shows that during NREMS the values of HP are positively correlated with previous values of BP, showing a spontaneous increase in blood pressure, which leads to a baroreflex-mediated decrease in HR. In contrast, during REMS, the central autonomic commands to the heart and the vessels produce hypertension and tachycardia.

In REMS, autonomic vascular control acts differentially on a regional basis. While MSNA increases on passing from NREMS to REMS [31], sympathetic activity decreases in visceral nerves [36, 37]. Accordingly, mesenteric and renal vasodilation is accompanied by muscular vasoconstriction [38]. Moreover, during phasic REMS, an inhibition of the MSNA occurs together with muscle twitches and phasic BP surges [31]. Simultaneous recording of sympathetic vascular activity in different peripheral districts was obtained by Futuro-Neto and Coote [39]. These authors showed that in mid-collicular decerebrate cats, during REMS-like periods, the activity of sympathetic vasoconstrictor fibers to muscle increases, whereas it decreases in the kidney, gastrointestinal tract, and pelvic viscera. It is notable that the integrated pattern of vasomotor sympathetic activity resulting from thermal stimulation is entirely preserved during NREMS, while it is abolished in REMS. During exposure to both low and high ambient temperatures, peripheral vasomotor changes on transitioning from NREMS to REMS are incompatible with thermoregulatory homeostasis [40] (see further on). During REMS, the loss of muscle tone that normally favors the maintenance of upper airway patency promotes the occurrence of obstructive sleep apneas (OSAs) which have a deep impact on cardiovascular regulation. Patients with OSAs show an increase in MSNA and BP variability even during wakefulness. During an apneic episode, there is a progressive increase in SNA due to the activation of chemoreceptors, which disappears at the onset of breathing. BP peaks at time of resumption of respiratory activity, often associated with an arousal [34]. Recurrent nocturnal episodes of hypoxia may produce oxidative stress and inflammation, with an increase in vascular sympathetic activity and BP [33].

Sleep-dependent changes in autonomic activity are modulated by circadian influences (see Fig. 5.1). In addition to circadian modulation of vigilance state, the hypothalamic SCN influences the cardiovascular system mainly via projections to pre-autonomic neurons (those projecting to preganglionic neurons) of PVN. Evident circadian rhythms of BP and HR, not dependent on sleep occurrence and on locomotory activity, have been described in mice [41, 42]. In humans, a circadian vagal influence on the heart has been reported [43, 44], while data on circadian sympathetic changes are not fully consistent [45, 46]. Even if the amplitudes of the circadian fluctuations of HR and BP are much smaller than those linked to the wake-sleep cycle, beside an alteration in the quantity and quality of sleep, a dysregulation of circadian rhythms can also promote an alteration of BP values. In this context, it is worth mentioning that an increase in the mean values of BP at nighttime is a major predictor of cardiovascular mortality [47].

Finally, it should be kept in mind that the relationship between behavioral state and autonomic regulation of cardiovascular function is a two-way relationship (see Fig. 5.1). While the state of the wake-sleep cycle modulates the level of activity of the sympathetic and parasympathetic nervous system (through changes in the baroreflex set point), the activation of the autonomic afferents can in turn modulate the behavioral state [30]. Mild baroreceptor stimulation may favor cortical synchronization [48], while strong changes in baroreflex activation can produce arousal in animal models [49] and human subjects [50]. NTS and parabrachial nuclei are strong candidates to be important mediators of this bidirectional interaction between autonomic control and vigilance state [30].

Sleep, Autonomic Function, and the Regulation of Body Temperature and Energy Expenditure

A strong interaction between sleep and the regulation of body temperature and energy expenditure has been shown and extensively reviewed in the last 50 years [51–54]. The basis of this interaction resides in the fact that, on a circadian basis, the most appropriate moment for sleep to occur is during the rest phase of the rest-activity cycle, when a centrally driven decrease of body temperature and energy expenditure is observed and the animal largely reduces interaction with the external environment. The relationship between sleep and thermoregulation appears to be reciprocal (see Fig. 5.1), since not only is it the case that thermoregulation is affected by the different sleep states, but also that thermoregulatory activation due to thermal challenges largely affects sleep occurrence [51, 52].

Overall, human adult body energy expenditure decreases during sleep. Although such a decrease is apparently modest compared to quiet wakefulness, it may be relevant for better energy conservation in infants or small mammals, which present an unfavorable surface to volume ratio [54]. Whole-body indirect calorimetry in humans has shown that energy expenditure progressively decreases in the first half of the night (up to a 35% decrease), and then remains almost stable until morning awakening [55]. Also, energy expenditure is a bit larger (2–4%) during REMS compared to NREMS. This effect is probably due to the relatively large size of the brain in humans, since brain energy metabolism, which decreases during NREMS, returns to levels around those of wakefulness during REMS. In fact, in small mammals, in which the size of the brain is rather modest, the decrease in energy expenditure due to REMS atonia is larger than the increase in brain metabolism and an overall decrease occurs on passing from NREMS to REMS.

Generally, thermoregulatory responses to thermal challenges can be either behavioral (posture and motor activity aimed at thermal comfort) or autonomic/physiological (piloerection, vasomotion, shivering, metabolic heat production, panting, and sweating). Although only the latter will be taken into account in this chapter, it is noteworthy that while during NREMS posture can be changed according to the thermal needs, during REMS this is no longer possible due to complete muscle atonia.

The use of constant routine protocols in humans brought evidence of the relevance of circadian-driven changes in body heat production and heat loss in the promotion of sleep onset [54]. In particular, in the hours preceding lights off, a decrease in metabolic heat production, which is accompanied by a decrease in heart rate, is followed by a vasodilation at the extremities, leading to an increase in heat loss and to a progressive decrease in core body temperature. Both effects are consequent to a decrease in sympathetic activity. Recent data point to a possible role of melatonin in the induction of peripheral vasodilation, but whether this occurs through its direct action on blood vessels or by means of a modulation of sympathetic activity remains unclear [56]. In the first hours after sleep onset, the constant heat transfer from the core to the shell of the body leads to a further decrease in body temperature. These processes are reversed in the morning during the transition to wakefulness. The mild warming of the extremities has been shown to shorten sleep latency in sleep onset insomniacs [57]. The hypothesis that this effect may be due to the thermal input from the skin to the centers where thermoregulation and sleep regulation overlap is supported by a recent study in mice [58], which showed that the selective activation of warm-sensitive glutamatergic/nitrergic neurons at the level of the median and medial preoptic areas promotes both NREMS onset and body cooling. Similar effects have been obtained in mice through the selective stimulation of galanin neurons in the VLPO [59].

Thus, the activity of the thermoregulatory system during the different wake-sleep states has been studied in conditions in which the subject has been thermally challenged through either the delivery of internal stimuli or the exposure to an ambient temperature far beyond the thermoneutral range. During quiet wakefulness, stimuli leading to central cooling increase body metabolism, induce shivering and cutaneous vasoconstriction, and promote heat-seeking behavior [60–65], while those leading to central warming induce grooming, panting and cutaneous vasodilation, and promote body relaxation [62–64, 66, 67]. Many studies have shown that while the autonomic/physiological responses are substantially maintained during NREMS, they are suppressed in animals and depressed in humans during REMS [52, 68]. Thus, as already introduced in the first paragraph, the regulatory modality of the preoptic-hypothalamic centers apparently shifts from a closed-loop to an open-loop one [1, 68].

In particular, during REMS, in animals kept at low Ta, peripheral vasoconstriction is replaced by a vasodilation [40, 67, 69–71] and shivering is suppressed [72]. The absence of shivering has also been observed in cats following a pontine lesion leading to the maintenance of muscle tone during REMS [73], showing that shivering suppression is not the mere consequence of muscle atonia. Reciprocally, in a warm environment peripheral vasoconstriction was observed on passing from NREMS to REMS [67, 69, 71] and thermal tachypnea is suppressed in cats [72]. In humans, sweating is suppressed at the beginning of the REMS episode, but a slow normalization of sweat production occurs in the course of the episode [74]. Recently, Tupone and coworkers [75] have proposed that at least part of this apparent reversal of the autonomic responses during REMS may be due to the activation of a central pathway which leads to inverted (i.e., positive instead of negative retroaction) thermoregulatory responses.

In small rodents, the direct preoptic-hypothalamic cooling during REMS is unable to increase oxygen consumption and body metabolism as it occurs in wakefulness and NREMS [65], and is not followed by the expected release of thyroid stimulating hormone (TSH) [76]. Likewise, direct preoptic-hypothalamic warming does not induce either thermal tachypnea [77], or cutaneous vasodilation in cats [67]. During REM sleep, thermal responsiveness of cold-sensitive neurons at the preoptic level is largely reduced, while inconsistent results come from studies on warm-sensitive neurons [78–80]. Because of such thermoregulatory impairment, during REMS body temperature slowly shifts toward that of the external environment [81].

The interaction between sleep and thermoregulatory process clearly emerges from studies in which the impact of thermoregulatory engagement on sleep occurrence has been studied [51, 52]. The activation of thermogenesis, driven by the sympathetic nervous system, appears to be incompatible with REMS occurrence, since, in different species, REMS is depressed in proportion to the environmental thermal load [82–84]. Likewise, REMS occurrence is largely depressed when animals are kept at a warm Ta well beyond the upper limit of thermoneutrality [85]. In rats kept at a very low Ta, NREMS-REMS cyclicity is also affected, and sleep is made just by a sequence of unsuccessful transitions from NREMS to REMS followed by a brief awakening [86]. In the presence of a mild environmental thermal load, a long-term metabolic and endocrine adaptation process may lead to a normalization of the wake-sleep cycle [87].

Sleep and Autonomic Function Within the Frame of Physiological Regulation

The sleep-dependent changes in autonomic function in different wake-sleep states may be better interpreted when discussed within the wider frame of the state-dependent changes in physiological regulation (i.e., the integrated neural control mechanisms underlying somatic and visceral activity or the behavior of the animal) [1, 2]. The integration of the activities of the somatic, autonomic and endocrine motor systems occurs at the hypothalamic level according to the needs of the different behaviors [13]. During wakefulness, different behaviors occur according to the homeostatic needs of the animal or to its motivation, for example, to flee from a danger, to fight to survive or to mate for species perpetuation. In this respect, it has recently been shown that thermogenesis is activated on ultradian basis as a part of a central program regulating the basic rest-activity cycle (BRAC), leading to a periodic increase in brain temperature that supports active waking [88]. This activation is always followed in few minutes by the ingestion of a meal, apparently independently from any specific homeostatic drive to food consumption.

During active wakefulness, the value of "instrumental" physiological variables (e.g., HR, stroke volume, cardiac output, BP, ventilation, muscle force and power) is continuously modulated in order to shape the behavior and to allow someone to reach its goal. In the meantime, the level of "primary" homeostatically regulated physiological variables (e.g., temperature, pH, O_2, CO_2, nutrients, water volume, osmolality) may fluctuate even over or below the normal physiological range but is promptly returned within this range during the following period of quiet wakefulness. Thus, during active wakefulness physiological regulation works to shape different behaviors and support their needs and goals. But quiet wakefulness is set to maintain the "primary" variables within their normal physiological range [1].

During NREMS, physiological regulation clearly operates according to the "homeostatic" modality. The ANS drives the "instrumental" variables toward lower limit of the physiological range in order to cope with the low somatic activity and reduced metabolic needs of this sleep state. Consequently, "primary" variables are kept near to their fixed value by well operant baroceptive, chemoceptive and thermoregulatory reflexes. Moreover, somatic activity allows the animal to find a proper posture to minimize any possible thermal discomfort.

On the contrary, REMS displays great variability in sympathetic activity associated with phasic changes in parasympathetic discharge, producing the appearance of BP surges, frequent irregularities in heart and breathing rhythmicity and thermoregulatory impairment. A phasic central nervous command has been shown to be able to drive the cardiovascular variables beyond the normal control of the baroceptive reflex [28]. Furthermore, muscle atonia does not allow the animal to adjust its posture according to different needs.

This operative modality of physiological regulation during REM sleep has been called "poikilostatic," since it is not visibly oriented to any goal or to maintenance of the stability of "primary" physiological variables, apparently allowing them to float as it occurs for body temperature in poikilothermic animals [1, 2, 68]. However, the finding that osmoregulation, a regulation that is physiologically more ancient than thermoregulation, is apparently preserved during REMS [89] and that a strong osmotic challenge does not substantially interfere with REMS occurrence [90] leads to the hypothesis that the loss of the integrative capacity at the hypothalamic level is substantially related to thermoregulation. Thus, at least part of the variability and instability of "instrumental" cardiovascular physiological variables during REMS may be due to the loss of the thermoregulatory control of such variables.

In conclusion, the changes in the ANS activity observed during sleep should be considered part of the integrated somatomotor, autonomic and neuroendocrine functional pattern, which defines any different state of waking and sleeping. This pattern appears to be clear and coherent for NREM sleep, but it is hardly explainable for REM sleep. While NREM sleep is regarded as a state that favors energy saving, recently it has been proposed that REMS represents a transient heterothermic state which allows endotherm animals to satisfy specific needs of their brain activity that cannot be fulfilled when thermoregulation is active [92]. This view appears to be in line with the remark that REMS and endothermy appeared concomitantly during evolution and somehow coevolved [91]. Such an evolutionary constraint may explain why the regulation of these two functions overlaps at the level of several brain areas (e.g., the medial and median preoptic area, the LH, and the periaqueductal gray), consequently leading to the mutual exclusivity in the occurrence of thermoregulation and REMS.

References

1. Parmeggiani PL. Physiologic regulation in sleep. In: Kryger MH, Roth T, Dement WC, editors. Principles and practice of sleep medicine. Philadelphia: Elsevier Saunders; 2005. p. 185–91.
2. Parmeggiani PL. Systemic homeostasis and poikilostasis in sleep. London: Imperial College Press; 2011. p. 1–38.
3. Khairandish A, Shapiro CM. Peripheral nervous system and sleep. In: Kushida CA, editor. The encyclopedia of sleep. Waltham: Academic Press; 2013. p. 494–502.
4. de Zambotti M, Trinder J, Silvani A, Colrain IM, Baker FC. Dynamic coupling between the central and autonomic nervous systems during sleep: a review. Neurosci Biobehav Rev. 2018;90:84–103.
5. Parmeggiani PL. Behavioral phenomenology of sleep (somatic and vegetative). Experientia. 1980;36(1):6–11.
6. Tobaldini E, Nobili L, Strada S, Casali KR, Braghiroli A, Montano N. Heart rate variability in normal and pathological sleep. Front Physiol. 2013;4:294.
7. Cardinali DP. The timed autonomic nervous system. In: Cardinali DP, editor. Autonomic nervous system: basic and clinical aspects. Cham: Springer International; 2018. p. 19–56.

8. Benarroch EE. Brainstem integration of arousal, sleep, cardiovascular, and respiratory control. Neurology. 2018;91(21):958–66.
9. Fukushi I, Yokota S, Okada Y. The role of the hypothalamus in modulation of respiration. Respir Physiol Neurobiol. 2019;265:172–9.
10. Geerling JC, Shin JW, Chimenti PC, Loewy AD. Paraventricular hypothalamic nucleus: axonal projections to the brainstem. J Comp Neurol. 2010;518(9):1460–99.
11. Kc P, Haxhiu MA, Tolentino-Silva FP, Wu M, Trouth CO, Mack SO. Paraventricular vasopressin-containing neurons project to brain stem and spinal cord respiratory-related sites. Respir Physiol Neurobiol. 2002;133(1–2):75–88.
12. Bondarenko E, Beig MI, Hodgson DM, Braga VA, Nalivaiko E. Blockade of the dorsomedial hypothalamus and the perifornical area inhibits respiratory responses to arousing and stressful stimuli. Am J Physiol Regul Integr Comp Physiol. 2015;308(10):R816–22.
13. Thompson RH, Swanson LW. Structural characterization of a hypothalamic visceromotor pattern generator network. Brain Res Brain Res Rev. 2003;41(2–3):153–202.
14. Li N, Li A, Nattie E. Focal microdialysis of CO(2) in the perifornical-hypothalamic area increases ventilation during wakefulness but not NREM sleep. Respir Physiol Neurobiol. 2013;185(2):349–55.
15. Yang CF, Feldman JL. Efferent projections of excitatory and inhibitory preBotzinger complex neurons. J Comp Neurol. 2018;526(8):1389–402.
16. Peyron C, Tighe DK, van den Pol AN, de Lecea L, Heller HC, Sutcliffe JG, et al. Neurons containing hypocretin (orexin) project to multiple neuronal systems. J Neurosci. 1998;18(23):9996–10015.
17. Gilbey MP, Jordan D, Richter DW, Spyer KM. Synaptic mechanisms involved in the inspiratory modulation of vagal cardioinhibitory neurones in the cat. J Physiol. 1984;356:65–78.
18. McAllen RM, Spyer KM. The baroreceptor input to cardiac vagal motoneurones. J Physiol. 1978;282:365–74.
19. Eckberg DL. The human respiratory gate. J Physiol. 2003;548(Pt 2):339–52.
20. Trinder J, Nicholas CL. Respiratory and cardiac activity at sleep onset. In: Douglas BT, Floras JS, editors. Sleep disorders and cardiovascular and cerebrovascular disease. New York: Marcel Dekker; 2000. p. 337–54.
21. Colrain IM, Trinder J, Fraser G, Wilson GV. Ventilation during sleep onset. J Appl Physiol (1985). 1987;63(5):2067–74.
22. Eckert DJ, Butler JE. Respiratory physiology: understanding the control of ventilation. In: Kryger MH, Roth T, Dement WC, editors. Principles and practice of sleep medicine. 6th ed. Philadelphia: Elsevier; 2017. p. 167–73.
23. Douglas NJ. Respiratory physiology: control of ventilation. In: Kryger MH, Roth T, Dement WC, editors. Principles and practice of sleep medicine. 4th ed. Philadelphia: Elsevier Saunders; 2005. p. 224–31.
24. Krieger J. Respiratory physiology: breathing in normal subjects. In: Kryger MH, Roth T, Dement WC, editors. Principles and practice of sleep medicine. 4th ed. Philadelphia: Elsevier Saunders; 2005. p. 232–44.
25. Silvani A. Sleep disorders, nocturnal blood pressure, and cardiovascular risk: a translational perspective. Auton Neurosci. 2019;218:31–42.
26. Lo Martire V, Silvani A, Alvente S, Bastianini S, Berteotti C, Valli A, et al. Modulation of sympathetic vasoconstriction is critical for the effects of sleep on arterial pressure in mice. J Physiol. 2018;596(4):591–608.
27. Silvani A, Dampney RA. Central control of cardiovascular function during sleep. Am J Physiol Heart Circ Physiol. 2013;305(12):H1683–92.
28. Silvani A. Physiological sleep-dependent changes in arterial blood pressure: central autonomic commands and baroreflex control. Clin Exp Pharmacol Physiol. 2008;35(9):987–94.
29. Nagura S, Sakagami T, Kakiichi A, Yoshimoto M, Miki K. Acute shifts in baroreflex control of renal sympathetic nerve activity induced by REM sleep and grooming in rats. J Physiol. 2004;558(Pt 3):975–83.
30. Silvani A, Calandra-Buonaura G, Benarroch EE, Dampney RA, Cortelli P. Bidirectional interactions between the baroreceptor reflex and arousal: an update. Sleep Med. 2015;16(2):210–6.
31. Somers VK, Dyken ME, Mark AL, Abboud FM. Sympathetic-nerve activity during sleep in normal subjects. N Engl J Med. 1993;328(5):303–7. Epub 1993/02/04
32. Pennestri MH, Montplaisir J, Colombo R, Lavigne G, Lanfranchi PA. Nocturnal blood pressure changes in patients with restless legs syndrome. Neurology. 2007;68(15):1213–8.
33. Lanfranchi PA, Pepin JL, Somers VK. Cardiovascular physiology: autonomic control in health and sleep disorders. In: Kryger MH, Roth T, Dement WC, editors. Principles and practice of sleep medicine. 6th ed. Philadelphia: Elsevier; 2017. p. 167–73.
34. Somers VK, Dyken ME, Clary MP, Abboud FM. Sympathetic neural mechanisms in obstructive sleep apnea. J Clin Invest. 1995;96(4):1897–904.
35. Silvani A, Asti V, Bojic T, Ferrari V, Franzini C, Lenzi P, et al. Sleep-dependent changes in the coupling between heart period and arterial pressure in newborn lambs. Pediatr Res. 2005;57(1):108–14.
36. Baust W, Weidinger H, Kirchner F. Sympathetic activity during natural sleep and arousal. Arch Ital Biol. 1968;106(4):379–90.
37. Miki K, Oda M, Kamijyo N, Kawahara K, Yoshimoto M. Lumbar sympathetic nerve activity and hindquarter blood flow during REM sleep in rats. J Physiol. 2004;557(Pt 1):261–71.
38. Mancia G, Baccelli G, Adams DB, Zanchetti A. Vasomotor regulation during sleep in the cat. Am J Phys. 1971;220(4):1086–93.
39. Futuro-Neto HA, Coote JH. Changes in sympathetic activity to heart and blood vessels during desynchronized sleep. Brain Res. 1982;252(2):259–68.
40. Cianci T, Zoccoli G, Lenzi P, Franzini C. Loss of integrative control of peripheral circulation during desynchronized sleep. Am J Phys. 1991;261(2 Pt 2):R373–7.
41. Bastianini S, Silvani A, Berteotti C, Lo Martire V, Zoccoli G. Mice show circadian rhythms of blood pressure during each wake-sleep state. Chronobiol Int. 2012;29(1):82–6.
42. Sheward WJ, Naylor E, Knowles-Barley S, Armstrong JD, Brooker GA, Seckl JR, et al. Circadian control of mouse heart rate and blood pressure by the suprachiasmatic nuclei: behavioral effects are more significant than direct outputs. PLoS One. 2010;5(3):e9783.
43. Burgess HJ, Trinder J, Kim Y, Luke D. Sleep and circadian influences on cardiac autonomic nervous system activity. Am J Phys. 1997;273(4):H1761–8.
44. Krauchi K, Wirz-Justice A. Circadian rhythm of heat production, heart rate, and skin and core temperature under unmasking conditions in men. Am J Phys. 1994;267(3 Pt 2):R819–29.
45. Carrington M, Walsh M, Stambas T, Kleiman J, Trinder J. The influence of sleep onset on the diurnal variation in cardiac activity and cardiac control. J Sleep Res. 2003;12(3):213–21.
46. Shea SA, Hilton MF, Hu K, Scheer FA. Existence of an endogenous circadian blood pressure rhythm in humans that peaks in the evening. Circ Res. 2011;108(8):980–4.
47. Yano Y, Kario K. Nocturnal blood pressure and cardiovascular disease: a review of recent advances. Hypertens Res. 2012;35(7):695–701.
48. Bridgers SL, Spencer SS, Spencer DD, Sasaki CT. A cerebral effect of carotid sinus stimulation. Observation during intraoperative electroencephalographic monitoring. Arch Neurol. 1985;42(6):574–7.
49. Horne RS, De Preu ND, Berger PJ, Walker AM. Arousal responses to hypertension in lambs: effect of sinoaortic denervation. Am J Phys. 1991;260(4 Pt 2):H1283–9.
50. Kesler B, Anand A, Launois SH, Weiss JW. Drug-induced arterial pressure elevation is associated with arousal from NREM sleep in normal volunteers. J Appl Physiol (1985). 1999;87(3):897–901.

51. Heller HC, Edgar DM, Grahn DA, Glotzbach SF. Sleep, thermoregulation, and circadian rhythms. In: Fregly MJ, Blatteis CM, editors. Handbook of physiology: environmental physiology. Oxford: Oxford University Press; 1996. p. 1361–74.
52. Parmeggiani PL. Thermoregulation and sleep. Front Biosci. 2003;8:s557–67.
53. Krauchi K, Deboer T. The interrelationship between sleep regulation and thermoregulation. Front Biosci (Landmark Ed). 2010;15:604–25.
54. Krauchi K, Deboer T. Body temperature, sleep, and hibernation. In: Kryger MH, Roth T, Dement WC, editors. Principles and practice of sleep medicine. 6th ed. Philadelphia: Elsevier; 2017. p. 220–8.
55. Katayose Y, Tasaki M, Ogata H, Nakata Y, Tokuyama K, Satoh M. Metabolic rate and fuel utilization during sleep assessed by whole-body indirect calorimetry. Metabolism. 2009;58(7):920–6.
56. Krauchi K, Cajochen C, Pache M, Flammer J, Wirz-Justice A. Thermoregulatory effects of melatonin in relation to sleepiness. Chronobiol Int. 2006;23(1–2):475–84.
57. Raymann RJ, Swaab DF, Van Someren EJ. Skin temperature and sleep-onset latency: changes with age and insomnia. Physiol Behav. 2007;90(2–3):257–66.
58. Harding EC, Yu X, Miao A, Andrews N, Ma Y, Ye Z, et al. A neuronal hub binding sleep initiation and body cooling in response to a warm external stimulus. Curr Biol. 2018;28(14):2263–73. e4
59. Kroeger D, Absi G, Gagliardi C, Bandaru SS, Madara JC, Ferrari LL, et al. Galanin neurons in the ventrolateral preoptic area promote sleep and heat loss in mice. Nat Commun. 2018;9(1):4129.
60. Hammel HT, Hardy JD, Fusco MM. Thermoregulatory responses to hypothalamic cooling in unanesthetized dogs. Am J Phys. 1960;198:481–6.
61. Satinoff E. Behavioral thermoregulation in response to local cooling of the rat brain. Am J Phys. 1964;206:1389–94.
62. Baldwin BA, Ingram DL. Effect of heating & cooling the hypothalamus on behavioral thermoregulation in the pig. J Physiol. 1967;191(2):375–92.
63. Gale CC, Mathews M, Young J. Behavioral thermoregulatory responses to hypothalamic cooling and warming in baboons. Physiol Behav. 1970;5(1):1–6.
64. Carlisle HJ, Ingram DL. The effects of heating and cooling the spinal cord and hypothalamus on thermoregulatory behaviour in the pig. J Physiol. 1973;231(2):353–64.
65. Glotzbach SF, Heller HC. Central nervous regulation of body temperature during sleep. Science. 1976;194(4264):537–9.
66. Roberts WW, Bergquist EH, Robinson TC. Thermoregulatory grooming and sleep-like relaxation induced by local warming of preoptic area and anterior hypothalamus in opossum. J Comp Physiol Psychol. 1969;67(2):182–8.
67. Parmeggiani PL, Zamboni G, Cianci T, Calasso M. Absence of thermoregulatory vasomotor responses during fast wave sleep in cats. Electroencephalogr Clin Neurophysiol. 1977;42(3):372–80.
68. Amici R, Bastianini S, Berteotti C, Cerri M, Del Vecchio F, Lo Martire V, et al. Sleep and bodily functions: the physiological interplay between body homeostasis and sleep homeostasis. Arch Ital Biol. 2014;152(2–3):66–78.
69. Franzini C, Cianci T, Lenzi P, Guidalotti PL. Neural control of vasomotion in rabbit ear is impaired during desynchronized sleep. Am J Phys. 1982;243(1):R142–6.
70. Palca JW, Walker JM, Berger RJ. Thermoregulation, metabolism, and stages of sleep in cold-exposed men. J Appl Physiol (1985). 1986;61(3):940–7.
71. Alfoldi P, Rubicsek G, Cserni G, Obal F Jr. Brain and core temperatures and peripheral vasomotion during sleep and wakefulness at various ambient temperatures in the rat. Pflugers Arch. 1990;417(3):336–41.
72. Parmeggiani PL, Rabini C. Shivering and panting during sleep. Brain Res. 1967;6(4):789–91.
73. Hendricks JC. Absence of shivering in the cat during paradoxical sleep without atonia. Exp Neurol. 1982;75(3):700–10.
74. Dewasmes G, Bothorel B, Candas V, Libert JP. A short-term poikilothermic period occurs just after paradoxical sleep onset in humans: characterization changes in sweating effector activity. J Sleep Res. 1997;6(4):252–8.
75. Tupone D, Cano G, Morrison SF. Thermoregulatory inversion: a novel thermoregulatory paradigm. Am J Physiol Regul Integr Comp Physiol. 2017;312(5):R779–86.
76. Martelli D, Luppi M, Cerri M, Tupone D, Mastrotto M, Perez E, et al. The direct cooling of the preoptic-hypothalamic area elicits the release of thyroid stimulating hormone during wakefulness but not during REM sleep. PLoS One. 2014;9(2):e87793.
77. Parmeggiani PL, Franzini C, Lenzi P, Zamboni G. Threshold of respiratory responses to preoptic heating during sleep in freely moving cats. Brain Res. 1973;52:189–201.
78. Glotzbach SF, Heller HC. Changes in the thermal characteristics of hypothalamic neurons during sleep and wakefulness. Brain Res. 1984;309(1):17–26.
79. Parmeggiani PL, Cevolani D, Azzaroni A, Ferrari G. Thermosensitivity of anterior hypothalamic-preoptic neurons during the waking-sleeping cycle: a study in brain functional states. Brain Res. 1987;415(1):79–89.
80. Alam MN, McGinty D, Szymusiak R. Preoptic/anterior hypothalamic neurons: thermosensitivity in rapid eye movement sleep. Am J Phys. 1995;269(5 Pt 2):R1250–7.
81. Parmeggiani PL, Franzini C, Lenzi P, Cianci T. Inguinal subcutaneous temperature changes in cats sleeping at different environmental temperatures. Brain Res. 1971;33(2):397–404.
82. Parmeggiani PL, Rabini C. Sleep and environmental temperature. Arch Ital Biol. 1970;108(2):369–87.
83. Haskell EH, Palca JW, Walker JM, Berger RJ, Heller HC. The effects of high and low ambient temperatures on human sleep stages. Electroencephalogr Clin Neurophysiol. 1981;51(5):494–501.
84. Cerri M, Ocampo-Garces A, Amici R, Baracchi F, Capitani P, Jones CA, et al. Cold exposure and sleep in the rat: effects on sleep architecture and the electroencephalogram. Sleep. 2005;28(6):694–705.
85. Sichieri R, Schmidek WR. Influence of ambient temperature on the sleep-wakefulness cycle in the golden hamster. Physiol Behav. 1984;33(6):871–7.
86. Cerri M, Morrison SF. Activation of lateral hypothalamic neurons stimulates brown adipose tissue thermogenesis. Neuroscience. 2005;135(2):627–38.
87. Kaushik MK, Kumar VM, Mallick HN. Hypothalamic temperature: a key regulator in homeostatic restoration of sleep during chronic cold exposure in rats. Indian J Physiol Pharmacol. 2012;56(4):301–13.
88. Blessing W, Mohammed M, Ootsuka Y. Brown adipose tissue thermogenesis, the basic rest-activity cycle, meal initiation, and bodily homeostasis in rats. Physiol Behav. 2013;121:61–9.
89. Luppi M, Martelli D, Amici R, Baracchi F, Cerri M, Dentico D, et al. Hypothalamic osmoregulation is maintained across the wake-sleep cycle in the rat. J Sleep Res. 2010;19(3):394–9.
90. Martelli D, Luppi M, Cerri M, Tupone D, Perez E, Zamboni G, et al. Waking and sleeping following water deprivation in the rat. PLoS One. 2012;7(9):e46116. Epub 2012/10/03
91. Lee KJ. REM and NREM sleep as natural accompaniments of the evolution of warm-bloodedness. Neurosci Biobehav Rev. 2002;26(8):889–906.
92. Cerri M, Luppi M, Tupone D, Zamboni G, Amici R. REM sleep and endothermy: potential sites and mechanism of a reciprocal interference. Front Physiol. 2017;8:624.

6 Brain–Heart Interaction: Cardiovascular Reflexes

Alessandro Silvani

Introduction

This chapter aims to provide readers with a succinct and updated overview of whether and how sleep entails changes in the properties of the arterial baroreceptor reflex (ABR), the cardiovascular reflex that is known to have a major impact on cardiovascular control during wakefulness. This question essentially addresses the nature and extent of the modulation of the ABR by central autonomic circuits, which is a core aspect of brain–heart interactions. Accordingly, sleep critically involves changes in brain activity, being, as it has been suggested [1], "of the brain, by the brain, and for the brain." This is not to disregard the long standing assumption that sleep is a phenomenon of the integral organism [2]. Sleep results in changes in body posture and a reduction in physical activity, both of which have deep impact on the cardiovascular system.

The discussion in this chapter shall focus on the ABR, which is arguably the most important and most amply studied cardiovascular reflex. For the sake of conciseness and clarity, this chapter shall not deal with other autonomic cardiovascular reflexes, whose involvement during sleep is still much less understood; these other reflexes include the cardiopulmonary baroreceptor reflex, the exercise pressor reflex, and the autonomic cardiovascular reflexes elicited by the arterial chemoreceptor afferents and by slowly adapting pulmonary receptors. Moreover, the chapter shall focus on data on healthy human subjects in physiological conditions, but evidence on experimental animal models shall also be discussed for greater mechanistic and causal insight.

A. Silvani (✉)
Department of Biomedical and Neuromotor Sciences (DIBINEM), University of Bologna, Bologna, Italy
e-mail: alessandro.silvani3@unibo.it

Sleep and Cardiovascular Control: A Matter of Time Scales

The Time Scale of Minutes: Sleep Macrostructure

Sleep is a widely heterogeneous behavior. Sleep in human subjects is classified with a time resolution of 30 s as stages N1, N2, N3, and R [3]. Collectively, the stages N1–N3 correspond to non-rapid-eye-movement (NREM) sleep in human subjects. The stages N2 and N3 translate to NREM sleep in experimental models, such as laboratory rodents. The stage R sleep corresponds to REM sleep both in human subjects and experimental mammalian models. With the 30-s time resolution of standard scoring, the alternation of episodes of wakefulness, NREM sleep, and REM sleep occurs at a time scale of minutes and may be referred to as sleep macrostructure.

Different aspects of the physiological cardiovascular changes associated with sleep macrostructure have been reviewed in recent years [4–8], and the interested reader is referred to these publications for full detail. In summary, compared to wakefulness, NREM sleep entails decreases in the mean values of arterial blood pressure, heart rate, and sympathetic nerve activity to the skeletal muscle, kidney, and skin of the extremities (hands/feet in humans, tail in rodents), which most likely targets the blood vessels of these tissues. During REM sleep, arterial blood pressure, heart rate, and sympathetic nerve activity to the skeletal muscles return to at or above their respective levels during wakefulness, whereas sympathetic nerve activity to the kidneys and the intestine decreases further below the level attained during NREM sleep. Recent evidence indicates that at least in mice, the modulation of sympathetic nerve activity to blood vessels is the critical mechanism for the occurrence of sleep-related changes in arterial blood pressure at the time scale of sleep macrostructure [9].

S. Chokroverty, P. Cortelli (eds.), *Autonomic Nervous System and Sleep*, https://doi.org/10.1007/978-3-030-62263-3_6

The Time Scale of Seconds: Sleep Microstructure

As remarked above, sleep is conventionally scored with a time resolution of 30 s [3]. Nonetheless, sleep is characterized by a well-known heterogeneity at a shorter time scale of few seconds. This heterogeneity is associated with a range of events including arousals, body movements, and apneas, which collectively constitute the so-called microstructure of sleep [4, 10]. In particular, a prominent cardiovascular variability has long been known to be associated with REM sleep at a time scale of seconds [11]. Arousals may occur during NREM sleep and REM sleep, causing concomitant increases in arterial blood pressure and heart rate in human subjects [12, 13]. The magnitude of the cardiovascular changes associated with arousals is similar in NREM sleep and REM sleep [14, 15]. Among the different types of arousal, phases of transitory activation including movements entail larger peak increases in heart rate than delta-bursts, kappa-bursts, and microarousals, which also show a later heart rate decrease [14]. The concomitance of increases in arterial blood pressure and heart rate also characterizes periodic leg movements during sleep (PLMS) in human subjects, at least during NREM sleep [16–19]. The association between PLMS and microarousals results in larger peak increases in arterial blood pressure and heart rate, and suppresses the delayed decrease in heart rate, which follows the heart rate peak in PLMS without microarousals [16, 18].

The available data thus point to a stereotyped sequence of cardiovascular events associated with arousals and PLMS: first, arterial blood pressure and heart rate increase; then, arterial blood pressure reaches a peak; then, heart rate returns to at or below baseline level; finally, arterial blood pressure also returns to baseline level [7]. The fundamental nature of this cardiovascular pattern is supported by its occurrence in temporal association with spontaneous increases in arterial blood pressure in wakefulness, NREM sleep, and REM sleep, regardless of the accompanying neurophysiological features, such as arousals or PLMS, in species as diverse as human subjects [20], rats [21, 22], mice [23–27], and sheep [28]. Notably, the magnitude of the peak increase in arterial blood pressure associated with arousals [13] and PLMS [16, 18] in human subjects is approximately 20 mm Hg, which is close to the modal decrease in arterial blood pressure from daytime wakefulness to nighttime sleep in human subjects [29]. Thus, the peak increase in arterial blood pressure associated with arousals and PLMS in human subjects essentially nullifies the physiological decrease in arterial blood pressure from wakefulness to NREM sleep.

Marked changes in arterial blood pressure and heart rate also characterize obstructive apneas during sleep in human subjects [30]. Airway obstruction entails relatively low values of heart rate and high values of sympathetic nerve activity to skeletal muscle blood vessels. Upon resumption of breathing, particularly in the case of arousal, sympathetic nerve activity to skeletal muscles shows a further transient increase, followed by a long-lasting suppression. At the same time, arterial blood pressure and heart rate undergo a transient dramatic rise [30]. Central sleep apneas may also be associated with increases in sympathetic nerve activity to skeletal muscles [31] and with increases in arterial blood pressure and heart rate, at least in children and in association with body movements during sleep [32].

The Time Scale of Hours: Circadian Sleep Rhythm

Sleep has a distinct 24-h distribution determined by a circadian rhythm, which is generally entrained to the daily light–dark cycle and is driven by a master body clock in the hypothalamic suprachiasmatic nuclei (SCN) [33]. The circadian control of sleep is effective on NREM sleep and on REM sleep, contributing to increasing the propensity to REM sleep at the end of the subjective rest period [34, 35].

Circadian rhythms of arterial blood pressure and heart rate, with peak values at a circadian time corresponding to the subjective activity period, have been demonstrated in human subjects even in the absence of sleep and other potential confounding factors [36], that is, under the so-called unmasking conditions [37]. Nonetheless, the amplitudes of the circadian rhythms of arterial blood pressure and heart rate under unmasking conditions in the absence of sleep appear small compared to those of the corresponding rhythms measured in usual living conditions that include sleep [29, 38]. The difference is particularly striking for arterial blood pressure, whose circadian rhythm under unmasking conditions has a peak–trough difference of 4–6 mm Hg [36], whereas the modal day–night arterial blood pressure difference in normal sleep conditions is approximately 20 mm Hg [29].

These results are consistent with the hypothesis that the circadian rhythm of arterial blood pressure and heart rate enhances the decreases in these variables during nighttime sleep compared to daytime wakefulness. Accordingly, circadian misalignment with mismatched behavioral and environmental cycles for three days significantly blunts the fall in arterial blood pressure and heart rate during daily sleep opportunities [39]. This conclusion is also supported by data on mice, which demonstrate the occurrence of circadian rhythms of arterial blood pressure during wakefulness, NREM sleep, and REM sleep [40]. The amplitude of the circadian rhythm of arterial blood pressure computed by averaging values during time periods when the mouse is spontaneously awake is significantly lower than the amplitude of the overall arterial blood pressure rhythm, computed by averaging over time regardless of the wake-sleep state. The same conclusion holds for the amplitude of the circadian rhythm of arterial blood pressure computed by averaging values during all time periods when the mouse is spontaneously sleeping in either NREM sleep or REM sleep. This overall arterial blood pressure rhythm in mice peaks during the subjective period of higher activity, similarly to what occurs in humans [40].

The Role of the ABR in the Hierarchic Organization of Cardiovascular Control

The ABR and Other Cardiovascular Reflexes Constitute the Intermediate Level of Cardiovascular Control

The ABR is triggered by the activity of mechanosensitive afferent neural fibers in the walls of the aortic arch and the carotid sinuses. These vessels are strategically located at the gates of the systemic and cerebral circulations. The relative contribution of carotid and aortic baroreceptor afferents to ABR functioning is still a matter of debate [41]. Nevertheless, bilateral denervation even of the sole carotid sinuses, as a consequence of carotid body tumor resection, is sufficient to prevent compensation of the hemodynamic consequences of upright posture, and leads to transient orthostatic hypotension even one year after denervation in human subjects [42]. This lack of redundancy demonstrates that the ABR is the most important of a set of neural and endocrine reflex mechanisms that allow for system-level integrated control of the cardiovascular system.

In response to decreases in aortic and carotid baroreceptor firing, the ABR increases heart rate and contractility and systemic vascular resistance. Increases in baroreceptor firing elicit the opposing effects [43]. The ABR control of the heart involves opposing changes in cardiac parasympathetic and sympathetic nerve activity [44], whereas that of vascular resistance involves the mesenteric, renal, skin, and particularly the skeletal muscle vascular beds [43, 45]. There is also evidence that decreases in arterial baroreceptor firing increase the secretion of arginine vasopressin [46] and renin, the latter by increasing sympathetic nerve activity to the kidney [46, 47]. The control of vascular resistance is the main mechanism by which the ABR controls arterial blood pressure at rest, and is thought to be the sole mechanism at stake during physical exercise [48]. Nevertheless, each of the neural and endocrine changes elicited by the ABR is directionally consistent with offsetting the change in baroreceptor firing that triggered the reflex. The ABR can thus be envisaged as a delayed closed-loop negative feedback control mechanism. The ABR tends to maintain the stretch of baroreceptor afferent fibers constant, with delays and time constants that depend on cardiac and vascular effector responses, on neural transmission, and on central integration. As the arterial baroreceptor stretch substantially depends on arterial blood pressure by Laplace's law, the ABR acts as a powerful mechanism that controls arterial blood pressure.

The ABR properties at steady state can be quantified with sigmoidal logistic functions of the form:

$$Y = A_1 / \{1 / \exp[A_2 (X - A_3)]\} + A_4$$

where X is the independent variable that indexes ABR input, such as arterial blood pressure within the carotid sinus; Y is the output variable controlled by the ABR, namely arterial blood pressure, or one of the instrumental output variables of the ABR, such as heart rate or sympathetic nerve activity to a specific vascular bed. The parameter A_1 indicates the responding range, which corresponds to the maximum to minimum change in Y. The operating range is, instead, the difference between the values of X at the threshold and saturation of the ABR. At rest, the operating point (the prestimulus value of X) and the centering point (the value of parameter A_3) are positioned together. The parameter A_2 is the gain coefficient. The maximal ABR gain or sensitivity is calculated as the gain value at A_3. Finally, the parameter A_4 indicates the minimum value of Y [43, 49].

The ABR Modulates Tissue-Specific Local Mechanisms That Constitute the Lowest Level of Cardiovascular Control

The local control of capillary blood flow by arteriolar resistance mainly consists of blood flow autoregulation, flow-metabolism coupling, and the local vascular effects of O_2 and CO_2. The local control of the heart mainly consists of the dependency of cardiac performance on cardiac filling, known as the Frank–Starling law of the heart. All these local mechanisms do not require long-range neural or endocrine transmission, and for this reason they can afford but a piecemeal control of the cardiovascular system. The ABR may modulate cardiac performance by affecting contractility, and may modulate blood flow regulation in the mesenteric, renal, skin, and skeletal muscle vascular beds by affecting vascular resistance.

In essence, blood flow autoregulation refers to the relative constancy of capillary blood flow despite changes in arterial blood pressure, as long as these changes are not excessively large [50]. For blood flow to remain relatively constant in the face of changes in arterial blood pressure, arteriolar vascular resistance needs to vary in the same direction as arterial blood pressure, so that arterioles constrict when arterial blood pressure increases and dilate when arterial blood pressure decreases. By Laplace's law, this implies the relative constancy of arteriolar wall stress, defined as the product of transmural pressure and vessel radius divided by vessel wall thickness [51]. These changes in arteriolar smooth muscle activity are the end result of myogenic and metabolic mechanisms, which add up with the effects of shear-stress and vascular compliance [50]. Myogenic mechanisms transduce changes in arteriolar wall stress into changes in the plasma membrane potential of arteriolar smooth muscle cells, whereas metabolic mechanisms involve paracrine signals that modulate vascular smooth muscle tone based on the mismatch between capillary blood flow and tissue metabolic rate. The nature of these signals is still the subject of debate. Supply-consumption mismatch signals as well as feed-forward signals directly associated with the rate of energy metabolism are thought to play a role [51]. These signals also mediate the correlation (flow-metabolism coupling) between local capillary blood flow and tissue energy metabolism, which is particularly strong in the cerebral [52] and the coronary [51] circulations. Hypoxia and hypercapnia are vasodilator stimuli for these circulations and in general for systemic vascular beds, with hypercapnia acting through changes in interstitial pH [51, 53]. The vascular effects of O_2 and, possibly, also those of CO_2 on systemic vascular beds thus bridge flow-metabolism coupling, when they result from mismatches between blood supply and energy needs, with the hemodynamic consequences of breathing alterations, such as respiratory insufficiency, apneas, and hypobaric hypoxia. Conversely, the pulmonary vascular reactivity to O_2 and CO_2 levels in the alveoli is in the opposing direction (i.e., with local hypoxia and hypercapnia eliciting vasoconstriction), which significantly contributes to ventilation–perfusion matching in the healthy human lung [54].

Local mechanisms also increase the systolic performance of cardiac ventricles in response to increases in preload and afterload. This is achieved by sarcomere length-induced changes in cardiac contractile protein responsiveness to activating calcium ions, which require the giant protein titin [55]. In general, the ventricular end-systolic pressure and volume depend on the combination of preload, afterload, and contractility [56]. This last term refers to the maximum ventricular systolic pressure attained at a given set of values of preload, afterload, and heart rate. In conditions of relatively low preload and high afterload, contractility is essentially the only determinant of the ventricular end-systolic pressure–volume relationship [56]. This implies that for a given level of contractility, stroke volume is essentially proportional to diastolic filling, and can be maintained in the face of increased aortic blood pressure simply by increasing diastolic filling [57].

Central Autonomic Commands Represent the Highest Level of Cardiovascular Control and Modulate the ABR

One limitation of the ABR is that it does not prevent perturbations in arterial blood pressure. These perturbations are needed to trigger the ABR and are not resolved instantaneously by the ABR once they occur. Another limitation of the ABR is that it is unable, in and by itself, to modify the arterial blood pressure baseline value to match the requirements associated with different behaviors. The main mechanism that overcomes these limitations of the ABR is represented by central autonomic commands, which are proactive open-loop mechanisms that control the cardiovascular system in anticipation of behavior.

Central autonomic commands are perhaps the least known of the cardiovascular control mechanisms [58]. The concept of central autonomic commands is linked to that of central motor patterns, which has long been employed to investigate the neural circuits that underlie locomotion [59]. Motor patterns are produced by hierarchical networks of interneurons called central pattern generators [60]. Central pattern controllers set the endogenous probability of manifestation of the motor patterns by controlling top-level pattern generators or pattern initiators [61].

The original concept of central motor pattern, which involved only somatic motor neurons targeting skeletal muscles, may be generalized to autonomic [62] and mixed autonomic and somatic motor patterns. This generalization fits well with the standard use of the central autonomic command construct, which refers to the cardiovascular correlates of physical exercise that cannot be explained by either reflex or local control mechanisms [63]. The central autonomic commands are thought to increase arterial blood pressure at the onset and at the steady state of exercise, at least in part by increasing sympathetic nerve activity to skeletal muscles and skin. The central autonomic commands of physical exercise also increase heart rate, due to parasympathetic withdrawal and possibly also to sympathetic activation [64–66]. These effects of the central autonomic commands help prevent hypotension due to local vasodilation associated with flow-metabolism coupling in exercising skeletal muscles.

The ABR During Sleep

Insights from the Relationship Between Controlled and Instrumental Variables of the ABR During Sleep at Different Time Scales

The relative contribution of the control of heart rate versus vascular resistance to the ABR control of arterial blood pressure is unclear during NREM sleep and REM sleep. As mentioned in the section "The ABR and Other Cardiovascular Reflexes Constitute the Intermediate Level of Cardiovascular Control," the ABR control of arterial blood pressure depends more on the control of vascular resistance than on that of heart rate during restful wakefulness [48]. It may be fair to assume as a working hypothesis that a similar conclusion holds during sleep.

The ABR control of heart rate may thus be largely redundant with the control of vascular resistance during sleep. Nevertheless, the study of the changes in heart rate as a function of those in arterial blood pressure during sleep may be of great value as a telltale sign of ABR function. As previously remarked, the ABR decreases heart rate in response to an increase in arterial blood pressure [43]. Heart rate can be measured noninvasively, unobtrusively, and relatively cheaply by electrocardiography. The parasympathetic control of heart rate is fast [44], being generally observed in one cardiac beat. The latency of the earliest cardiac ABR response is thus shorter than 1 s [67]. Taken together, these considerations indicate that changes in arterial blood pressure and heart rate which occur in the same direction are either unrelated to the ABR or driven by a change in ABR properties. While this argument also holds concerning the directional correspondence between changes in arterial blood pressure and sympathetic nerve activity, the availability of sympathetic nerve activity recordings during sleep is very limited due to the invasiveness of microneurography. As detailed above, sleep is associated with changes in arterial blood pressure and heart rate in the same direction at the time scales of minutes (sleep macrostructure), seconds (sleep microstructure), and hours (circadian sleep rhythms). At the time scale of sleep macrostructure, there is also evidence that NREM sleep is associated with changes in arterial blood pressure in the same direction as those in sympathetic nerve activity to skeletal muscles [68] and kidneys [69] compared to wakefulness.

The relationship between changes in arterial blood pressure and those in heart rate can be quantified mathematically by a range of techniques including linear cross-correlation functions (CCF). This approach has been mostly applied during sleep at the microstructural time scale, investigating the relationship between systolic arterial blood pressure and heart period, which is the reciprocal of heart rate. There is evidence that heart period varies linearly with the frequency of cardiac sympathetic and parasympathetic nerve activity, whereas this is not the case for heart rate [70]. The CCF between arterial blood pressure and heart period yields the linear correlation coefficient between these variables as a function of their time shift. The sign of the correlation coefficient indicates the direction of the linear relationship between the variables, which may be direct (e.g., increases in arterial blood pressure associated with increases in heart period) or inverse (e.g., increases in arterial blood pressure associated with decreases in heart period). The absolute value of the correlation coefficient indicates the strength of the linear relationship between arterial blood pressure and heart period and is bounded between 0 (i.e., no linear relationship) and 1 (i.e., perfect linear relationship).

Being a delayed negative feedback control, the ABR is expected to lengthen heart period after an increase in arterial blood pressure, thereby causing a positive correlation between heart period and the previous values of arterial blood pressure. This CCF pattern shall hereafter be called CCF pattern I for ease of reference. Experimental work on spontaneous cardiovascular fluctuations at the time scale of seconds (sleep microstructure) has demonstrated that CCF pattern I is stronger during NREM sleep than either during quiet wakefulness or during REM sleep in species as diverse as sheep [28], rats [22, 71], and mice [23–27]. Conversely, a different CCF pattern of negative correlation between arterial blood pressure and heart period, which shall hereafter be called CCF pattern II for simplicity, was found to prevail during REM sleep in rats [22, 71] and in mice, albeit only at thermoneutrality in this latter species [23–27]. In humans, CCF pattern II prevails during wakefulness in the lying position, whereas CCF pattern I prevails during sitting, NREM sleep, and standing, and is the strongest in the latter posture [20, 72, 73].

Sleep Modifies the Integration Between the ABR and Central Autonomic Commands at Different Time Scales

The occurrence of changes in arterial blood pressure in the same direction as those in heart rate or sympathetic nerve activity cannot be explained based on the local mechanisms of cardiovascular regulation, which, as detailed above, do not involve these variables. As discussed previously, these changes cannot be readily attributed to the ABR, either, at least under the assumption that the ABR properties remain constant. An explanation may be represented by hemodynamic mechanisms, whereby increases in heart rate or sympathetic nerve activity raise arterial blood pressure by increasing cardiac output or vascular resistance, respectively. However, this explanation would leave unexplained the regulatory mechanisms underlying the increases in heart rate and sympathetic nerve activity in the first place.

I have previously proposed that the construct of central autonomic commands is apt to also describe the open-loop proactive control of the cardiovascular system associated with sleep at different time scales [4, 6, 7]. The mechanisms of anticipatory autonomic regulation that manifest as circadian rhythms, those that characterize the macrostructure of each wake–sleep state, and those that are associated with arousals and other transient sleep events, may all be qualified as central autonomic commands. Together, these mechanisms may contribute to matching cardiovascular system activity to a continuum of somatic motor activity at multiple time scales. The traditional concept of central autonomic commands associated with physical exercise during wakefulness would then lie at one of the extremes of this continuum at the time scale of minutes.

At least for what concerns the time scale of sleep microstructure, this hypothesis is quantitatively coherent with the available evidence, as demonstrated with mathematical modeling of the cardiovascular system [74]. A simple linear summation of central autonomic commands and ABR on parasympathetic and sympathetic nerve activity to the heart proved sufficient to simulate the biphasic sequential increases/decreases in heart rate which characterize transient sleep events such as microarousals and PLMS [74]. This suggests that central autonomic commands may transiently override the ABR control at the onset of microarousals or PLMS. The central autonomic commands would then fade away, but the return of arterial blood pressure to baseline levels would lag behind due to the relative sluggishness of arterial blood pressure response to sympathetic nerve activity [75]. The ABR response to elevated arterial blood pressure, consisting of reduced heart rate, would then manifest. In this scenario, longer-lasting central autonomic commands may mask the decrease in heart rate driven by the ABR, potentially explaining its lack after phases of transitory activation or PLMS associated with microarousals (cf. The Time Scale of Seconds: Sleep Microstructure).

Mathematical modeling also suggested that a simple summation of the effects of central autonomic commands and ABR on the heart may explain the peculiar features of the coupling between spontaneous fluctuations in arterial blood pressure and heart period [74], which have been uncovered with CCF analyses during sleep. Simulations indicated that CCF pattern I (cf. "The ABR During Sleep") ensues as a result of ABR buffering of the arterial blood pressure fluctuations generated by changes in vascular resistance irrespective of their cause. Conversely, CCF pattern II requires central autonomic commands to the heart. Thus, the prevalence of CCF pattern I versus II depends on the balance between the cardiac ABR response to changes in arterial blood pressure caused by changes in vascular resistance, on one hand, and the central autonomic commands to the heart, on the other hand. In this light, the empirical results presented in "The ABR During Sleep" indicate that NREM sleep entails a prevalence of ABR control of the heart over central autonomic commands, which is strikingly robust across species. The ABR contribution to cardiac control decreases from NREM sleep to REM sleep in all species studied and may become negligible in rodents. This interpretation agrees with the conclusions obtained with a linear model of the ABR applied to the empirical data obtained during sleep in rats [76]. The ABR contribution to cardiac control also decreases from NREM sleep to quiet wakefulness in the lying position in all species studied. Recent evidence indicates that the enhanced ABR coupling between arterial blood pressure and heart period in humans in the upright position is not triggered by decreased central venous pressure, but rather reflects buffering of enhanced fluctuations of vascular resistance [72]. Conversely, the enhancement of CCF pattern I during NREM sleep compared to wakefulness in the supine position is accompanied by a significant decrease in the low-frequency variability of arterial blood pressure. The occurrence of enhanced CCF pattern I in subjects lying supine during NREM sleep compared to wakefulness may, therefore, be related to weaker central autonomic commands to the heart associated with the lack of active engagement with the external environment [72].

Central Autonomic Commands Change ABR Properties During Sleep

Another hypothesis to explain the observed relationship between arterial blood pressure and heart period during sleep at different time scales is that central autonomic commands act on the cardiovascular system indirectly by modulating ABR properties. One possibility to differentiate direct cardiovascular effects of central autonomic commands during sleep from effects mediated by changes in ABR properties would be to analyze sleep-related cardiovascular changes after an experimental surgical lesion of the arterial baroreceptors. Unfortunately, as previously reviewed [4], the experiments that performed sinoaortic denervation in animal models [77–80] did not yield consistent results on sleep-related cardiovascular control at the time scale of sleep macrostructure; these findings are possibly due to the arterial blood pressure instability after denervation and to the confounding effects of the concomitant deafferentation of the arterial chemoreceptors. The development of more refined surgical techniques for selective baroreceptor and chemoreceptor denervation may open the way to clarification of this issue [81]. Information is also missing on whether modulation of the ABR by central autonomic commands is necessary for the occurrence of sleep-related cardiovascular changes at the sleep microstructure time scale. On the other hand, limited available evidence obtained with sinoaortic denervation in rats suggests that the sleep-related changes in arterial blood pressure at the circadian time scale require modulation of ABR properties, whereas those in heart rate do not [82]. The sleep-related changes in heart rate at the circadian time scale may therefore result from central autonomic commands that do not modulate the ABR. To summarize, the central autonomic commands during sleep may act on the cardiovascular system at different time scales both directly, without changing ABR properties, and indirectly, by modulating ABR properties.

A resetting of the ABR by central autonomic commands has long been recognized to occur during physical exercise. With reference to the ABR sigmoid function curves mentioned in the section "The ABR and Other Cardiovascular Reflexes Constitute the Intermediate Level of Cardiovascular Control", this resetting essentially involves an upward shift of the curves along the *Y* variable axis, where *Y* correspons to the output variable controlled by the ABR, and a rightward shift to higher operating values of *X*, where *X* is the independent variable that indexes ABR input, such as arterial blood pressure within the carotid sinus. For what concerns heart rate as the *Y* variable, the rightward shift of the ABR sigmoid functions exceeds that of the operating point, which corresponds to the pre-stimulus value of X. As a result, the operating point shifts leftward away from the centering point, ie, from the the value of parameter A_3 of the baroreflex sigmoidal logistic function, and closer to the ABR threshold, to a location of reduced gain, whereas the ABR gain around the centering point varies little [49]. The decreased gain of the ABR control of heart rate around the operating point is associated with decreased ABR gain as assessed with the analysis of spontaneous cardiovascular fluctuations, and reflects exercise intensity-related decreases in cardiac parasympathetic tone and modulation [49, 64].

The available evidence on shifts of ABR sigmoid function curves associated with sleep is restricted to the sleep macrostructure time scale in rat models, likely due to the prohibitive technical difficulties involved in these experiments. The sigmoid functions relating arterial blood pressure to ABR-driven changes in heart rate and renal sympathetic nerve activity during NREM sleep in rats were found shifted downward and leftward compared to those during grooming, a form of spontaneously active wakefulness [83]. For what concerns the ABR control of heart rate, NREM sleep entailed a significant increase in parameter A_1 and significant decreases in parameters A_2, A_3, and A_4 (cf. section above), indicating significant decreases in maximum heart rate response, arterial blood pressure threshold, and gain at the centering point, and a significant increase in the ABR operating range. Significant decreases in parameters A_3 and A_4 also occurred during NREM sleep compared to grooming for the ABR control of renal sympathetic nerve activity, indicating significant decreases in maximum sympathetic nerve activity response, arterial blood pressure threshold, and arterial blood pressure saturation. During REM sleep, the sigmoid function corresponding to the ABR control of heart rate was virtually superimposed to that during NREM sleep. The sigmoid function corresponding to the ABR control of sympathetic nerve activity during REM sleep had significantly lower values of parameter A_1 compared to NREM sleep, corresponding to a significantly lower maximum response. Finally, the operating point was located to the left of the centering point for heart rate control during grooming, NREM sleep, and REM sleep. Conversely, the ABR operating point was located near the centering point of the curve for the ABR control of sympathetic nerve activity during grooming and NREM sleep, and was shifted rightward of the centering point during REM sleep [83].

These detailed findings on rats [83] would predict the lack of substantial differences in the ABR gain computed with the analysis of spontaneous cardiovascular fluctuations during either NREM sleep or REM sleep compared to wakefulness. Accordingly, a review of the evidence on human subjects and animal models published before 2008 concluded that the reported effects of sleep on the gain of the ABR control of heart rate and sympathetic nerve activity were inconsistent and/or insubstantial [4]. This conclusion essentially still holds also for more recent studies that explicitly analyzed differences in the gain of the ABR control of heart rate between wake–sleep states. In particular, one study published in 2008 employing the sequence technique on healthy adult human subjects reported no significant differences in the ABR gain between either NREM sleep or REM sleep and quiet wakefulness [73]. Another study published in 2009 with the sequence technique on normotensive adults reported increases in ABR gain during sleep compared to wakefulness [84]. However, the significance of these changes depended on sleep macrostructural and circadian factors (first vs. last sleep episodes during the night, wakefulness pre-sleep vs. post-sleep) and on the direction of the triggering changes in arterial blood pressure [84]. A study on human infants published in 2011 employing spectral analysis and the sequence technique reported that the ABR gain was higher in quiet sleep than in active sleep in infants aged five to six months sleeping in the supine position, whereas this was not the case for infants of that age sleeping in the prone position, nor for younger infants aged two weeks to three months [85]. Concerning experimental animal models, a study published in 2012 employing the sequence technique on wild-type mice reported a higher ABR gain during NREM sleep than either during quiet wakefulness or REM sleep [25]. A study published in 2010 employing the sequence technique on wild-type rats found increased ABR gain during sleep compared to wakefulness, but the significance of the differences was limited to REM sleep and to decreases in arterial blood pressure as ABR triggers [86].

The Functional Neuroanatomy of the ABR and Central Autonomic Commands in Different Wake–Sleep States

Functional Neuroanatomy of the ABR and Central Autonomic Commands During Wakefulness

The ABR control of parasympathetic nerve activity to the heart involves excitatory projections from sinoaortic baroreceptor afferents to the nucleus of the solitary tract (NTS) in the medulla, and from the NTS to parasympathetic preganglionic neurons in the nucleus ambiguus of the medulla [44]. On the other hand, the ABR control of sympathetic nerve activity involves an excitatory projection from the NTS to the caudal ventrolateral medulla (CVLM), and an inhibitory projection from the CVLM to neurons in the rostral ventrolateral medulla (RVLM). These pre-sympathetic neurons, which send monosynaptic projections to sympathetic preganglionic neurons in the spinal cord, are mainly adrenergic neurons of the C1 group, and likely constitute different subgroups controlling sympathetic nerve activity to the heart and different vascular beds [44, 87].

The central neural pathways of the central commands associated with physical exercise during wakefulness are still unclear [58]. These are thought to include not only cortical areas, such as the anterior cingulate cortex [88], but also a vast array of other diencephalic and brainstem structures of the central autonomic network [44, 64, 89].

Functional Neuroanatomy of the Direct Cardiovascular Effects of Sleep-Related Central Autonomic Commands

A parsimonious hypothesis for the neural pathways associated with the sleep-related central autonomic commands at the time scale of sleep circadian rhythms is that they originate directly from the master circadian clock in the SCN. The SCN controls separate populations of pre-sympathetic and pre-parasympathetic neurons in the hypothalamic paraventricular nucleus (PVN) [8, 90].

On the other hand, direct experimental evidence demonstrating the neural pathways of central autonomic commands associated with the macro- and microstructural features of NREM sleep is still lacking. Based on the available neuroanatomical and electrophysiological evidence, these pathways may include at least four targets of projections from neurons of the hypothalamic ventrolateral preoptic nucleus (VLPO) that are active during NREM sleep. One of these targets is the median preoptic nucleus (MnPO) of the hypothalamus. The MnPO modulates the thermoregulatory pathways for heat generation and retention, which control sympathetic nerve activity to the skin and critically include the medullary raphe pallidus and dorsomedial nucleus of the hypothalamus. Another VLPO target is the hypothalamic PVN, a master switch of the autonomic and endocrine systems, which may bridge sleep-dependent central autonomic commands at time scales from minutes to hours. The third VLPO target is the pedunculopontine nucleus (PPT) between the caudal midbrain and rostral pons, which is associated with the central locomotor region, and may underlie the continuum between sleep-related and exercise-related central autonomic commands. The fourth VLPO target is the parabrachial nucleus (PBN) of the pons. As detailed below, this pathway may play a key role in the interactions between sleep-related central autonomic commands and the ABR.

The peculiar features of cardiovascular control during REM sleep at the time scale of sleep macrostructure (summarized in "The Time Scale of Minutes: Sleep Macrostructure") suggest that their underlying central autonomic commands operate with an original regulatory modality extraneous to the rest-activity continuum that apparently spans from NREM sleep to physical exercise. Remarkable examples of these peculiarities of REM sleep include the mismatch between a brain metabolic rate similar to that during wakefulness [52, 91] and behavioral inactivity with skeletal muscle atonia [3], and the mismatch between increases in sympathetic nerve activity to skeletal muscles [68] and, probably, to the heart [9], and decreases in sympathetic nerve activity to the kidneys and intestine [4].

A working hypothesis of the central neural pathways underlying central autonomic commands during REM sleep has been formulated based on a review of the available evidence [7]. In particular, the increases in sympathetic nerve activity to skeletal muscle and the heart during REM sleep may result from direct excitatory projections from REM sleep-promoting brain circuits, including the pontine sublaterodorsal nucleus (SLD), to the RVLM, the PPT, and PBN. As it was previously remarked concerning NREM sleep, this last pathway may be key for the modulation of the ABR by central autonomic commands. The disparate changes in sympathetic nerve activity to different vascular beds, such as that of skeletal muscles versus kidney, may reflect modulation of the activity of the medullary raphe obscurus and the ventrolateral and lateral regions of the midbrain periaqueductal gray (PAG) by REM sleep-promoting brain circuits. Both the raphe obscurus and the PAG include neurons that excite and others that inhibit sympathetic nerve activity [7]. The enhanced cardiovascular variability, typical of REM sleep at the time scale of sleep microstructure [4, 11], may result from the activity of the medial and inferior vestibular nuclei of the medulla [7]. These nuclei may receive REM sleep-related inputs from the hypothalamic VLPO and modulate autonomic cardiovascular activity through the same pathways that include the PPT and PBN neurons (see above). This arrangement would explain why the transient cardiovascular activations during REM sleep follow the same stereotyped sequence of changes in arterial blood pressure and heart rate as noted during arousals and body movements during NREM sleep (see The Time Scale of Seconds: Sleep Microstructure).

Functional Neuroanatomy of the Modulation of ABR Properties by the Central Autonomic Commands During Sleep

A testable hypothesis for the neural circuits responsible for modulation of the ABR properties during NREM sleep has been proposed [7]. This hypothesis is based on evidence that neurons within the PBN, including its Koelliker-Fuse (KF) subnucleus, are capable of modulating the ABR, the most prominent effect being inhibition (see "Functional Neuroanatomy of Direct Cardiovascular Effects of Sleep-Related Central Autonomic Commands"). This modulation may be achieved by direct projections from the PBN and KF to the NTS, which is the first relay for baroreceptor afferents. Through this pathway, decreases in PBN activity during NREM sleep, possibly due to inhibition by the VLPO, may disinhibit the ABR at the sleep macrostructure time scale. Conversely, the loss of this VLPO-driven decrease in PBN activity may inhibit the ABR during REM sleep compared to NREM sleep at this time scale. Transient increases in PBN activity during arousals in NREM sleep or during the phasic neurophysiological events of REM sleep (the latter possibly through projections from the medial vestibular nucleus) may also inhibit the ABR transiently at the sleep microstructure time scale. The pathways that mediate the ABR modulation at the circadian time scale are less clear, and might include projections from the SCN to the PVN [90], and, thence, to the NTS [92].

Based on a recent conceptual model of ABR resetting [93], the changes in ABR sigmoid functions observed during sleep in rats [83] suggest that sleep-related central autonomic commands act in parallel on the NTS and on other central autonomic network structures (see section "The Functional Neuroanatomy of the ABR and Central Autonomic Commands in Different Wake–Sleep States"). In particular, the leftward shift of ABR function curves observed during sleep compared to grooming [83] may be driven by decreased inhibitory inputs to second-order barosensitive neurons in the NTS [93]. The decrease in the maximum gain of the ABR control of heart rate observed during sleep compared to grooming [83] may be due to a decrease in facilitatory inputs to CVLM neurons that indirectly control sympathetic nerve activity to the heart [93] and to decreased modulation of neurons in the nucleus ambiguus. The decreases in maximum ABR responses of heart rate and sympathetic nerve activity noted during sleep [83] may be attributed to decreases in the activation of RVLM pre-sympathetic neurons and spinal sympathetic preganglionic neurons [93] and to the activation of parasympathetic preganglionic neurons in the nucleus ambiguus.

It is worth mentioning that neural pathways that involve the NTS, PBN, and RVLM may mediate not only the effects of sleep on the ABR, but also effects of the ABR on sleep. As recently reviewed [10], arterial baroreceptor stimulation, if very mild or performed under anesthesia, may inhibit cortical arousal, whereas substantial increases or decreases in arterial baroreceptor stimulation cause arousal in animal models and human subjects in physiological conditions. These interactions may constitute a positive feedback loop that facilitates coordinated brain state transitions upon awakening, with the arterial blood pressure increase caused by central autonomic commands stabilizing arousal by loading baroreceptors [5, 10]. Based on the available neuroanatomical and neurophysiological evidence, it has been hypothesized that baroreceptor unloading in conscious conditions may promote arousal by a circuitry involving decreased NTS activity, disinhibition of adrenergic C1 neurons of the RVLM, and activation of noradrenergic neurons in the pontine locus coeruleus. On the other hand, arterial baroreceptor loading in conscious conditions may promote arousal by a circuitry which involves increased activity of the NTS, the PBN, the basal forebrain, and intralaminar nuclei of the thalamus [10].

References

1. Hobson JA. Sleep is of the brain, by the brain and for the brain. Nature. 2005;437(7063):1254–6.
2. Hess WR. Sleep as a phenomenon of the integral organism. Prog Brain Res. 1965;18:3–8.
3. American Academy of Sleep Medicine AASM Manual for the Scoring of Sleep and Associated Events. American Academy of Sleep Medicine, 2018, v. 2.5.0.
4. Silvani A. Physiological sleep-dependent changes in arterial blood pressure: central autonomic commands and baroreflex control. Clin Exp Pharmacol Physiol. 2008;35(9):987–94.
5. Silvani A. Orexins and the cardiovascular events of awakening. Temperature (Austin). 2017;4(2):128–40.
6. Silvani A. Night, darkness, sleep, and cardiovascular activity. In: Govoni S, Politi P, Vanoli E, editors. Brain and heart dynamics. In: Springer International Publishing; 2020; 585-602.
7. Silvani A, Dampney RA. Central control of cardiovascular function during sleep. Am J Physiol Heart Circ Physiol. 2013;305(12):H1683–92.
8. de Zambotti M, Trinder J, Silvani A, Colrain IM, Baker FC. Dynamic coupling between the central and autonomic nervous systems during sleep: a review. Neurosci Biobehav Rev. 2018;90:84–103.
9. Lo Martire V, Silvani A, Alvente S, Bastianini S, Berteotti C, Valli A, Zoccoli G. Modulation of sympathetic vasoconstriction is critical for the effects of sleep on arterial pressure in mice. J Physiol. 2018;596(4):591–608.
10. Silvani A, Calandra-Buonaura G, Benarroch EE, Dampney RA, Cortelli P. Bidirectional interactions between the baroreceptor reflex and arousal: an update. Sleep Med. 2015;16(2):210–6.
11. Snyder F, Hobson JA, Goldfrank F. Blood pressure changes during human sleep. Science. 1963;142(3597):1313–4.

12. Morgan BJ, Crabtree DC, Puleo DS, Badr MS, Toiber F, Skatrud JB. Neurocirculatory consequences of abrupt change in sleep state in humans. J Appl Physiol (1985). 1996;80(5):1627–36.
13. Goff EA, O'Driscoll DM, Simonds AK, Trinder J, Morrell MJ. The cardiovascular response to arousal from sleep decreases with age in healthy adults. Sleep. 2008;31(7):1009–17.
14. Sforza E, Jouny C, Ibanez V. Cardiac activation during arousal in humans: further evidence for hierarchy in the arousal response. Clin Neurophysiol. 2000;111(9):1611–9.
15. Bangash MF, Xie A, Skatrud JB, Reichmuth KJ, Barczi SR, Morgan BJ. Cerebrovascular response to arousal from NREM and REM sleep. Sleep. 2008;31(3):321–7.
16. Pennestri MH, Montplaisir J, Colombo R, Lavigne G, Lanfranchi PA. Nocturnal blood pressure changes in patients with restless legs syndrome. Neurology. 2007;68(15):1213–8.
17. Siddiqui F, Strus J, Ming X, Lee IA, Chokroverty S, Walters AS. Rise of blood pressure with periodic limb movements in sleep and wakefulness. Clin Neurophysiol. 2007;118(9):1923–30.
18. Pennestri MH, Montplaisir J, Fradette L, Lavigne G, Colombo R, Lanfranchi PA. Blood pressure changes associated with periodic leg movements during sleep in healthy subjects. Sleep Med. 2013;14(6):555–61.
19. Sieminski M, Pyrzowski J, Partinen M. Periodic limb movements in sleep are followed by increases in EEG activity, blood pressure, and heart rate during sleep. Sleep Breath. 2017;21(2):497–503.
20. Silvani A, Grimaldi D, Barletta G, Bastianini S, Vandi S, Pierangeli G, Plazzi G, Cortelli P. Cardiovascular variability as a function of sleep-wake behaviour in narcolepsy with cataplexy. J Sleep Res. 2013;22(2):178–84.
21. Berteotti C, Franzini C, Lenzi P, Zoccoli G, Silvani A. Surges of arterial pressure during REM sleep in spontaneously hypertensive rats. Sleep. 2008;31(1):111–7.
22. Silvani A, Bastianini S, Berteotti C, Franzini C, Lenzi P, Lo Martire V, Zoccoli G. Central and baroreflex control of heart period during the wake-sleep cycle in consomic rats with different genetic susceptibility to hypertension. Clin Exp Pharmacol Physiol. 2010;37(3):322–7.
23. Silvani A, Bastianini S, Berteotti C, Franzini C, Lenzi P, Lo Martire V, Zoccoli G. Dysregulation of heart rhythm during sleep in leptin-deficient obese mice. Sleep. 2010;33(3):355–61.
24. Lo Martire V, Silvani A, Bastianini S, Berteotti C, Zoccoli G. Effects of ambient temperature on sleep and cardiovascular regulation in mice: the role of hypocretin/orexin neurons. PLoS One. 2012;7(10):e47032.
25. Silvani A, Bastianini S, Berteotti C, Lo Martire V, Zoccoli G. Control of cardiovascular variability during undisturbed wake-sleep behavior in hypocretin-deficient mice. Am J Physiol Regul Integr Comp Physiol. 2012;302(8):R958–64.
26. Silvani A, Bastianini S, Berteotti C, Cenacchi G, Leone O, Lo Martire V, Papa V, Zoccoli G. Sleep and cardiovascular phenotype in middle-aged hypocretin-deficient narcoleptic mice. J Sleep Res. 2014;23(1):98–106.
27. Silvani A, Berteotti C, Bastianini S, Cohen G, Lo Martire V, Mazza R, et al. Cardiorespiratory anomalies in mice lacking CB1 cannabinoid receptors. PLoS One. 2014;9(6):e100536.
28. Silvani A, Asti V, Bojic T, Ferrari V, Franzini C, Lenzi P, et al. Sleep-dependent changes in the coupling between heart period and arterial pressure in newborn lambs. Pediatr Res. 2005;57(1):108–14.
29. Staessen JA, Bieniaszewski L, O'Brien E, Gosse P, Hayashi H, Imai Y, et al. Nocturnal blood pressure fall on ambulatory monitoring in a large international database. The Ad Hoc Working Group Hypertension. 1997;29(1 Pt 1):30–9.
30. Somers VK, Dyken ME, Clary MP, Abboud FM. Sympathetic neural mechanisms in obstructive sleep apnea. J Clin Invest. 1995;96(4):1897–904.
31. Shimizu T, Takahashi Y, Kogawa S, Takahashi K, Saito Y, Hishikawa Y, Broughton RJ. Muscle sympathetic nerve activity during central, mixed and obstructive apnea: are there any differences? Psychiatry Clin Neurosci. 1997;51(6):397–403.
32. O'Driscoll DM, Foster AM, Ng ML, Yang JS, Bashir F, Wong S, et al. Central apnoeas have significant effects on blood pressure and heart rate in children. J Sleep Res. 2009;18(4):415–21.
33. Easton A, Meerlo P, Bergmann B, Turek FW. The suprachiasmatic nucleus regulates sleep timing and amount in mice. Sleep. 2004;27(7):1307–18.
34. Daan S, Beersma DG, Borbély AA. Timing of human sleep: recovery process gated by a circadian pacemaker. Am J Phys. 1984;246(2 Pt 2):R161–83.
35. Wehr TA, Aeschbach D, Duncan WC Jr. Evidence for a biological dawn and dusk in the human circadian timing system. J Physiol. 2001;535(Pt 3):937–51.
36. Shea SA, Hilton MF, Hu K, Scheer FA. Existence of an endogenous circadian blood pressure rhythm in humans that peaks in the evening. Circ Res. 2011;108(8):980–4.
37. Minors DS, Waterhouse JM. Masking in humans: the problem and some attempts to solve it. Chronobiol Int. 1989;6(1):29–53.
38. Ben-Dov IZ, Kark JD, Ben-Ishay D, Mekler J, Ben-Arie L, Bursztyn M. Blunted heart rate dip during sleep and all-cause mortality. Arch Intern Med. 2007;167(19):2116–21.
39. Morris CJ, Purvis TE, Hu K, Scheer FA. Circadian misalignment increases cardiovascular disease risk factors in humans. Proc Natl Acad Sci U S A. 2016;113(10):E1402–11.
40. Bastianini S, Silvani A, Berteotti C, Lo Martire V, Zoccoli G. Mice show circadian rhythms of blood pressure during each wake-sleep state. Chronobiol Int. 2012;29(1):82–6.
41. Ishii K, Idesako M, Matsukawa K. Differential contribution of aortic and carotid sinus baroreflexes to control of heart rate and renal sympathetic nerve activity. J Physiol Sci. 2015;65(5):471–80.
42. Smit AA, Timmers HJ, Wieling W, Wagenaar M, Marres HA, Lenders JW, et al. Long-term effects of carotid sinus denervation on arterial blood pressure in humans. Circulation. 2002;105(11):1329–35.
43. Dampney RA. Central neural control of the cardiovascular system: current perspectives. Adv Physiol Educ. 2016;40(3):283–96.
44. Silvani A, Calandra-Buonaura G, Dampney RA, Cortelli P. Brain-heart interactions: physiology and clinical implications. Philos Trans A Math Phys Eng Sci. 2016;374(2067):20150181.
45. Vatner SF, Franklin D, Van Citters RL, Braunwald E. Effects of carotid sinus nerve stimulation on blood-flow distribution in conscious dogs at rest and during exercise. Circ Res. 1970;27(4):495–503.
46. Leimbach WN Jr, Schmid PG, Mark AL. Baroreflex control of plasma arginine vasopressin in humans. Am J Phys. 1984;247(4 Pt 2):H638–44.
47. Gross R, Hackenberg HM, Hackenthal E, Kirchheim H. Interaction between perfusion pressure and sympathetic nerves in renin release by carotid baroreflex in conscious dogs. J Physiol. 1981;313:237–50.
48. Ogoh S, Fadel PJ, Nissen P, Jans Ø, Selmer C, Secher NH, Raven PB. Baroreflex-mediated changes in cardiac output and vascular conductance in response to alterations in carotid sinus pressure during exercise in humans. J Physiol. 2003;550(Pt 1):317–24.
49. Raven PB, Fadel PJ, Ogoh S. Arterial baroreflex resetting during exercise: a current perspective. Exp Physiol. 2006;91(1):37–49.
50. Carlson BE, Arciero JC, Secomb TW. Theoretical model of blood flow autoregulation: roles of myogenic, shear-dependent, and metabolic responses. Am J Physiol Heart Circ Physiol. 2008;295(4):H1572–9.
51. Goodwill AG, Dick GM, Kiel AM, Tune JD. Regulation of coronary blood flow. Compr Physiol. 2017;7(2):321–82.

52. Madsen PL. Blood flow and oxygen uptake in the human brain during various states of sleep and wakefulness. Acta Neurol Scand Suppl. 1993;148:3–27.
53. Hoiland RL, Bain AR, Rieger MG, Bailey DM, Ainslie PN. Hypoxemia, oxygen content, and the regulation of cerebral blood flow. Am J Physiol Regul Integr Comp Physiol. 2016;310(5):R398–413.
54. Dorrington KL, Balanos GM, Talbot NP, Robbins PA. Extent to which pulmonary vascular responses to P_{CO2} and P_{O2} play a functional role within the healthy human lung. J Appl Physiol (1985). 2010;108(5):1084–96.
55. Ait-Mou Y, Hsu K, Farman GP, Kumar M, Greaser ML, Irving TC, de Tombe PP. Titin strain contributes to the Frank-Starling law of the heart by structural rearrangements of both thin- and thick-filament proteins. Proc Natl Acad Sci U S A. 2016;113(8):2306–11.
56. Han JC, Pham T, Taberner AJ, Loiselle DS, Tran K. Solving a century-old conundrum underlying cardiac force-length relations. Am J Physiol Heart Circ Physiol. 2019;316(4):H781–93.
57. de Tombe PP, Mateja RD, Tachampa K, Ait Mou Y, Farman GP, Irving TC. Myofilament length dependent activation. J Mol Cell Cardiol. 2010;48(5):851–8.
58. Williamson JW. Autonomic responses to exercise: where is central command? Auton Neurosci. 2015;188:3–4.
59. Grillner S. Biological pattern generation: the cellular and computational logic of networks in motion. Neuron. 2006;52(5):751–66.
60. Grillner S. Neurobiological bases of rhythmic motor acts in vertebrates. Science. 1985;228(4696):143–9.
61. Swanson LW. Cerebral hemisphere regulation of motivated behavior. Brain Res. 2000;886(1–2):113–64.
62. Saper CB. The central autonomic nervous system: conscious visceral perception and autonomic pattern generation. Annu Rev Neurosci. 2002;25:433–69.
63. Goodwin GM, McCloskey DI, Mitchell JH. Cardiovascular and respiratory responses to changes in central command during isometric exercise at constant muscle tension. J Physiol. 1972;226(1):173–90.
64. Fisher JP, Young CN, Fadel PJ. Autonomic adjustments to exercise in humans. Compr Physiol. 2015;5(2):475–512.
65. Doherty CJ, Incognito AV, Notay K, Burns MJ, Slysz JT, Seed JD, Nardone M, Burr JF, Millar PJ. Muscle sympathetic nerve responses to passive and active one-legged cycling: insights into the contributions of central command. Am J Physiol Heart Circ Physiol. 2018;314(1):H3–H10.
66. Victor RG, Secher NH, Lyson T, Mitchell JH. Central command increases muscle sympathetic nerve activity during intense intermittent isometric exercise in humans. Circ Res. 1995;76(1):127–31.
67. Baskerville AL, Eckberg DL, Thompson MA. Arterial pressure and pulse interval responses to repetitive carotid baroreceptor stimuli in man. J Physiol. 1979;297(0):61–71.
68. Somers VK, Dyken ME, Mark AL, Abboud FM. Sympathetic-nerve activity during sleep in normal subjects. N Engl J Med. 1993;328(5):303–7.
69. Miki K, Kato M, Kajii S. Relationship between renal sympathetic nerve activity and arterial pressure during REM sleep in rats. Am J Physiol Regul Integr Comp Physiol. 2003;284(2):R467–73.
70. Berntson GG, Cacioppo JT, Quigley KS. The metrics of cardiac chronotropism: biometric perspectives. Psychophysiology. 1995;32(2):162–71.
71. Berteotti C, Asti V, Ferrari V, Franzini C, Lenzi P, Zoccoli G, Silvani A. Central and baroreflex control of heart period during the wake-sleep cycle in spontaneously hypertensive rats. Am J Physiol Regul Integr Comp Physiol. 2007;293(1):R293–8.
72. Silvani A, Calandra-Buonaura G, Johnson BD, van Helmond N, Barletta G, Cecere AG, et al. Physiological mechanisms mediating the coupling between heart period and arterial pressure in response to postural changes in humans. Front Physiol. 2017;8:163.
73. Silvani A, Grimaldi D, Vandi S, Barletta G, Vetrugno R, Provini F, et al. Sleep-dependent changes in the coupling between heart period and blood pressure in human subjects. Am J Physiol Regul Integr Comp Physiol. 2008;294:R1686–92.
74. Silvani A, Magosso E, Bastianini S, Lenzi P, Ursino M. Mathematical modeling of cardiovascular coupling: central autonomic commands and baroreflex control. Auton Neurosci. 2011;162(1–2):66–71.
75. Briant LJ, Burchell AE, Ratcliffe LE, Charkoudian N, Nightingale AK, Paton JF, et al. Quantifying sympathetic neuro-haemodynamic transduction at rest in humans: insights into sex, ageing and blood pressure control. J Physiol. 2016;594(17):4753–68.
76. Berteotti C, Franzini C, Lenzi P, Magosso E, Ursino M, Zoccoli G, Silvani A. The baroreflex contribution to spontaneous heart rhythm assessed with a mathematical model in rats. Auton Neurosci. 2008;138(1–2):24–30.
77. Junqeira FL Jr, Krieger EM. Blood pressure and sleep in the rat in normotension and in neurogenic hypertension. J Physiol. 1976;259(3):725–35.
78. Sei H, Morita Y, Tsunooka K, Morita H. Sino-aortic denervation augments the increase in blood pressure seen during paradoxical sleep in the rat. J Sleep Res. 1999;8(1):45–50.
79. Guazzi M, Baccelli G, Zanchetti A. Reflex chemoceptive regulation of arterial pressure during natural sleep in the cat. Am J Phys. 1968;214(5):969–78.
80. Silveira NP, Moreira ED, Drager LF, Silva GJ, Krieger EM. Effects of sinoaortic denervation on hemodynamic parameters during natural sleep in rats. Sleep. 2008;31(3):328–33.
81. Castania JA, Katayama PL, Brognara F, Moraes DJA, Sabino JPJ, Salgado HC. Selective denervation of the aortic and carotid baroreceptors in rats. Exp Physiol. 2019;104(9):1335–42.
82. Makino M, Hayashi H, Takezawa H, Hirai M, Saito H, Ebihara S. Circadian rhythms of cardiovascular functions are modulated by the baroreflex and the autonomic nervous system in the rat. Circulation. 1997;96(5):1667–74.
83. Nagura S, Sakagami T, Kakiichi A, Yoshimoto M, Miki K. Acute shifts in baroreflex control of renal sympathetic nerve activity induced by REM sleep and grooming in rats. J Physiol. 2004;558(Pt 3):975–83.
84. Drager LF, Ueno LM, Lessa PS, Negrão CE, Lorenzi-Filho G, Krieger EM. Sleep-related changes in hemodynamic and autonomic regulation in human hypertension. J Hypertens. 2009;27(8):1655–63.
85. Yiallourou SR, Sands SA, Walker AM, Horne RS. Baroreflex sensitivity during sleep in infants: impact of sleeping position and sleep state. Sleep. 2011;34(6):725–32.
86. Schwimmer H, Stauss HM, Abboud F, Nishino S, Mignot E, Zeitzer JM. Effects of sleep on the cardiovascular and thermoregulatory systems: a possible role for hypocretins. J Appl Physiol (1985). 2010;109(4):1053–63.
87. McAllen RM, May CN, Shafton AD. Functional anatomy of sympathetic premotor cell groups in the medulla. Clin Exp Hypertens. 1995;17(1–2):209–21.
88. Gillies MJ, Huang Y, Hyam JA, Aziz TZ, Green AL. Direct neurophysiological evidence for a role of the human anterior cingulate cortex in central command. Auton Neurosci. 2019;216:51–8.
89. Benarroch EE. The central autonomic network: functional organization, dysfunction, and perspective. Mayo Clin Proc. 1993;68(10):988–1001.
90. Buijs RM, la Fleur SE, Wortel J, Van Heyningen C, Zuiddam L, Mettenleiter TC, et al. The suprachiasmatic nucleus balances sympathetic and parasympathetic output to peripheral organs through separate preautonomic neurons. J Comp Neurol. 2003;464(1):36–48.

91. Silvani A, Asti V, Berteotti C, Ferrari V, Franzini C, Lenzi P, et al. Sleep-dependent changes in cerebral oxygen consumption in newborn lambs. J Sleep Res. 2006;15(2):206–11.
92. Furlong TM, McDowall LM, Horiuchi J, Polson JW, Dampney RA. The effect of air puff stress on c-Fos expression in rat hypothalamus and brainstem: central circuitry mediating sympathoexcitation and baroreflex resetting. Eur J Neurosci. 2014;39(9):1429–38.
93. Dampney RAL. Resetting of the Baroreflex control of sympathetic vasomotor activity during natural behaviors: description and conceptual model of central mechanisms. Front Neurosci. 2017;11:461.

Sleep and Circadian Regulation of the Autonomic Nervous System

7

Massimiliano de Zambotti and Fiona C. Baker

Sleep from an Integrated Perspective: Central and Autonomic Nervous System Interactions

Sleep is an active process. Although it is mainly referred to and defined as a central nervous system (CNS) phenomenon, i.e., a state of brain activation, the entire organism undergoes profound changes during sleep, from a molecular to a system level. Phasic and tonic changes in autonomic nervous system (ANS) activity during sleep are critical. In fact, the ANS acts in regulating most of our bodily functions, exerting control over the cardiovascular (CV) system, via afferent and efferent sympathetic and parasympathetic pathways, guaranteeing system homeostasis.

During sleep, the brain dynamically communicates bidirectionally with most of bodily systems, resulting in a coordinated cascade of central and peripheral events, following their specific temporal dynamics [1]. The communication (coupling) between cortical and ANS rhythms during sleep is among the most studied [1], due to the key role of cortical and ANS function during sleep, their temporal resolution, their closed anatomy and physiology, and accessibility.

Sleep is under control of homeostatic and circadian processes that respectively dictate the "*need for sleep*" and "*when to sleep.*" Polysomnography (PSG) is the gold standard to measure sleep in the laboratory and consists of the evaluation of cortical electroencephalographic (EEG), electrooculographic (EOG), and electromyographic (EMG) activities. This information is used to visually score wake and sleep (N1, N2, N3 or slow wave sleep [SWS], and rapid-eye-movement [REM] sleep) and thus determine sleep macrostructure [2]. Sleep comprises two main states, non-REM (NREM) and REM sleep. REM or EEG desynchronized *wake-like* sleep state accounts for 20–25% of the sleep period. NREM sleep is characterized by a progressive EEG synchronization or *deepening* of sleep (N1 → N2 → N3), accounting overall for 75–80% of the sleep period. NREM and REM stages alternate cyclically (every ~90 min) across the night. At the microstructural level (quantitative EEG analysis, i.e., power spectral analysis of the EEG signals), several sleep EEG features have been shown to be fundamental for health and associated with ANS functioning. EEG slow wave activity (SWA; cortical activity in the range of 0.4–4 Hz which includes slow oscillations [SOs, <1 Hz] and delta waves [1–4 Hz]) has received the most attention. SWA is maximal in the first part of the night and declines over sequential NREM-REM cycles, reflecting a dissipation of homeostatic pressure across the night [3].

Sleep and the ANS system are intimately connected with the ANS being under circadian and sleep-dependent influences [4, 5]. ANS activity fluctuates across 24 h, within the night according to stages of sleep and time of the night, and as a function of phasic sleep events such as transient EEG desynchronizations (e.g., spontaneous arousals) and synchronization (e.g., k-complexes), lip movements, and respiratory events [1].

During sleep, the interaction between EEG SWA and cardiac ANS function (e.g., R-R intervals and/or measures of high frequency heart rate [HR] variability [HRV] as indicators of vagal functioning) is probably one of the major expressions of the central-autonomic nervous system interaction [1]. Converging evidence from observational studies indicates that cortical EEG and cardiac ANS measures not only covary across the night, with high vagal dominance being associated with increases in cortical synchronization, but they mutually influence each other with precise temporal dynamics. However, the nature and directionality of brain-heart communication during sleep remain unclear due to the bidirectional nature of the interaction between sleep and the ANS [1].

M. de Zambotti (✉) · F. C. Baker
SRI International, Menlo Park, CA, USA
e-mail: massimiliano.dezambotti@sri.com

S. Chokroverty, P. Cortelli (eds.), *Autonomic Nervous System and Sleep*, https://doi.org/10.1007/978-3-030-62263-3_7

Sleep ANS Control: Sleep Stage Modulation

The ANS is strongly influenced by the sleep-wake cycle, and its activity changes across the night in response to sleep stage shifting. During NREM sleep, sympathetic ANS activity[1] reduces (decreases in cardiac sympathetic activity and sympathetic vascular tone), while cardiac vagal activity[2] and baroreflex sensitivity increase, as compared to wake. In contrast, REM sleep is characterized by a return of this activity approximately to wake levels (Fig. 7.1). A change in ANS innervation of the heart and vasculature drives wake-to-sleep reductions in blood pressure (BP; typically reaching its minimum in the first hour of sleep), HR, and systemic vascular resistance, which are further reduced as NREM sleep persists. On entry to REM sleep, HR and BP become more variable and show an overall increase relative to NREM sleep [5, 7, 8]. Of note, these sleep-stage-dependent ANS changes occurring during night-time sleep also seem to be evident during daytime napping [9–11]. Within NREM periods, ANS and CV activities are relatively stable. The variability in ANS activity during REM is possibly due to repeated transient activations (e.g., tachycardia, BP rises) associated with phasic REM events.

Changes in CV and ANS function across the night largely reflect changes in sleep stage distribution across the night (e.g., progressive increases in the time spent in REM sleep over subsequent NREM-REM cycles across the night). However, as discussed later, circadian influences also play a role in influencing these measures, particularly HR.

Overall, the reduction in CV activity during sleep, and particularly during NREM sleep (which, as highlighted above, occupies the majority of the sleep period), plays a key role in maintaining CV health providing a period of CV quiescence, what has been described as a *"holiday"* for the CV system [5]. For example, the extent to which BP falls during the sleeping period, characterizing the individual's *dipping profile,* as compared to waking values (~10–20% BP reduction during sleep), is considered a clinically important marker for CV health [12].

Insufficient nocturnal CV recovery could have repercussions for health, increasing the risk for several adverse outcomes, including CV disease [13, 14]. Arousals from sleep, accompanied by vagal withdrawal, SNS activation, peripheral vasoconstriction, and abrupt BP surges, are the major determinant in altering an individuals' nocturnal ANS and CV profile.

Sleep ANS Control: Circadian Modulation

Techniques like forced desynchrony[3] or constant routine[4] have been used to isolate circadian-specific influences on ANS. Evidence indicates that HR is under strong circadian influence, reflecting the tight correlation between HR and metabolic heat production. In absence of sleep, the 24-h rhythm of HR approximates a sine wave, with HR being higher during the "normal daytime wake" period and reaching its lowest at night, in the second-half of the "normal sleep period" [5, 8]. Similarly, cardiac vagal ANS activity, as determined by the variability in the beat-to-beat intervals (respiratory sinus arrhythmia), also shows circadian influences, with rises in vagal modulation even anticipating the onset of sleep, reaching its maximum at night, and being generally suppressed during the "normal waking hours." It is possible that this rise in vagal activity preceding the onset of sleep may contribute to the occurrence of sleep. Differently, cardiac sympathetic ANS activity seems to be mainly influenced by the sleep system, showing little or no circadian variations [5, 8].

The 24-h profile of BP resembles a square wave function with high and constant BP values during the waking hours, which is followed by an abrupt BP drop in association with the onset of sleep, a constant lower BP during sleep relative to wake, and a rapid rise in BP at morning awakening (which seems to be more related to postural and ambulatory changes rather than an effect of the sleep/wake transition). These

[1]Cardiac sympathetic nervous system activity can be non-invasively determined during sleep using impedance cardiography. This technique in combination with ECG allows measurement of beat-to-beat changes in chest electrical impedance. It allows the assessment of the pre-ejection period, i.e., the timing between the onset of the electrical depolarization of the left ventricle and the mechanical opening of the aortic valve, considered a valid index of cardiac sympathetic nervous system function. A direct measure of peripheral sympathetic activity can be obtained via microneurography, an invasive technique directly recording from sympathetic nerve fibers (e.g., peroneal or tibial nerves at the knee) using intraneural microelectrodes. However, due to its invasiveness, microneurography has limited application in sleep studies [1].

[2]Cardiac vagal functioning is commonly determined non-invasively during sleep via heart rate variability (HRV) analysis techniques using electrocardiographic (ECG) signals. In particular, ECG HRV in the high frequency range (0.15–0.40 Hz, which comprises the normal respiratory frequency) reflects respiratory sinus arrhythmia, i.e., the variation in the beat-to-beat intervals in synchrony with respiration (beat-to-beat intervals are shortening during inspiration and lengthening during expiration), which is widely accepted as a measure of cardiac vagal modulation [6].

[3]Forced desynchrony is used to study the interaction between sleep homeostasis and circadian rhythmicity. Forced desynchrony protocols impose on individuals very short (about 20 h) or very long (about 28 h) cycles of rest-activity, which are outside the range of entrainment of the circadian pacemaker (about 24 h). This allows disruption of the alignment between the environment and the intrinsic circadian rhythm.

[4]Constant routine protocols are also commonly used in sleep circadian science to isolate the effect of circadian (endogenous) rhythms from the influence of confounding factors like sleep, temperature, light, food intake, postural changes, and physical activity. In constant routine protocols, individuals are kept awake for at least 24 h under controlled laboratory conditions.

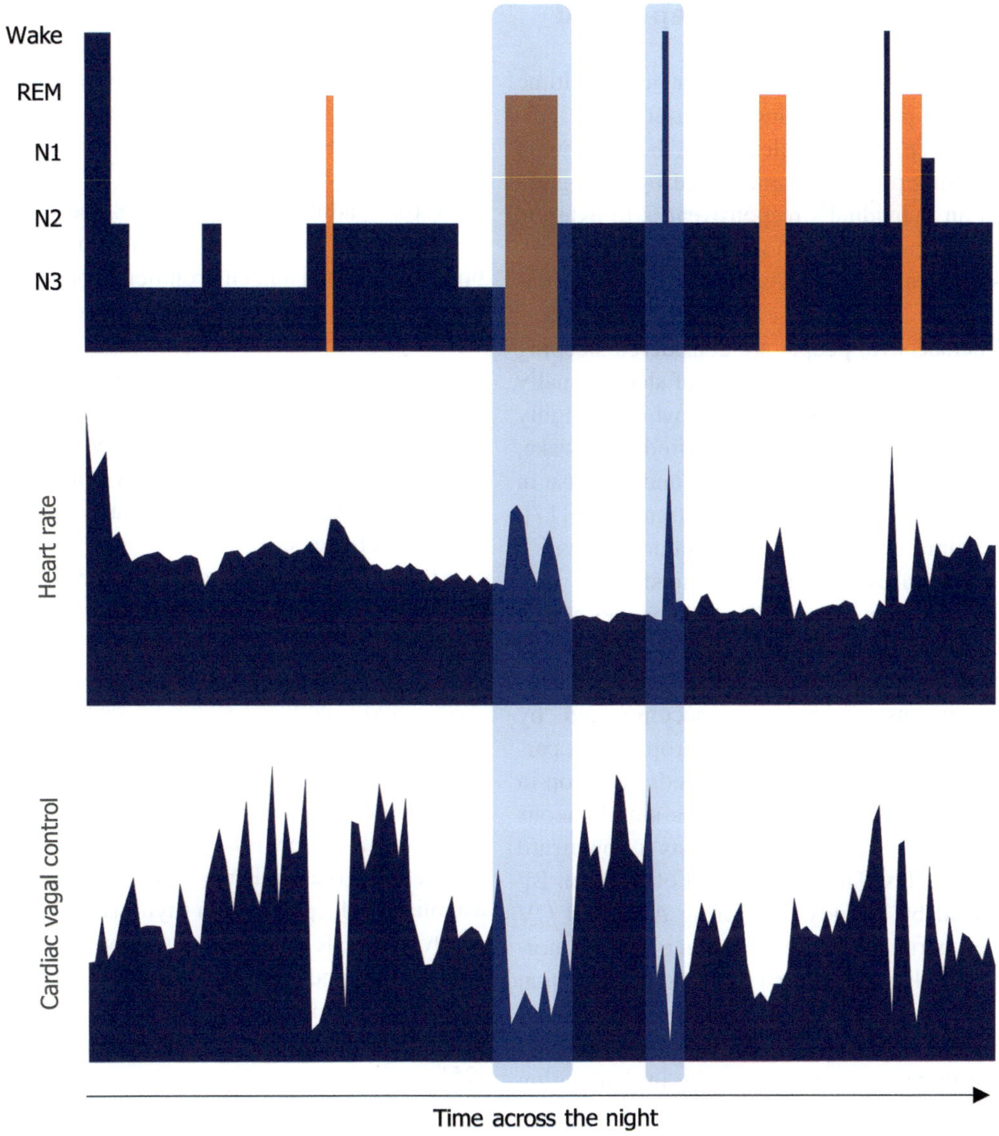

Fig. 7.1 The graph highlights a typical shifting in sleep autonomic nervous system (ANS) control across the night, as a function of sleep/wake state and sleep stages. In the top panel, sleep stages (wake, rapid-eye-movement [REM] sleep, N1, N2, and N3) are plotted as a function of time across the night. This graphic representation is called a "sleep hypnogram," which provides a graphical picture of an individual's sleep macrostructure. The middle panel reflects the variation of electrocardiographic-derived heart rate across the night. Finally, the bottom panel represents the variation in cardiac vagal control (determined by the frequency analysis of heart rate variability as the proportion of high frequency heart rate variability relative to total heart rate variability) across the night. In the graph, readers can notice a wake-to-sleep drop in heart rate and increases in cardiac vagal control across the falling asleep period, with the opposite pattern in association with awakenings at night. Cardiac acceleration and reduced vagal control characterize REM periods when compared to non-REM (N1, N2, and N3) sleep. Data are from a young adult who underwent a polysomnographic recording at the SRI Human Sleep Laboratory

changes are strongly influenced by the sleep system. The circadian influences over BP are less clear, with some studies showing some circadian effects and some others not [8]. It is possible that confounding effects, like the extent to which individuals are sleep deprived, may have accounted for possible discrepancies among studies. See also [15], for a further discussion about endogenous and exogenous factors affecting the 24-h BP profile.

Circadian influences on the ANS are of potential clinical relevance, since CV events (e.g., ischemic stroke and myocardial infarction) display a circadian distribution with higher incidence in the morning hours [16].

Sleep ANS Control: The Falling Asleep Period

Sleep onset marks the wake-to-sleep transition, after bedtime (or *lights-off*, the time point reflecting the onset of the individual's attempt to sleep). Falling asleep could be considered a dynamic de-arousing process characterized by a progressive reduction in an individual's responsiveness to external stimuli and by an increase in behavioral quiescence, accompanied by physiological changes that involve most of our biological systems.

From a PSG perspective, people are considered sleeping when first reaching any PSG-marked stage of sleep (usually N1 or N2). The individuals' cortical activity, which is highly desynchronized and of low voltage amplitude in wake, moves to an overall decrease in complexity and increase in synchronization across the wake-to-sleep transition [17]; core body temperature drops, distal temperature increases, and respiration rate reduces in the approach to sleep.

The ANS and CV systems show profound changes across the wake-to-sleep transition, which is typically characterized by a shifting from sympathetic to parasympathetic regulation. The sleep onset process is accompanied by peripheral vasodilation, and by an abrupt drop in BP, particularly evident when stable sleep is achieved. The drop in BP is coupled with a reduction in HR. This simultaneous drop in BP and, to a less extent, HR suggests a downward resetting of the baroreflex. The strong effect of sleep on BP is further elucidated by a study comparing ANS and CV measures between participants going to sleep at their normal time vs. after a delay of 3 hours [18]. Results show that a delayed sleep onset is associated with a delayed BP fall. In the same study, a strong influence of sleep on vagal activity was evident, with increases in vagal activity in association with sleep onset.

Sleep ANS Control: Developmental Maturation and Sex Differences

Profound changes in sleep occur from birth to adolescence, particularly in the first year of life and across the adolescent period.

Newborns spend about 64% of their time sleeping, which is characterized by a polyphasic sleep/wake pattern. Circadian rhythms are not yet fully expressed, and sleep stages consist of active (adult REM-like sleep; lasting about 50% of their total sleep time) and quiet sleep (adult NREM-like sleep; lasting about 14% of their total sleep time), alternating two to three times within a single sleep period [19]. Across the first year of life, the sleep periods lengthen with a reduction in the total sleep duration (due to a reduction in daytime sleep), and there is a shift in the proportion of quiet and active sleep. By the end of the first year, the amount of quiet sleep is greater than 50%. Also, sleep progressively shifts from polyphasic to monophasic, due to a maturation of the circadian processes and becomes more consolidated (less awakenings). To a less extent, sleep maturation progresses across the pre-school years (~1–5 years) and middle childhood (~6–12 years) [19].

Across adolescence (~12–18 years), sleep duration decreases due to changes in bioregulatory processes combined with social and environmental pressures, which lead to later bedtimes and early morning awakenings (mainly dictated by school schedules), reducing the time available for sleep. In particular, dramatic changes occur in sleep structure with SWA showing a dramatic reduction (>50%) starting between age 11 and 12 [20]. Given the central-autonomic nervous system's interdependency during sleep [1], it is not surprising that sleep ANS function is also affected by developmental changes.

Sleep ANS control in children and adolescents is largely unexplored and primarily based on cross-sectional data employing HRV analyses techniques. Further, sex differences in development are poorly understood. Shifting in ANS activity between stages of sleep (e.g., quiet vs. active sleep) is evident in newborns and infants, and even in fetuses [21–23], despite not fully resembling the sleep-dependent changes in ANS activity seen in adults. Circadian variation in ANS activity seems to appear in late infancy [24] which is in line with the evidence that newborns do not have fully established sleep circadian rhythms.

Overall, HR progressively slows across childhood and adolescence and HRV increases (reflecting increases in cardiac vagal dominance) until reaching a peak between the ages of 15 and 18 years and then declines with advancing age [25].

Intriguing results from our cross-sectional study of nocturnal HR and HRV in adolescents indicated that developmental differences in nocturnal HR and HRV were not equivalent between the sexes: older boys showed a lower HR than younger boys, across the age range of 12–22 years, an age effect not evident in girls, such that older girls had a faster nocturnal HR than older boys [26]. Differently, only girls showed a significant age-related drop in cardiac vagal ANS activity. HR and HRV showed the same pattern of change across the sleep period in adolescents, as seen in adults, with a drop in HR and increase in vagal activity across the night, and higher HR in REM sleep versus NREM sleep [26]. However, boys showed a greater increase in HRV across the night than did girls, which could reflect a sex difference in circadian regulation of the ANS, although further study is needed. An apparent sex difference in sleep stage shifting in ANS control was also apparent, with girls exhibiting a greater NREM-to-REM HR increase than boys. Sedentary activity (increasing with age in girls) partially mediated the age- and sex divergencies in HR [26].

Sleep ANS functioning changes with aging in adults, toward an overall decline in vagal control and faster heart rate during sleep in older vs. younger adults [27, 28], even when age-related changes in respiratory patterns and sleep quality (declining in older age) are considered. Sleep stage shifting in ANS activity is preserved in older adults, but it appears to be blunted (reduced magnitude of NREM-REM changes in ANS activity), as compared to younger adults [27]. The overall age-related decline in sleep cardiac vagal control parallels the age-related sleep deterioration characterized by marked drops in SWA, although the relationship between vagal functioning and SWA across the night is maintained with aging [28], suggesting that these cortical-cardiac interactions during sleep are preserved.

Adult women have generally higher HR paired with greater cardiac vagal control, as compared to men [29] but sex-specific differences in sleep ANS control are less clear. For example, studies are conflicting, with some indicating greater NREM-to-REM cardiac ANS excitatory responses (toward sympathetic dominance) in men compared to women, and others showing the opposite [30–32].

Sleep ANS Control: Female-Specific Hormonal Factors

Across their lifespan, from puberty to post-menopause, women experience fluctuations in reproductive hormones. When evaluating sleep ANS control, female-specific hormonal factors need to be accounted for, since hormones interact with sleep and the ANS. For example, estrogen receptors are present in many systems including the CV system. Estradiol is considered a cardioprotective factor, with evidence indicating that it acts centrally in modulating the ANS via increasing vagal outflow and decreasing sympathetic drive [33]. Opposite ANS effects seem to be driven by progesterone.

Cyclical changes in reproductive hormones across the menstrual cycle influence sleep and ANS regulation during sleep. Sleep ANS control shifts toward a greater HR and reduced cardiac vagal ANS control in the luteal phase (where progesterone is high) compared with the follicular phase of the menstrual cycle. However, NREM-REM shifting in ANS control is maintained across phases of the menstrual cycle [34, 35]. An increased HR and reduced vagal activity in the luteal phase are not specific to sleep, being evident when analyzing short periods of ECG recording during wake, or across 24 h [36]. Body temperature changes across the menstrual cycle, with a higher temperature in the luteal phase compared to the follicular phase, may be implicated in the menstrual phase-related ANS changes.

Changes in the hormonal environment across the menopause transition in midlife, when women experience variable menstrual cycle lengths and then amenorrhea, have also been linked to changes in ANS control toward a reduction in cardiac vagal activity and a shifting to sympathetic dominance in post- compared to pre-menopause. These changes need to be considered in addition to age-related changes in ANS control. Shifting in ANS control according to menopausal stage seems to be attenuated in women taking estrogen replacement therapy, but not when estrogens are combined with progestins [36]. However, studies are based on 24 h or short daytime assessment of ANS function, and there is a lack of evidence about changes in ANS activity during sleep across the menopause transition. Menopause specific symptoms, i.e., nocturnal hot flashes,[5] impact sleep [38] and sleep ANS control [39, 40] in symptomatic women. Overall, hot flashes are associated with transient tachycardia, increases in cardiac sympathetic activity and vagal withdrawal. They are also associated with blood pressure drops when flashes are occurring in undisturbed sleep; differently, hot flashes are associated with sudden and transient BP rises when accompanied by arousals [40], reflecting the strong sleep/wake modulation of BP. Despite the evidence of transient shifting in sleep ANS control, it is unclear if these changes affect tonic sleep ANS control across the night, and whether the nocturnal ANS profile and CV restoration are altered.

Potential Advancements in Understanding Sleep ANS Control: Sleep-Tracking Technology

Over recent years, there has been substantial growth in consumer sleep-tracking technologies (CSTs) (e.g., wearables and nearables) and sophisticated inexpensive multisensory devices (most commonly, wristwatches) that can track users' behavior and physiology. Of relevance, they can provide information about an individuals' sleep/wake state, and most recently, sleep stages (NREM "light" and "deep" sleep, and REM sleep), together with the recording of the functioning of other body systems such as the ANS [41], and thus potentially providing a window on an individuals' sleep-related ANS functioning. Beat-to-beat HR is usually recorded by these devices via analysis of blood flow as measured by photoplethysmogram sensor, and similarly to the HR detected via ECG, its variability can be analyzed and features reflecting ANS control can be extracted [42, 43] (an example of the nocturnal profile for HR as detected by a

[5]Hot flashes are a hallmark of the menopausal transition, affecting up to 80% of women. Hot flashes are a sensation of heat, sweating, flashing, anxiety, and chills lasting 3–10 min. They are a thermoregulatory phenomenon described as a heat dissipation response (peripheral vasodilation → increases in heat loss → increases in sweating → evaporative cooling). The frequency and perceived intensity of the flash can vary widely, and they can occur both day and night [37].

commercial sleep-tracking device and gold standard ECG can be found in [44]).

While originally designed as fitness trackers, targeting the general consumers as recreational devices with claims of general wellness, CSTs are now being increasingly used in clinical and research protocols [42]. CSTs allow collection and processing of information about sleep and cardiac function 24/7 over time, from a few months to years. They can be integrated with the use of ecologic momentary assessments, at-home collection of biospecimens, etc., which could potentially allow the investigation of sleep and cardiac function in relation to a myriad of biopsychosocial factors and conditions (e.g., sleep deprivation, jet lag, stress, demographic factors such as age and sex, hormones, substance use). This could be extremely valuable in mapping the normal development of sleep cardiac function, under which circumstances and how sleep ANS regulation is impacted, and which factors can promote sleep ANS and CV restoration. Also, deviating sleep HR profiles can be used in disease recognition and management, and potentially in predicting the onset of CV conditions.

The use of CSTs is currently facing several challenges, including questions on the level of accuracy and reliability of these devices [41], as well as privacy and ethical issues; however, in the near future, CSTs may play a role in advancing the understanding of sleep-dependent and circadian regulation of ANS.

References

1. de Zambotti M, Trinder J, Silvani A, Colrain IM, Baker FC. Dynamic coupling between the central and autonomic nervous systems during sleep: a review. Neurosci Biobehav Rev. 2018;90:84–103.
2. Iber C, Ancoli-Israel S, Chesson A, Quan S. The AASM manual for the scoring of sleep and associated events: rules, terminology, and technical specification. 1st ed. Westchester: American Academy of Sleep Medicine; 2007.
3. Dijk D-J. Regulation and functional correlates of slow wave sleep. J Clin Sleep Med. 2009;5(2 Suppl):S6–15.
4. Burgess H, Trinder J, Kim Y, Luke D. Sleep and circadian influences on cardiac autonomic nervous system activity. Am J Phys. 1997;273(4):H1761–H8.
5. Trinder J, Waloszek J, Woods M, Jordan A. Sleep and cardiovascular regulation. Pflugers Arch. 2012;463(1):161–8.
6. Heart rate variability. Standards of measurement, physiological interpretation and clinical use. Task Force of the European Society of Cardiology and the North American Society of Pacing and Electrophysiology. Circulation. 1996;93(5):1043–65.
7. Trinder J, Kleiman J, Carrington M, Smith S, Breen S, Tan N, et al. Autonomic activity during human sleep as a function of time and sleep stage. J Sleep Res. 2001;10(4):253–64.
8. Trinder J. Cardiac activity and sympathovagal balance during sleep. Sleep Med Clin. 2007;2(2):199–208.
9. Cellini N, Whitehurst LN, McDevitt EA, Mednick SC. Heart rate variability during daytime naps in healthy adults: autonomic profile and short-term reliability. Psychophysiology. 2016;53(4):473–81.
10. Cellini N, Torre J, Stegagno L, Sarlo M. Cardiac autonomic activity during daytime nap in young adults. J Sleep Res. 2018;27(2):159–64.
11. Whitehurst LN, Naji M, Mednick SC. Comparing the cardiac autonomic activity profile of daytime naps and nighttime sleep. Neurobiol Sleep Circadian Rhythms. 2018;5:52–7.
12. Staessen JA, Wang JG, Thijs L. Cardiovascular protection and blood pressure reduction: a meta-analysis. Lancet. 2001;358(9290):1305–15.
13. Wolk R, Gami AS, Garcia-Touchard A, Somers VK. Sleep and cardiovascular disease. Curr Probl Cardiol. 2005;30(12):625–62.
14. Yano Y, Kario K. Nocturnal blood pressure and cardiovascular disease: a review of recent advances. Hypertens Res. 2012;35(7):695.
15. Smolensky MH, Hermida RC, Portaluppi F. Circadian mechanisms of 24-hour blood pressure regulation and patterning. Sleep Med Rev. 2017;33:4–16.
16. Thosar SS, Butler MP, Shea SA. Role of the circadian system in cardiovascular disease. The J Clin Invest. 2018;128(6):2157–67.
17. Marzano C, Moroni F, Gorgoni M, Nobili L, Ferrara M, De Gennaro L. How we fall asleep: regional and temporal differences in electroencephalographic synchronization at sleep onset. Sleep Med. 2013;14(11):1112–22.
18. Carrington M, Walsh M, Stambas T, Kleiman J, Trinder J. The influence of sleep onset on the diurnal variation in cardiac activity and cardiac control. J Sleep Res. 2003;12(3):213–21.
19. Crabtree VM, Williams NA. Normal sleep in children and adolescents. Child Adolesc Psychiatr Clin N Am. 2009;18(4):799–811.
20. Colrain IM, Baker FC. Changes in sleep as a function of adolescent development. Neuropsychol Rev. 2011;21(1):5–21.
21. Takatani T, Takahashi Y, Yoshida R, Imai R, Uchiike T, Yamazaki M, et al. Relationship between frequency spectrum of heart rate variability and autonomic nervous activities during sleep in newborns. Brain and Development. 2018;40(3):165–71.
22. Massin MM, Withofs N, Maeyns K, Ravet F, Gérard P. Normal ranges for the variability in heart rate in young infants while sleeping. Cardiol Young. 2001;11(6):619–25.
23. Van Laar J, Peters C, Vullings R, Houterman S, Oei S. Power spectrum analysis of fetal heart rate variability at near term and post term gestation during active sleep and quiet sleep. Early Hum Dev. 2009;85(12):795–8.
24. Massin MM, Maeyns K, Withofs N, Ravet F, Gerard P. Circadian rhythm of heart rate and heart rate variability. Arch Dis Child. 2000;83(2):179–82.
25. Eyre E, Duncan M, Birch S, Fisher J. The influence of age and weight status on cardiac autonomic control in healthy children: a review. Auton Neurosci. 2014;186:8–21.
26. de Zambotti M, Javitz H, Franzen PL, Brumback T, Clark DB, Colrain IM, et al. Sex- and age-dependent differences in autonomic nervous system functioning in adolescents. J Adolesc Health. 2018;62(2):184–90.
27. Brandenberger G, Viola AU, Ehrhart J, Charloux A, Geny B, Piquard F, et al. Age-related changes in cardiac autonomic control during sleep. J Sleep Res. 2003;12(3):173–80.
28. Jurysta F, van de Borne P, Lanquart J, Migeotte P, Degaute J, Dumont M, et al. Progressive aging does not alter the interaction between autonomic cardiac activity and delta EEG power. Clin Neurophysiol. 2005;116(4):871–7.
29. Koenig J, Thayer JF. Sex differences in healthy human heart rate variability: a meta-analysis. Neurosci Biobehav Rev. 2016;64:288–310.
30. Valladares EM, Eljammal SM, Motivala S, Ehlers CL, Irwin MR. Sex differences in cardiac sympathovagal balance and vagal tone during nocturnal sleep. Sleep Med. 2008;9(3):310–6.
31. Elsenbruch S, Harnish MJ, Orr WC. Heart rate variability during waking and sleep in healthy males and females. Sleep. 1999;22(8):1067–71.

32. Richard M, LeBlanc A, Pennestri M, Montplaisir J, Carrier J, Lavigne G, et al. The effect of gender on autonomic and respiratory responses during sleep among both young and middle-aged subjects. Sleep Med. 2007;8(7–8):760–7.
33. Saleh TM, Connell BJ. Role of oestrogen in the central regulation of autonomic function. Clin Exp Pharmacol Physiol. 2007;34(9):827–32.
34. de Zambotti M, Nicholas CL, Colrain IM, Trinder JA, Baker FC. Autonomic regulation across phases of the menstrual cycle and sleep stages in women with premenstrual syndrome and healthy controls. Psychoneuroendocrinology. 2013;38(11):2618–27.
35. de Zambotti M, Trinder J, Colrain I, Baker F. Menstrual cycle-related variation in autonomic nervous system functioning in women in the early menopausal transition with and without insomnia disorder. Psychoneuroendocrinology. 2017;75:44–51.
36. von Holzen JJ, Capaldo G, Wilhelm M, Stute P. Impact of endo- and exogenous estrogens on heart rate variability in women: a review. Climacteric. 2016;19(3):222–8.
37. Baker FC, de Zambotti M, Colrain IM, Bei B. Sleep problems during the menopausal transition: prevalence, impact, and management challenges. Nat Sci Sleep. 2018;10:73–95.
38. de Zambotti M, Colrain IM, Javitz HS, Baker FC. Magnitude of the impact of hot flashes on sleep in perimenopausal women. Fertil Steril. 2014;102(6):1708–15 e1.
39. de Zambotti M, Colrain IM, Sassoon SA, Nicholas CL, Trinder J, Baker FC. Vagal withdrawal during hot flashes occurring in undisturbed sleep. Menopause. 2013;20(11):1147–53.
40. Baker F, Forouzanfar M, Goldstone A, Claudatos S, Javitz H, Trinder J, et al. Changes in heart rate and blood pressure across nocturnal hot flashes associated with or without arousal from sleep. Sleep. 2019;42(11):pii: zsz175.
41. de Zambotti M, Cellini N, Goldstone A, Colrain I, Baker F. Wearable sleep technology in clinical and research settings. Med Sci Sports Exerc. 2019;51(7):1538–57.
42. de Zambotti M, Cellini N, Menghini L, Sarlo M, Baker FC. Sensors capabilities, performance, and use of consumer sleep technology. Sleep Med Clin. 2020;15(1):1–30. PMID: 32005346. PMCID: PMC7482551 (available on 2021-03-01). https://doi.org/10.1016/j.jsmc.2019.11.003.
43. Schäfer A, Vagedes J. How accurate is pulse rate variability as an estimate of heart rate variability?: a review on studies comparing photoplethysmographic technology with an electrocardiogram. Int J Cardiol. 2013;166(1):15–29.
44. de Zambotti M, Baker F, Willoughby A, Godino J, Wing D, Patrick K, et al. Measures of sleep and cardiac functioning during sleep using a multi-sensory commercially-available wristband in adolescents. Physiol Behav. 2016;158:143–9.

Nocturnal Arousal Phenomenon and the Autonomic Nervous System

8

Liborio Parrino

The heart asks pleasure first,
And then, excuse from pain;
And then, those little anodynes
That deaden suffering,
And then, to go to sleep;
And then, if it should be
The will of its Inquisitor,
The liberty to die.

—Emily Dickinson

The House of Sleep

According to the rules recommended by the American Academy of Sleep Medicine (AASM), sleep analysis is centered on the recognition of rapid eye movement (REM) sleep and non-REM sleep (NREM), the latter divided into three stages (N1, N2, N3) [1]. Stages N1 and N2 represent light sleep, and stage N3 corresponds to deep sleep. These stages and their temporal succession constitute the macrostructure of sleep.

Sleep macrostructure may also be called the architecture of sleep. Sleep macrostructure may be likened to the construction of a house with rooms, stairs, and functional spaces in addition to the openings in the external walls to let light and air inside, allowing interaction between the outward and the internal habitat (Fig. 8.1). In sleep, arousals may be considered as the windows of the house allowing integration between inner and environmental influences. Conventional electroencephalographic (EEG) arousals are transient intrusions (about 10 seconds) of wakefulness in sleep. As short-duration events, individuals retain no memory of nocturnal arousals but the body and the brain do not remain neutral to these transient interruptions: sleep EEG is abruptly replaced by a wake path, the muscle tone is activated, heart rate accelerates, and arterial pressure rises [2].

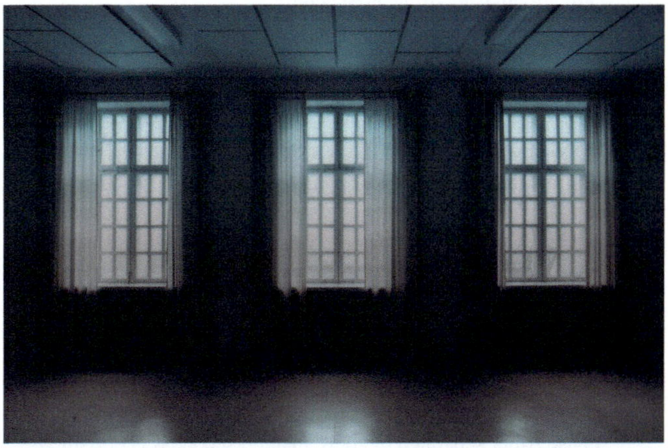

Fig. 8.1 A relaxing home setting as a metaphor of sleep architecture. Arousals are expressed by the windows that offer a two-way interaction with the outside world. (Photo courtesy of Hans Eiskonen on Unsplash)

Arousal is therefore an oxymoron, a lucid contradiction, which manages to combine the main characteristics of activity (dominance of the orthosympathetic nervous system) within a framework of quietness and rest (dominance of the vagal system). Being a fleeting activation, the impact of a single arousal tends to leave limited consequences on sleep continuity and on the health of the individual. However, in the context of physiological sleep, arousals rarely appear as isolated phenomena, while they are often aggregated to other arousals and organized like flying swarms (Fig. 8.2). These periodic EEG events become the choreography of sleep, a sequence named the cyclic alternating pattern or CAP (Box 8.1) [3].

During CAP, fluctuations in the level of vigilance swing in harmony with changes in the autonomic nervous system. The heart rhythm accelerates during phase A and slows down during phase B (Fig. 8.3). Similarly, muscle tone is activated during phase A and is attenuated during phase B.

L. Parrino (✉)
Sleep Disorders Center, Department of Medicine and Surgery, University Hospital Parma, Parma, Italy
e-mail: liborio.parrino@unipr.it

S. Chokroverty, P. Cortelli (eds.), *Autonomic Nervous System and Sleep*, https://doi.org/10.1007/978-3-030-62263-3_8

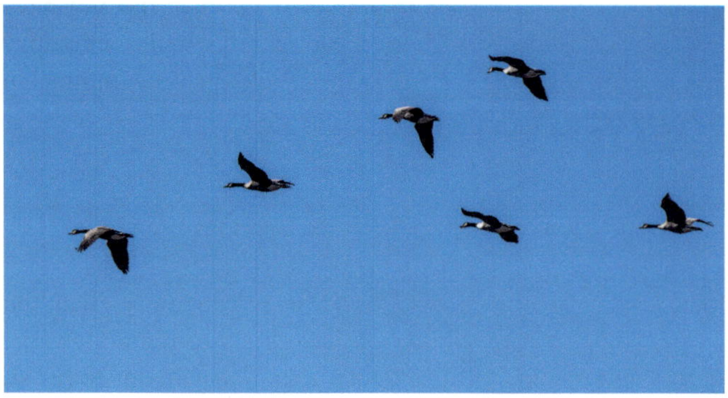

Fig. 8.2 In non-rapid eye movement (NREM) sleep, arousals rarely appear as scattered events but are lumped together in the organized cyclic alternating pattern (CAP) just like a flock of birds. (Photo courtesy of https://www.goodfreephotos.com)

Box 8.1 The Rules of the Cyclic Alternating Pattern (CAP)

In all non-rapid eye movement (NREM) stages, CAP is organized in sequences:

A CAP sequence consists of a succession of CAP cycles.

Each CAP cycle consists of a phase A (activation) and the following phase B (interval).

At least two consecutive CAP cycles are required to define a CAP sequence.

Each CAP phase has a duration of 2–60 seconds.

The absence of CAP for>60 seconds is defined as non-CAP.

An isolated phase A (i.e., preceded or followed by another phase A but separated by more than 60 seconds) is classified as non-CAP.

Non-CAP coincides with a condition of physiological stability.

Non-CAP and CAP sequences constitute the microstructure of sleep.

The A phases of CAP are identified by specific EEG features and reflect different degrees of cerebral, vegetative, and behavioral activation [2]:

- Subtypes A1: Dominated by K-complexes and delta bursts generally accompanied by a weak autonomic and motor enhancement.
- Subtypes A3: Consisting of alpha and beta EEG activities associated with powerful autonomic and behavioral impact.
- Subtypes A2: A mixture of A1 and A3 EEG features with intermediate vegetative and motor consequences.

Beyond the Sleep Stages

Under physiological conditions, subtypes A1 are involved in the buildup and consolidation of slow wave sleep (homeostatic process), while subtypes A2 and A3 mostly prepare the transition from NREM to REM sleep (ultradian process) [4]. This means that conventional arousals (CAP phases A2 and A3) and arousal-equivalents (CAP phases A1) play an active role in the dynamic organization of sleep. They become detrimental only when their amount exceeds certain limits or when they occur outside the operational sleep model.

The inability of conventional rules to capture the differences in EEG patterns within epochs and between epochs of the same stage is a puzzling issue. As pointed out by Younes et al. [5], a 30-s epoch is scored awake whether the EEG pattern is fully awake throughout or contains one or more brief sleep patterns (microsleep), so long as the duration of the sleep pattern is <15 seconds. Once the 15-s threshold is exceeded, the stage becomes sleep (N1, N2, N3, REM).

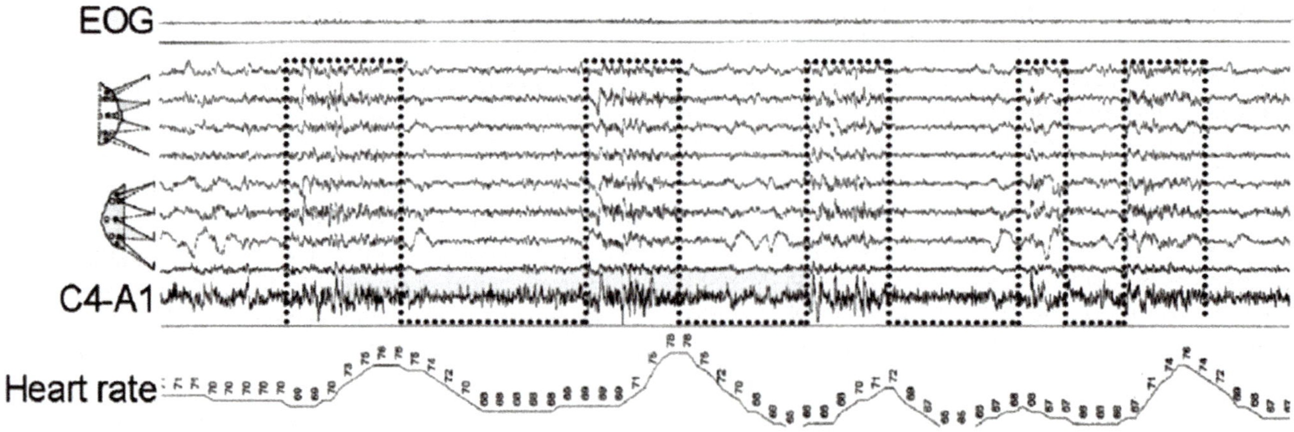

Fig. 8.3 When the cyclic alternating pattern (CAP) appears on the electroencephalogram, the autonomic system undergoes tempered synchronized oscillations with the A phases generally preceding the onset of cardiac rhythm increases

Likewise, sleep in any stage can be interrupted by EEG patterns associated with wakefulness, but the whole epoch is scored as sleep, so long as the awake patterns are <15 s in duration. It is also known that fast (beta) and slow (delta) EEG features oscillate reciprocally across NREM and REM sleep even within the same stage [6].

The phase A subtypes of CAP offer a more flexible interpretation of these dynamic shifts within and between the scoring epochs. High-amplitude slow rhythms or K-complexes are associated with the same kind of motor and vegetative changes typically accepted as arousal signs. Both spontaneous and evoked K-complexes are associated with a significant acceleration of heart rate compared to baseline conditions. According to Kokkinos et al. [7], "K-complex embodies an arousal with subsequent sleep guarding counteraction that might on one hand serve monitoring of the environment with basic information processing and on the other hand protect continuity of sleep and thus its restoring effect."

In children and young adults, CAP subtypes A1 become dominant. As we age, this subtype gradually becomes less frequent in elderly individuals. Conversely, A3 subtypes rise linearly from adulthood to senescence, reflecting an age-related decline of sleep resilience [8, 9].

In addition, CAP A phases enhance the hierarchic range of arousal responses in relation to the ongoing behavioral and autonomic conditions. In healthy individuals [10], CAP phases A3 remain unmodified under increasing sound pressure levels, while subtypes A1 and A2 parallel the rise of noise intensity applied throughout the night [11]. In sleep pathologies [12], subtypes A2 and A3 are increased in periodic limb movement disorders while all CAP subtypes are increased in sleep-related hypermotor epilepsy (SHE). In obstructive sleep apnea syndrome (OSAS) patients, 60.3% of hypopneas and 28.4% of apneas terminate with an A1 subtype during NREM sleep [13, 14], suggesting that weaker respiratory events require weaker EEG reactions to restore effective breathing. Analysis of sleep recordings carried out in OSAS patients also showed no difference in the arousal index between mild and moderate-severe OSAS patients, while CAP time underwent a progressive enhancement ($p < 0.0001$) from normal subjects (152.5 ± 20.76 min) to mild (180.64 ± 34.76 min) and moderate to severe (282.27 ± 58.02 min) conditions. Although only 41.1% of intermittent flow limitation (FL) events met the AASM criteria for the definition of RERA (respiratory effort-related arousal), 75.5% of FL events ended with a CAP A phase terminating in most cases (69.1%) with a phase A3 subtype [14]. Once again, micro-events related to sleep EEG or breathing patterns remain inadequately explored without the support of CAP metrics.

Surrogate Markers of Cortical Arousals

The use of portable monitoring has become a reliable cost-effective alternative to standard polysomnography, although this method lacks information on EEG activities. Analysis of polysomnographic recordings from 20 male individuals with OSAS quantified the combined (interval of 4 s before and 4 s after breathing recovery) or separate occurrence of CAP A-phases (cortical activation), and pulse wave amplitude (PWA) drops (below 30%) in relation to apneas, hypopneas and FL events. Across the night, 71.8% of all types of respiratory events were followed by a dual response (A phase associated with a PWA drop). The combined cortical and autonomic activation confirms that the perturbed sleeping brain reacts in most cases with a simultaneous activation of both EEG and vegetative subsystems and suggests a possible role of PWA as a marker of the EEG response to airflow reduction or increased upper airway resistance. Overall, 90% of apneas, 83% of hypopneas, and 69% of FL events were associated with a PWA drop, without significant differences between NREM and REM sleep. The study also showed a progressive increase of dual responses from FL to hypopneas and apneas indicating that the arousal response evolves into a more powerful and extensive activation as airway obstruction increases [15].

Measuring Heart Rate Variability: The R-R Interval

According to the polyvagal theory [16], a physiological state, characterized by a vagal withdrawal, would support the mobilization behaviors of fight and flight. In contrast, when the environment is perceived as safe, the bodily state promotes growth and restoration (e.g., visceral homeostasis) through an increase in the influence of myelinated vagal motor pathways on the cardiac pacemaker that slows the heart, inhibits the fight or flight mechanisms of the sympathetic nervous system, dampens the stress response system of the *hypothalamo-pituitary-adrenocortical* (HPA) axis (e.g., cortisol), and reduces inflammation by modulating immune reactions (e.g., cytokines).

The beat-to-beat variability is the superimposed sum of different rhythmic heart rate oscillations. The two main heart rate periodicities occur at a "fast" high-frequency (HF) associated with spontaneous breathing (i.e., respiratory sinus arrhythmia [RSA]) and a slower or "low" frequency (LF) assumed to be related to the endogenous rhythm of blood pressure regulation via the baroreceptors and spontaneous vasomotor activity.

The frequency of RSA is generated by the same brainstem mechanisms involved in generating the frequency of respiration, while the amplitude of RSA represents the functional impact of vagal efferent pathways originating in the nucleus ambiguus on the cardiac pacemaker [17–19].

RR intervals (RRI) are quantified by measuring the distance between ECG-derived R-waves. The LF component of RRI (LFRR) is considered a marker of sympathetic cardiac modulation, whereas the HF component of RRI variability reflects respiratory-driven vagal modulation to the sinoatrial node. During sleep, RRI increases in comparison to wakefulness, with concomitant decrease in low-frequency RRI and increases in high-frequency RRI oscillations.

R-R

In normal young adults, exposure to repetitive acoustically induced arousals during sleep produces cumulative effects on autonomic control characterized by significant increases in LF oscillations of systolic blood pressure. Moreover, the RSA gains that accompany progressive sleep depth in normal sleep are prevented from occurring [20].

In NREM sleep, the RRI increases before the A phase and decreases in the post-phase A epoch suggesting a relation between CAP and autonomic modulation. Although both sympathetic and parasympathetic pathways are involved during the occurrence of A phases, the increase of sympatho-vagal ratio LF/HF appears more relevant during post-epochs in A2 and A3 phases, commonly associated with visible sleep fragmentation. However, a significant increase in LF/HF and LF% also in both pre- and post-epochs of A1 subtypes is reported in *nocturnal frontal lobe epilepsy* (now renamed SHE), suggesting that these patients have continuously higher levels of arousal activity during NREM sleep [21]. Assessment of the cardiovascular system during sleep in normal controls and NFLE patients shows that all the activations (A phases) present a similar latency (4 seconds) at the minimum of the RR interval with respect to the A-phase onset [22].

Cardiopulmonary Coupling and CAP

During the respiratory cycle, the heart-to-electrode distance changes due to the movement of the ECG electrodes in relation to the heart. Accordingly, the QRS morphology and amplitude vary in concordance with the changes in the transthoracic impedance as the lungs fill and empty. Modulation of the respiratory signal obtained from a single-lead ECG is a technique known as ECG-derived respiration (EDR). Cardiopulmonary coupling (CPC) is a frequency-based method that captures the phase differences (or degree of coupling) between the EDR and the RRI [23].

Analyzing ratios between CPC and the main heart rate frequency bands, the preponderance of power ratio in the LF is correlated with CAP periods and can be an indication of periodic respiration during sleep disordered breathing. In contrast, a preponderance of power in the HF is associated with deep sleep, physiologic respiratory sinus arrhythmia, and non-CAP periods [24, 25]. In patients with severe OSAS, where CAP rate is heavily enhanced, the phase coupling is significantly lower compared to controls [24]. On the contrary, during continuous positive airway pressure (CPAP) therapy, which increases the amount of non-CAP, coupling shows a strengthened frequency [26]. The consistent association between EEG features (CAP vs non-CAP) and LF/HF modulation confirms that CPC can be used as a surrogate measure of sleep quality, OSA severity, and successful treatment. More extensively, these findings endorse the entangled interaction between rapid autonomic adjustments and the CAP system in the adaptive preservation of sleep against internal or environmental menaces.

Sleep Protection Insurance

Modern homes rely on a number of key systems (water supply, power, electronics, heating, and cooling) that influence the quality of our domestic lives. Although the architectural project of our sleep cannot be personally designed, we may try to understand the flexible solutions that the brain-body connection seeks to maintain survival during 8 hours of unconscious rest (Fig. 8.4). Resilience is the ability of a substance or object to spring back into shape, the capacity to recover quickly from adverse or sudden changes. Manifold guardians including circadian, ultradian, and homeostatic processes, brain networking, muscle tone, gravity, and dreams warrant sleep resilience, and CAP is one of these basic sentinels [9]. Unexpected perturbations require communication between the brain and body. An acoustic stimulus administered during sleep is elaborated at a microscale level (CAP) before inducing relevant macrostructural changes. Due to anatomic connectivity, assessment of the noise input inevitably spreads across the neural pathways carrying information to motor, sensorial, and vegetative networks. This sharing process enables the nervous system to evaluate the potential risk of the perturbing factor and generate suitable counter-actions. A transient noise can be perceived as trivial (e.g., a car passing by under the window) or relevant (a child crying in the night). In the first case, sleep will be reversibly interrupted by an arousal. In the second scenario, the parent will adopt a more complex behavior—processing the acoustic message, and rising to console the child. In both cases, EEG activation and autonomic activation must be coupled: one cannot stand and walk without ade-

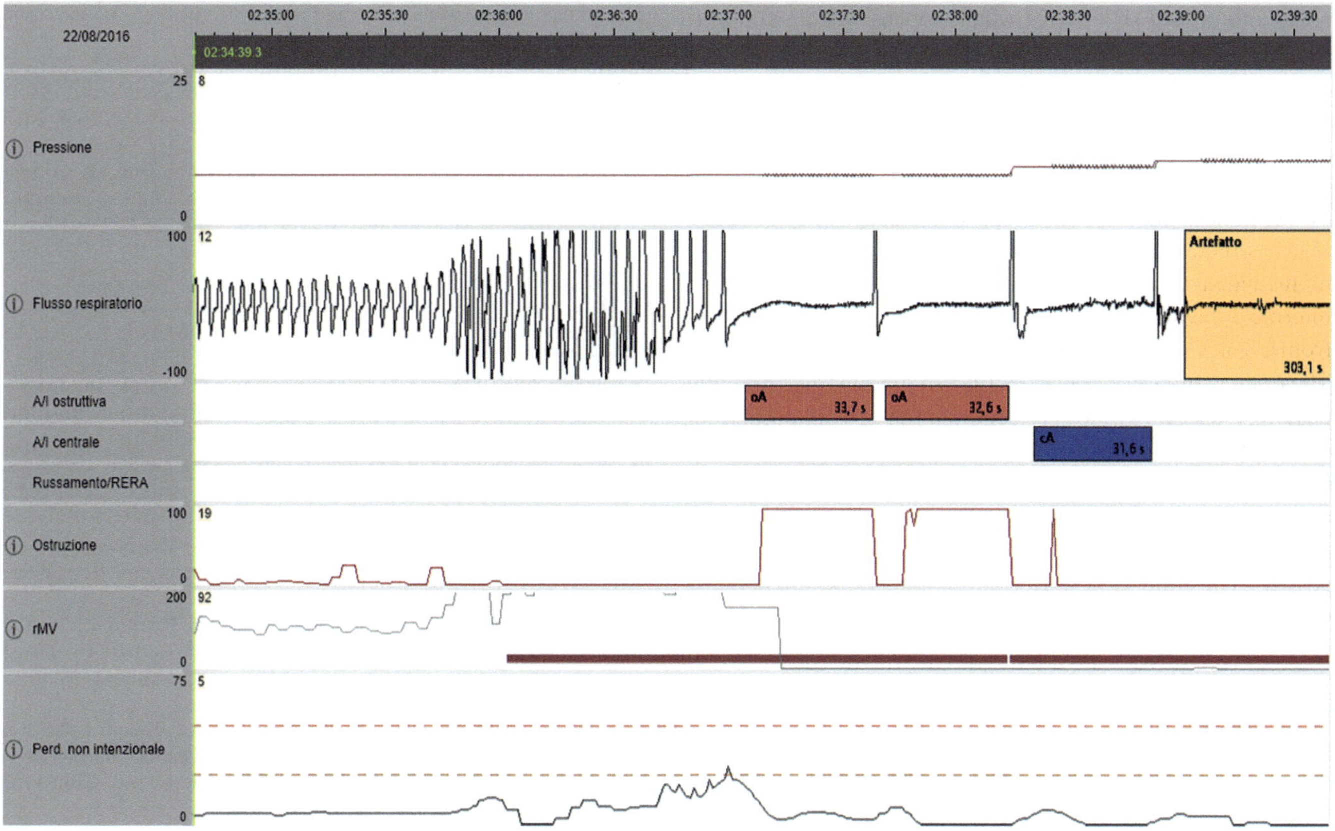

Fig. 8.4 The exact moment a man dies. This is the final nocturnal recording of an 80-year-old male effectively treated with continuous positive airway pressure (CPAP) therapy for severe sleep apnea syndrome. At 2:35 AM, the breathing flow shows a regular pattern indicating lack of respiratory trouble or menaces. Suddenly, an error occurs (likely a cardiac arrest) that is probably perceived by the patient who starts a powerful breathing to overcome the life-threatening condition. Whether the patient is fully awake or hyperventilation occurs automatically while asleep currently remains unknown. What is dramatically evident is the strenuous autonomic activation that a human being exploits before dying in the extreme effort to cling to life

quate values of blood pressure and heart rate. Moreover, if it is decided to maintain a passive strategy, at least for a number of seconds, the vegetative nervous system will be in an alert mode ready to shift from passive to active behavior. The restless flow of information between brain, body, and environment indicates that sleep is not only the autonomous development of a rigid internal algorithm, but it is also the product of the interaction between sleep and psychic and organic and external factors.

Every single arousal response is a cooperative phenomenon involving several interactions taking place in a coupled manner. According to the cybernetic law of requisite variety [27], availability of different arousal reactions (phase A subtypes of CAP) is mandatory to assure maintenance of sleep regulation when the system may undergo a wide spectrum of aggressions.

In neurodegenerative disorders [28, 29] where CAP rate is pathologically reduced, the lack of appropriate options (phase A subtypes) makes the system insufficient to respond to potential internal or environmental disruptors. In these conditions, the sleeping brain offers a fragile interface against ongoing menaces as the paucity of EEG arousal responses parallels a shortage of autonomic reactions. Besides motor impairment, patients with amyotrophic lateral sclerosis (ALS) show a typical unbalanced autonomic modulation. In ALS patients, EEG activity and vegetative functions during sleep are less reactive, as shown by a decreased CAP rate and a reduction in HRV features, both in time and frequency domain, influenced by sympathetic and vagal systems. In particular, full-night analysis shows reduced values of pNN20 (dependent on parasympathetic activity), LF (dependent on sympathetic activity), and LF/HF ratio [30].

In conclusion, nocturnal arousal phenomena are not a single all-or-nothing reaction but are expressed by a variety of adaptative processes during sleep. Variety means the total number of possible macro- and microstates of a system. Because redundancy increases systemic stability, sleep can survive when the number of states is greater than or equal to the number of potential or unexpected factors that need to be controlled. During sleep, a healthy brain can also transform noise into order [31]. This is what happens when a stimulus triggers a CAP sequence: a succession of EEG arousals and arousal-equivalents aiming to preserve sleep continuity. This protective reaction is accompanied by intermittent autonomic activation ensuring a higher readiness for awakening by enhancing sensory transmission. A special microstate that avoids useless interruptions of sleep and adaptively reduces a potentially dangerous sensory deafferentation [32]. A brain-body reaction that transforms a trivial noisy input into a meaningful cascade of events which increases systemic complexity and information during sleep [31]. Siclari et al. [33] identified large slow waves in the frontal regions (possibly CAP A1 subtypes), which occurred on a background of reduced SWA and were associated with high-frequency power increases (local "microarousals") heralding the successful recall of dream content. Does this mean that arousal events are also associated with elementary cognitive processes? The time is now ripe to explore these challenging issues.

References

1. Iber C, Ancoli-Israel S, Chesson AL, Quan SF. The AASM manual for the scoring of sleep and associated events: rules, terminology, and technical specifications. 1st ed. Westchester: American Academy of Sleep Medicine; 2007.
2. Sforza E, Jouny C, Ibanez V. Cardiac activation during arousal in humans: further evidence for hierarchy in the arousal response. Clin Neurophysiol. 2000;111(9):1611–9.
3. Smerieri A, Parrino L, Agosti M, Ferri R, Terzano MG. Cyclic alternating pattern sequences and non-cyclic alternating pattern periods in human sleep. Clin Neurophysiol. 2007;118(10):2305–13.
4. Terzano MG, Parrino L, Smerieri A, Carli F, Nobili L, Donadio S, Ferrillo F. CAP and arousals are involved in the homeostatic and ultradian sleep processes. J Sleep Res. 2005;14(4):359–68.
5. Younes M, Ostrowski M, Soiferman M, Younes H, Younes M, Raneri J, Hanly P. Odds ratio product of sleep EEG as a continuous measure of sleep state. Sleep. 2015;38(4):641–54.
6. Uchida S, Maloney T, Feinberg I. Beta (20–28 Hz) and delta (0.3–3 Hz) EEGs oscillate reciprocally across NREM and REM sleep. Sleep. 1992 Aug;15(4):352–8.
7. Kokkinos V, Koupparis AM, Kostopoulos GK. An intra-K-complex oscillation with independent and labile frequency and topography in NREM sleep. Front Hum Neurosci. 2013;7:163.
8. Parrino L, Boselli M, Spaggiari MC, Smerieri A, Terzano MG. Cyclic alternating pattern (CAP) in normal sleep: polysomnographic parameters in different age groups. Electroencephalogr Clin Neurophysiol. 1998;107(6):439–50.
9. Parrino L, Vaudano AE. The resilient brain and the guardians of sleep: new perspectives on old assumptions. Sleep Med Rev. 2018;39:98–107.
10. Halász P, Bódizs R, Parrino L, Terzano M. Two features of sleep slow waves: homeostatic and reactive aspects—from long term to instant sleep homeostasis. Sleep Med. 2014;15(10):1184–95.
11. Terzano MG, Parrino L. Functional relationship between micro- and macrostructure of sleep. In: Terzano MG, Halasz P, Declerck AC, editors. Phasic events and dynamic organization of sleep. New York: Raven Press; 1991. p. 101–19.
12. Parrino L, Ferri R, Bruni O, Terzano MG. Cyclic alternating pattern (CAP): the marker of sleep instability. Sleep Med Rev. 2012;16(1):27–45.
13. Thomas RJ. Arousals in sleep-disordered breathing: patterns and implications. Sleep. 2003;26(8):1042–7.
14. Milioli G, Bosi M, Grassi A, Riccardi S, Terzano MG, Cortelli P, et al. Can sleep microstructure improve diagnosis of OSAS? Integrative information from CAP parameters. Arch Ital Biol. 2015 Jun-Sep;153(2–3):194–203.
15. Bosi M, Milioli G, Riccardi S, Melpignano A, Vaudano AE, Cortelli P, et al. Arousal responses to respiratory events during sleep: the role of pulse wave amplitude. J Sleep Res. 2018;27(2):259–67.
16. Porges SW. The polyvagal perspective. Biol Psychol. 2007;74(2):116–43.
17. Haselton JR, Solomon IC, Motekaitis AM, Kaufman MP. Bronchomotor vagal preganglionic cell bodies in the dog: an anatomic and functional study. J Appl Physiol. 1992;73:1122–9.
18. Richter DW, Spyer KM. Cardiorespiratory control. In: Loewy AD, Syper KM, editors. Central regulation of autonomic function. New York: Oxford University Press; 1990. p. 189–207.
19. Spye KM, Jordan D. Electrophysiology and the nucleus ambiguus. In: Hainsworth R, McWilliam PN, Mary D, editors. Cardiogenic reflexes. London: Oxford; 1987. p. 237–49.
20. Chaicharn J, Carrington M, Trinder J, Khoo MC. The effects on cardiovascular autonomic control of repetitive arousal from sleep. Sleep. 2008;31(1):93–103.
21. Dorantes-Méndez G, Mendez MO, Alba A, Parrino L, Milioli G. Time-varying analysis of the heart rate variability during A-phases of sleep: healthy and pathologic conditions. Biomed Signal Process Control. 2018;40:111–6.
22. Dorantes G, Méndez M, Alba A, Gonzaáez JS, Parrino L, Milioli G. Heart rate variability in cyclic alternating pattern during sleep in healthy and Nocturnal Front Lobe Epilepsy patients. Conf Proc IEEE Eng Med Biol Soc. 2015;2015:5944–7.
23. Thomas RJ, Mietus JE, Peng CK, Goldberger AL. An electrocardiogram-based technique to assess cardiopulmonary coupling during sleep. Sleep. 2005;28(9):1151–61.
24. Ibrahim LH, Jacono FJ, Patel SR, Thomas RJ, Larkin EK, Mietus JE, Peng CK, Goldberger AL, Redline S. Heritability of abnormalities in cardiopulmonary coupling in sleep apnea: use of an electrocardiogram-based technique. Sleep. 2010;33(5):643–6.
25. Kabir MM, Dimitri H, Sanders P, Antic R, Nalivaiko E, Abbott D, Baumert M. Cardiorespiratory phase-coupling is reduced in patients with obstructive sleep apnea. PLoS One. 2010 May 13;5(5):e10602.
26. Chang JS, Lee SD, Ju G, Kim JW, Ha K, Yoon IY. Enhanced cardiorespiratory coupling in patients with obstructive sleep apnea following continuous positive airway pressure treatment. Sleep Med. 2013;14(11):1132–8.
27. Ashby WB. Requisite variety and its implications for the control of complex systems. Cybernetica. 1958;1(2):83–99.
28. Carnicelli L, Maestri M, Di Coscio E, Tognoni G, Fabbrini M, Schirru A, et al. A longitudinal study of polysomnographic variables in patients with mild cognitive impairment converting to Alzheimer's disease. J Sleep Res. 2019;28(5):e12821.
29. Melpignano A, Parrino L, Santamaria J, Gaig C, Trippi I, Serradell M, et al. Isolated rapid eye movement sleep behavior disorder and cyclic alternating pattern: is sleep microstructure a predictive parameter of neurodegeneration? Sleep. 2019;42(10):zsz142.
30. Congiu P, Mariani S, Milioli G, Parrino L, Tamburrino L, Borghero G, et al. Sleep cardiac dysautonomia and EEG oscillations in amyotrophic lateral sclerosis. Sleep. 2019;42(11):zsz164.
31. Atlan HL. Organisation biologique et la théorie de l'information. Paris: Hermann; 1972.
32. Halasz P, Ujszaszi J. Spectral features of evoked micro-arousals. In: Terzano MG, Halasz P, Declerck AC, editors. Phasic events and dynamic organization of sleep. New York: Raven Press; 1991. p. 85–100.
33. Siclari F, Bernardi G, Cataldi J, Tononi G. Dreaming in NREM sleep: a high-density EEG study of slow waves and spindles. J Neurosci. 2018;38(43):9175–85.

Part II

Laboratory Evaluation

Methods of Laboratory Evaluation of the Autonomic Nervous System in Wakefulness and Sleep

9

Jacquie Baker and Kurt Kimpinski

Laboratory Evaluation of the Autonomic Nervous System (ANS) in Wakefulness

Clinically Validated Methods for Evaluation of Sudomotor Function

Quantitative Sudomotor Axon Reflex Test (QSART)

Equipment To obtain accurate and reliable sweat volumes the following are required: (1) sudorometer, (2) multi-compartmental sweat capsules, and (3) acetylcholine (ACh) preparation.

Sudorometer QSART was originally validated at the Mayo Clinic (Rochester, MN) using a Mayo-built sudorometer and nitrogen gas to calculate relative humidity changes. However, because the Mayo-built sudorometer was not commercially available, another QSART device, namely Q-Sweat (WR Medical, Maplewood MN, USA), has since been manufactured and is commercially available. In contrast to the Mayo-built sudorometer, Q-Sweat uses dehumidified room air drawn in from an intake pump and channeled through desiccant. Air returning from the skin, consisting of evaporated sweat, causes a relative humidity change that is calculated and interpreted as a sweat response [1]. Studies directly comparing the two devices show similar sweat responses [2, 3].

J. Baker (✉)
University Hospital, London Health Sciences Centre, London, ON, Canada
e-mail: jbaker62@alumni.uwo.ca

K. Kimpinski
School of Kinesiology, Western University, London, ON, Canada

Department of Clinical Neurological Sciences, University Hospital, London Health Sciences Centre, London, ON, Canada

Schulich School of Medicine & Dentistry, Western University, London, ON, Canada

Acetylcholine Two different ACh preparations have been validated: either a solution-based vehicle consisting of a 10% weight:volume ratio or a gel-based preparation consisting of 0.55 M ACh in a 2.4 weight/volume agarose gel [3]. The advantage of the solution is that it is quick and easy to mix, whereas gel preparation must be done in advance. However, there are some technical challenges to working with the solution, which can cause the liquid to leak into the recording compartment of the multi-compartmental sweat capsule [2]. In contrast, the consistency of the gel helps to maintain constant contact at the skin–capsule interface, which not only prevents leaking across compartments but also avoids air leaks that can interrupt volume recordings. In an early study, directly comparing gel- versus solution-based methods, there were no remarkable differences [3]. Furthermore, sweat volumes have been further compared using both the gel-based delivery with the commercially available Q-Sweat device. Normative data using these methods compared favorably to the volumes originally validated at the Mayo Clinic [2].

Protocol Throughout testing, individuals should remain supine in a quiet room maintained at a relatively constant temperature (~23.5–25.5°C). Prior to testing, the skin must be prepared using the following four-step process: First, acetone is used to remove excess oils, followed by alcohol to remove acetone and water to remove alcohol, and the preparation is finished by using a dry paper towel to remove any excess moisture [1]. This process is performed at the following four standard sites: forearm (ulnar nerve: ~3/4 the distance between the ulnar epicondyle and pisiform), proximal leg (peroneal nerve: ~5 cm distal to the fibular head), distal leg (saphenous nerve: ~5 cm proximal to the medial malleolus) and the dorsal foot (sural nerve: flat surface over the extensor digitorum brevis) [1]. To complete the circuit, adhesive ground electrodes are placed ~3–5 cm proximal to the sweat gland. Once all sweat capsules are in place and a flat baseline is achieved, ACh is trans-dermally iontophoresed at

S. Chokroverty, P. Cortelli (eds.), *Autonomic Nervous System and Sleep*, https://doi.org/10.1007/978-3-030-62263-3_9

a constant current of 2 mA for 5 minutes. Following stimulation, an additional 5-minute post-stimulation period is completed to record residual sweat responses. Software programs, that is, WR Testworks (WR Medical Electronics, Maplewood, MN, USA), can calculate total sweat volumes from the integrated area under the curve for the entire 10-minute protocol.

Physiology Quantitative Sudomotor Axon Reflex Test (QSART) evaluates the integrity of post-ganglionic sympathetic axons. The neural pathway consists of an axon reflex mediated by the post-ganglionic sympathetic sudomotor axon. ACh binds to nicotinic receptors to activate the axon terminal, creating an antidromic impulse that travels to a branch point. Subsequently, an orthodromic impulse travels to a secondary nerve terminal whereby ACh is released. ACh released from the secondary axon terminal binds to M3 muscarinic receptors on eccrine sweat glands to evoke a reflexive sweat response [1, 4]. Total sweat volumes provide an assessment of the integrity of this reflex pathway. Normative sweat volume data collected both in the United States and Canada report a significant effect of sex and age on sweat volumes [2, 3]. Generally speaking, males sweat more than females and total sweat volumes significantly decline with age. To control for technical differences and geographical regions, it is encouraged for individual labs to generate their own normative data. For those laboratories just starting out, normative data are available [3]. A normal sweat response is indicative of an intact post-ganglionic sympathetic axon reflex.

Clinical Interpretation Absent or reduced sweat volumes indicate a lesion to the post-ganglionic axon (Fig. 9.1a). In peripheral neuropathies, the distribution of sweat volume responses is of particular importance as length dependent change can provide insight into the severity of impairment. Diabetic autonomic neuropathies and other small fiber neuropathies will show absent or reduced sweat volumes at more distal sites, and as the severity of the disease progresses, evidence of more proximal impairment will emerge (Fig. 9.1b).

In disorders of autonomic dysfunction consisting of a preganglionic lesions (i.e. multiple system atrophy [MSA]) QSART may appear normal; however, up to 30% of MSA patients can have abnormal QSART responses [5]. In contrast, patient with post-ganglionic lesions (pure autonomic failure [PAF], Parkinson disease [PD] + autonomic failure, etc.) will show evidence of reduced or absent sweat responses indicative of post-ganglionic sympathetic sudomotor failure (see Fig. 9.1a). Although not widely available, thermoregulatory sweat testing (TST) is another clinically validated tool that, when used in conjunction with QSART, can delineate impairment of pre- versus post-ganglionic sympathetic pathways. For example, TST stimulates a rise in core body temperature (CBT), a reflexive sympathetic response mediated by both pre- and post-ganglionic nerves [4]. Therefore, abnormal TST + normal QSART would indicate a preganglionic lesion. For a more in-depth discussion of TST, see the studies by Low and colleagues [6].

Sympathetic Skin Response

Protocol Sympathetic Skin Response (SSR) can be done using a standard electromyography (EMG) machine with silver-silver chloride electrodes. Electrodes should be placed where there is a high density of eccrine sweat glands. Typically, recordings are taken from the palm and sole of the foot, with a reference electrode placed on the dorsum of the respective body parts [7, 8]. Similar to QSART, subjects should be supine in a laboratory setting maintained at a constant temperature (22–24°C). In addition, skin temperature should be maintained between 32 and 36°C [7]. SSR can be evoked using a variety of stimuli; however, the most common is electrical stimulation delivered at a peripheral nerve, frequently the median and tibial, respectively. A single-square wave electrical pulse, 0.1–0.2 ms in duration delivered at an intensity of 10–50 mA, is frequently applied to both the contralateral and ipsilateral sides relative to the site of recording. Inter-stimulus intervals should typically be >60 seconds to minimize habituation [7, 8].

Physiology Similar to QSART, SSRs originate by activation of a polysynaptic reflex arc. Efferent sympathetic c-fibers activate eccrine sweat glands through a cholinergic pathway, as the response can be blocked with atropine [9]. SSR measures the change in potential on the surface of the skin, which represents sudomotor sympathetic nerve function. SSR evoked responses can be triphasic, biphasic, and, although rare, monophasic. The shape consists usually of positive and negative deflections with inter- and intra-individual variations in shape, latency, and amplitude. Two similar, yet opposing responses have been reported: P-type and N-type although P-type is most common [8], (Fig. 9.2). Latency of the SSR response is measured from the onset of stimulation to the first deflection from baseline. Amplitude is measured from the peak of the first deflection to the peak of the second deflection (peak-to-peak amplitude). Normative values for latency and amplitude have been quantified from upper and lower extremities [8]. Factors that can influence SSR include body temperature, type of stimulus used (i.e., cough, loud noise, inspiratory gasp), habituation, and individual demographics such as sex, age, and height.

Clinical Interpretation SSR is most frequently used to assess relative impairment of post-ganglionic sudomotor sympathetic fibers in peripheral neuropathies. However,

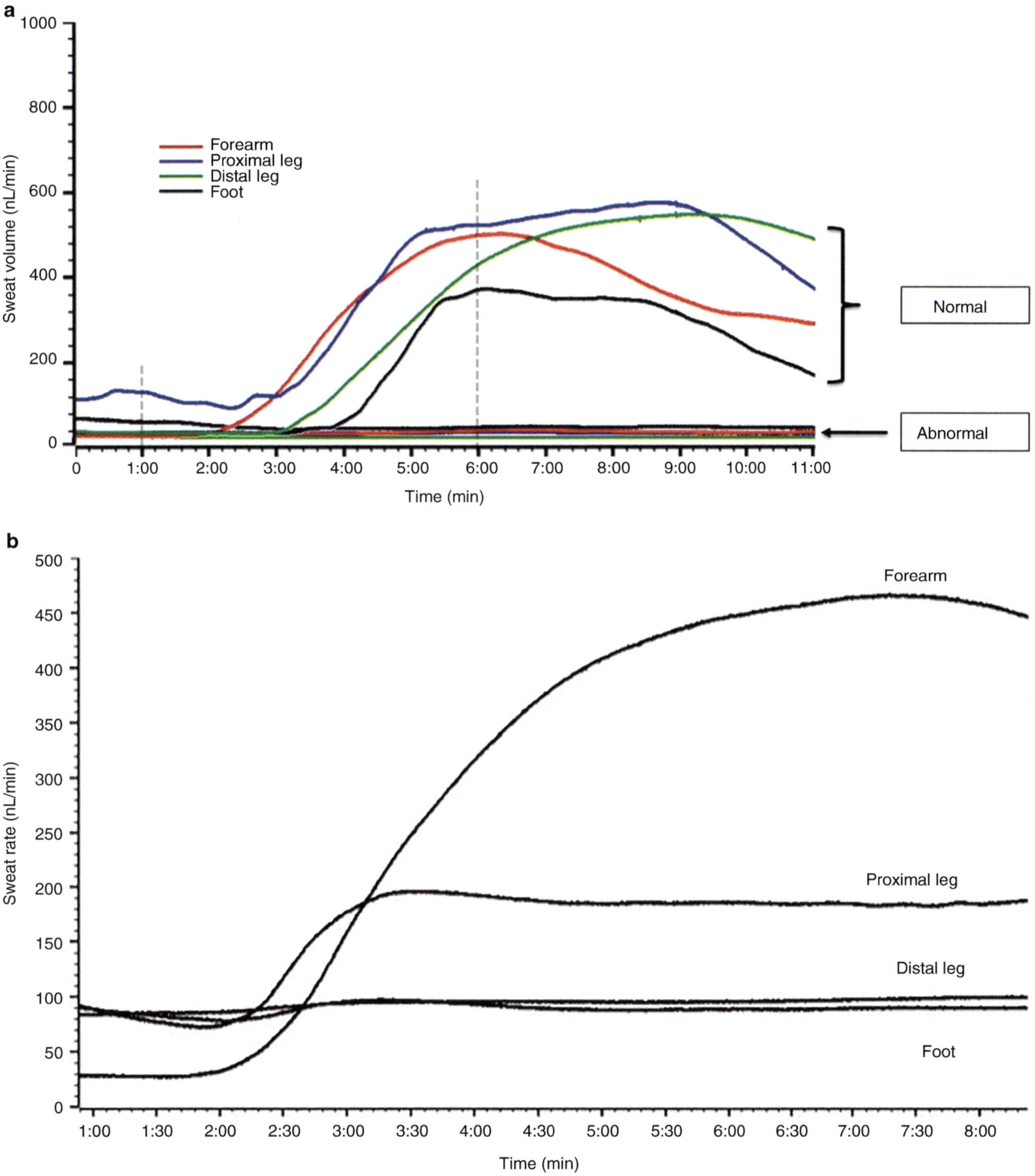

Fig. 9.1 Normal, abnormal (**a**) and length-dependent (**b**) sweat changes during QSART

there is little consensus on proper methods for evaluating SSR responses for detecting pathological states. Some laboratories use a qualitative approach, for example, absence of an SSR at one or more sites is indicative of a pathological state. In contrast, other laboratories favor quantitative evaluation of the latency and amplitude parameters [8].

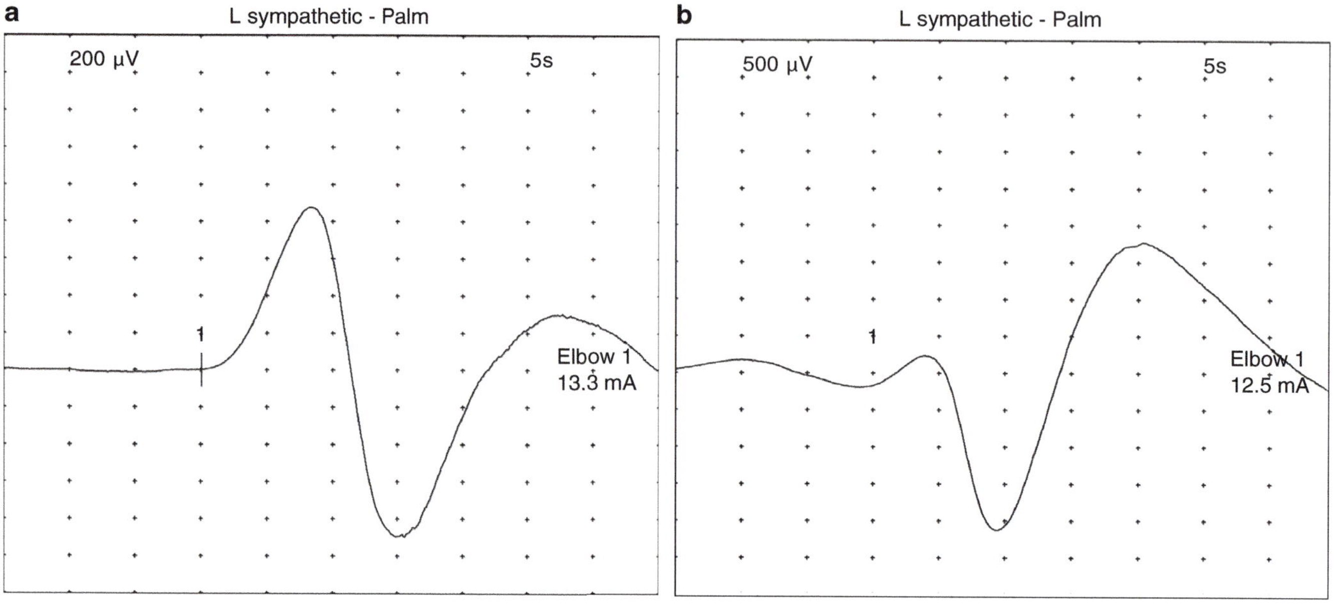

Fig. 9.2 Sympathetic skin response waveforms: (**a**) N-wave (scaled) and (**b**) P-wave (scaled)

Heart Rate Response to Deep Breathing (HRDB)

Equipment: ECG Autonomic testing can be completed with a standard three-lead electrocardiography. To ensure good contact and limit electrical impedance, avoid placing electrodes over any bony prominences. In addition, the skin should be prepared such that the electrodes remain intact at the site of placement. To enhance contact, ensure the skin is dry, removed of any excess oils, hair, and/or dead skin. Following adequate skin preparation, place chest electrodes below each clavicle within the ribcage. Place the lower lead on the left side below the lower edge of the left ribcage.

Beat-to-Beat Recording of Blood Pressure While the Korotkoff method remains the clinical gold standard for non-invasive blood pressure (BP) monitoring. This technique, along with the automated oscillometric method, is largely limited in autonomic assessments by the non-continuous nature of the recordings. The ability to measure beat-to-beat blood pressure (BP) remains an essential component for autonomic testing. While arterial catheterization remains the gold standard, this technique is invasive, requires trained personnel and introduces addition risk to the patient [10]. Therefore, the Penaz technique was the first to offer a non-invasive method for continuous blood pressure monitoring. The technique applies a volume-clamp approach using a small finger cuff containing a photoplethysmograph. Using a light source on one side of the cuff and an infrared receiver on the other side, blood volume could be estimated based on absorbance of the infrared light. "Finapres" (finger arterial pressure) (Finapres Medical Systems BV, Enschede, The Netherlands) was the first to modify the Penaz technique and is currently one of the most widely used devices for continuous blood pressure monitoring [10]. Furthermore, Finapres BP measurements accurately reflect blood pressure when calibrated against intra-arterial measurements, and notably, the calibration is maintained throughout autonomic maneuvers [1].

Protocol To produce the maximal variation between breaths, individuals are asked to complete eight breaths at a rate of six breaths/minute.

[11]. Participants should be encouraged to breathe slow and steady so that breaths are smooth, but maximal. Visual feedback can be provided using an oscillatory bar set at a period of 10 seconds. Under ideal testing conditions, the maneuver should be repeated at minimum, two times in order to see two consistent responses. Standard analysis consists of calculating the five highest consecutive peak-to-trough heart rate (HR) differences (maximum–minimum) and averaging these values to provide an average heart rate response to deep breathing.

Physiology Breathing naturally causes a pattern of discharge from the vagus nerve, and the rate of discharge can be influenced by the rate and depth of respiration. The vagus nerve to the heart contains both the afferent and efferent pathways for this reflex arc, and therefore a robust heart rate change during deep breathing is regarded as a measure of healthy cardiovagal functioning. In contrast, reduced HR responses to deep breathing suggest cardiovagal impairment. To accurate interpret cardiovagal impairment, normative data for HRDB have been generated across different laboratories [2, 3]. In general, a consistent effect of age but not sex has been reported [2, 3] such that the average heart rate response progressively declines with age. However, as with all normative datasets it is encouraged for individual labs to generate their own set of control values. As with QSART, normative data have been generated and are available for reference. Other significant factors that may influence heart rate outcomes include: rate and depth of breathing, hypocapnia, medications, and obesity [3].

Clinical Interpretation Based on the generation of normative datasets, a physiological "normal" can be determined for different age groups. Reduced/absent heart rate responses relative to a healthy age- and sex-matched cohort provide evidence of cardiovagal impairment (Fig. 9.3).

Valsalva Maneuver (VM)

Protocol While in the supine position, participants are instructed to perform a deep inhalation with the mouthpiece out of their mouth. Immediately following inhalation, participants should then be instructed to put the mouthpiece in their mouth, create a tight seal around the mouthpiece, and subsequently exhale into the mouthpiece. Exhalation should be maintained at an expiratory pressure of 40 mm Hg held for 15 seconds. Following release of the maneuver, participants should be encouraged not to talk for 30 seconds while a recovery phase is completed.

Physiology Valsalva maneuver (VM) is a simple, noninvasive test ideal for providing information regarding adrenergic and cardiovagal health. The response consists of beat-to-beat changes in blood pressure that, when properly executed, produce the following quadriphasic blood pressure response (Fig. 9.4a).

- Phase I: Phase I is mechanical in nature, upon inhalation there is a large increase in intra-thoracic pressure that causes compression of the aorta and a subsequent small increase in systolic blood pressure (SBP).
- Phase II_Early: In early phase II, there is a transient decline in SBP due to a reduced stroke volume and consequently a reduction in cardiac output (Q).
- Phase II_Late: The drop in SBP is arrested and begins to rise as a result of increased plasma concentration of norepinephrine (NE) and increased sympathetic discharge. This response is alpha-adrenergically mediated and together increase total peripheral resistance (TPR).
- Phase III: Phase III, similar to Phase I, is mechanical. Upon release of the maneuver, the drop in intra-thoracic pressure results in a rapid drop in SBP.
- Phase IV: In response to the sudden drop in SBP in Phase III, there is a burst in sympathetic activity to increase Q. Increased Q in conjunction with the increased TPR from Phase II_Late results in a large SBP overshoot above baseline levels.

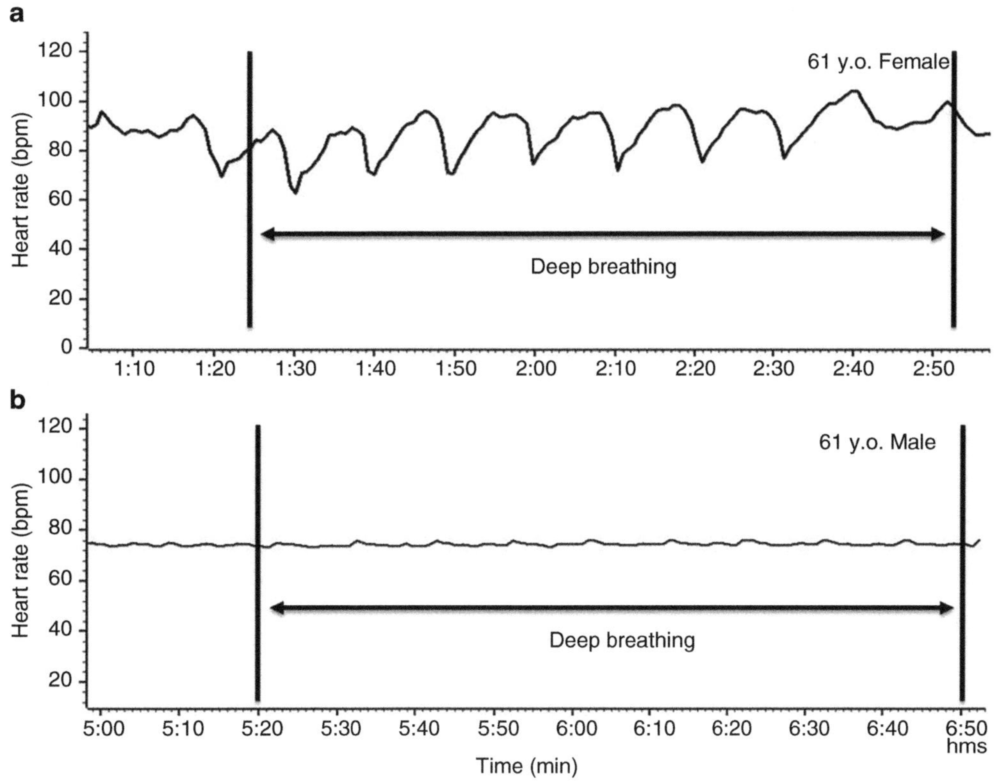

Fig. 9.3 Normal (**a**) and severely reduced (**b**) heart rate responses to deep breathing

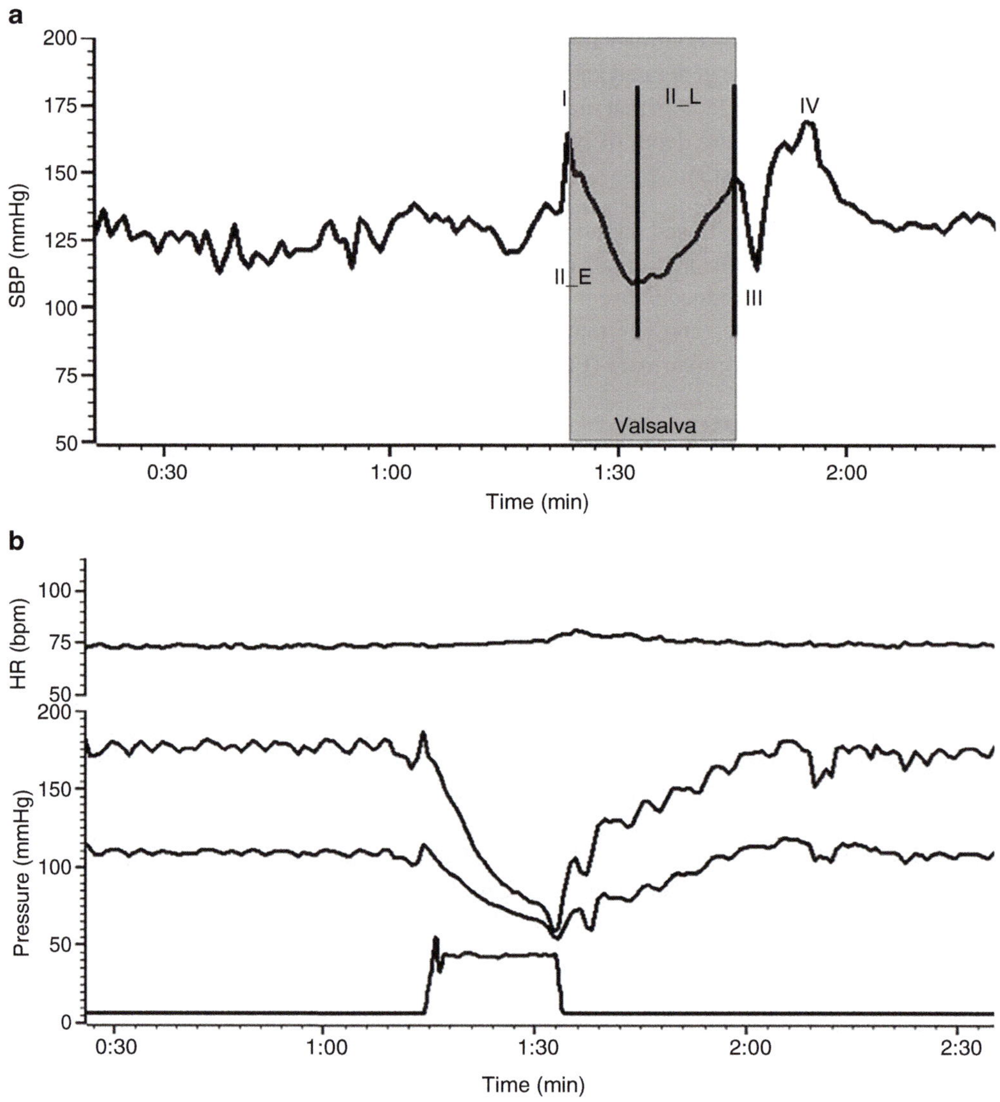

Fig. 9.4 Normal (**a**) and impaired (**b**) hemodynamic responses to Valsalva maneuver

Clinical Interpretation When properly executed, this maneuver provides immediate qualitative interpretation of cardiovagal (Valsalva ratio [VR]), alpha-adrenergic (late phase II) and beta-adrenergic (phase IV) health. Physically the vagus nerve is a long nerve, and as such shows impairment in the early stages of diabetic autonomic neuropathies. Reduced VRs indicate evidence of cardiovagal impairment, which can be present before adrenergic impairment. In contrast, patients with peripheral adrenergic failure will have an absent late phase II, but intact phase IV. When both late phase II and phase IV are absent, this indicates both peripheral and cardiac sympathetic innervation is impaired (Fig. 9.4b).

It is important to note that in healthy individuals the classic quadriphasic response previously described can be variable. For example, in a study of over 100 healthy individuals, only 40% displayed the classic hemodynamic response (Fig. 9.5a). Among the remaining 60%, two other blood pressure patterns emerged [12]. In some cases, late phase II can be so efficient that by the end of the maneuver, systolic blood pressure is already at or above baseline levels. As a result, the phase IV overshoot will be less profound (Fig. 9.5b). A third pattern, predominantly evident in females, revealed a blood pressure pattern with a large rise in SBP during phase I. As a result, SBP does not fall below baseline levels during Phase II_Early. This response can obscure the physiological need for an overshoot and as such has been called a flat-top response (Fig. 9.5c). Previous studies have either omitted these responses from data analysis or corrected them by tilting individuals upward ~20° [13, 14]. However, given the prevalence in healthy populations, the data argue that these responses represent healthy variability. Despite the variable phase IV overshoot, late phase II is

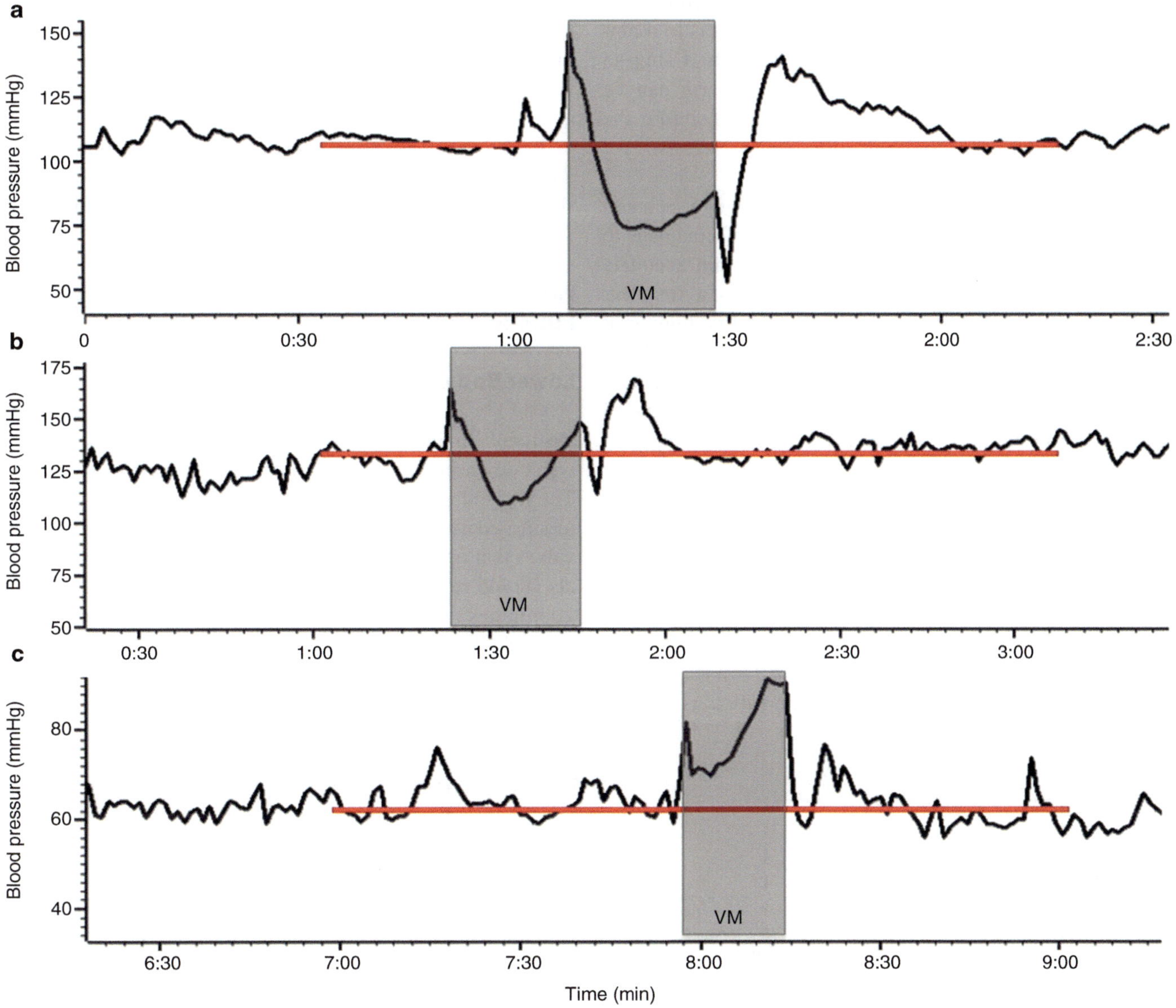

Fig. 9.5 Three blood pressure profiles in response to Valsalva maneuver in healthy individuals. Black lines represent systolic blood pressure; red lines represent average baseline blood pressure levels

always evident in healthy populations and together provides important clinical information.

Valsalva Ratio During the maneuver, there is a progressive compensatory tachycardia due to the decrease in SBP starting from Phase II_Early. Subsequently, the Phase IV SBP overshoot is accompanied by a transient bradycardia following release of the maneuver. As a result, in addition to detecting adrenergic dysfunction/failure, proper VM execution can provide an additional measure of cardiovagal functioning derived from this heart rate response, known as the Valsalva ratio. A VR is calculated by dividing the highest heart rate generated from the maneuver by the lowest heart rate achieved within 30 seconds following maneuver release.

Head-Up Tilt (HUT)

Protocol Beat-to-beat heart rate and blood pressure responses to an orthostatic challenge, such as passive head-up tilt (HUT) provide key insight into adrenergic function. Individuals should remain in the supine position for a minimum of 20 minutes prior to tilt. Following baseline, passively tilt the angle of the bed to a minimum of 60° from the horizontal. An angle below 60° does not generate sufficient orthostatic stress; therefore 70° is often used to produce sufficient orthostatic stress, while simultaneously minimizing large muscle contraction. During tilt it is important to ensure that the arm or hand recording BP remains at heart level, as position can influence measurements. Methods for maintaining the hand at the appropriate level includes the following: (1) Individual participation: if capable ask patients to maintain their hand at the axillary line. (2) Armrests: Using an armrest that attaches to the bed, a patient's arm can be abducted, placed in the armrest, and remain therefore the duration of testing.

Physiology In response to an orthostatic challenge such as a passive head-up tilt (HUT), there are natural mechanisms to counteract the effects of gravity and to maintain adequate blood pressure. Upon the initial tilt, there is a transient decline in SBP that often recovers within the first minute of HUT (Fig. 9.6a). This recovery is mediated by sympathetic activation resulting in reflexive tachycardia, increased release of norepinephrine and increased total peripheral resistance via vasoconstriction. Therefore, measuring the changes in HR and SBP in response to HUT provides a measure of sympathetic function.

Clinical Interpretation In patients with adrenergic failure, there is a marked and progressive fall in blood pressure and pulse pressure. Patients with concurrent cardiac sympathetic impairment will also not demonstrate an appropriate compensatory tachycardia in response to the BP fall (Fig. 9.6b). In contrast, if cardiac sympathetic innervation is spared, patients can mount a compensatory heart rate response (Fig. 9.6c). In postural orthostatic tachycardia syndrome, there is evidence of an excessive postural tachycardia with very little changes to orthostatic blood pressure (Fig. 9.6d).

In vasovagal syncope, early hemodynamic responses may appear normal; however, with prolonged tilt, patients will show progressive BP, pulse pressure, and HR reductions.

Non-clinically Validated Tests of Autonomic Functioning

Lower Body Negative Pressure (LBNP)

Protocol In the supine position, patients are sealed from the waist down in an airtight container connected to a vacuum. The level of suction (i.e. negative pressure) can be precisely monitored using a manometer and rapidly controlled through valves that open to room pressure. Similar to HUT, individuals should remain in the supine position for a minimum of 20 minutes prior to testing. LBNP provides a unique orthostatic challenge, especially for patients with limited mobility, as the testing can be executed entirely in the supine position while still producing a similar orthostatic challenge to that of

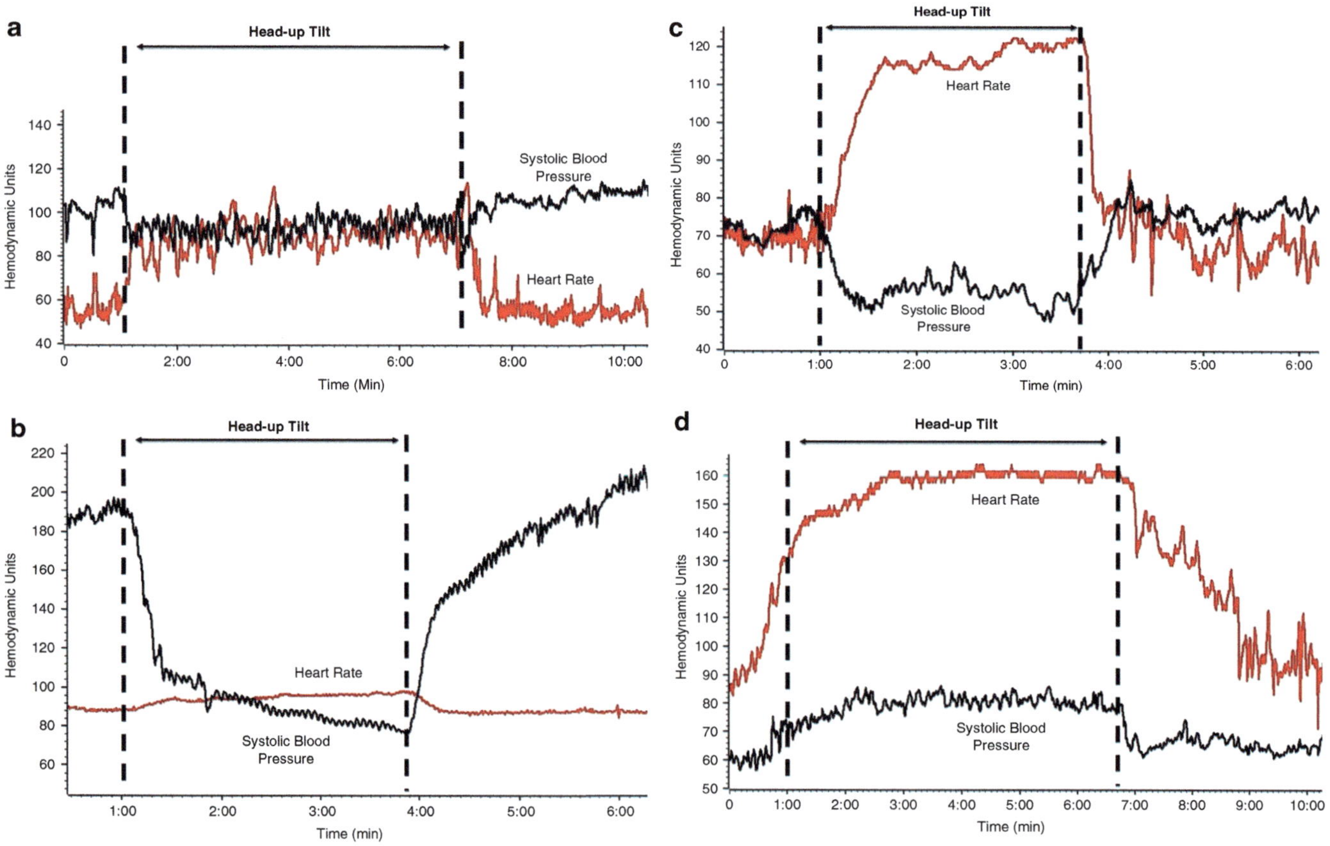

Fig. 9.6 Hemodynamic responses to head-up tilt in (**a**) healthy, (**b**) neurogenic orthostatic hypotension, (**c**) autoimmune autonomic ganglionopathy, and (**d**) postural orthostatic tachycardia syndrome

HUT. However, as this test is not clinically validated, there are no set guidelines for testing. Despite the lack of validation studies, LBNP remains a unique method as the level of negative pressure can be graded to produce an uncoupling of cardiopulmonary and arterial baroreceptor reflexes. For example, at lower negative pressures (i.e. <15 mm Hg), baroreflex unloaded produces peripheral sympathetic activation without a heart rate change, whereas higher negative pressure (i.e. > 30 mm Hg) elicits both sympathetic activation and tachycardia [15, 16].

Physiology LBNP investigates the effects of blood volume displacement to reliably activate the baroreflex through baroreceptor unloading. Negative pressure applied to the lower half of the body redistributes blood from the upper to the lower extremities resulting in relative central hypovolemia. When applied at lower levels, LBNP reduces central blood volume (CBV) and increases peripheral sympathetic activity primarily by unloading cardiopulmonary baroreceptors. At higher levels of suction, there is additional arterial baroreceptor unloading, to cause further reductions in CBV, accompanied by reduced cardiac filling and stroke volume. As a result, these changes produce reflex tachycardia and even greater levels of peripheral sympathetic activity [15–17].

Isometric (Static) Handgrip

Isometric (static) handgrip (HG) elicits a continuous increase in arterial blood pressure, sympathetic outflow, and vasoconstriction. Additionally, there is an early rise in heart rate (and cardiac output) mediated by efferent cardiac vagal withdrawal, whereas the later tachycardic response stems from increased sympathetic activity [3, 18] (Fig. 9.7). The stimulus is driven by both the metaboreflex and central commands. Handgrip has been adapted for clinical evaluation of sympathetic autonomic function; however, the test is of limited sensitivity and specificity. Typical recommendations are such that it is performed at 30% of an individual's maximal voluntary contraction maintained between 3 and 5 minutes. A normal response consists of an arterial pressor response greater than 16 mm Hg diastolic [19].

Techniques for Measuring Sympathetic Nerve Activity (Autonomic Functioning)

Microneurography

Microneurography is a unique modality for obtaining direct sympathetic nerve activity (SNA). Sympathetic microneurography requires the insertion of an electrode (typically tungsten) percutaneously into an underlying peripheral nerve. Peripheral nerves contain fascicles surrounded by the high-impedance perineurium, which acts to prevent noise between neighboring fascicles [20]. Sympathetic fibers typical exist as bundles, and all fibers within a fascicle are destined for the same tissue (i.e. skin or muscle). Therefore, microneurography can be used to obtain sympathetic nerve activity from both muscle (MSNA) and skin (SSNA). In studies of autonomic regulation, MSNA is used to measure efferent sympathetic nerve activity innervating vascular smooth muscle within the skeletal muscle.

Equipment To record MSNA signals, the following are needed: (1) recording and reference electrodes, (2) amplifiers, (3) integrator, and (4) output system.

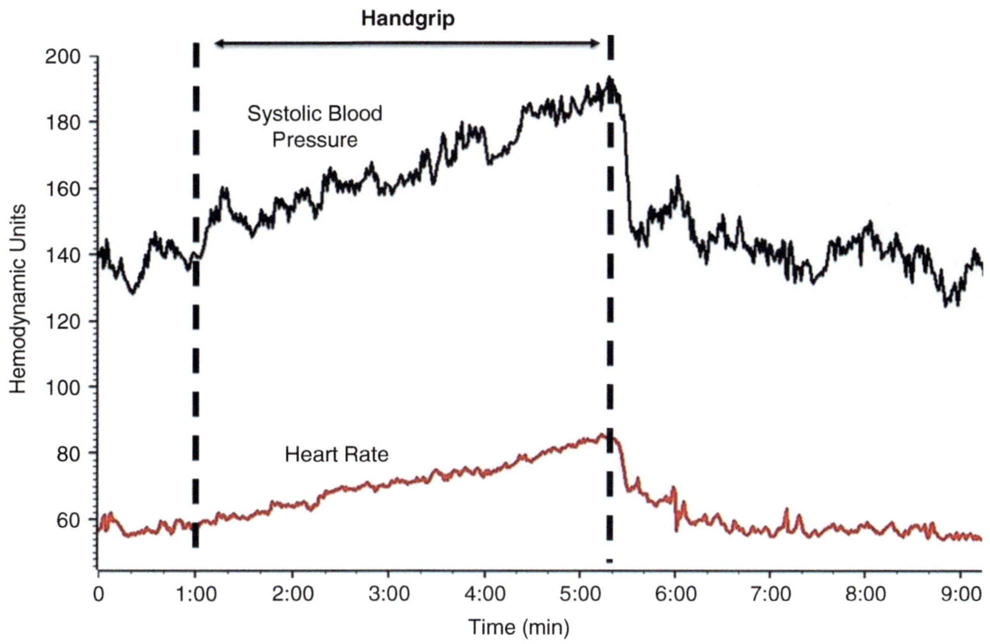

Fig. 9.7 Hemodynamic responses to isometric handgrip exercise at submaximal (30%) of maximal voluntary contraction

Getting Started When choosing a nerve for recording, the nerve should be large and relatively superficial. In the arm, the median, ulnar, and radial nerves have all been used for sympathetic recordings. For electrodes placement along with advantages and disadvantages of each recording site, we provide a brief description based on the review by White et al. The peroneal (fibular) nerve, at or proximal to the fibular head is the most commonly used site in microneurography studies. Recording from the peroneal is advantageous as it is superficial, easy to identify and recordings can be obtained in a variety of positions (i.e. supine, semi-recumbent, seated upright) [21].

For peroneal recordings, the lower limb should be extended in a comfortable position with a slight bend at the knee (~30–45°). This can be accomplished by placing foam padding under the thigh such that the lower limb is relaxed. The foot should be supported at 90°. It is important that subjects are comfortable to ensure the limb remains as still and stable as possible.

Different laboratories use different techniques to help identify the nerve, including manual palpation [22], electrical stimulation [23] and ultrasound imaging [24]. Following nerve identification, the uninsulated tungsten reference microelectrode is inserted percutaneously ~1–3 cm from the recording sites. Next, the insulated recording electrode (with an uninsulated tip [~5 um]) is inserted through the skin and into the nerve bundle (Fig. 9.8). The recording electrode usually requires manipulation until an adequate recording signal is found. High quality signals can be assessed by the following criteria: (1) increased burst frequency in response to a breath hold, (2) lack of bursts associated with a startle or sensory stimuli, such as lightly brushing the skin, and (3) pulse synchronous bursts, characterized by a burst ~1.2 seconds after an ECG R spike [25].

Once a high-quality MSNA site is obtained, the raw signal is passed through a pre-amplifier to amplify the signal by ~×1000 before being routed to another main amplifier (~×75) (typical amplification ranges from ~50,000 to 100,000). The amplified signal is then band-pass filtered (300–2000 Hz), rectified, and integrated at a time constant of 0.1 seconds using a resistance-capacitance circuit. Finally, the signal can be directed to a computer software program or as an analog signal (Absolute Design NTA; ADI NeuroAmp) for recording, storing, and later analysis. For a more in-depth look at microneurography details and discussions of the technique, including signal normalization, quantification, and standardization, readers are directed to the following reviews [21, 25, 26].

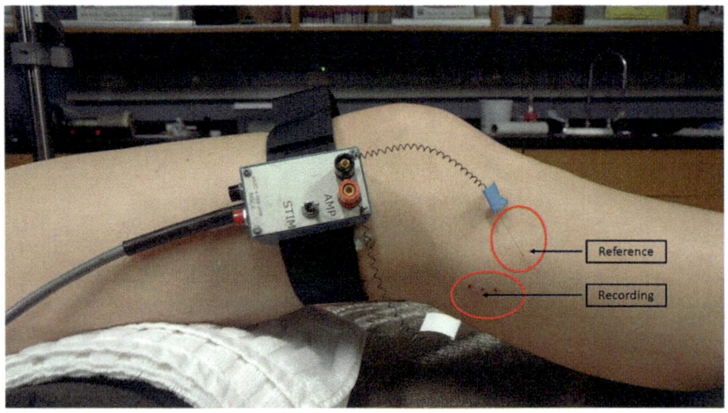

Fig. 9.8 Microneurography setup. (Photo courtesy of J. Kevin Shoemaker, PhD, CAHS, Laboratory for Brain and Heart Health at the University of Western Ontario, London, Ontario, Canada)

Tests of Sympathetic Integrity

Neuroimaging Tests

Neuroimaging can be employed to provide an assessment of cardiac sympathetic integrity. Imaging techniques such as 6-[18F]Fluorodopamine positron emission tomographic scans and [123I]metaiodobenzylguanidine ([123I]MIBG) have been used to identify cardiac sympathetic innervation in various disorders of autonomic failure [27, 28]. General findings have demonstrated that patients with primarily peripheral autonomic lesions have cardiac sympathetic impairment, whereas central autonomic disorders maintain intact cardiac sympathetic innervation. MIBG is a widely available technique with an abundance of literature to support MIBG as a quantitative measure of cardiac sympathetic integrity [29, 30].

Neuropharmacological Tests

Cardiovascular and plasma catecholamine responses to neuropharmacological drugs, such as yohimbine, trimethaphan, norepinephrine and isoproterenol also can provide an assessment of sympathetic nerve integrity.

A normal physiological response to α_2-receptor antagonist such as yohimbine includes a large pressor response and increased plasma catecholamine levels. In contrast, sympathetic nerve transmission blockers, such as trimethaphan, cause a large drop in blood pressure and reduced catecholamine levels [31–33]. Non-selective β-adrenoceptor agonist, isoproterenol, reflexively elevates sympathetic nerve trafficking in response to systemic vasodilation. As a result, there is a significant increase in plasma NE in response to isoproterenol infusions. Low et al. used two infusions at a dose of 0.01 and 0.02 mg/kg/min with a minimum recovery period of 10 minutes between infusions [3].

Similar to yohimbine and trimethaphan, isoproterenol can be used to differentiate intact versus impaired post-ganglionic sympathetic nerves. Individuals with sympathetic denervation will show significantly blunted increases in plasma NE [33–36]. In addition, isoproterenol infusions combined with head-up tilt can increase the likelihood of presyncope/syncope during tilt. The combination is thought to provoke a vagally mediated cardioinhibitory reflex by activating ventricular mechanoreceptor afferents [3].

Patients with sympathetic denervation, norepinephrine responses to isoproterenol, and blood pressure responses to trimethaphan and yohimbine are all significantly blunted [31–39].

Tests to support evidence of hypersensitivity can also be used to detect post-ganglionic denervation. For example, in patients with post-ganglionic adrenergic denervation, the BP and HR response to intravenous phenylephrine, at low doses, will demonstrate a large BP response as a result of α-receptor up-regulation. In contrast, a healthy individual would lack the aforementioned pressor response [3, 40, 41].

Neurochemical Tests

Sympathetic integrity can be further assessed through plasma catecholamines and their metabolites. Norepinephrine is the main sympathetic neurotransmitter derived from sympathetic nerves, and therefore is widely used to evaluate sympathetic nerve activity. Commonly blood draws are taken from the antecubital vein following a minimum rest period of 30 minutes. The supine value provides an index of net sympathetic activity [42]. Additionally, comparison between supine and standing has been used as an index to separate pre- versus post-ganglionic denervation.

Generally speaking, in post-ganglionic autonomic failure, resting catecholamine levels will be considerably reduced compared to individuals with pre-ganglionic disorders, which will demonstrate normal levels. Upon standing, both clinical populations show blunted elevations in the upright position [43]. Standing norepinephrine levels provide a more sensitive index of adrenergic function. However, these results have also been shown to be quite variable in differentiating pre- versus post-ganglionic denervation in autonomic failure. For example, Goldstein and colleague (2003) showed that PAF patients had low NE and EPI level, while the MSA + NOH and PD+NOH had normal mean levels of NE and EPI [44]. Furthermore, this same group has highlighted a number of limitations regarding plasma norepinephrine that must be considered when making interpretations regarding peripheral versus central pathology [45]. One such limitation pertaining to the relationship between plasma NE and actual sympathetic nerve transmission is complex. The plasma concentration depends not only on the rate of release but also the rate removal. Therefore, a high plasma NE concentration could mean a high rate of sympathetic nerve traffic, or it could be the result of slower uptake, metabolism or general removal. Therefore, if available, measures of its primary metabolite, plasma dihydroxyphenylglycol are encouraged.

Laboratory Evaluation of the ANS During Sleep (Rationale and Measurement Techniques for Studying ANS Functions During Sleep)

Mammals, including humans, operate on a 24-hour cycle. Circadian timing is regulated by our biological pacemaker located in the suprachiasmatic nuclei of the hypothalamus. The hypothalamus is the primary cortical structure involved in proper homeostatic regulation of many physiological functions related to the ANS. Functions regulated by the hypothalamus include, but are not limited to, thermoregulation, neuroendocrine modulation, and cardiovascular functioning. As the ANS is highly integrated with many physiological systems, it is not surprising that there is also a measurable circadian influence on the sympathetic and parasympathetic divisions of the ANS. During sleep, there is a shift in dominance toward parasympathetic over sympathetic activity [46, 47]. Not surprising then, the processes under autonomic control show similar circadian shifts. For example, for healthy individuals it is well established that heart rate and blood pressure increase during the day and decrease throughout the night. In contrast, evidence of suboptimal regulation may be indicative of compromised adaptation. While it is not clear whether rhythmic disruption results in illness or illness causes disruption, there is a clear and well-documented relationship between disrupted biological rhythms and illnesses [48, 49]. Therefore, techniques for objectively evaluating basic physiological phenomena may provide key insight into autonomic neural function during sleep. Direct measures of sympathetic and parasympathetic activity are often difficult, require active participation or are invasive, and as such are not ideal for measuring ANS function during sleep. Therefore, practical measures of ANS function must rely primarily on indirect measures based on biological rhythms under autonomic control. In practice, biological rhythms can be investigated via core body temperature, blood pressure profiling, measurements or changes in respiration, and biological markers of neuroendocrine fluctuations.

Respiration (See Also Chap. 11)

Respiration is intimately linked with cardiovascular and autonomic function to ensure an optimal relationship between ventilation and perfusion. Breathing naturally causes a pattern of discharge from the vagus nerve, and the rate of discharge can be influenced by the rate and depth of respiration. Respiratory sinus arrhythmia describes a phenomenon in which heart rate increases during inspiration and decreases during expiration. Therefore, measuring respiration with concurrent heart rate changes provides a reliable measure of parasympathetic innervation of the heart. Respiratory sinus arrhythmia is also linked with the high frequency domain of heart rate variability, which is primarily thought to reflect parasympathetic activity [50, 51].

Therefore, measuring respiratory changes at rest, as well as pattern shifts from sleep versus wake, may provide indirect evaluation of autonomic shifts in parasympathetic versus sympathetic dominance. Several non-invasive techniques can be applied to measure respiration. Techniques such as airflow sensing, respiratory effort, and blood gas measurements provide just some of the current methods used in both research and clinical settings. A summary of respiratory techniques is provided in Table 9.1.

Airflow Sensing

Pneumotachography The most widely used technique for pneumotachographical recordings measures differential pressure airflow, which can accurately quantify airflow volume [52]. Patients usually wear a facemask to allow airflow to be passed through a resistive field. The passage of airflow creates a pressure drop, which is measured using a simple differential manometer [52]. The flow is typically laminar, which facilitates a linear relationship between pressure difference and flow. Of note, the resistive element should be heated to prevent condensation. Other factors that influence the pressure–flow relationship, and therefore need to be corrected for, include viscosity, density, and temperature [52]. If these physical properties are corrected for, a pneumotachograph can give quantitative measures of flow, which can also be used to determine volume; the technique is, however, somewhat cumbersome.

Some devices for airflow detection take advantage of physical differences between inspired versus expired air. For example, expiratory air is warmer, more humid, and contains higher carbon dioxide (CO_2) levels compared to inhaled air. Therefore, devices capable of measuring temperature, humidity, and/or CO_2 can be used for qualitative assessment of airflow. For temperature and humidity, sensors are typically placed in or in front of the nasal/oral region.

Nasal Airway Pressure Relative to ambient air pressure, nasal airway pressure is negative during inspiration and positive during expiration. Based on these pressure differentials, nasal airway pressure (NAP) provides a surrogate estimate of airflow and thus respiration. Notably, NAP correlates well with pneumotachographic signals [53] and, when an individual breathes through their nose, NAP offers a greater sensitivity to subtle flow changes compared to thermography [54].

Temperature and Humidity Air in the lungs is warmed by core body temperature and subsequently expired air is warmer than ambient air. Consequently, measuring the temperature of expired air provides a surrogate measure of airflow. Thermistors are thermally sensitive resistors that, when connected in circuit, produce voltage alterations. When thermistors detect temperature changes, it produces large changes in resistance, which translates into voltage changes [52]. For this reason, it is essential for thermistors to remain below body temperature, otherwise the expired air will not produce a detectable temperature change and, in turn, no change in resistance. Thermocouples also measure temperature changes, and like thermistors they need to be placed in

Table 9.1 Methods for measuring airflow, blood gas concentrations, and respiratory effort

Airflow sensing device/parameter	Sensor(s)	Placement	Reference
Differential pressure airflow	Pneumotachograph	Facemask: mouth and nose	[52]
Nasal airway pressure	Nasal cannula	Nares	[53, 54]
Temperature	Thermistor Thermocouples	Nasal/oral region	[52]
Humidity	Hygrometer Fiber-optic	Nasal/oral region	[52, 55, 56]
Carbon dioxide	Infrared Mass-spectrometry	Nasal/oral sampling	[57, 58]
Blood gas measurements			
Arterial oxygen saturation with pulse oximetry	Fiber-optic sensor	Periphery—Usually finger or toe	[58, 59]
End-tidal CO_2 concentration	Infrared Mass-spectrometry	Nasal/oral sampling	[60, 61]
End-tidal oxygen concentration	Mass-spectrometry Electric analyzer Oxygen sensor	Nasal/oral sampling	[52, 61]
Transcutaneous CO_2 concentration	Chemical skin sensor	Skin	[58, 61–63]
Respiratory effort: movement/volume			
Abdomen and thoracic strain-gauge transducers	Resistive strain-gauge	Abdomen and chest	[52, 58, 60, 61]
Respiratory inductance plethysmography	Transducer	Abdomen and thoracic	[61, 64]

front of the nares or mouth. Expired air will heat the sensors and change the resistance. The transducer will produce an oscillatory tracing based on voltage alterations associated with the detectable changes in warmer expired air versus cooler inspired air to provide a measure of respiratory airflow.

Additionally, fiber optic techniques can measure humidity using water vapor condensation that forms on the tip of a fiber optic sensor placed in front of the mouth and nose. During expiration, there is a relative increase in humidity and condensation which alters the optic signal. This change is recorded as a breath and enables an easy measurement of humidity [55, 56]. Of note, some studies have reported an overestimation of the respiratory rate using the fiber optic sensors, whereas more recent developments in the technique show more promising results demonstrating good precision, speed, and repeatability [56].

Measure Carbon Dioxide (CO_2) Expired air is comprised of a much higher concentration of carbon dioxide (CO_2) relative to ambient air, and therefore a large CO_2 difference exists between inspired versus expired air. For carbon dioxide sensing, infrared analyzers or mass-spectrometry of gases from the nasal/oral region provide a measure of CO_2 concentration. Carbon dioxide sensing offers several useful advantages relative to thermal sensing. First, end-tidal CO_2 concentrations can provide useful insights into PCO_2 [52]. Furthermore, a typical CO_2 curve will plateau when there is evidence of a steady-state baseline. Changes in an individual's breathing pattern will be evident by a loss of this plateau [52]. Finally, measures of expired CO_2 can detect central apneas and provide evidence of hypoventilation, which are not detectable using thermistors or thermocouples [52].

Important Considerations Methods for airflow detection that involve air collection can introduce several limitations. For example, Folke et al., found that subtle differences in the design of the collecting device could result in large differences in sensor performance [57]. Furthermore, the use of air collectors can affect breathing activity such as respiratory rate and CO_2 production. Other considerations include how well individuals tolerate a mouthpiece or facemask. Therefore, non-contact methods for monitoring respiration have been introduced. For example, one study used a thermal camera centered on the tip of the nose to monitor skin temperature changes, from which an algorithm was applied for respiratory rate monitoring [58].

Blood Gas Measurement

Pulse Oximetry See also section "Methods for Evaluating Asleep Blood Pressures". Blood gas measurements offer indirect measures of respiratory activity. Pulse oximetry provides an indirect means to measure differences in oxygen saturation. In brief, pulse oximetry uses infrared technology to determine the amount of oxygen saturation in the blood, which indirectly relates to the amount of oxygen entering the lungs, and thus respiration. Furthermore, the oximeter provides a percentage of blood oxygen saturation (SpO_2), pulse rate, and plethysmogram. In both healthy adults as well as infants, studies have extracted respiratory waves/respiratory rates based on a wavelet transformation of the plethysmogram [58, 59].

End-Tidal Measurements End-tidal O_2 and CO_2 concentrations provide a direct measure of gas exchange on a breath-by-breath basis [60, 61]. Similar to carbon dioxide sensing for airflow detection, end-tidal CO_2 can be measured using mass-spectrometry/infrared sensors from nasal/oral samples. During hypoventilation, end-tidal O_2 concentrations change more rapidly than end-tidal CO_2, whereas decreased end-tidal CO_2 concentrations precede low pulse oximetry readings [52].

Transcutaneous CO_2 Transcutaneous CO_2 sensors do not provide any information on breath-to-breath respiratory activity, but they do offer an estimate of arterial CO_2 concentration and therefore allow for measurements as a result of abnormal ventilation [58]. Transcutaneous monitors (usually applied on the arm) provide an overall estimate of CO_2 changes based on the diffusion of gas to the skin. Notably, the accuracy of these devices is impacted by several factors, including cardiovascular function, skin thickness, impaired perfusion, and age [62]. This technique also requires monitoring to avoid burns in the case of sensitive and neonatal skin [63].

Respiratory Effort (Movement and Volume)

Qualitative airflow detection and expiratory gas concentrations cannot reliably differentiate central apneas, obstructive apneas and prolonged inspirations [52]. Therefore, airflow detection is often combined with measures of respiratory effort. The most common techniques for measuring respiratory effort is the use of abdominal and ribcage movements. Strain gauges and respiratory inductance plethysmography (RIP) provide safe and reliable measures of abdominal and chest movement.

Strain Gauges Strain gauges are capable of measuring breathing patterns based on stretch imposed on the strap by inflation and deflation of the torso. The bands are typically elasticized tubes filled with conducting material. When current is passed through the bands and the length is held constant, so too is the resistance and current. Current is inversely related to gauge length and therefore provides an index of length changes associated with the chest/abdominal expansion during respiration. When stretched, there is a proportional increase in resistance and inverse change in current. An amplifier transduces this signal into a measurable and recordable voltage output.

Respiratory Inductance Plethysmography Respiratory inductance plethysmography (RIP) provides a relatively non-invasive, semi-quantitative assessment of thoracic and abdominal pressure changes related to ventilation. RIP requires two bands (thoracic and abdominal) placed around the ribcage and over the abdomen at the level of the umbilicus, respectively. Each elasticized band has a transducer, consisting of an insulated wire sewn onto it. Based on measurable changes in cross-sectional area, the transducers determine changes in inductance or resistance to flow. When properly calibrated, these measures reflect chest and abdominal volume changes associated with inspiration and expiration. The sum of the two signals provides an estimate of tidal volume [64]. Accurate initial calibrations are imperative for valid measurements. Additionally, inaccuracies can be introduced by band displacement and body position change.

Finally, if properly calibrated against a volume measuring system, these devices can also be used to provide quantitative assessments of lung volume. Using the two measurements, thoracic and abdominal, lung volume can be determined based on displacement/length changes detectable by the transducers. Therefore, for a given change in ribcage and abdominal volume (and the assumption that the individual contributions remain constant) one can infer lung volume changes. Unfortunately, this technique also assumes that the thoracic and abdominal expansion will occur together. Asynchronous motion can be indicative of partial or complete upper airway obstruction. However, other considerations for asynchronous movement include the following: loss of diaphragm tone, loss of accessory respiratory muscle tone, body position changes, snoring, and device migration [52].

Blood Pressure

24-Hour Ambulatory Blood Pressure

Twenty-four-hour ambulatory blood pressure monitors (ABPM) provide BP readings during the day and particularly during sleep. In healthy, normotensive individuals, circadian blood pressure follows a reproducible profile, which includes a characteristic "dip" throughout the night. The dip is expressed as a percentage of change relative to the diurnal BP {[(mean day BP – mean night BP)/day BP] × 100} [65].

A 10–20% nocturnal dip is a normal range and accepted measure of a healthy circadian BP profile (Fig. 9.9a), while deviations from this dipping response have become acceptable measures of cardiovascular risk [66, 67]. Other patterns include, non-dipping (<10% reduction) (Fig. 9.9b), extreme dipping (>20%) and reverse dipping (increased nocturnal BP) (Fig. 9.9c) [65]. Although the underlying mechanisms producing each pattern have yet to be fully elucidated, there are an increasing number of studies to support a link between the alternative blood pressure profiles and increased cardiovascular risk and mortality [49, 65, 68–71]. Notably, altered autonomic rhythms may play a key role as non-dipping patterns have been reported in patients with autonomic failure [72, 73].

Methods for Evaluating Asleep Blood Pressures

Oscillometric Technique Home monitors and 24-hour ABPM commonly use the automated oscillometric technique. For this approach, the center of the cuff is placed over the brachial artery on the non-dominant arm. The cuff inflates to suprasystolic pressures followed by a slow deflation. Pressure sensors detect oscillations electronically, which indirectly estimate systolic, diastolic, and mean arterial pressures [10]. Monitors can be set to take measurements at predetermined intervals (i.e. every 20 minutes) throughout the day and night, which can provide key insights into circadian blood pressure profiles. However, in the event that patients are woken by the cuff inflation throughout the night, then true asleep and circadian blood pressure measurements will not be captured. Therefore, a new technological wave of cuffless blood pressure devices is emerging to measure 24-hour blood pressure and, particularly, asleep blood pressures.

Arterial Tonometry Arterial tonometry provides a non-invasive cuffless technique for measuring blood pressure. Similar to the Penaz technique, tonometry produces a blood pressure waveform that can either provide beat-to-beat continuous blood pressures or an ambulatory monitor for blood pressure measurements outside a clinical setting.

In practice, the tonometer sensor is placed over a superficial artery close to an underlying bone. The radial artery is most frequently used due to its large diameter and easy access; however, other arterial measures have been captured from the dorsalis pedis and temporal arteries [74].

Arterial tonometry estimates blood pressure by slightly compressing, but not occluding, the artery. Blood pressure is estimated based on the "hold down pressure" [10], which is the amount of pressure required to flatten the artery. This pressure is calculated based on an algorithm, which includes systolic, diastolic, and pulse pressures [10].

Due to the large arterial diameter (i.e., compared to finger cuffs), arterial tonometry is thought to better represent central pressures, and is less sensitive to inaccuracies related to vascular disease [10]. The primary disadvantage of this technique is the possibility of human error as it can be difficult to manually place the sensor precisely over the artery and

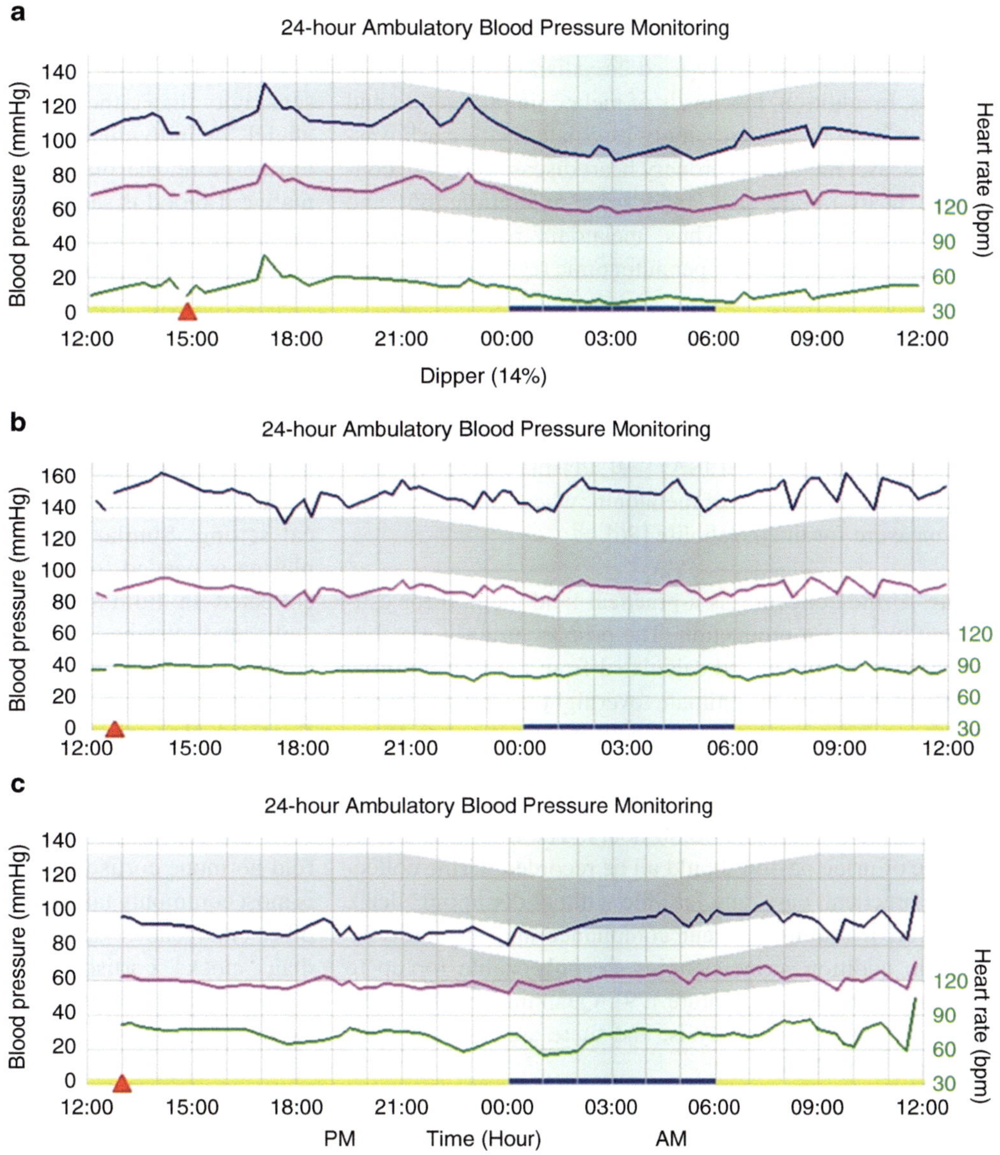

Fig. 9.9 24-hour blood pressure profiles of (**a**) healthy dipping pattern 14%, (**b**) non-dipping pattern (1%), and (**c**) reverse dipper (−3%)

ensure that it does not move over the course of the recording period. In addition, arterial tonometry typically requires initial calibration, by another technique, which can introduce additional inaccuracies and variability [10].

Pulse Oximetry Pulse oximetry is a widely used and relatively inexpensive technique for monitoring hemoglobin oxygenation. Using spectrophotometrics, the technique takes advantage of the physical changes in light absorption between oxygenated and deoxygenated blood [75].

For blood pressure recordings, pulse oximetry can be used to derive pulse transit time (PTT), also known as the photometric method, which is one of the newest methods receiving attention. PTT is based on pulse wave velocity, which uses pulse transducers at two separate sites and measures the time between arterial pulses between the two sites [10]. Alternatively, PTT can be measured from the ECG R-wave to a peripheral pulse. Finger pulse oximetry can be incorporated to detect the arrival of a pulse at a peripheral site. PTT is inversely related to systolic blood pressure [76]. However, the relationship between PTT and diastolic and mean pressure are more complicated, and therefore more work is needed [76].

Neuroendocrine

Melatonin

In mammals, melatonin synthesis is regulated by the suprachiasmatic nuclei and is secreted by the pineal gland under low light conditions [77, 78]. In normal entrained individuals, melatonin levels will begin to increase throughout the evening (20:00–23:00 hours), reaching peak values between 02:00 and 04:00 hours before returning to baseline levels throughout the morning 08:00–10:00 hours [79]. This circadian pattern of melatonin production has been shown to reliably estimate the timing of the internal circadian clock, and thus is the most commonly used circadian phase marker in humans. In addition, low levels of melatonin production and secretion have been increasingly associated with cardiovascular disease, including coronary heart disease [80–83], congestive heart failure [84], myocardial infarction [85] and nocturnal hypertension. Thus, melatonin provides a link between melatonin and proper autonomic regulation of blood pressure [78].

Melatonin (IUPAC name: N-[2-(5-methoxy-1H-indol-3-yl)ethyl]acetamide) and its major metabolite (6-sulphatoxymelatonin (aMT6s)) can be routinely sampled and analyzed by radioimmunoassay (RIA) or enzyme-linked immunosorbent assay (ELISA) [79]. Plasma and saliva samples provide an estimate of melatonin, whereas urinary samples measure for the metabolite [86].

Urine Urine collection is a practical field method for estimating melatonin production. The primary urinary metabolite, aMT6s, sampled and calculated from the first morning void can be used to estimate overnight excretion levels. Alternatively, urinary samples collected every 2–8 hours across a 24-hour period can provide an estimate of timing and global melatonin production [86]. aMT6s levels usually peak between 04:00 and 08:00 hours. The timing and total volume of urine passed should all be recorded. Urine collection is practical, easy, and feasible without disrupting sleep. However, it requires patient compliance and an ability to void. In addition, urine samples are only stable for up to five days at room temperature [79]. Quantitative RIA is the principle method for analysis, and there are also commercially available ELISA kits.

Saliva Similar to urine samples, saliva sampling offers a relatively easy and practical method for measuring melatonin both in a clinical setting and field studies. Saliva samples should be collected every 30–60 minutes in low light conditions starting at least 1 hour prior to the expected rise [86]. However, unlike urinary samples, the feasibility of measuring melatonin throughout the night is impractical and thus limits its overnight utility. Saliva melatonin levels have been shown to peak around 22:00 hours when collected between 18:00–22:00 hours [86]. Saliva melatonin is roughly 30% of plasma levels, but offers a non-invasive method for collection. Most assays require a minimum of 0.4 mL per tube, or a minimum of 1.5 mL for duplicates [79, 86]. For accurate analysis, it is important for individuals to follow careful instructions to ensure the sample is not contaminated with food particulates, food dyes or blood. Samples should be frozen immediately after collection and centrifuged prior to analysis. Commercial saliva collection tubes and saliva ELISA and RIA kits are available [79].

Plasma One benefit to plasma melatonin concentrations is that the plasma levels are roughly three times that of saliva [79, 86]. Therefore, the higher levels allow for a greater sensitivity than either saliva or urine, and thus may be beneficial for individuals with low melatonin concentrations. Furthermore, the plasma approach can be the most informative if blood is sampled at frequent intervals throughout the night (i.e. every 30 minutes). However, to make frequent blood draws throughout the night, the use of an intravenous catheter with long-line tubing are recommended. With this approach, melatonin concentrations reach a maximum between roughly 02:00 and 05:00 hours [86]. While this approach does allow for frequent samples without disrupting sleep, it is also invasive, requires trained medical personnel, and increases risk to the patient. Together these disadvantages limit the use of plasma melatonin to a clinical setting. Similar to saliva, a minimum of 1.5 mL of plasma is needed for duplicate assays. Samples should be collected in lithium/heparin tubes, centrifuged immediately, and plasma should be separated and kept frozen (−20 °C) until analysis [79].

Cortisol, Norepinephrine, and Epinephrine

Human plasma contains several measurable markers that provide indirect measures of autonomic activity, including catecholamines, epinephrine (EPI), norepinephrine, and steroid hormone cortisol. For human research, blood sampling is most commonly taken from the antecubital vein. Similar to other endogenous variables influenced by the body's circadian "clock," cortisol along with catecholamines (norepinephrine [NE] and epinephrine [EPI]) secretion and excretion exhibit characteristic peak-to-trough rhythmicity.

Cortisol Cortisol levels are typically very low between 23.00 and 2.00 hours. This is followed by a sharp rise between 5.00 and 8.00 hours [87]. Plasma and urine excretion both provide a measure of circadian cortisol oscillations. However, it is important to note that plasma levels begin to rise and reach a peak long before waking, suggesting the biological mechanism is separate from that of active awakening. In contrast, the morning rise in urinary cortisol excretion is roughly 3 hours later compared to plasma levels, whereas the evening fall shows considerable less lag [88].

Catecholamines Similarly, plasma catecholamines can be collected to provide characteristic circadian oscillations. However, urinary excretion is more easily obtained under normal environmental conditions. Epinephrine (EPI) excretion is often very low during sleep, and roughly quadruples throughout the day until reaching a maximum in the early afternoon. EPI patterns oscillate in a stable sinusoidal pattern, and have been shown to maintain this pattern despite exogenous conditions, including sleep deprivation [88].

These patterns also demonstrate persistence under conditions of constant light, activity, and food intake [88], suggesting EPI circadian rhythmicity is highly influenced by endogenous factors. Typically, plasma epinephrine levels reflect neural outflow to the adrenal medulla as these cells secrete their contents directly into the bloodstream [45].

Similar to EPI and cortisol, norepinephrine also displays clear circadian rhythmicity under normal sleep/wake conditions, peaking around noon and reaching a nadir during sleep. However, unlike EPI, NE patterns can be largely disrupted by various exogenous stimuli, such as sleep deprivation, activity, and light exposure. Age and sex should be considered as factors that can affect cortisol [89]. NE is the main neurotransmitter of the sympathetic nervous system regulating cardiovascular functions. However, a number of factors can affect the rate of NE release and the rate of NE removal from the plasma, and therefore the relationship between plasma NE and sympathetic activity is not simple [45].

Body Temperature

Proper thermoregulation represents another major homeostatic function that integrates hypothalamic and autonomic processes. Core body temperature is maintained within a narrow window (0.2–0.5 °C) [90] primarily through vasomotor skin response such as vasodilation and vasoconstriction facilitated by the ANS. Larger CBT fluctuations outside this window make corrections through activation of sweating or shivering [90]. Of note, impaired thermoregulation can be indicative of brainstem/spinal lesions or autonomic failure.

Core body temperature (CBT), cortisol and melatonin all represent robust markers of biological rhythms. However, unlike neuroendocrine markers, CBT is perhaps the easiest and most amenable to continuous measurements in a wide variety of subjects, settings and conditions.

Choosing a Site

The term *core* body temperature is somewhat of a misnomer. CBT assumes to represent internal or deep tissue temperatures that are less influenced by variations in ambient and environmental factors. However, it is important to note that even within specific regions, tissues, and even organs, there is temperature variation [91]. CBT can be measured at a variety of sites, including rectal, oral, esophageal intra-vascular, tympanic, bladder, and axillary. With the rectal temperatures as a reference point, Table 9.2 provides comparable clinical temperatures from commonly used sites in an afebrile individual. Additionally, Table 9.3 provides advantages and disadvantages of various sites for measuring CBT.

Table 9.2 Comparable temperature variations relative to rectal temperature

Site	Temperature variation (°C)
Rectal ~37 °C	–
Oral	0.3–0.5° lower
Esophageal	0.2° lower
Pulmonary artery	0.2–0.3° lower
Tympanic membrane	0.05–0.25° lower
Bladder	0.1–0.2° lower
Axillary	0.6–0.8° lower

Data adapted from Holtzclaw [86]

Table 9.3 Advantages and disadvantages of various sites for measuring core body temperature

Site	Advantages	Disadvantages
Oral	Convenient Reasonable safe Relatively non-invasive Familiar to patient	Not ideal for patients with: Mucositis/mouth irritations Receiving heated respiratory gases Nasal packing Patient who are: Unconscious Restless Disoriented
Esophageal	More reliable Proper placement yields temperatures close to that of the heart	Placement is crucial (lower 4th) Nasopharyngeal trauma Risk of tracheoesophageal fistula Unsafe for prolonged monitoring
Tympanic	Proximal to hypothalamus Convenient Comfortable Safe and familiar to patients	Risk of eardrum trauma or rupture May be influenced by environmental temperatures
Pulmonary artery	Obtains central temperatures Considered a "gold standard" Exceptional sensitivity and accuracy Resistant to drift	Invasive Requires trained personnel for catheter insertion Required manufacturer calibration Requires testing by hospital bioengineers ~every six months
Bladder	Exceptional sensitivity and accuracy Resistant to drift	Invasive Requires trained personnel for catheter insertion Required manufacturer calibration Requires testing by hospital bioengineers ~every six months
Rectal	Provide important information about thermal status Track closely (but slower) with pulmonary artery temperature	Patient discomfort and embarrassment Risk of rectum trauma/perforation

(continued)

Table 9.3 (continued)

Site	Advantages	Disadvantages
Skin	Non-invasive Safe Convenient	Highly variable Affected by environmental factors Affected by vasoconstriction and dilation Not reliable for measuring circadian rhythms
Axillary	Enclosure within axillary pocket prevents environmental influence Tracks well with central temperatures Relatively safe and easy for use in pediatric and neonatal patients	Affected by vasoconstriction and dilation Not reliable for chilled/hypothermic patients Long-time requirement for accurate readings (~3 minutes) Not reliable for measuring circadian rhythms

Equipment

Most studies using animal models use radio telemetry. In practice, this technique requires a transmitter that is implanted into the peritoneal cavity along with a receiver [92]. The transmitter consists of sensors and wires connected to an amplifier used to modulate radio frequency waves. The receiver detects the radio waves and reconstructs the original amplified signal, which includes body temperature [92]. Other telemetry systems include (1) sensors hardwired to recording devices and (2) battery operated system that log and store data for later download. Ideally, the thermometry system should have a resolution < 0.1 °C, flexible sampling intervals, measure a wide temperature range, and have extensive memory capacity for measuring over a long period of time with frequent intervals [93].

Finally, when choosing a sampling interval, it is important that the intervals are not too large (i.e. hours) as they do not allow for an accurate reconstruction of the biological variations. In contrast, frequent sampling intervals can result in data redundancy. Therefore, most investigators opt for a sampling frequency no less than a 6-minute interval, which provides reliable temperature changes over time [93]. For a more in-depth reading of experimental methods, including constant routine, forced desynchronization and purification, along with data analysis components, please see the excellent review by Hanneman [93].

It is important to note that, in addition to site, several other factors can affect temperature resulting in relatively marked temperature variations. These factors include, but are not limited to, age [94], activity level [95] and sex [96]. For example, menstrual cycle temperature variations, known as circamensal, are predictable and well recognized, such that they are often used in fertility planning. Circamensal rhythms have a period approximately equal to one menstrual cycle, with measurable temperature fluctuations throughout the ovulation, follicular, and luteal phases [96].

References

1. Low PA. Testing the autonomic nervous system. Semin Neurol. 2003;23(4):407–21.
2. Baker J, Kimpinski K. An updated normative data set from the autonomic reflex screen representative of southwestern Ontario. Can J Physiol Pharmacol. 2019;97(2):107–11.
3. Low PA, Sletten DM. Laboratory evaluation of autonomic failure. In: Low PA, Benarroch EE, editors. Clinical autonomic disorders. 3rd ed. Philadelphia: Wolters Kluwer Health/Lippincott Williams & Wilkins; 2008. p. 130–63.
4. Low P, Opfer-Gehrking TL. The autonomic laboratory. Am J Electroneurodiagnostic Technol. 1999;39(2):65–76.
5. Coon EA, Fealey RD, Sletten DM, Mandrekar JN, Benarroch EE, Sandroni P, et al. Anhidrosis in multiple system atrophy involves pre- and postganglionic sudomotor dysfunction. Mov Disord. 2016;32(3):397–404.
6. Low P, Benarroch E, editors. Clinical autonomic disorders. 3rd ed. Philadelphia: Wolters Kluwer Health/Lippincott Williams & Wilkins; 2008.
7. Vetrugno R, Liguori R, Cortelli P, Montagna P. Sympathetic skin response: basic mechanisms and clinical applications. Clin Auton Res. 2003;13(4):256–70.
8. Kucera P, Goldenberg Z, Kurca E. Sympathetic skin response: review of the method and its clinical use. Bratisl Lek Listy. 2004;105(3):108–16.
9. Elie B, Guiheneuc P. Sympathetic skin response: normal results in different experimental conditions. Electroencephalogr Clin Neurophysiol. 1990;76(3):258–67.
10. Chung E, Chen G, Alexander B, Cannesson M. Non-invasive continuous blood pressure monitoring: a review of current applications. Front Med. 2013;7(1):91–101.
11. Angelone A, Coulter NAJ. Respiratory sinus arrhythemia: a frequency dependent phenomenon. J Appl Physiol. 1964;19:479–82.
12. Palamarchuk I, Baker J, Kimpinski K. Non-invasive measurement of adrenergic baroreflex during Valsalva maneuver reveals three distinct patterns in healthy subjects. Clin Neurophysiol. 2016;127(1):858–63.
13. Huang CC, Sandroni P, Sletten DM, Weigand SD, Low PA. Effect of age on adrenergic and vagal baroreflex sensitivity in normal subjects. Muscle Nerve. 2007;36(5):637–42.
14. Schrezenmaier C, Singer W, Swift NM, Sletten D, Tanabe J, Low PA. Adrenergic and vagal baroreflex sensitivity in autonomic failure. Arch Neurol. 2007;64(3):381–6.
15. Floras JS, Butler GC, Ando SI, Brooks SC, Pollard MJ, Picton P, et al. Differential sympathetic nerve and heart rate spectral effects of nonhypotensive lower body negative pressure. Am J Physiol Regul Integr Comp Physiol. 2001;281(2):R468–75.
16. Kimmerly DS, Shoemaker JK. Hypovolemia and neurovascular control during orthostatic stress. Am J Physiol Heart Circ Physiol. 2002;282(2):645–55.
17. Kimmerly DS. A review of human neuroimaging investigations involved with central autonomic regulation of baroreflex-mediated cardiovascular control. Auton Neurosci-Basic. 2018;207:10–21.
18. Shoemaker JK, Badrov MB, Al-Khazraji BK, Jackson DN. Neural control of vascular function in skeletal muscle. Compr Physiol. 2016;6(1):303–29.
19. Ewing DJ, Irving JB, Kerr F, Wildsmith JA, Clarke BF. Cardiovascular responses to sustained handgrip in normal subjects and in patients with diabetes mellitus: a test of autonomic function. Clin Sci Mol Med. 1974;46(3):295–306.
20. Charkoudian N, Wallin BG. Sympathetic neural activity to the cardiovascular system: integrator of systemic physiology and interindividual characteristics. Compr Physiol. 2014;4(2):827–50.
21. White DW, Shoemaker JK, Raven PB. Methods and considerations for the analysis and standardization of assessing muscle

sympathetic nerve activity in humans. Auton Neurosci Basic Clin. 2015;193:12–21.
22. Steinback CD, Salmanpour A, Breskovic T, Dujic Z, Shoemaker JK, Shoemaker JK. Sympathetic neural activation: an ordered affair. J Physiol. 2010;588(Pt 23):4825–36.
23. Macefield VG. Sympathetic microneurography. Handb Clin Neurol. 2013;117:353–64.
24. Curry TB, Charkoudian N. The use of real-time ultrasound in microneurography. Auton Neurosci-Basic. 2011;162(1–2):89–93.
25. Hart EC, Head GA, Carter JR, Wallin BG, May CN, Hamza SM, et al. Recording sympathetic nerve activity in conscious humans and other mammals: guidelines and the road to standardization. Am J Physiol Heart Circ Physiol. 2017;312(5):H1031–51.
26. Shoemaker JK, Klassen SA, Badrov MB, Fadel PJ, Shoemaker JK. Fifty year of microneurography: learning the language of the peripheral sympathetic nervous system in humans. J Neurophysiol. 2018;119(5):1731–44.
27. Goldstein AOD, Holmes CTC, Stuhlmuller JE, Lenders JW, Kopin IJ, Goldstein DS. 6-[18F]fluorodopam i ne positron emission tomographic scanning in the assessment of cardiac sympathoneural function—studies in normal humans. Clin Auton Res. 1997;7(1):17–29.
28. Satoh A, Serita T, Tsujihata M. Total defect of metaiodobenzylguanidine (MIBG) imaging on heart in Parkinson's disease: assessment of cardiac sympathetic denervation. Nihon Rinsho. 1997;55(1):202–6.*(Article in Japanese)*
29. Goldstein DS, Holmes C, Li S-T, Bruce S, Metman LV, Cannon RO. Cardiac sympathetic denervation in Parkinson disease. Ann Intern Med. 2000;133(5):338.
30. Tipre DN, Goldstein DS. Cardiac and extracardiac sympathetic denervation in Parkinson's disease with orthostatic hypotension and in pure autonomic failure. J Nucl Med. 2005;46(11):1775–81.
31. Sharabi Y, Eldadah B, Li S-T, Dendi R, Pechnik S, Holmes C, et al. Neuropharmacologic distinction of neurogenic orthostatic hypotension syndromes. Clin Neuropharmacol. 2006;29(3):97–105.
32. Grossman E, Rea RF. Hoffman a, Goldstein DS. Yohimbine increases sympathetic nerve activity and norepinephrine spillover in normal volunteers. Am J Phys. 1991;260(1 Pt 2):R142–7.
33. Sharabi Y, Imrich R, Holmes C, Pechnik S, Goldstein DS. Generalized and neurotransmitter-selective noradrenergic denervation in parkinson disease with orthostatic hypotension. Mov Disord. 2008;23(12):1725–32.
34. Goldstein DS, Zimlichman R, Stull R, Keiser HR. Plasma catecholamine and hemodynamic responses during isoproterenol infusions in humans. Clin Pharmacol Ther. 1986;40(2):233–8.
35. Imrich R, Eldadah BA, Bentho O, Pechnik S, Sharabi Y, Holmes C, et al. Functional effects of cardiac sympathetic denervation in neurogenic orthostatic hypotension. Parkinsonism Relat Disord. 2009;15(2):122–7.
36. Robertson D, Goldberg MR, Tung C-S, Hollister AS, Robertson RM. Use of alpha 2 adrenoreceptor agonists and antagonists in the functional assessment of the sympathetic nervous system. J Clin Invest. 1986;78(2):–576, 81.
37. Senard J, Rascol O, Durrieu G, Tran M, Berlan M, Rascol A, et al. Effects of Yohimbine on plasma catecholamine levels in orthostatic hypotension related to Parkinson disease or multple system atrophy. Clin Neuropharmacol. 1993;16(1):70–6.
38. Goldberg MR, Hollister AS, Robertson D. Influence of yohimbine on blood pressure, autonomic reflexes, and plasma catecholamines in humans. Hypertension. 1983;5(5):772–8.
39. Shibao C, Okamoto LE, Gamboa A, Yu C, Diedrich A, Raj SR, et al. Comparative efficacy of yohimbine against pyridostigmine for the treatment of orthostatic hypotension in autonomic failure. Hypertension. 2010;56(5):847–51.
40. Smith AA, Dancis J. Exaggerated response to infused norepinephrine in familial dysautonomia. N Engl J Med. 1964;270(14):704–7.
41. Low PA, Walsh JC, Huang CY, McLeod JG. The sympathetic nervous system in diabetic neuropathy: a clinical and pathological study. Brain. 1975;98(3):341–56.
42. Polinsky RJ, Kopin IJ, Ebert MH, Weise V. Pharmacologic distinction of different orthostatic hypotension syndromes. Neurology. 1981;31(1):1–7.
43. Goldstein DS, Sharabi Y. Neurogenic orthostatic hypotension: a pathophysiological approach. Circulation. 2009;119(1):139–46.
44. Goldstein DS, Holmes C, Sharabi Y, Brentzel S, Eisenhofer G. Plasma levels of catechols and metanephrines in neurogenic orthostatic hypotension. Neurology. 2003;60(8):1327–32.
45. Goldstein DS, Eisenhofer G, Kopin IJ. Sources and significance of plasma levels of catechols and their metabolites in humans. J Pharmacol Exp Ther. 2003;305(3):800–11.
46. Biaggioni I. Circadian clocks, autonomic rhythms and blood pressure dipping. Hypertension. 2008;52(5):797–8.
47. Bristow J, Honour A, Pickering T, Sleight P. Cardiovascular and respiratory changes during sleep in normal and hypertensive subjects. Cardiovasc Res. 1969;3(4):476–85.
48. Kario K, Pickering TG, Matsuo T, Hoshide S, Schwartz JE, Shimada K. Stroke prognosis and abnormal nocturnal blood pressure falls in older hypertensives. Hypertension. 2001;38(4):852–7.
49. Pickering TG. The clinical significance of diurnal blood pressure variations. Dippers and nondippers. Circulation. 1990;81(2):700–2.
50. Malik J, Bigger J, Camm A, Kleiger R, Moss A, Schwartz P. Heart rate variability. Standards of measurement, physiological interpretation, and clinical use. Task force of the European Society of Cardiology and the north American Society of Pacing and Electrophysiology. Eur Heart J. 1996;17(3):354–81.
51. Pomeranz B, Macaulay RJB, Caudill MA, Kutz I, Adam D, Gordon D, et al. Assessment of autonomic function by heart rate spectral analysis in humans. Am J Phys. 1985;248(1 Pt 2):H151–3.
52. Hirshkowitz M, Kryger M. Monitoring techniques for evaluating suspected sleep-disordered breathing. In: Kryger M, Roth T, Dement W, editors. Principles and practice of sleep medicine. 5th ed. St. Louis: Elsevier; 2011. p. 1610–23.
53. Montserrat JM, Farre R, Ballester E, Felez MA, Pasto M, Navajas D. Evaluation of nasal prongs for estimating nasal flow. Am J Respir Crit Care Med. 1997;155(1):211–5.
54. Norman RG, Ahmed MM, Walsleben JA, Rapoport DM. Detection of respiratory events during NPSG: nasal cannula/pressure sensor versus thermistor. Sleep. 1997;20(12):1175–84.
55. Larsson C, Staun P. Evaluation of a new fibre-optic monitor for respiratory rate monitoring. J Clin Monit Comput. 1999;15(5):295–8.
56. Limodehi HE, Légaré F. Fiber optic humidity sensor using water vapor condensation. Opt Express. 2017;25(13):15313–21.
57. Folke M, Granstedt F, Ho B, Kan Scheer H. Comparative provocative test of respiratory monitoring methods. J Clin Monit Comput. 2002;17(2):97–103.
58. Al-Khalidi FQ, Saatchi R, Burke D, Elphick H, Tan S. Respiration rate monitoring methods: a review. Pediatr Pulmonol. 2011;46(6):523–9.
59. Leonard P, Beattie F, Addison PS. Standard pulse oximeters can be used to monitor respiratory rate. Emerg Med J. 2003;20(6):524–5.
60. Eriksson I, Berggren L, Hallgren S. CO2 production and breathing pattern during invasive and non-invasive respiratory monitoring. Acta Anaesthesiol Scand. 1986;30(6):438–43.
61. Folke M, Cernerud L, Ekström M, Hök B. Critical review of non-invasive respiratory monitoring in medical care. Med Biol Eng Comput. 2003;41(4):377–83.
62. Santos LJ, Varon J, Pic-Aluas L, Combs AH. Practical uses of end-tidal carbon dioxide monitoring in the emergency department. J Emerg Med. 1994;12(5):633–44.
63. Lee-Chiong T. Sleep: a comprehensive handbook. Hoboken: John Wiley & Sons; 2006.

64. Mehra R, Strohl K. Evaluation and monitoring of respiratory effort. In: Sleep disorders medicine. 3rd ed: Elsevier; Philadelphia, PA 2009. p. 188–97.
65. Friedman O, Logan AG. Can nocturnal hypertension predict cardiovascular risk? Integr Blood Press Control. 2009;2:25–37.
66. Bloomfield D, Park A. Night time blood pressure dip. World J Cardiol. 2015;7(7):373–6.
67. Chobanian AV, Bakris GL, Black HR, Cushman WC, Green LA, Izzo JL, et al. Seventh report of the joint national committee on preventon, detection, evaluation, and treatment of high blood pressure. Hypertension. 2003;42:1206–52.
68. Cuspidi C, Meani S, Salerno M, Valerio C, Fusi V, Severgnini B, et al. Cardiovascular target organ damage in essential hypertensives with or without reproducible nocturnal fall in blood pressure. J Hypertens. 2004;22(2):273–80.
69. Portaluppi F, Tiseo R, Smolensky MH, Hermida RC, Ayala DE, Fabbian F. Circadian rhythms and cardiovascular health. Sleep Med Rev. 2012;16(2):151–66.
70. Ohkubo T, Imai Y, Tsuji I, Nagai K, Watanabe N, Minami N, et al. Relation between nocturnal decline in blood pressure and mortality: the Ohasama study. Am J Hypertens. 1997;10(11):1201–7.
71. Verdecchia P, Porcellati C, Schillaci G, Borgioni C, Ciucci A, Battistelli M, et al. Ambulatory blood pressure. An independent predictor of prognosis in essential hypertension. Hypertension. 1994;24(6):793–801.
72. Mann S, Altman DG, Sc B, Raftery EB, Sc B, Bannister R. Circadian variation of blood pressure in autonomic failure. Circulation. 1983;68(3):477–83.
73. Omboni S, Smit AAJ, van Lieshout JJ, Settels JJ, Langewouters GJ, Weiling W. Mechanisms underlying the impairment in orthostatic tolerance after nocturnal recumbency in patients with autonomic failure. Clin Sci. 2001;101:609–18.
74. Kemmotsu O, Uedo M, Otsuka H, Yamamura T, Winter D, Eckerle J. Arterial tonometry for noninvasive, continuous blood pressure monitoring during anesthesia. Anesthesiology. 1991;75:333–40.
75. Jubran A. Pulse oximetry. Crit Care. 2015;19:272.
76. Lane J, Greenstadt L, Shapiro A, Rubinstein E. Pulse transit time and blood pressure: an intensive analysis. Psychophysiology. 1983;20(1):45–9.
77. Moore R. Neural control of the pineal gland. Behav Brain Res. 1996;73:125–30.
78. Baker J, Kimpinski K. Role of melatonin in blood pressure regulation: an adjunct anti-hypertensive agent. Clin Exp Pharmacol Physiol. 2018;45(8):755–66.
79. Hutchinson JSM. Measurement of melatonin and 6-sulphatoxymelatonin. In: Wheeler M, Hutchinson JSM, editors. Hormone assays in biological fluids. Totowa: Humana Press; 2008. p. 235–54.
80. Brugger P, Marktl W, Herold M. Impaired nocturnal secretion of melatonin in coronary heart disease. Lancet. 1995;345(8962):1408.
81. Yaprak M, Altun A, Vardar A, Aktoz M, Ciftci S, Ozbay G. Decreased nocturnal synthesis of melatonin in patients with coronary artery. Int J Cardiol. 2003;89:103–7.
82. Sakotnik A, Liebmann PM, Stoschitzky K, Lercher P, Schauenstein K, Klein W, et al. Decreased melatonin synthesis in patients with coronary artery disease. Eur Heart J. 1999;20(18):1314–7.
83. Girotti L, Lago M, Ianovsky O, Carbajales J, Elizari MV, Brusco LI, et al. Low urinary 6-sulphatoxymelatonin levels in patients with coronary artery disease. J Pineal Res. 2000;29(3):138–42.
84. Girotti L, Lago M, Ianovsky O, Elizari MV, Dini A, Lloret SP, et al. Low urinary 6-sulfatoxymelatonin levels in patients with severe congestive heart failure. Endocrine. 2003;22(3):245–8.
85. Dominguez-Rodriguez A, Abreu-Gonzalez P. Myocardial ischemia-reperfusion injury: possible role of melatonin. World J Cardiol. 2010;2(8):233–6.
86. Benloucif S, Burgess HJ, Klerman EB, Lewy AJ, Middleton B, Murphy PJ, et al. Measuring melatonin in humans. J Clin Sleep Med. 2008;4(1):66–9.
87. Bailey SL, Heitkemper MM. Circadian rhythmicity of cortisol and body temperature: morningness-eveningness effects. Chronobiol Int. 2001;18(2):249–61.
88. Akerstedt T, Levi L. Circadian rhythms in the secretion of cortisol, adrenaline and noradrenaline. Eur J Clin Investig. 1978;8(2):57–8.
89. Van Cauter E, Leproult R, Kupfer DJ. Effects of gender and age on the levels and circadian rhythmicity of plasma cortisol. J Clin Endocrinol Metab. 1996;81(7):2468–73.
90. Benarroch EE. Thermoregulation recent concepts and remaining questions. Neurology. 2007;69(12):1293–7.
91. Holtzclaw B. Monitoring body temperature. AACN Clin Issues. 1993;4(1):44–55.
92. Gegout-Pottie P, Phillippe L, Simonin M, Guingamp C, Gillet P, Netter P, et al. Biotelemetry: an original approach to experimental models of inflammation. Inflamm Res. 1999;48(8):417–24.
93. Hanneman SK. Measuring circadian temperature rhythm. Biol Res Nurs. 2001;2(4):236–48.
94. Van Someren EJ. More than a marker: interaction between the circadian regulation of temperature and sleep, age-related changes, and treatment possibilities. Chronobiol Int. 2000;17(3):313–54.
95. Waterhouse J, Weinert D, Minors D, Atkinson G, Reilly T, Folkard S, et al. The effect of activity on the waking temperature rhythm in humans. Chronobiol Int. 1999;16(3):343–57.
96. Kelly G. Body temperature variability (Part 1): A review of the history of body temperature and its variability due to site selection, biological rhythms, fitness, and aging. Altern Med Rev. 2006;11(4):278–93.

Interpreting Heart Rate Variability in Sleep: Why, When, and How?

10

Massimo Pagani, Pietro Guaraldi, Francesca Baschieri, Daniela Lucini, and Pietro Cortelli

Introduction

...he ascertained by his pulse, now stronger, now weaker, what his malady was.

—J. R. Pinault [1]

The interplay between emotions, consciousness, and behavior with the purpose of improving health and combating disease has roots in ancient wisdom. A large body of empirical observations, often reflected in popular writing, particularly highlight the mind-heart-disease continuum, elegantly alluded to by William Harvey's words: "*...For every passion of the mind which troubles men's spirits, either with grief, joy, hope, or anxiety, and gets access to the heart, there makes it to change from its natural constitution, by distemperature, pulsation, and the rest...*" [2].

Throughout history there was also interest in the underlying mechanisms of this connection, as hinted by Lower [3]: "*...within the brain [there is] a perpetual storeroom of animal spirits, so that there may be a continuous inflow of them into the heart ...and so the movement of the heart will be very greatly changed by variation in their inflow.*" Accordingly, heart movements could be influenced by the "*incorrect nature*" of these spirits or a "*diminution of their inflow*" [4]. The subsequent vivid description of the cardiac nerves by Antonio Scarpa in 1794 [5] offered a credible pathway through which those *spirits* could reach the heart. However, seeing the nerves was not enough. It was necessary to combine observations with a method to assess with accuracy and reliability the *movement of the heart* and the *change from its natural constitution*, in order to unravel their relationship.

Although the observation of arterial pulses was reported by Hales in the early 1700s [6], it was only at the turn of nineteenth century that quartz string galvanometers gave Einthoven the sensitivity necessary to accurately study the normal and abnormal electrical activities of the heart [7]. Furthermore, it took until the late 1960s for digital computers culture to join in with novel initiatives such as the birth of the *Journal of Electrocardiology* (the *Official Journal of the International Society for Computerized Electrocardiology*). The employment of analog and digital computers combined with advanced mathematical modeling permitted scientists to focus on the potential importance of the relationship between autonomic innervation and cardiac performance (see e.g., finally giving substance to the classical *spirits* of old [8]).

A seminal, game-changing approach derived from shifting the focus of inquiry from average heart rate to the small beat-by-beat variations in heart period (i.e., heart rate variability [HRV]) that the new digital technology permitted scientists to assess with accuracy. This variability could be the result of the *balance* between parasympathetic and sympathetic activity and may respond to specific stimuli, such as stress at work [9]. However, the influence of additional physiological factors, such as respiration, could confound early interpretation of changes in HRV.

A few years later, Akselrod et al. [10] tried to unravel the hidden determinants of the small spontaneous changes in the inter-beat interval (i.e., the tachogram) with specific experiments in conscious dogs, in which the autonomic balance was altered experimentally. They suggested that the spontaneous "frequency specific contributions" extracted

M. Pagani (✉)
Department of Medical Biotechnology and Translational Medicine (BIOMETRA), University of Milan, Milan, Italy

P. Guaraldi
IRCCS Istituto di Scienze Neurologiche, Bologna, Italy

F. Baschieri
Department of Biomedical and NeuroMotor Sciences (DIBINEM), University of Bologna, Bologna, Italy

D. Lucini
Department of Medical Biotechnology and Translational Medicine (BIOMETRA), Istituto Clinico Humanitas, University of Milan, Milan, Italy

P. Cortelli
IRCCS Istituto di Scienze Neurologiche, Bologna, Italy

Department of Biomedical and NeuroMotor Sciences (DIBINEM), University of Bologna, Bologna, Italy

S. Chokroverty, P. Cortelli (eds.), *Autonomic Nervous System and Sleep*, https://doi.org/10.1007/978-3-030-62263-3_10

from the tachogram could furnish a proxy of "the functioning of the principal ...cardiovascular control system: the sympathetic [and] parasympathetic systems" [10]. This investigation thus represented a first step into cracking the mysterious link *between movement of the heart* and *variation of ...brain spirits*, or, using a more modern terminology: heartbeat and autonomic regulation. Needless to say "parasympathetic and sympathetic nervous activity" implicitly corresponded to the time sequence of neural spikes running through relevant nerve fibers [11] and releasing chemical transmitters at the periphery [9].

Historically, a *change from natural pulsations* of the heart was linked to disparate conditions, such as lovesickness in the case of Antioch and his stepmother [2] or sudden death for fear of God's wrath in the case of Ananias and his wife because of a fraud in the sale of a field [12]. More recently, alterations of heart rhythm alone or combined with other conditions, in particular coronary artery disease and heart failure, gained growing epidemiological and clinical interest [13]. That interest was furthered by the development of microelectronics and previously unprecedented computer power, rendering the time-consuming task of rhythm assessment amenable to automatic analysis and artificial intelligence [14]. Improvement of technology, such as the addition of functional magnetic resonance imaging (fMRI), may help further pinpoint the widespread nature of the functional anatomy of autonomic cardiovascular regulation [15]. Moreover, the easier access to simple biological signals, such as the electrocardiogram (ECG), rendered possible by wearable electronics, is likely to further individual applications, favored by a growing market, which is set to grow from $70.06 million in 2017 to reach $435.11 million by 2025 with a growth of 25.7% from 2018 to 2025 [16].

A discussion on **heart rate variability (HRV),** particularly over large scales cannot disregard the different potentially interacting domains that must be considered simultaneously: medicine, physiology, statistics, and computer science [17]. The risk of misunderstanding and confounding of language is real, sometimes unrecognized and frequently just incomprehensible as highlighted by some investigators, rhetorically asking: HRV: why do spectral analysis? [18]. Here, we deal with "reciprocal mutual connections ... between the sympathetic-ergotropic and the parasympathetic-trophotropic areas, ... at each moment they produce a dynamic equilibrium adapted to the situation at any given moment of the organism as a whole" [19]. This combination may be difficult to interpret if assessed strictly within the physiological domain. We may, however, increase our capacity of understanding conflicting data thanks to the enormous compression of information rendered possible by considering dynamic self-organization from micro to macro structures [20].

Is the Autonomic Nervous System Really Autonomous?

Conflicts are frequently over semantics, not substance.

—D. Brown [21]

The awareness of a rich nerve network close to the heart can be dated to near the end of the eighteenth century with the publication of the beautiful anatomical engravings by Scarpa [5]. Subsequently, and largely following Langley's suggestions [22], autonomic (vegetative and involuntary) innervation was divided into sympathetic and parasympathetic systems.

Pharmacological experiments with catecholamines mimicking sympathetic stimulation and physostigmine-simulating parasympathetic excitation would support a monolithic view of "autonomic" innervation; in essence functioning as an overall efferent structure, consisting of two "fundamentally different systems" [22]. In consequence, afferent fibers from visceral organs were not considered to have a physiological function because "all autonomic nerves [are] motor" [22]. However, a physiological function was observed for visceral neural reflexes, organized as simple reflexes [23], of both negative and positive feedback sign [24] (Fig. 10.1) and essentially organized as a continuous vagal-sympathetic balance. By cybernetically focusing on the control and regulation of complex functions, the model underlying neural cardiac regulation considers a complex structure in which both efferent and afferent information travels through visceral nerves. Cardiac innervation would, therefore, be characterized by a dual innervation (sympathetic and parasympathetic) made up of mixed (afferent and efferent [i.e., sensory and motor]) nerves [24]. The neural innervation of the cardiovascular system may remain a laboratory curiosity until new experimental needs suggest an

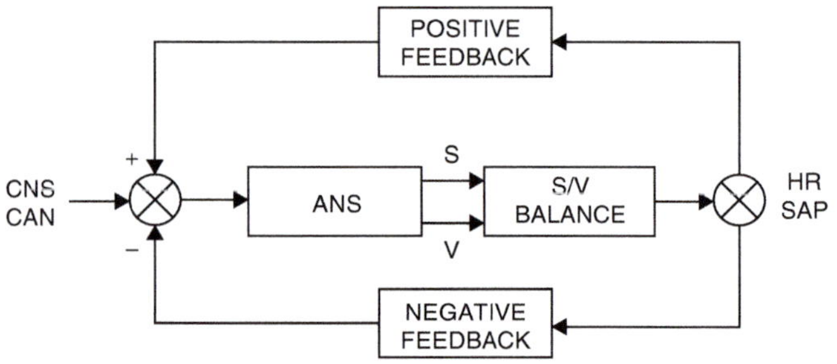

Fig. 10.1 Schematic representation of opposing feedback mechanisms that, in addition to central integration, subserve neural control of the cardiovascular system. Baroreceptive and vagal afferent fibers from the cardiopulmonary region mediate negative feedback mechanisms (exciting the vagal outflow and inhibiting the sympathetic outflow), whereas positive feedback mechanisms are mediated by sympathetic afferent fibers (exciting the sympathetic outflow and inhibiting the vagal outflow) [24]

appropriate technique of investigation [19] or users' needs might lead to innovative applications (e.g., electroceuticals).

It may also be argued that the "autonomic nervous system (ANS)" is not really autonomous, given the important reliance on reflexes initiated by visceral afferents, and the critical hierarchical organization connecting the periphery to the spinal cord, the brain stem up to a central neuronal network that includes the hypothalamus [25]. Notably, groups of neurons located in the brain stem reticular formation play a critical role in coordination between reflexes and elemental behavior, supporting homeostasis and life [26]. The level and quality of task performance are context dependent and contingent upon regulatory inputs from specialized nuclei such as the locus coeruleus. Usually, the relationship between performance and attention is represented by an inverse U curve (umbrella type), indicating that at the extremes (low and high) of attention performance is low, while it reaches a maximum approximately at mid-attention, as proposed several decades ago by Moruzzi and Hobs.

Regarding the cardiovascular system, vagal and arterial pressure afferents subserve the major cardiovascular homeostatic regulatory mechanisms by way of a negative feedback organization, which are intertwined with an opposite positive feedback loop [24]. Thus, the quality of the dynamic matching between local, end organ demands and beat-by-beat performance of the overall system is dependent upon the interplay of these peripheral (neural) loops with control signals generated from higher "central" structures which are intimately connected with the hypothalamus and the central autonomic network (CAN) [27]. Motor and visceral regulations both have somatic and visceral behavior [28] that cannot be functionally separated (Fig. 10.2) [11, 29, 30]. Moreover, they are simultaneously the result of concerted firing of organized groups of neurons. Within this design, the same (neural) channel may carry time-varying information of post-synaptic control of effectors through a simple amplitude code (more spikes translate into more quantal release and a greater target function response) [29], as well as more complex coding based on frequency, phase, and coherence between multiple oscillators providing aggregated information on the integrated performance of the overall control system. Further, the fine-tuned regulation of sympathetic–parasympathetic balance is also under a strict cellular and molecular control governing the adaptation to changing physiological and pathological demands [31, 32].

On the other hand, the importance of visceral afferents, particularly vagal afferents, is increasingly recognized as an obligatory constituent of newly discovered circuits regulating diverse functions (e.g., the inflammatory reflex [33] or food intake [34] and ultimately obesity treatment [34]) .

This complexity of neural (autonomic) organization is frequently overlooked, and the efferent only ("pharmacological") model is utilized [22]. This potentially unrecognized bias may significantly influence the field of HRV, limiting the range of information that can be handled by the system, particularly if we deal with everyday clinical problems, which usually are long-term issues requiring attention to real-life behavior away from the hospital [28]. In this context, a primary role is played by the autonomic nervous system in governing the dual nature of emotions, as superbly synthesized by Aristotle [35]: *"In answer to the question what is anger, the logician will call it a crave for retaliation, while the natural philosopher will describe it as a surge of blood and heat round the heart. Clearly the affections of the soul are formulae expressed in matter."*

Heart Rate Variability: The Modelling Approach

> *...it is necessary to know which disease states arise from powers and which from structures.*
>
> —Hippocrates [36]

To understand the clinical potentialities of heart rate variability (HRV), particularly in long-term conditions, like hypertension, coronary artery disease, obesity, inflammatory bowel diseases, cancer, or stress it is necessary to recognize, in analogy with psychosomatic medicine, its ubiquity [28] and, radical dyadic separation in physiological and bioengineering domains [37]. Starting to rise in the late 1960s, the number of yearly published studies on "heart rate variability or HRV" as of 2020 total to over 50,000 hits in the Medline database. Of these about 13,000 focused on autonomic nervous system, near 8000 on methodological aspects, about 2000 on nerve activity rhythm, less than 200 on neurophysiology, and only 5 on "neural code."

Given the clinical importance of techniques capable of decrypting data on autonomic cardiac and vascular innervation which would be potentially useful in a majority of conditions, particularly in the cardiovascular field [38] and considering a range of activity and arousal (e.g., from rest to stress and exercise), as well as a part of cardiovascular risk assessment, it is understandable why several investigators sought to confirm the practical value of HRV. As a caveat, it is important to recall that neural visceral regulation is based on a multiplicity of circuits and reflexes whereby multiple organs are coordinated toward a unitary functional aim [19], even during extreme excitatory (fight-or-flight [39]) responses (often colloquially equated to an *adrenaline rush*). Moreover, "the parts of the brain communicating directly with the spinal cord at the upper end of the medulla oblongata, and the segment lying directly beneath the cerebrum, the so-called diencephalon, exert a decisive influence on the vegetative controlling mechanisms" [19, 40, 41]. Consequently, somato-motor behavior is inextricably intertwined with viscero-(i.e., autonomic) motor behavior

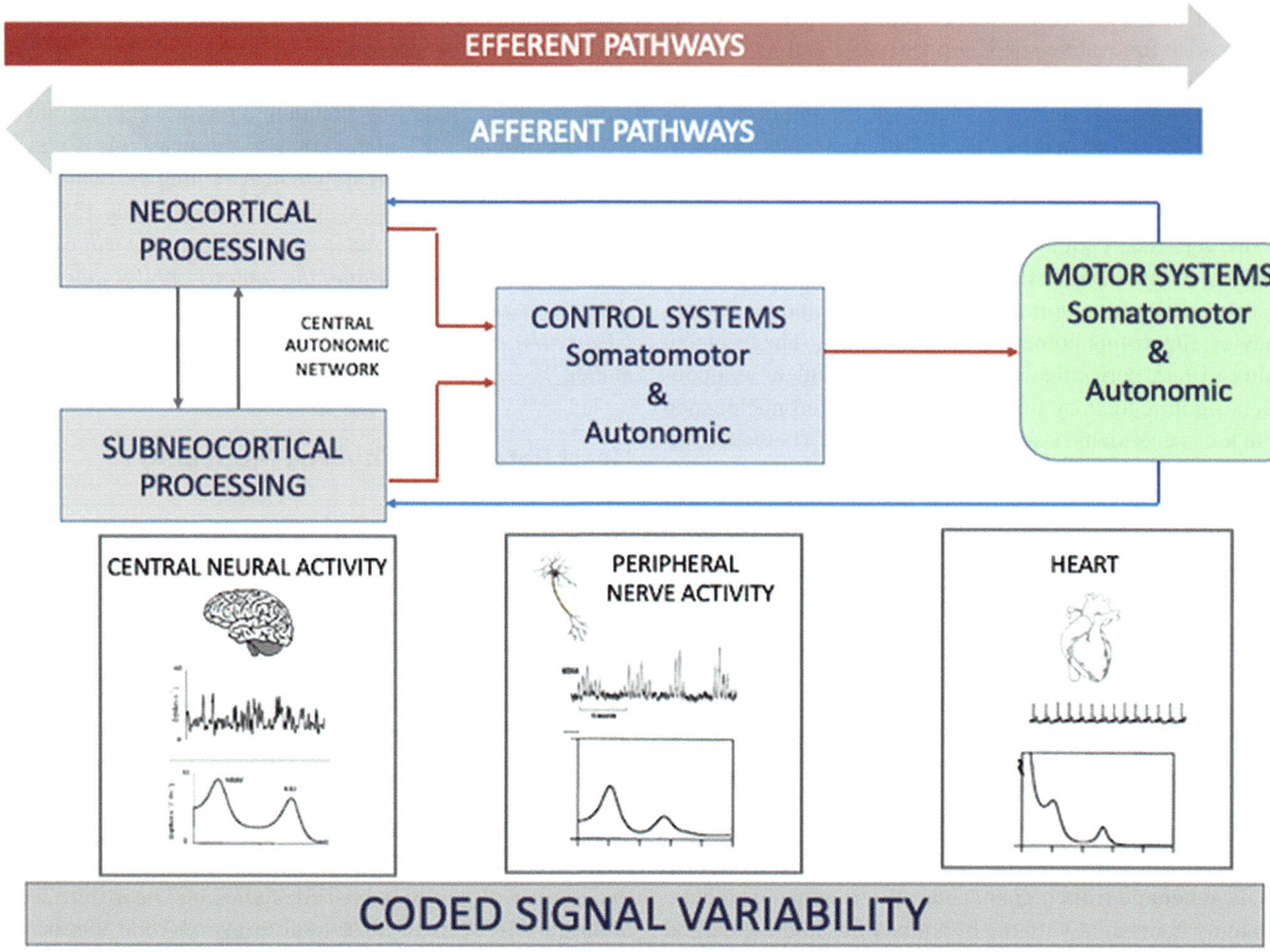

Fig. 10.2 Idealized, schematic representation of the circuitry responsible for generating simultaneous autonomic and somatomotor behavior as derived from motoneuron pools' activity comprised of neocortical and subneocortical processes, based upon a group of interconnected nuclei constituting the CAN. These are dynamically linked to more distal control systems eventually governing the somatomotor and visceromotor effectors. Overall, the integrated functional performance of the individual depends on a continuous flow of afferent and efferent information continuously channeled across the entire hierarchical structure. Notice that somatic and autonomic regulatory activities are inextricably intertwined. In parallel, it is possible to extract central (e.g., thalamic), efferent peripheral (e.g., muscular) sympathetic nerve activity, and peripheral (RR) time in msec between two successive R wave peaks of the electrocardiogram interval coding from selected variability signals. Notice the similarity of patterns across different domains, suggesting the possibility of common coding [29]. (Data from Pagani et al. [11] and Massimini et al. [30])

[25] (see Fig. 10.2). In clinical applications, such as in risk assessment [42], focus is particularly on the properties of individual reflex circuits. One example being the gain of cardiac baroreflex, possibly combined with other functional indicators, (e.g., metrics from HRV [43]). These indices are frequently treated as proxies to underlying autonomic regulation, not always with clear definition of attendant neural model, thus generating a still unresolved debate [18, 44–47].

We will now report a brief overview of the vagal and sympathetic effects on the activity of the SA node. In spite of experimental evidence to the contrary [48, 49], these are considered to be purely efferent [50]. Furthermore, they are usually modeled as linear and additive, while experimental data show strong non-linearities of cardiac responsiveness to changes in vagal and sympathetic neural activity [51, 52]. As a consequence, "a slow heart rate does not preclude the presence of a high frequency of action potentials in the efferent sympathetic nerves to the heart" [51]. Moreover, changes in the effector site milieu (e.g., accumulation of cytosolic adenosine 3′, 5′-cyclic monophosphate, cAMP) might contribute to the sympathetic augmentation of dynamic vagal control of the SA node [52].

However, while it might seem practical to simply conceive autonomic regulation of the heart as depending solely on efferent activities [22] of the sympathetic and parasympathetic nerves, animal and clinical studies in the last few decades have clearly shown that cardiac neural regulation is complex. In fact, cardiac neural regulation is based not only on a dual antagonistic innervation [19] but the system also heavily relies on information relayed from the periphery to the centers via afferent vagal and sympathetic sensory fibers

[53], subserving a double (positive and negative sign) feedback mechanism [24]. The functional basis is provided by simple (sympatho-sympathetic and vago-vagal) reflexes [48, 49] already involving the spinal level. A complex hierarchy of structures integrates spinal with supraspinal centers, functionally connecting the periphery with a CAN [27], constituting in essence a fully functional brain–heart axis (see Fig. 10.2) [54]. The operation of the system depends on a complex organization starting from dynamic molecular interactions between efferent nerve endings and target cells [31] at the periphery and cranially integrating multiple neural circuits operating in concert with somatic motor control [25]. In spite of the complexity of the circuitry, the ample dynamics of the system can be simplified by a unitary function relating the brain stem reticular formation with overall performance. A nonlinear, "umbrella" like relationship was in fact proposed several decades ago by Moruzzi [54] as the representation of the effectiveness of cue function versus arousal of reticular activation (Fig. 10.3) [55–57]. This schema implies an activation continuum, starting from low levels, well below conscious wakefulness (e.g., sleep or coma where performance is at a minimum), through intermediate levels of arousal (with optimal performance), up until extreme arousal (such as maximal stress or fatal insomnia [58]) that disturbs performance, which reaches a minimum. It may be easy to graphically demonstrate (see Fig. 10.3) the parallel behavior of synchronous signals such as the electroencephalogram (EEG) and electrocardiogram (ECG), thus offering the opportunity to simultaneously appreciate the work of the brain and ANS. Of note, we recently described such an umbrella shape in the dynamics of the strength of the relationship between baroreflex gain and HRV indices against the continuum of arterial pressure levels in a relatively large population [17]. Our data suggested a tighter systematic link in pre-hypertensive patients. Following this reasoning, it may be tempting to simplify the dynamics of

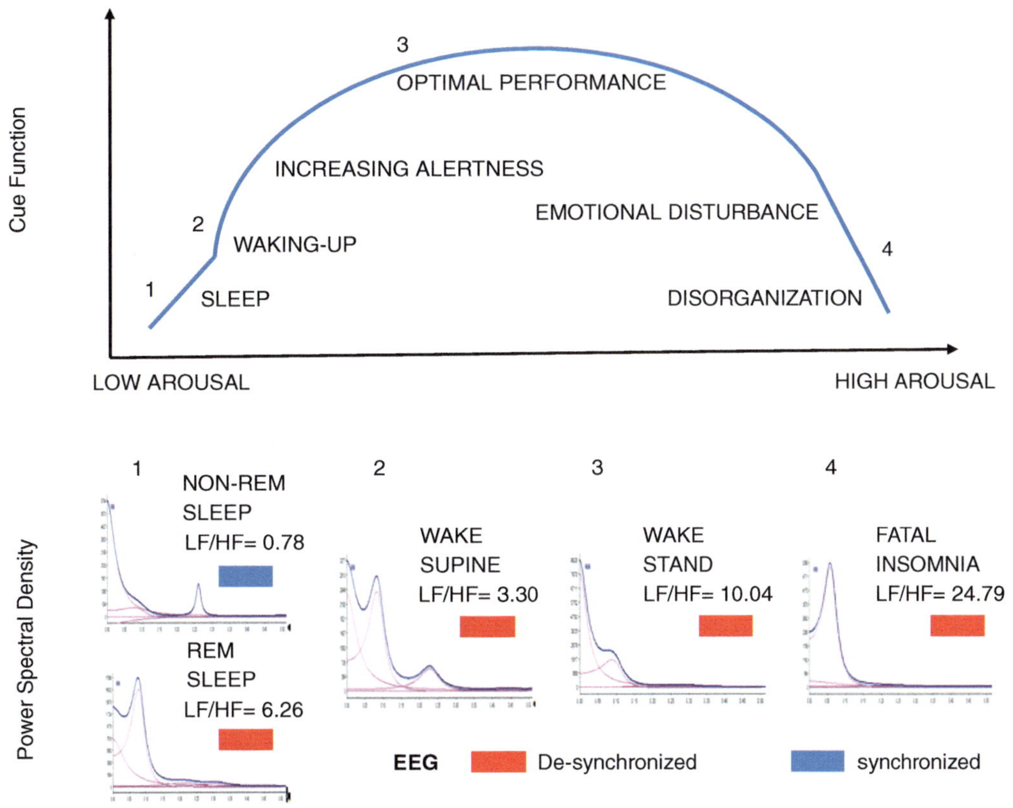

Fig. 10.3 Schematic representation of the umbrella like continuous cue function of the brain stem reticular formation from low arousal (step 1) to high arousal (step 4) showing *that there is an optimal level of arousal for effective behavior* (Moruzzi [55] and Hebb [56]). Power spectral density from RR (i.e. ECG derived interbeat) variability may simultaneously provide a proxy of the cue function as expressed by the LF/HF ratio of RR V. Notice that, in this example, LF/HF reaches the smallest value (0.78) during non-REM sleep. During wakefulness LF/HF increases to 3.3 at wake up (supine posture), and further to 10.04 while obtaining the standing position. During sleep, arousal is indicated by the increase of LF/HF to 6.26. An example of the marked increase of LF/HF (24.79) in conditions characterized by extreme arousal (fatal insomnia) is also presented. Notably, the significant information as a proxy of the autonomic sympatho-vagal balance, is provided numerically by LF/HF and graphically by the RR variability autospectra. A qualitative description of EEG pattern is also presented with red and blue color coding (for desynchronized and synchronized, respectively). This cue function is similar to the (also umbrella like) relationship between activity of locus-caeruleus-neurons and attentiveness in monkeys. The task execution performance is minimal at the extremes of arousal (low or high attentiveness), maximal with moderate, focused attention [57]

autonomic regulation as resulting from the instantaneous balance between excitatory and inhibitory circuits (sympatho-vagal) [24]. The brain stem, through a multiplicity of neural structures and monoaminergic and cholinergic mediators, maintains and controls arousal [59] by modulating neurons in the thalamus and cortex. A special role may be played by the locus coeruleus–norepinephrine system whose neurons optimize task performance through phasic or tonic coded activity [57]. The poor performance at the extremes of arousal (low or high) with a maximum performance at mid-arousal would thus correspond to the umbrella like function. It should also be mentioned that specific signals reaching the brain stem from the vascular periphery may induce complex behaviors [60], e.g., carotid sinus stimulation causes prolonged pyramidal relaxation in conscious dogs [61] and chemoreceptor stimulation induces a *sham rage* response in decorticated cats [62].

We may thus conclude that behavioral reflex responses [28] would result from the dynamic interplay between (at least) two simultaneous and opposed mechanisms. Accordingly, negative and positive feedback circuits interact continuously (see Fig. 10.1) under the restraining or facilitating influence of central command (i.e., CAN) in order to achieve an optimal behavioral control [24]. This model accounts for different conditions or context (rest, microgravity, unloading of baroreceptors, exercise, fight, flight, and coronary artery disease) (Fig. 10.4) that may be characterized by various levels of excitation in the cue function [55]

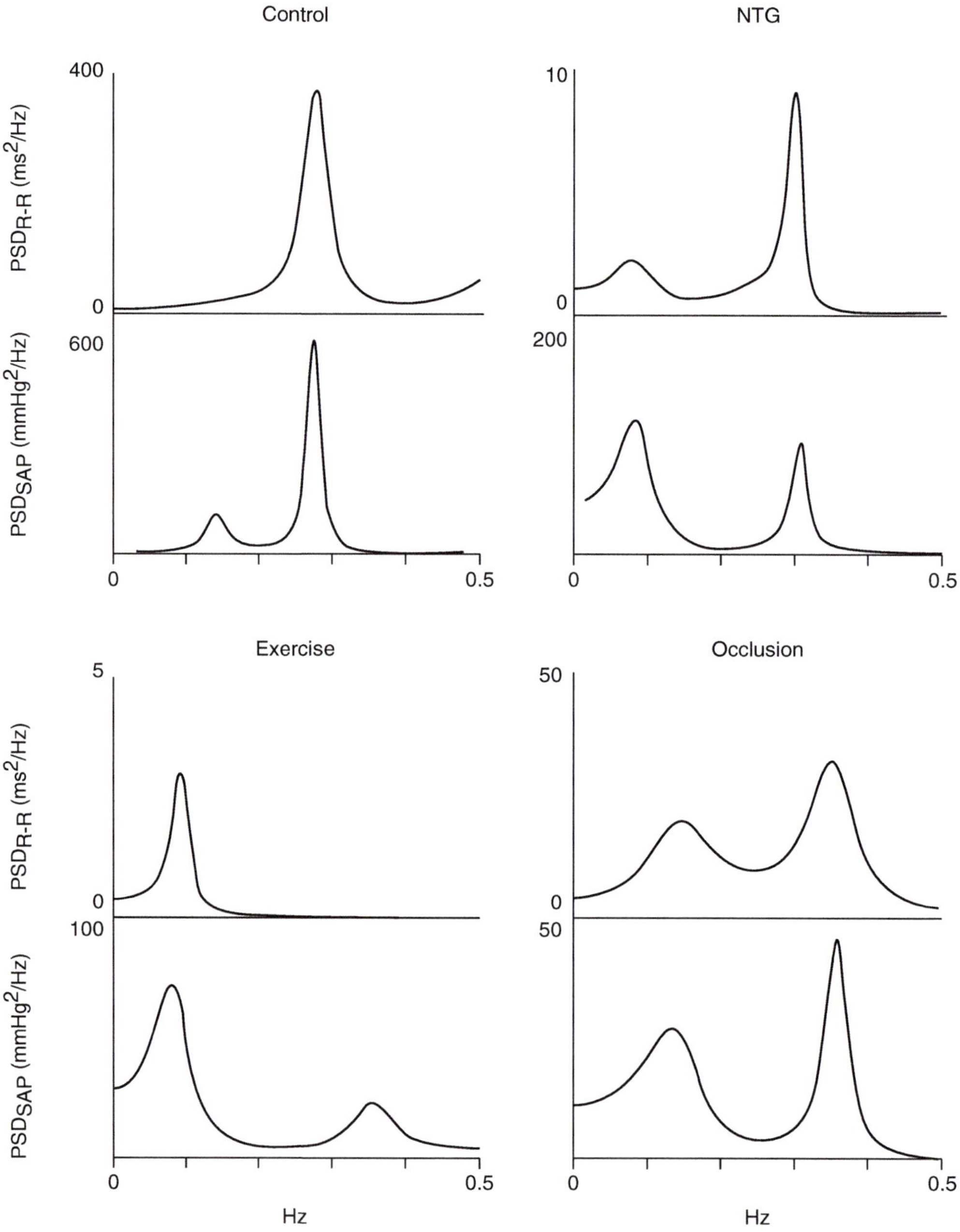

Fig. 10.4 Spectral analysis of RR interval (*upper tracings in each panel*) and systolic arterial pressure (SAP) (*lower tracings in each panel*) variabilities in conscious dogs at rest (Control) and during experimental maneuvers leading to a sympathetic predominance (i.e., nitroglycerin infusion [NTG], treadmill exercise [Exercise], and transient acute coronary artery occlusion [Occlusion]). Note, at control, the presence of a single major high-frequency component in the RR interval autospectrum; in SAP, a smaller low-frequency component is also evident. During sympathetic activation, spectral distribution is altered in favor of low frequency determining a leftward shift; simultaneously, a drastic reduction in RR variance occurs (notice different scales on ordinates). Schematically, a sympathetic excitatory condition is characterized by a simultaneous reduction of RR Variance (amplitude domain) and leftward shift (frequency domain). PSD, power spectral density. (From Malliani et al. [24], with permission Wolters Kluwer) (Fig. 3 in original paper)

and different settings of target organ physiology, such as the average RR interval or sympathetic nerve activity [11]. For clinical applications, it may be convenient to consider an overall set of the autonomic motor system subserving functional activation (i.e., arousal) or inhibition, and easily translated into a unitary autonomic nervous system index (ANSI) defining a rank from 0 to 100 benchmarked against a large reference population [63]. We would renounce the capacity of measuring sympathetic or parasympathetic activity, but we would gain an assessment of the continuous (opposite) dynamics of the cue function [55]. As shown in Fig. 10.5 [63], the physiological continuum from the sympathetic–parasympathetic balanced condition of rest versus the excitatory sympathetic condition of tilt or active standing can be approximately appreciated by spectral analysis of RR interval variability, which shows a clear relative increase of the power of the low frequency (LF) component (and a simultaneous decrease of high frequency [HF]) during tilt. A more detailed description of the methodological aspects of HRV as studied in our laboratory can be found in Ref. [17].

In summary, for ease of recording and simplicity of analysis, the majority of investigations focus specifically on time domain aspects of HRV [43] thought to reflect particularly vagal efferent control of the SA node. However, to what extent HRV might carry information about other autonomic control systems, such as the inflammatory reflex [64] or body weight balance [65] currently remains unclear. Autonomic regulation is also frequently treated as an all-or-nothing (on–off) global modality disregarding the large body of evidence showing a rather selective organization of autonomic regulation [66].

In this context, new investigations, taking advantage of progressive improvements in wearable electronics and artificial intelligence [67] show a rapidly growing utilization of HRV either alone or combined with other signals (e.g., arterial pressure and respiration) to assess autonomic cardiac regulation in behavioral long-term conditions (e.g., sleep) [68]. However, as a caveat, this model is implicitly based on a dynamic balance between paired antagonistic [19] reflexes, while in several circumstances (e.g., the diving reflex) vagal and sympathetic motor nerves might be activated in parallel [69].

Heart Rate Variability: A Synopsis

> *A central task consists in finding ways…to make unbiased estimates leading to probabilities that are in agreement with all the possible knowledge available about the system*
>
> —H. Haken [20]

We begin with the seminal idea [10] that "sympathetic and parasympathetic nervous activity make frequency-specific contributions to the heart rate power spectrum" proposing a strong interaction between physiology and information domains. Accordingly, HR fluctuations could furnish a probe (i.e., proxy) of short-term neural cardiac reg-

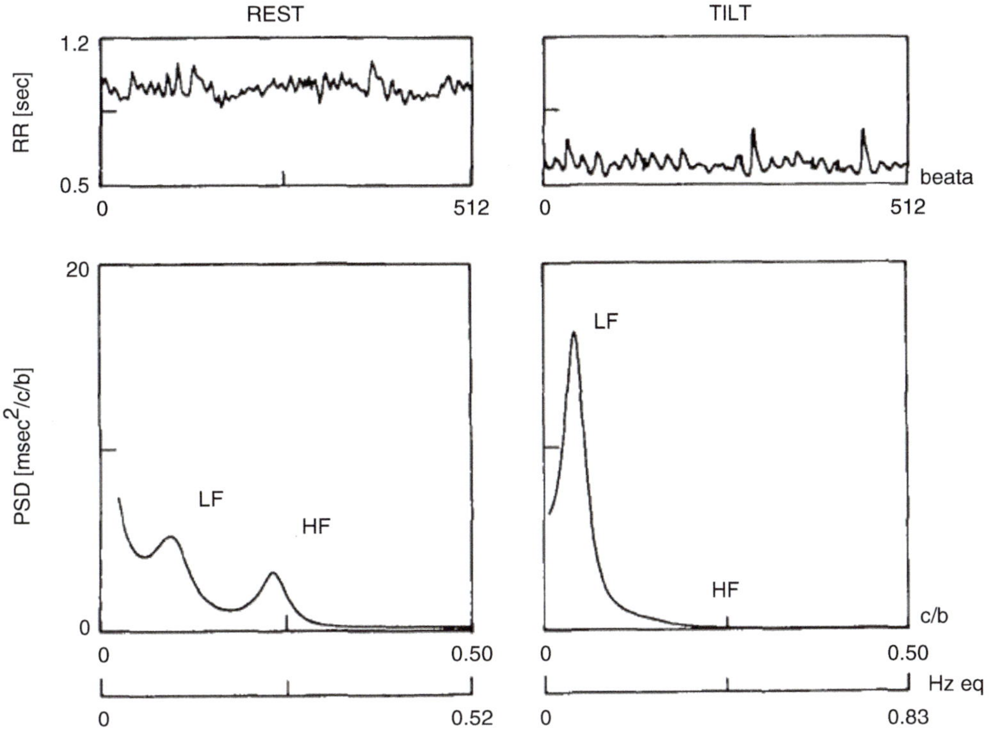

Fig. 10.5 Example of the spectral analysis of RR-interval Variability in a control subject. RR interval series (i.e., tachogram) at rest and during passive upright 90° tilt are reported in top panels. In the autospectra (*bottom panels*), two clearly separated low- and high-frequency components are presented at rest. During the sympathetic excitatory state induced by tilt, the low-frequency component becomes preponderant. Notice the change of pattern from leftward shift to rightward shift. (From Pagani et al. [63], with permission Wolters Kluwer)

ulation. A critical task, however, consists in *finding ways* to make estimates that are both *unbiased* and in *agreement with all* possible *knowledge* [20]. The focus on the speed of oscillations (as opposed to amplitude) as a provider of specific information [29], and time versus frequency domain as computational methods [70], or phasic versus tonic activity of the central neural governing structures [57] was implicit and far reaching.

It is important to consider that model-based mathematical descriptions of complex physiology (e.g., left ventricle cardiac dynamics) rely on a combination of indicators, comprised of an adimensional metric (e.g., ejection fraction percentage) along with their physical companions (e.g., ventricular volumes). Since a ratio between quantities is usually present as adimensional, the term "ratiology" has been used to identify this process [71]. A similar approach can be used to describe RR variability spectral analysis, combining an adimensional indicator (e.g., ANSI) [39] with an established physical measure (e.g., HR).

The model should also account for the obligatory neural interaction between the two branches of the ANS, one example being electrophysiological experiments on single cardiac vagal or sympathetic efferent fibers [48], considering also the mixed (afferent and efferent) nature of cardiac vagal and sympathetic nerves [24], as well as the possibility that the relative powers of low- (LF) and high-frequency (HF) oscillations by shifting the attention from raw (numerical) spectral data to **patterns** of oscillations might furnish additional details about coded information, such as the arousal–performance relationship [55]. These latter patterns are simply approximated by the LF/HF ratio or using normalized units to indicate (relative) oscillatory activity [63]. This corresponds to a/the shift from simple quantitative appraisal of autonomic cardiac regulation, based on amplitude of sympathetic and vagal motor activity (reflected into a raw quantification of modulatory oscillations of RR intervals) to multiple levels of encoding the overall control of autonomic motor function via several feedback circuits (from peripheral sensory inputs to CAN inputs [25, 27]). Accordingly, in addition to providing an adrenergic–cholinergic visceromotor system [72] in the role of the final common pathway regulating (one way) visceral performance, we must deal with a complex (two way, multicomponent) control system. Information must, therefore, be distributed throughout the system at various levels suggesting the value of more complex analysis [73], rather than simple raw amplitude (number of spikes/sec; amount of raw RR variability), various patterns may be addressed. Information bits may thus change meaning according to the specific distribution throughout the control network [29] (see **Figs. 10.2** and **10.3**). Pattern analysis carries the additional advantage that information embedded across multiple indices may be retrieved with an efficiency greater than using single indices [20]. In line with this, we reported recently that HRV combined with cardiac baroreflex can increase the predictive capacity to recognize the hypertensive state [74]. Functionally, the autonomic motor drive is carried by the efferent sympathetic and parasympathetic pathways (governing beat-by-beat cardiac function), which, in addition, encode autonomic information (at least) in amplitude and frequency [75]. As a behavioral example [28], response to a recognized threat might activate an excitatory reflex (fight or flight [38]), producing an increase in the amount of synaptic transmitter release, corresponding to an increase of the number of spikes that could be recorded from sympathetic motor nerves (in parallel with a reduction of vagal release of acetylcholine). As a first approximation activation of the system could thus be assessed by the amplitude of the changes (e.g., an increase in HR accompanied by a reduction in time domain measures of HRV) in controlled parameters. Simultaneously, the excitatory response is thought to be expressed into a leftward shift of oscillatory power in the chain from the CAN, to autonomic motor nerves and in the beat-by-beat changes in RR interval (with a change in oscillatory balance: increase of LF and decrease of HF normalized oscillatory components of RR variability (see Fig. 10.5).

Linear and nonlinear encoding may thus suggest the specifics of autonomic motor setting. Again, we are dealing with simultaneously with physiology (extent and directionality of the response, with amplitude coding of hemodynamics, biochemistry, and nerve firing) and information (regarding the autonomic neural setting), with frequency coding whereby activation is indicated by a/the leftward shift of oscillations in nerve firing and RR variability (for example, Fig. 10.6 [11]). In essence, we introduce pattern as code, travelling together with amplitude control signal in peripheral nerves (sympathetic and parasympathetic [29]).

Accordingly, following the general hypothesis that HRV is a proxy of cardiac neural information [24], we might label patients with the probability of belonging to a specific pattern (either a disease, such as hypertension, diabetes, and coronary artery disease, or a physiological condition, such as high-level athletes) using a single purpose-built index [76]. Individual labeling will thus depend on a benchmark derived from a large population utilizing multivariete techniques for the statistical analysis [77]. This approach builds on the observation that multiple variables may be reduced to few significant hidden components, each belonging to an informational ontology, whereby amplitude and oscillations might define different aspects of autonomic (dys)regulation, including (adimensional) pattern specific modalities [37].

For the purpose of this review, it may be relevant to recall that in a large group of patients the most informative clusters of HRV variables consisted of amplitude and oscillations of HRV, pulse rate, and arterial pressure [77].

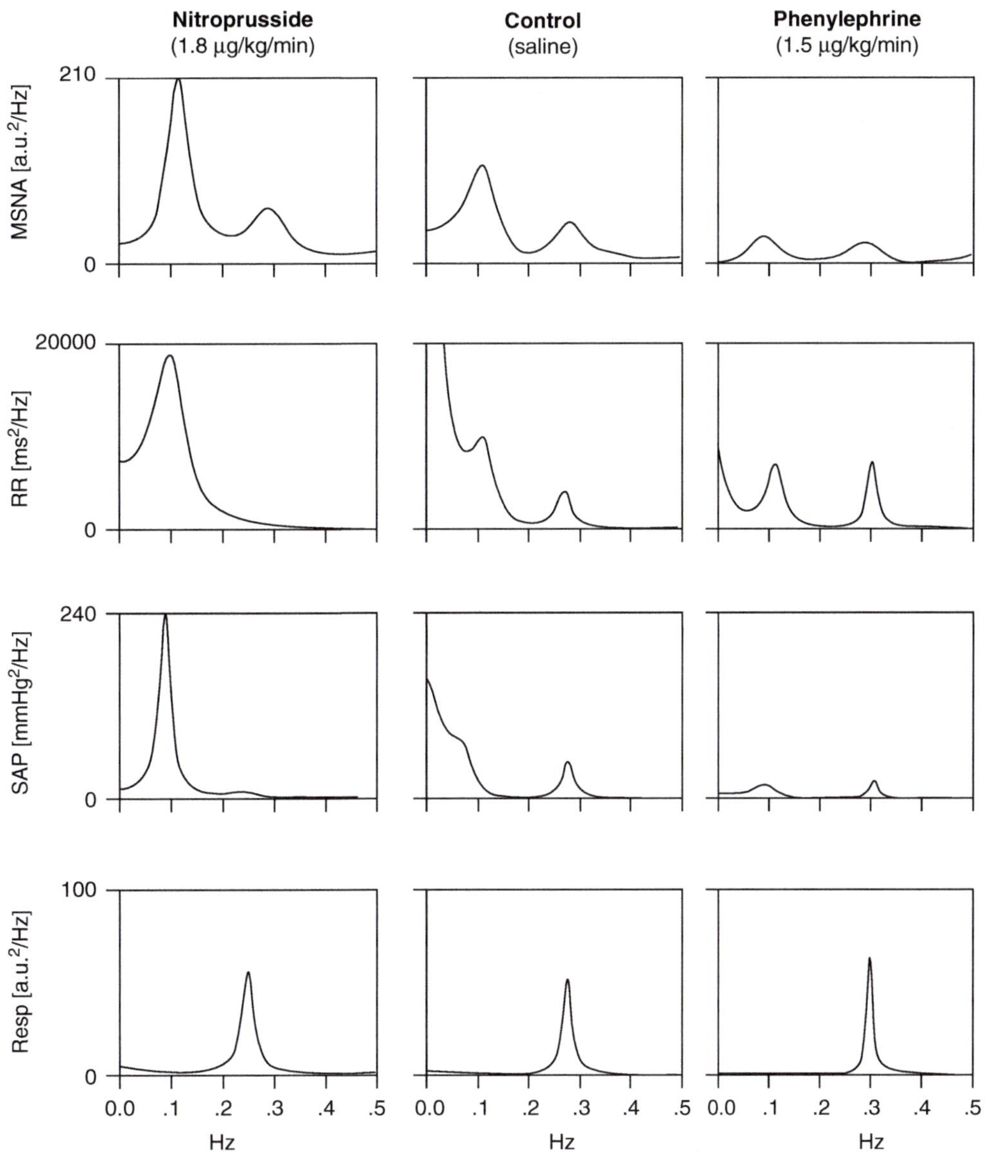

Fig. 10.6 Power spectra of muscle sympathetic nerve activity (MSNA), RR interval, and respiration (Resp) in a single subject during infusions of saline (Control), nitroprusside, and phenylephrine. During sympathetic activation induced by nitroprusside (left), the LF component of neural and cardiovascular variability signals predominates relative to the HF component (i.e., leftward shift). Conversely, during sympathetic inhibition and vagal activation induced by phenylephrine (right), there is an increase of the HF component relative to the LF component (i.e., rightward shift). a.u. indicates arbitrary units. Notice the change of patterns. (From Pagani et al. [11], with permission Wolters Kluwer)

Sleep: A Simplified View

Sleep is the intermediate state between wakefulness and death; wakefulness being regarded as the active state of all the animal and intellectual functions, and death as that of their total suspension.

—R. Macnish [78]

Not simply the absence of waking, sleep is a special activity of the brain, controlled by elaborate and precise mechanisms.

—J.A. Hobson [79]

The deepest sleep resembles death.

—I Samuel 26:12

Sleep and death are similar . . . sleep is one-sixtieth [i.e., one piece] of death.

—*The Talmud*, Berachoth 576

There she [Aphrodite] met sleep, the brother of death.

—Homer, *The Iliad*

To sleep: perchance to dream ...;
For in that sleep of death what dreams may come

—Shakespeare, *Hamlet*

How wonderful is death;
Death and his brother sleep

—Shelley, *Queen Mab*

Sleep has classically been considered as a passive process, an inactive state of the brain originating from reduced sensory inputs, reduced blood flow to the brain (vascular theories), or accumulation of various "hypnotoxins" with the consequent diminishment of brain activity. No real distinction was seen between sleep and other state of quiescence (coma/anesthesia) and sleep was considered closely related to death.

Nowadays, we know that sleep is an active and dynamic process comprising two clearly distinct types, rapid eye movement (REM) and non-REM sleep, which have different neurophysiological characteristics, subserve different functions, and are organized in different regions of the brain and by different neural networks.

The first evidence of sleep as an active process came in the second decade of the twentieth century when the Baron Constantin von Economo, an Austrian psychiatrist and neurologist of Romanian origin and Greek descent, documented that in patients with epidemic encephalitis ("the Spanish flu"), who appeared clinically agitated and insomniac, the anatomical lesion was located in the anterior hypothalamus and basal forebrain [80]. In contrast, if patients were hypersomnolent or stuporous, the predominant lesion was in the posterior hypothalamus and rostral midbrain. He concluded that the anterior hypothalamus contained the *Schlafzentrum* (sleep center) and the posterior hypothalamus the *Wachzentrum* (wake center).

A few years later, Walter Rudolf Hess, a Swiss physiologist, confirmed these findings in intact free moving cats. In this preparation electrical stimulation of the anterior region of the hypothalamus led to a behavior of quiescence due to the activation of trophotropic structures, while the stimulation of the posterior hypothalamus led to active behaviors and, therefore, hosted ergotropic structures [81]. However, true sleep appeared with a short latency only upon stimulating the anteromedial region of the thalamus. Hess, therefore, believed that it was the thalamus and not the hypothalamus that contained the true sleep center.

In 1928, the German psychiatrist Hans Berger [82] for the first time recorded the electrical activity of the human brain and named it electroencephalogram (EEG). For the first time, sleep could be continuously and qualitatively measured without disturbing the sleeper.

All the major elements of sleep brain wave patterns were described by Harvey, Hobart, Davis, and others at Harvard University in a series of papers published in 1937 and 1938 [83–85]. Blake, Gerard, and Kleitman added to this from their studies at the University of Chicago [86, 87]. In human EEG, sleep was characterized by high-amplitude slow waves and spindles, whereas wakefulness was characterized by low-amplitude waves and alpha rhythm. The image of the sleeping brain completely "turned off" gave way to the image of the sleeping brain engaged in slow, synchronized, "idling" neuronal activity.

The 1930s also saw a series of investigations that seemed to establish conclusively both the passive theory of sleep and the notion that it occurred in response to reduction of stimulation and activity. These were the investigations of Belgian physiologist Frederick Bremer reported in 1935 [88] and 1936 [89]. Bremer documented that slicing the brain along the line between the medulla and spinal cord (so-called encephale isolé preparation) did not impair the animal's ability to stay awake [88]. In contrast, if the slice was made along the line joining the mesencephalon and diencephalon (*cerveau isolé* preparation), the animal no longer presented EEG signs of wakefulness [89]. He concluded that sleep was a passive phenomenon due to a loss of peripheral (visceral and somatic) stimuli reaching the cerebral cortex through the brain stem. Although incorrectly interpreted, Bremer's experimental findings were historically important because they shifted physiologists' attention away from the diencephalon to the brain stem. Studying the brain stem reticular formation, Moruzzi, first with Magoun [90] and then with his collaborators, discovered that the upper brain stem contains an arousing (desynchronizing) system whereas the dearousing (synchronizing) structures are located in the lower brain stem [90, 91].

Between 1953 and 1957, Kleitman's laboratory in Chicago made a discovery which revolutionized sleep physiology unequivocally demonstrating sleep as an active process. Aserinsky and Kleitman discovered that there are two types of sleep: one identified by EEG tracings alone since the 1930s and characterized by high amplitude EEG waves (sleep spindles and slow or delta waves), the other one identified by recording eye movements that had been ignored until this time because its EEG features (low amplitude fast EEG activity) could not be distinguished from those characterizing active wakefulness and drowsiness [92]. Sleep associated with eye movements and vivid dream activity was called REM sleep.

Between 1958 and 1962, the French physiologist Michel Jouvet demonstrated that the executive mechanisms responsible for REM sleep are located in the rostral part of the pontine reticular formation [93, 94]. Jouvet called REM sleep "paradoxical sleep" because it represented a strange neuropsychological situation: a "waking" (dreaming) brain in a "sleeping" body (skeletal muscles are functionally blocked during REM sleep).

Modern sleep researchers [95, 96] define sleep on the basis of both behavior while asleep and the related physiologic changes that occur to the brain's electrical rhythm. The behavioral criteria include lack of mobility or slight mobility, closed eyes, a characteristic species-specific sleeping posture, reduced response to external stimulation, quiescence, increased reaction time, elevated arousal threshold, impaired cognitive function, and a reversible unconscious state. The physiologic criteria are based on the findings from EEG, electro-oculo-graphy (EOG), and electromyography (EMG) as well as other physiologic changes in ventilation and circulation. Based on these criteria, sleep is divided into two states: REM sleep (or desynchronized sleep) and non-REM sleep (synchronized sleep, which has three different stages N1, N2, N3). Each is linked to specific brain waves and neuronal activity. Table 10.1 reports synthetically key elements of NREM and REM sleep states combined with essential HRV proxies of cardiac autonomic regulation.

In an ideal situation (which may not be seen in all normal individuals), NREM and REM alternate in a cyclic manner, each cycle lasting on average from 90 to 110 minutes. During a normal sleep period in adults, four to six such cycles are

Table 10.1 The key elements of non-rapid eye movement (NREM) sleep and rapid eye movement (REM) sleep states and heart rate variability (HRV) proxies of cardiac autonomic regulation

Function	Wakefulness	NREM	REM
Posture	Normal	Recumbent	Recumbent
Mobility	Normal	Slightly reduced or immobile; postural shifts	Moderately reduced or immobile; myoclonic jerks
Response to stimulation	Normal	Mildly to moderately reduced	Moderately reduced to no response
Level of alertness	Alert	Unconscious but reversible	Unconscious but reversible
Eyelids	Open	Closed	Closed
Eye movements	Waking eye movements	Slow rolling eye movements	Rapid eye movements
Electroencephalogram	Alpha waves; desynchronized	Synchronized	Theta or sawtooth waves; desynchronized
Electro-oculography	Normal	Mildly reduced	Moderately to severely reduced or absent
	Waking eye movements	Slow rolling eye movements	Rapid eye movements
HRV amplitude	Reduced	Increased	Reduced
HRV oscillations	Low-frequency shift	High-frequency shift	Low frequency shift
Cardiac baroreflex	Reduction of gain	Increase of gain	Reduction of gain

noted. The first two cycles are dominated by slow-wave sleep (SWS) [97] (Rechtschaffen and Kales stages 3 and 4 NREM and AASM stage N3 sleep); subsequent cycles contain less SWS, and sometimes SWS does not occur at all. In contrast, the REM sleep cycle increases from the first to the last cycle and the longest REM sleep episode toward the end of the night may last for an hour. Thus, in human adult sleep, the first third is dominated by the SWS and the last third is dominated by REM sleep. This is in line with Moruzzi's view [55] that physiological sleep is characterized: (a) by the presence of a short- or long-lasting appetitive phase, possibly corresponding to the subjective feeling of drowsiness; (b) by the complete reversibility of all hypnic manifestations, as shown by the arousal produced by sensory and cortical stimulation; and finally (c) by the alternation between synchronized and desynchronized episodes of sleep, the presence of short lasting paradoxical episodes and of the corresponding hallucinations, the dreams, being an indispensable manifestation of every type of physiological mammalian sleep. Once the instinctive behavior of sleep has started, a chain of consummatory actions with complex reverberations between brain stem and cerebrum will prevent a further fall of reticular tone to levels that would lead to a coma, a situation that would by definition abolish physiological sleep (see Fig. 10.3). A change in the opposite direction occurs at the moment of arousal, since all manifestations of sleep disappear when the reticular tone reaches the critical levels for consciousness.

The Close Link Between Sleep and the Autonomic Nervous System

REM sleep triggers marked increases in sympathetic-nerve activity. —VK Somers et al. [98]

Sleep and ANS are closely associated on both biological and clinical grounds. Neuronal pathways located in the brain stem and basal forebrain responsible for the wake–sleep transition are connected with areas of the central nervous system regulating ANS activity (i.e., the CAN) [71, 99]. Indeed, sleep itself may be considered one of the most highly integrated autonomic functions at the forebrain diencephalic level, where the behavioral and homeostatic integration occurs. The close and bidirectional interconnection with hierarchical levels (i.e., state of consciousness) [100] supports this assertation. Hence, sleep disorders may cause or be associated with an unbalanced shift of autonomic modulation of the cardiovascular functions during sleep and wakefulness. On the other hand, general medical and neurologic disorders that determine cardiovascular autonomic dysfunction may also provoke sleep disturbances. Cardiovascular autonomic dysfunction is also an important risk factor for cerebrovascular and cardiovascular disease. Therefore, many studies addressed changes in ANS activity associated with sleep disorders and *vice versa* [101].

In normal circumstances, the day–night circadian rhythm of the sleep–wake cycle is characterized by excitatory–inhibitory alternations. Recalling the "unitary" multi component organization of autonomic control [19], HRV oscillations parallel analogous oscillations in other cardiovascular reflexes, such as the baroreflex that shows higher gain during the night and lower values during daily wakefulness [102]. The circadian modification of the autonomic function also has implications for clinical practice, considering the higher occurrence of cardiovascular and cerebrovascular events in early morning hours [103].

The concept that the ANS is differently modulated according to the wake or sleep state (i.e., the state-dependent modulation) is relatively recent. By simultaneous recording of cardiovascular and respiratory autonomic parameters during sleep, it was possible first to describe their profile during sleep, and second to investigate the implications of such connections in clinical practice. In this regard, Coccagna and colleagues [104] demonstrated for the first time the dramatic effects of apneas on systemic and pulmonary blood pressure

(BP) in patients with obstructive sleep apnea. Lugaresi and coworkers described the motor and autonomic characteristics of sleep, reporting a progressive reduction of autonomic activation from stage 1 throughout stage 3 of NREM sleep, and an irregular pattern of cardiovascular and respiratory parameters during REM sleep, which also presented abolished motor activity, leading to the fascinating condition of a very active autonomic brain (corresponding to an excitatory shift) in an inactive body (characterized by an inhibitory shift) [104, 105].

Subsequent extensive studies have better elucidated autonomic changes according to sleep stage [106], which can be summarized as follows:

(a) During NREM sleep, there is a predominance of the parasympathetic inhibitory setting, and the ANS regulatory responses to internal or external stimuli may be activated in order to maintain homeostasis. Coherently with this view, the pattern of integrated automatic regulation minimizing energy expenditure includes the BP and HR fall, the lowering of metabolic heat production and body temperature and the lowering of the breathing rate. In this phase, the HRV profile is characterized by a "vagal shift," that is, increase in amplitude and relative prevalence of HF oscillations. In this stage, the cardiovascular risk is decreased.
(b) REM sleep is characterized by a disruption of the homeostatic physiologic equilibrium leading to effector responses of great instability with alteration of temperature, cardiovascular and breathing regulation resulting in excitatory efferent activation [98]. During REM, the HRV profile mimics a sympathetic predominance: low HRV amplitude and leftward shift of frequency distribution. We know that in this condition the cardiovascular risk is increased (Table 10.2).

Table 10.2 Autonomic changes according to sleep stage

Function	NREM sleep	REM sleep
Main feature	Homeostatic Autonomic stability	Not homeostatic Autonomic instability
ANS effectors	Parasympathetic predominance	Phasic fluctuations of parasympathetic and sympathetic/sympathetic predominance
Cardiovascular system	Decreased HR, decreased BP, increased BRS CV risk decreased	Wide fluctuations in BP and HR, impaired BRS Risk increased
Respiration	Dominated by chemical control	Irregular, impaired respiratory reflexes, atonia

NREM = non-rapid eye movement; *REM* = rapid eye movement; *ANS* = autonomic nervous system; *HR* = heart rate; *BP* = blood pressure; *BRS* = baroreceptor reflex sensitivity; *CV* = cardiovascular.

Heart Rate Variability in Sleep Disorders

At the beginning of all experimental work stands the choice of the appropriate technique of investigation.

—W. R. Hess [19]

Important insights on autonomic function during wake and sleep were obtained in the early 1990s by the work of Somers and colleagues, by means of muscle sympathetic nerve activity (MSNA) recordings [98]. However, MSNA depends largely on specific codes, describing single or multiunit firing, amplitude, frequency, phase, or correlation between circuits and is invasive. Even if the interpretation of HRV is still far from established and largely depends on the underlying model of autonomic functions [107], HRV components may be used to study how autonomic function is modulated during sleep stages and in response to arousal.

Obstructive sleep apnea is an example of a sleep disorder causing autonomic dysfunction. It is characterized by repetitive episodes of complete or partial upper-airway obstruction during sleep, resulting in blood oxygen desaturation and often terminating by a brief arousal [108].

Each apneic episode induces dramatic changes on cardiovascular parameters, which are BP increase and HR decrease, followed by tachycardia on resuming of breathing [104]. These alterations are secondary to an overactivity of the sympathetic nervous system due to a hypoxia-induced tonic activation of excitatory chemoreflex afferents [109, 110] and depression of spontaneous baroreceptor reflex sensitivity [111].

Sympathetic overactivity was demonstrated also during wakefulness in patients with obstructive sleep apnea. Circadian rhythm analysis of HRV showed lower parasympathetic and higher sympathetic activity from morning to noon in obstructive sleep apnea patients compared to controls [112]. Moreover, normotensive obstructive sleep apnea patients have higher HR and norepinephrine plasma levels at rest during wakefulness and a higher BP response to head-up tilt compared to controls [113]. Further, these patients presented significantly lower values of respiratory arrhythmia and Valsalva ratio associated with a greater decrease in HR induced by cold face test, suggesting blunted reflex responses dependent on baroreceptor or pulmonary afferents and normal or increased cardiac parasympathetic efferent activity.

The sympathetic activation functional to halt the apnea, when repeated several times for an extended period may induce remodeling of central neuronal circuits that in turn lead to a sustained chronic peripheral sympathetic overactivity. This is responsible for the increased risk of developing cardiovascular and cerebrovascular diseases (hypertension, myocardial infarction, arrhythmias, heart failure, and stroke) in patients affected by this condition.

A different profile of autonomic dysfunction marks REM sleep behavior disorder (RBD), a sleep parasomnia characterized by dream-enacting behaviors, often violent and injurious, occurring during REM sleep and associated with loss of the physiological REM muscle atonia [108]. Since its first description, Schenck and colleagues noted the lack of HR changes which would have been expected in association with the vigorous behaviors during REM sleep in such patients [114]. Several subsequent studies reported reduced HRV during night-time, reduced HR response to arousals and leg movements, and lack of the decrease in RR interval and HF components from NREM to REM sleep transition that is the absence of the physiologic parasympathetic withdrawal and sympathetic increase observed during REM sleep compared to NREM sleep in these patients [115]. HRV analysis during tilt test showed lower LF and higher HF components as well as significant reduction of LF/HF ratio in RBD patients compared to controls, suggesting an impaired autonomic response to orthostatic stress during wakefulness in RBD [116].

Pathogenesis of idiopathic RBD is yet to be fully understood; however, degeneration of areas involved in sleep regulation and REM promotion located in the brain stem seem to play a role. The close vicinity with the CAN suggests that autonomic circuits are also directly involved in the degenerative process and are thus associated with this condition.

In summary, to interpret the autonomic changes occurring during sleep it may be useful to abandon the traditional view of parasympathetic and sympathetic efferent control (often indicated as sympatho-vagal balance) and substitute it with a more dynamic (cybernetic) view, synthesized in the balance of opposing negative and positive feedbacks, as the former is inhibitory and the latter is excitatory functionally. The change is not cosmetic, but substantial, since it gives a critical role to autonomic afferents and to reflexes interacting with the central command (better indicated as CAN), rendering the ANS "connected" (not autonomous) in various ways to the rest of the neural circuitry.

Generally, autonomic regulation is implicitly considered a "functional unity" resulting in dynamical changes in efferent (motor) sympathetic or parasympathetic activity; an important possibility that is usually disregarded depicts possible changes in functional organization, resulting in a cybernetic reset. As an example, we may recall the disconnection between autonomic and somatomotor circuits during REM sleep. Operationally, it is noteworthy that an increase in HR might result from an increase in sympathetic activity, or a reduction in vagal activity depending upon the integrated balance of various regulatory circuits. This balance is the end result of the physiological dynamics of "software" or of anatomical disruption, whereby severing an excitatory input may result in inhibition overall.

HRV and Sleep in the Clinic

The finger pointing at the moon is not the moon.

—Thich Nhat Hanh [117]

Given the still incomplete agreement about the clinical value of HRV as a reliable autonomic measure [118, 119], we should start from the a priori consideration that the importance of HRV during various conditions, such as during sleep, varies according to the specific questions that are addressed.

Regarding the present review, clinical studies should be preferred to experimental ones, recognizing the importance of estimating model parameters in individual patients [120] and of selecting the proper metrics to serve as patient oriented (bio) markers [68] among a multiplicity of (quarreling) contenders. Multiple studies since historical findings of the 1980s to 1990s [10, 70, 121] have been largely interpreted as indication that some metrics from HRV (in particular HF spectral components of RR variance linked to respiration) may reliably assess vagal influences to the SA node, while sympathetic influences are more difficult to glean from LF components [43]. Of note, more complex indices (e.g., the bivariate baroreflex gain) might prove more reliable indicators of overall neurovisceral regulation (inhibitory and excitatory) [17]. Conversely, the interpretation of other indices (such as the lower frequency oscillations) derived from spectral analysis of RR V or MSNA [11] receives a weaker consensus of interpretation [44]. Finally, recent evidence seems to provide much needed genetic support to the link between reduced vagal control (as reflected by low HRV) and greater risk of cardiac mortality [122].

HRV and the Clinic: Importance of Models

The supreme art of war is to subdue the enemy without fighting.

—Sun Tzu [123]

Considering that neural control of cardiac functions is engrained in dynamics of changing requests from the periphery, one might also consider the capacity of HRV (and derived indices) of signaling variations in autonomic drive (modeling either only peripheral efferent activity or more correctly the complex hierarchy of the entire control system). Following this integrated (closed loop, sensory and motor, dynamical) model, unitary indices of HRV gain a more compelling value than the separated vagal or sympathetic (motor only) hypothesis. The dynamics of RR V (RR variability?) implies a focus on large, fast changes in raw (e.g., RR variance measured in m/s^2) and computed (e.g., the ratio LF/HF) indices. The combination of both raw and derived variables might in addition represent a better approach to cardiovascular metrics [68] helping integrate clinical research with medical care [124]. Consensus on the use of HRV in sleep medicine should thus be viewed as a progressive journey rather than a magical, single revealing step.

Conclusion: HRV, Sleep, and Digital Medicine

Although the autonomic motor system is largely involuntary, the behaviours controlled by it are tightly integrated with voluntary movements controlled by the somatic motor system.

—J.P. Horn and L.W. Swanson [25]

Medicine has evolved from the time of Hippocrates to become mostly digitalized. Technology largely pervades all medical fields to help doctors in a major shift from diagnoses and treatment of groups of patients, to maintain health in a longer, happier life according to individually titrated procedures [125]. Technology has furthered research and hopefully will continue to do so. Yet, it is important to avoid being overwhelmed by the digital data provided in large numbers, but to learn to correctly interpret such results in light of the multifarious clinical settings.

Sleep is one of the most fascinating and integrated human functions to study, and technology has provided us with a great chance to dig more deeply in to its physiology and pathophysiology. HRV is an easy and reliable parameter useful to clinicians to assess autonomic function dynamics also during sleep. A comprehensive evaluation of sleep requires a structured, complete video-polysomnography, in a dedicated environment, generating huge amounts of data, thus allowing deep evaluations of all its multiple components. HRV, conversely, may be of particular interest because of its technical simplicity. Ease of measure is, however, coupled to a still debated interpretation, which falls short of providing measures of sympathetic or parasympathetic efferent activity but seems to furnish an index of activation/inhibition balance [30] of the autonomic neural organization and therefore of arousal [55] and attendant link with performance. In accordance with system medicine, HRV does not provide direct information regarding the pathogenesis of individual autonomic dysfunctions but correlates with multiple parameters of different domains such as motor control in various ways in line with the underlying background, condition, and environment.

In conclusion, oriented longitudinal intervention studies using benchmarked simple HRV indices [76] on large populations might support methods to assess (**How?**) the role of autonomic (dys)regulation in dynamic conditions such as during normal or abnormal sleep (**When?**) and furnish stronger rational motives for a more cogent clinical use of a relatively simple technique, useful also in dire times, when keeping distance may be advisable (**Why?**).

References

1. Pinault JR. Hippocratic lives and legends. Studies in ancient medicine, vol. 4. EJ Brill: Leiden; 1992.
2. Harvey W. The anatomical exercises: de motu cordis and de circulatione sanguinis. English translation. Keynes G, editor. New York: Dover; 1995.
3. Lower R. Tractatus de corde. Item de motu & colore sanguinis et chyli in eum transitu. London: Typis Jo Redmayne, impensiss Jacobi Allestry; 1669.
4. Wooley CF. Palpitation: brain, heart, and 'spirits' in the seventeenth century. J R Soc Med. 1998;91(3):157–60.
5. Fye WB. Profiles in cardiology. Antonio Scarpa. Clin Cardiol. 1997;20(4):411–2.
6. Eknoyan G. Stephen Hales: the contributions of an enlightenment physiologist to the study of the kidney in health and disease. G Ital Nefrol. 2016;33(Suppl 66):33.S66.5.
7. Rivera-Ruiz M, Cajavilca C, Varon J. Einthoven's string galvanometer: the first electrocardiograph. Tex Heart Inst J. 2008;35(2):174–8.
8. Warner HR, Cox A. A mathematical model of heart rate control by sympathetic and vagus efferent information. Simulation. 1964;3(1):63–71.
9. McSayers BA. Analysis of heart rate variability. Ergonomics. 1973;16(1):17–32.
10. Akselrod S, Gordon D, Ubel FA, Shannon DC, Berger AC, Cohen RJ. Power spectrum analysis of heart rate fluctuation: a quantitative probe of beat-to-beat cardiovascular control. Science. 1981;213(4504):220–2.
11. Pagani M, Montano N, Porta A, Malliani A, Abboud FM, Birkett C, et al. Relationship between spectral components of cardiovascular variabilities and direct measures of muscle sympathetic nerve activity in humans. Circulation. 1997;95(6):1441–8.
12. Bible Gateway. New international version. Acts 5 Ananias and Sapphira. https://www.biblegateway.com/passage/?search=Acts.5&version=NIV. Accessed 2 Aug 2020.
13. La Rovere MT, Bigger JT, Marcus FI, Mortara A, Schwartz PJ. Baroreflex sensitivity and heart-rate variability in prediction of total cardiac mortality after myocardial infarction. Lancet. 1998;351(9101):478–84.
14. Breakspear M, Heitmann S, Daffertshofer A. Generative models of cortical oscillations: neurobiological implications of the Kuramoto model. Front Hum Neurosci. 2010;4:190.
15. Gerlach DA, Manuel J, Hoff A, Kronsbein H, Hoffmann F, Heusser K, et al. Novel approach to elucidate human baroreflex regulation at the brainstem level: pharmacological testing during fMRI. Front Neurosci. 2019;13:193.
16. Dooley D. Wearable electronics market development status, emerging technologies, regional trends and comprehensive research study 2025. Press release. 1 Jul 2020. America news hour. https://www.americanewshour.com/2020/07/01/wearable-electronics-market-development-status-emerging-technologies-regional-trends-and-comprehensive-research-study-2025-2/375399. Accessed 2 Sep 2020.
17. Solaro N, Malacarne M, Pagani M, Lucini D. Cardiac baroreflex, HRV, and statistics: an interdisciplinary approach in hypertension. Front Physiol. 2019;10:478.

18. Karemaker JM. Heart rate variability: why do spectral analysis? Heart. 1997;77(2):99–101.
19. Hess WR. The central control of the activity of internal organs. In: The Nobel Foundation, editor. Nobel lecture physiology or medicine 1942–1962. Amsterdam: Elsevier; 1964.
20. Haken H. Synergetics: an introduction: nonequilibrium phase transitions and self-organization in physics, chemistry and biology (Springer series in Synergetics). 3rd ed. Berlin: Springer Verlag; 1983.
21. Brown D. Origin. New York: Doubleday/Penguin Random House; 2017.
22. Langley JN. The autonomic nervous system. Cambridge: W. Heffer & Sons; 1921.
23. Sherrington CS. The integrative action of the nervous system. New Haven: Yale University Press; 1911.
24. Malliani A, Pagani M, Lombardi F, Cerutti S. Cardiovascular neural regulation explored in the frequency domain. Circulation. 1991;84(2):482–92.
25. Horn JP, Swanson LW. The autonomic motor system and the hypothalamus. In: Kandel ER, Schwartz JH, Jessell TM, Siegelbaum SA, Hudspeth AJ, editors. Principles of neural science. 5th ed. New York: McGraw Hill; 2013. p. 1056–78.
26. Kandel ER, Schwartz JH, Jessell TM, Siegelbaum SA, Hudspeth AJ, editors. Principles of neural science. 5th ed. New York: McGraw Hill; 2013.
27. Cersosimo MG, Benarroch EE. Central control of autonomic function and involvement in neurodegenerative disorders. Handb Clin Neurol. 2013;117:45–57.
28. Engel BT. Psychosomatic medicine, behavioral medicine, just plain medicine. Psychosom Med. 1986;48(7):466–79.
29. Pagani M, Malliani A. Interpreting oscillations of muscle sympathetic nerve activity and heart rate variability. J Hypertens. 2000;18(12):1709–19.
30. Massimini M, Porta A, Mariotti M, Malliani A, Montano N. Heart rate variability is encoded in the spontaneous discharge of thalamic somatosensory neurones in cat. J Physiol. 2000;526(Pt 2):387–96.
31. Fukuda K, Kanazawa H, Aizawa Y, Ardell JL, Shivkumar K. Cardiac innervation and sudden cardiac death. Circ Res. 2015;116(12):2005–19.
32. Zaglia T, Mongillo M. Cardiac sympathetic innervation, from a different point of (re)view. J Physiol. 2017;595(12):3919–30.
33. Tracey KJ. The inflammatory reflex. Nature. 2002;420(6917):853–9.
34. Yao G, Kang L, Li J, Long Y, Wei H, Ferreira CA, et al. Effective weight control via an implanted self-powered vagus nerve stimulation device. Nat Commun. 2018;9(1):5349.
35. Aristotle. On the soul. Parva naturalia. On breath. Trans. Hett WS. Loeb Classical Library 288. Cambridge, MA: Harvard University Press; 1957.
36. Hippocrates. Ancient medicine. Airs, waters, places. Epidemics 1 and 3. The Oath. Precepts. Nutriment. Trans. Jones WHS. Loeb Classical Library 147. Cambridge, MA: Harvard University Press; 1923.
37. Sassi R, Cerutti S, Lombardi F, Malik M, Huikuri HV, Peng CK, et al. Advances in heart rate variability signal analysis: joint position statement by the e-cardiology ESC working group and the European heart rhythm association co-endorsed by the Asia Pacific Heart Rhythm Society. Europace. 2015;17(9):1341–53.
38. La Rovere MT, Porta A, Schwartz PJ. Autonomic control of the heart and its clinical impact. A personal perspective. Front Physiol. 2020;11:582.
39. Abboud FM. The Walter B. Cannon memorial award lecture, 2009. Physiology in perspective: the wisdom of the body. In search of autonomic balance: the good, the bad, and the ugly. Am J Physiol Regul Integr Comp Physiol. 2010;298(6):R1449–67.
40. Beissner F, Meissner K, Bär KJ, Napadow V. The autonomic brain: an activation likelihood estimation meta-analysis for central processing of autonomic function. J Neurosci. 2013;33(25):10503–11.
41. Valenza G, Sclocco R, Duggento A, Passamonti L, Napadow V, Barbieri R, Toschi N. The central autonomic network at rest: uncovering functional MRI correlates of time-varying autonomic outflow. NeuroImage. 2019;197:383–90.
42. La Rovere MT, Pinna GD, Hohnloser SH, Marcus FI, Mortara A, Nohara R, et al. Barorefiex sensitivity and heart rate variability in the identification of patients at risk for life-threatening arrhythmias: implications for clinical trials. Circulation. 2001;103(16):2072–7.
43. Heart rate variability: standards of measurement, physiological interpretation and clinical use. Task force of the European society of cardiology and the North American society of pacing and electrophysiology. Circulation. 1996;93(5):1043–65.
44. Billman GE. The LF/HF ratio does not accurately measure cardiac sympatho-vagal balance. Front Physiol. 2013;4:26.
45. Eckberg D. Sympathovagal balance: a critical appraisal. Circulation. 1997;96(9):3224–32.
46. Sleight P, Bernardi L. Sympathovagal balance (letter). Circulation. 1998;98(23):2640.
47. Malliani A, Pagani M, Montano N, Mela GS. Sympathovagal balance: a reappraisal. Circulation. 1998;98(23):2640–3.
48. Pagani M, Pizzinelli P, Bergamaschi M, Malliani A. A positive feedback sympathetic pressor reflex during stretch of the thoracic aorta in conscious dogs. Circ Res. 1982;50(1):125–32.
49. Schwartz PJ, Pagani M, Lombardi F, Malliani A, Brown AM. A cardiocardiac sympathovagal reflex in the cat. Circ Res. 1973;32(2):215–20.
50. Prechtl JC, Powley TL. B-afferents: a fundamental division of the nervous system mediating homeostasis? Behav Brain Sci. 1990;13(2):289–300.
51. Warner HR, Russell RO. Effect of combined sympathetic and vagal stimulation on heart rate in the dog. Circ Res. 1969;24(4):567–73.
52. Sunagawa K, Kawada T, Nakahara T. Dynamic nonlinear Vago-sympathetic interaction in regulating heart rate. Heart Vessel. 1998;13(4):157–74.
53. Malliani A, Pagani M. Afferent sympathetic nerve fibres with aortic endings. J Physiol. 1976;263(2):157–69.
54. Jänig W. The integrative action of the autonomic nervous system: neurobiology of homeostasis. Cambridge: Cambridge University Press; 2006.
55. Moruzzi G. Sleep and instinctive behavior. Arch Ital Biol. 1969;107(2):175–216.
56. Hebb DO. A textbook of psychology. 3rd ed. Philadelphia: Saunders; 1966.
57. Aston-Jones G, Cohen JD. An integrative theory of locus coeruleus-norepinephrine function: adaptive gain and optimal performance. Annu Rev Neurosci. 2005;28:403–50.
58. Cortelli P, Parchi P, Contin M, Pierangeli G, Avoni P, Tinuper P, et al. Cardiovascular dysautonomia in fatal familial insomnia. Clin Auton Res. 1991;1(1):15–21.
59. Richerson GB, Aston-Jones G, Saper CB. The modulatory functions of the brain stem. In: Kandel ER, Schwartz JH, Jessell TM, Siegelbaum SA, Hudspeth AJ, editors. Principles of neural science. 5th ed. New York: McGraw Hill; 2013. p. 1038–55.
60. Guazzi M, Malliani A, Zanchetti A. Reflex regulation of consciousness and emotional behaviour. Acta Neurochir. 1964;12(2):198–214.
61. Koch E. Die Irradiation der pressoreceptorischen Kreislaufreflexe. KlinWschr. 1932;11:225–7.
62. Bizzi E, Libretti A, Malliani A, Zanchetti A. Reflex chemoceptive excitation of diencephalic sham rage behavior. Am J Physiol Content. 1961;200(5):923–6.
63. Pagani M, Lombardi F, Guzzetti S, Rimoldi O, Furlan R, Pizzinelli P, et al. Power spectral analysis of heart rate and arterial pressure

variabilities as a marker of sympatho-vagal interaction in man and conscious dog. Circ Res. 1986;59(2):178–93.
64. Williams DWP, Koenig J, Carnevali L, Sgoifo A, Jarczok MN, Sternberg EM, et al. Heart rate variability and inflammation: a meta-analysis of human studies. Brain Behav Immun. 2019;80:219–26.
65. Föhr T, Pietilä J, Helander E, Myllymäki T, Lindholm H, Rusko H, et al. Physical activity, body mass index and heart rate variability-based stress and recovery in 16 275 Finnish employees: a cross-sectional study. BMC Public Health. 2016;16:701.
66. Abboud FM, Thames MD. Interaction of cardiovascular reflexes in circulatory control. In: Terjung R, editor. Compr physiol. Hoboken: Wiley; 2011. p. 675–753.
67. Milani RV, Bober RM, Lavie CJ. The role of technology in chronic disease care. Prog Cardiovasc Dis. 2016;58(6):579–83.
68. Chouchou F, Desseilles M. Heart rate variability: a tool to explore the sleeping brain? Front Neurosci. 2014;8:402.
69. Kollai M, Koizumi K. Reciprocal and non-reciprocal action of the vagal and sympathetic nerves innervating the heart. J Auton Nerv Syst. 1979;1(1):33–52.
70. Malik M, John Camm A, Thomas Bigger J, Breithardt G, Cerutti S, Cohen RJ, et al. Heart rate variability: standards of measurement, physiological interpretation, and clinical use. Circulation. 1996;93(5):1043–65.
71. Kerkhof PLM, Peace RA, Handly N. Ratiology and a complementary class of metrics for cardiovascular investigations. Physiology. 2019;34(4):250–63.
72. Benarroch EE. The central autonomic network: functional organization, dysfunction, and perspective. Mayo Clin Proc. 1993;68(10):988–1001.
73. Ahn AC, Tewari M, Poon CS, Phillips RS. The clinical applications of a systems approach. PLoS Med. 2006 Jul;3(7):e209.
74. Lucini D, Solaro N, Pagani M. May autonomic indices from cardiovascular variability help identify hypertension? J Hypertens. 2014;32(2):363–73.
75. Gerstner W, Kreiter AK, Markram H, Herz AVM. Neural codes: firing rates and beyond. Proc Natl Acad Sci USA. 1997;94(24):12740–1.
76. Sala R, Malacarne M, Solaro N, Pagani M, Lucini D. A composite autonomic index as unitary metric for heart rate variability: a proof of concept. Eur J Clin Investig. 2017;47(3):241–9.
77. Lucini D, Solaro N, Pagani M. Autonomic differentiation map: a novel statistical tool for interpretation of heart rate variability. Front Physiol. 2018;9:401.
78. Macnish R. The philosophy of sleep. 1st American ed. New York: Appleton; 1834.
79. Hobson JA. Sleep. Scientific American library series, no. 27. New York: Scientific American Library: distributed by W.H. Freeman; 1989.
80. Von Economo C. Die Encephalitis lethargica. Leipzig/Wein: Franz Deuticke; 1918.
81. Hess WR. Das Schlafsyndrom als Folge diencephaler Reizung. Helv Physiol Pharmacol Acta. 1944;2:305–44.
82. Berger H. Über das Elektrenkephalogramm des Menschen. Arch f Psychiatrie. 1929;87:527–70.
83. Davis H, Davis PA, Loomis AL, Harvey EN, Hobart G. Changes in human brain potentials during the onset of sleep. Science. 1937;86(2237):448–50.
84. Davis H, Davis PA, Loomis AL, Harvey EN, Hobart G. Human brain potentials during the onset of sleep. J Neurophysiol. 1938;1(1):24–38.
85. Loomis AL, Harvey EN, Hobart GA. Cerebral states during sleep, as studied by human brain potentials. J Exp Psychol. 1937;21(2):127–44.
86. Blake H, Gerard RW. Brain potentials during sleep. Am J Phys. 1937;119(4):692–703.
87. Blake H, Gerard RW, Kleitman N. Factors influencing brain potentials during sleep. J Neurophysiol. 1939;2(1):48–60.
88. Bremer F. Cerveau 'isolé' et physiologie du sommeil. Comptes rendus des séances et mémoires de la Société de biologie. 1935;118:1235–41.
89. Bremer F. Cerveau. Nouvelles recherches sur le mecanisme du sommeil. Comptes rendus des séances et mémoires de la Société de biologie. 1936;122:460–4.
90. Moruzzi G, Magoun HW. Brain stem reticular formation and activation of the EEG. Electroencephalogr Clin Neurophysiol. 1949;1(4):455–73.
91. Batini C, Moruzzi G, Palestini M, Gf R, Zanchetti A. Presistent patterns of wakefulness in the pretrigeminal midpontine preparation. Science. 1958;128(3314):30–2.
92. Aserinsky E, Kleitman N. Regularly occurring periods of eye motility, and concomitant phenomena, during sleep. 1953. J Neuropsychiatry Clin Neurosci. 2003;15(4):454–5.
93. Jouvet M, Michel F, Courjon J. On a stage of rapid cerebral electrical activity in the course of physiological sleep. C R Seances Soc Biol Fil. 1959;153:1024–8. (*Article in French*)
94. Jouvet M. Research on the neural structures and responsible mechanisms in different phases of physiological sleep. Arch Ital Biol. 1962;100:125–206. (*Article in French*)
95. Jones BE. The mysteries of sleep and waking unveiled by Michel Jouvet. Sleep Med. 2018;49:14–9.
96. Gutiérrez-Rivas E, de Andrés I, Gómez-Montoya J, Reinoso-Suárez F. The influence of the rostropontine-ventrolateral region on the sleep-wakefulness cycle. Experientia. 1978;34(1):61–2.
97. Chokroverty S. An overview of normal sleep. In: Chokorverty S, editor. Sleep disorders medicine: basic science, technical considerations, and clinical aspects. 3rd ed. Philadelphia: Saunders/Elsevier; 2009.
98. Somers VK, Dyken ME, Mark AL, Abboud FM. Sympathetic-nerve activity during sleep in normal subjects. N Engl J Med. 1993;328(5):303–7.
99. Benarroch EE. Autonomic neurology. (contemporary neurology series). New York: Oxford University Press; 2014.
100. Tononi G, Koch C. Consciousness: here, there and everywhere? Philos Trans R Soc Lond Ser B Biol Sci. 2015;370(1668):20140167.
101. Calandra-Buonaura G, Provini F, Guaraldi P, Plazzi G, Cortelli P. Cardiovascular autonomic dysfunctions and sleep disorders. Sleep Med Rev. 2016;26:43–56.
102. Pagani M, Somers V, Furlan R, Dell'Orto S, Conway J, Baselli G, et al. Changes in autonomic regulation induced by physical training in mild hypertension. Hypertension. 1988;12(6):600–10.
103. Muller JE, Ludmer PL, Willich SN, Tofler GH, Aylmer G, Klangos I, et al. Circadian variation in the frequency of sudden cardiac death. Circulation. 1987;75(1):131–8.
104. Coccagna G, Mantovani M, Brignani F, Parchi C, Lugaresi E. Continuous recording of the pulmonary and systemic arterial pressure during sleep in syndromes of hypersomnia with periodic breathing. Bull Physiopathol Respir. 1972;8(5):1159–72.
105. Lugaresi E, Coccagna G, Mantovani M. Pathophysiological, clinical and nosographic considerations regarding hypersomnia with periodic breathing. Bull Physiopathol Respir. 1972;8(5):1249–56.
106. Tobaldini E, Nobili L, Strada S, Casali KR, Braghiroli A, Montano N. Heart rate variability in normal and pathological sleep. Front Physiol. 2013;4:294.
107. de Zambotti M, Trinder J, Silvani A, Colrain IM, Baker FC. Dynamic coupling between the central and autonomic nervous systems during sleep: a review. Neurosci Biobehav Rev. 2018;90:84–103.
108. Academy of Sleep Medicine. International classification of sleep disorders. 3rd ed. Darien: American Academy of Sleep Medicine; 2014.

109. Hedner J, Ejnell H, Sellgren J, Hedner T, Wallin G. Is high and fluctuating muscle nerve sympathetic activity in the sleep apnoea syndrome of pathogenetic importance for the development of hypertension? J Hypertens Suppl. 1988;6(4):S529–31.
110. Vanninen E, Tuunainen A, Kansanen M, Uusitupa M, Lansimies E. Cardiac sympathovagal balance during sleep apnea episodes. Clin Physiol. 1996;16(3):209–16.
111. Parati G, Di Rienzo M, Bonsignore MR, Insalaco G, Marrone O, Castiglioni P, et al. Autonomic cardiac regulation in obstructive sleep apnea syndrome: evidence from spontaneous baroreflex analysis during sleep. J Hypertens. 1997;15(12 Pt 2):1621–6.
112. Noda A, Yasuma F, Okada T, Yokota M. Circadian rhythm of autonomic activity in patients with obstructive sleep apnea syndrome. Clin Cardiol. 1998;21(4):271–6.
113. Cortelli P, Parchi P, Sforza E, Contin M, Pierangeli G, Barletta G, et al. Cardiovascular autonomic dysfunction in normotensive awake subjects with obstructive sleep apnoea syndrome. Clin Auton Res. 1994;4(1–2):57–62.
114. Schenck CH, Bundlie SR, Ettinger MG, Mahowald MW. Chronic behavioral disorders of human REM sleep: a new category of parasomnia. Sleep. 1986;9(2):293–308.
115. Chiaro G, Calandra-Buonaura G, Cecere A, Mignani F, Sambati L, Loddo G, et al. REM sleep behavior disorder, autonomic dysfunction and synuclein-related neurodegeneration: where do we stand? Clin Auton Res. 2018;28(6):519–33.
116. Rocchi C, Placidi F, Liguori C, Del Bianco C, Lauretti B, Diomedi M, et al. Daytime autonomic activity in idiopathic rapid eye movement sleep behavior disorder: a preliminary study. Sleep Med. 2018;52:163–7.
117. Nhat HT. Old path, white clouds : walking in the footsteps of the Buddha. Berkeley: Parallax Press; 1991.
118. Pagani M, Lucini D, Porta A. Sympathovagal balance from heart rate variability: time for a second round? Exp Physiol. 2012;97(10):1141–2.
119. Heathers JA. Sympathovagal balance from heart rate variability: an obituary. Exp Physiol. 2012;97(4):556.
120. Pant S, Corsini C, Baker C, Hsia TY, Pennati G, Vignon-Clementel IE. Inverse problems in reduced order models of cardiovascular haemodynamics: aspects of data assimilation and heart rate variability. J R Soc Interface. 2017;14(126):20160513.
121. Schwartz PJ, La Rovere MT, Vanoli E. Autonomic nervous system and sudden cardiac death. Experimental basis and clinical observations for post-myocardial infarction risk stratification. Circulation. 1992;85(1 Suppl):177–91.
122. Nolte IM, Munoz ML, Tragante V, Amare AT, Jansen R, Vaez A, et al. Genetic loci associated with heart rate variability and their effects on cardiac disease risk. Nat Commun. 2017;8:15805.
123. Tzu S, Giles L. The art of war. New York: Open Road Integrated Media, LLC; 2014. p. 64.
124. Sacristan JA. Clinical research and medical care: towards effective and complete integration. BMC Med Res Methodol. 2015;15:4.
125. Steinhubl SR. The future of individualized health maintenance. Nat Med. 2019;25(5):712–4.

Laboratory Evaluation of Sleep Disorders: PSG, MSLT, MWT, and Actigraphy

11

Sushanth Bhat and Sudhansu Chokroverty

Introduction

A physician dealing with patients suffering from autonomic dysfunction must have a basic knowledge about a variety of sleep disorders that may occur in such patients. For this particular reason, it is essential to know when to order sleep laboratory tests, the rationale behind these tests, and the essential sleep laboratory findings in major conditions with autonomic failure manifesting significant sleep-related symptoms. It is incumbent upon the autonomic specialist to remember that there is an intimate relationship among the central autonomic network (CAN) in the brainstem with its reciprocal ascending and descending connections, hypnogenic neurons (located in the brainstem and hypothalamus), and brainstem respiratory neurons. Sleep has a profound effect on the function of the autonomic nervous system (ANS). Furthermore, dysfunction of the ANS significantly impacts human sleep and particularly breathing during sleep. It is, therefore, logical to expect sleep dysfunction and sleep disordered breathing (SDB) in patients with autonomic failure. In many patients with primary autonomic failure (e.g., multiple system atrophy [MSA], primary autonomic failure [PAF], familial dysautonomia [FD], idiopathic subtype of postural tachycardia syndrome [POTS]) and in some patients with secondary autonomic failure (e.g., diabetic autonomic neuropathy, Guillain-Barre syndrome, central neurodegenerative diseases, such as Parkinson's disease [PD] and diffuse Lewy body disease with dementia [DLBD]), sleep dysfunction and SDB have been noted. In addition, Fatal Familial Insomnia, a rare prion disease, presents with severe sleep disturbances and dysautonomia. In this chapter, we will briefly describe a variety of sleep laboratory tests (e.g., overnight polysomnography [PSG], Home Sleep Apnea Test [HSAT], Multiple Sleep Latency Test [MSLT], Maintenance of Wakefulness Test [MSWT], and actigraphy) which are important for the diagnosis and monitoring of sleep dysfunction as well as SDB. Finally, we will briefly allude to consumer-oriented sleep technology (not of much practical use currently) and list sleep laboratory findings in some of the conditions with both autonomic and sleep dysfunction mentioned above.

S. Bhat (✉)
Neuroscience Institute, Hackensack Meridian Health, JFK Medical Center, Seton Hall University, Edison, NJ, USA

S. Chokroverty
Hackensack Meridian Health, Neuroscience Institute at JFK, JFK University Medical Center, Edison, NJ, USA

Seton Hall University & Hackensack Meridian School of Medicine at Seton Hall, South Orange, NJ, USA

Rutgers Robert Wood Johnson Medical School, New Brunswick, NJ, USA

Techniques to Measure Sleep-Disordered Breathing

Polysomnography

Clinical Utility Attended overnight in-laboratory PSG remains the gold standard in the evaluation of OSA and other types of SDB including central sleep apnea and Cheyne-Stokes respirations (seen in many patients with autonomic failure) as well as ataxic breathing that may be seen in patients on opioid therapy or those with neurodegenerative diseases (e.g., MSA, DLBD, and PD) and demyelinating diseases such as multiple sclerosis [1]. In addition, the routine recording of multiple physiological characteristics in addition to respiratory function simultaneously during sleep, including electroencephalography (EEG), electrooculography (EOG), and chin and limb muscle electromyography (EMG), allows for the evaluation of unusual behavior in sleep (parasomnias), including rapid eye movement (REM) sleep behavior disorder (RBD), as well as epileptiform activity and clinical seizures during sleep [2], especially when additional EEG and EMG channels are employed.

S. Chokroverty, P. Cortelli (eds.), *Autonomic Nervous System and Sleep*, https://doi.org/10.1007/978-3-030-62263-3_11

In general, during PSG recording, patients spend one entire night in the sleep laboratory with the goal of capturing a typical night's sleep. Figure 11.1 depicts a typical 30-s epoch from an overnight PSG. The study assesses wakefulness and sleep stages, respiration, cardiopulmonary function, and body movements. Airflow and respiratory effort channels are used to score respiratory events including apneas and hypopneas. The finger pulse oximetry channel allows for scoring of event-related oxygen desaturations as well as sleep hypoxemia independent of apneic and hypopneic events. In patients undergoing continuous positive airway (CPAP) or bilevel titration for OSA, the C-flow channel provides the airflow signal, and PAP pressure is continuously adjusted during the night to eliminate respiratory events. EEG, EOG, and chin EMG channels are used to stage sleep, and limb (EMG) electrodes are typically placed on the legs (usually the tibialis anterior muscle) for scoring and evaluation of limb movements. Additional EMG channels may be used in special montages, especially when it is necessary to determine the presence of REM sleep without atonia in patients with RBD. A single channel electrocardiography (EKG) channel and a snore channel are part of the typical PSG setup. Video and audio recording are essential for recording position and evaluating abnormal movements and behavior in sleep (such as bruxism, catathrenia, and various other parasomnias). Table 11.1 presents a standard set of montages for PSG recording, modified from the American Academy of Sleep Medicine (AASM) recommendations [3].

Technical Considerations Biological signals recorded during PSG are of very small amplitude (EEG, EOG, and EMG activities are in the microvolt range) and need to be amplified to be displayed and analyzed. Additionally, these waveforms also need to be filtered in order to best visualize activity of interest and exclude artifact. PSG equipment is, thus, a series of amplifiers that record and amplify this activity and then pass it through adjustable filters for display at different sensitivity settings.

PSG equipment uses differential amplifiers, which amplify the potential difference between the two amplifier inputs. The result of this is that unwanted extraneous environmental noise, which is likely to be seen at the two electrodes, is subtracted out and therefore cannot contaminate the recording.

The amplifiers used consist of both alternating current (AC) and direct current (DC) amplifiers. The AC amplifiers are used to record physiological characteristics showing high frequencies such as EEG, EOG, EMG, and EKG. The AC amplifier contains both high- and low-frequency filters. DC amplifiers have no low-frequency filters and are typically used to record potentials with slow frequency such as the output from the oximeter, the output from the pH meter, CPAP titration used for upper airway pressurization to eliminate apneic events, and for some special techniques such as intraesophageal pressure readings. AC or DC amplifiers may be used to record respiratory flow and effort. Sensitivity and filter settings vary according to the physiological characteristics recorded (Table 11.1 and 11.2).

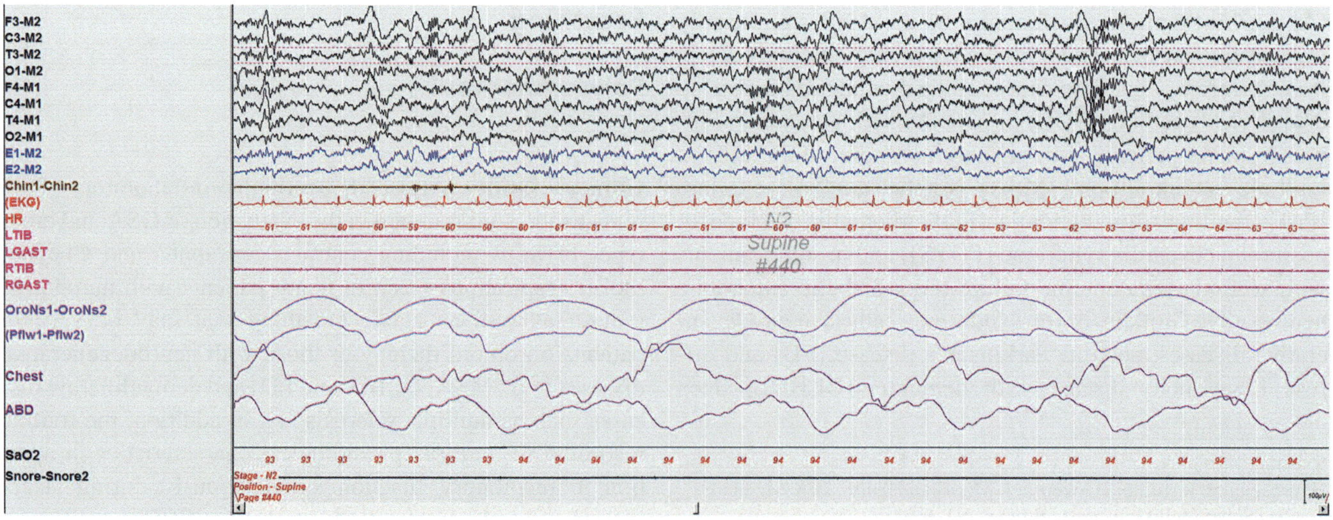

Fig. 11.1 A 30-s epoch depicting N2 sleep from the overnight polysomnogram of a 24-year-old woman with insomnia and snoring. Top eight channels; EEG recording with electrodes placed according to the 10–20 international electrode placement system. E1-M2, E2-M2; electro-oculogram channels. Chin1-Chin2; submental electromyogram (EMG). EKG; electrocardiogram. HR; heart rate. LTIB, RTIB; left and right tibialis anterior EMG. LGAST, RGAST; left and right gastrocnemius EMG. OroNs1-OroNS2; oronasal airflow. Pflw1-Pflw2; nasal pressure transducer recording. Chest and ABD; effort belts. SaO_2; arterial oxygen saturation by finger oximetry. Also included is a snore channel

Table 11.1 Typical overnight polysomnographic montage used in our laboratory

Channel number	Name
1.	F3-M2
2.	C3-M2
3.	T3-M2[a]
4.	01-M2
5.	F4-M1
6.	C4-M1
7.	T4-M1[a]
8.	02-M1
9.	Left electro-oculogram (E1-M2)
10.	Right electro-oculogram (E2-M2)
11.	Chin electromyogram (EMG)
12.	EKG
13.	Heart rate
14.	Left gastrocnemius EMG[b]
15.	Left tibialis anterior EMG
16.	Right gastrocnemius EMG[b]
17.	Right tibialis anterior EMG
18.	Intercostal EMG[b]
19.	Oronasal thermistor[c]
20.	Nasal pressure transducer[c]
21.	Chest
22.	Abdomen
23.	Snoring
24.	Arterial oxygen saturation

Channels 1–8 record electroencephalogram activity from bilateral cerebral hemispheres in a referential chain; electrode designation per the 10–20 International System of electrode placement. M1 and M2, left and right mastoid, respectively. Channel 19 and 20 record airflow ("flow channels"). Channels 21 and 22 record respiratory effort ("effort channels") (see also Fig. 11.1)

[a]Temporal EEG channels are not part of the standard recommendations of the American Academy of Sleep Medicine (AASM) but included in our laboratory to increase the potential yield for epileptiform activity

[b]Additional EMG channels (not part of the standard AASM recommendations) used in our laboratory

[c]In a CPAP titration study, flow channels are replaced by a CPAP signal (C-flow signal)

Table 11.2 Filter and sensitivity settings for polysomnographic studies

Characteristics	High-frequency filter (Hz)	Time constant (s)	Low-frequency filter (Hz)
Electroencephalogram 5–7 μV/mm	70 or 35	0.4	0.3
Electro-oculogram 5–7 μV/mm	70 or 35	0.4	0.3
Electromyogram 2–3 μV/mm	90	0.04	5.0
Electrocardiogram 1 mV/cm to start	15	0.12	1.0
Airflow and effort 5–7 μV/mm; adjust	15	1	0.1

The standard speed for recording traditional PSG is 10 mm/s, so that each monitor screen is a 30-s epoch, making sleep staging easy to identify. A 30 mm/s speed is the traditional speed at which EEGs are analyzed, as they allow for easy identification of epileptiform activities. While reviewing the PSG at the traditional 10 mm/s speed, the polysomnographer may pick up EEG abnormalities that can be better analyzed by slowing the recording down to 30 mm/s. On the other hand, with experience, polysomnographers may choose a 5 mm/s speed, rendering a 60-s epoch, to better visualize respiratory events.

Electroencephalography The main purpose of EEG recording incorporated into PSGs is twofold: to distinguish between wakefulness and the various stages of sleep and to recognize an arousal. EEG electrodes are placed as per the ten-twenty international electrode placement system (Fig. 11.2) [4–7]. The AASM recommends a minimum of three channels (F4-M1, C4-M1, 02-M1) representing the right frontal, central, and occipital electrodes referenced to the contralateral mastoid. While the above montage would theoretically be sufficient to detect a posterior dominant rhythm in wakefulness (best seen in occipital leads) and major sleep architecture (vertex waves, sleep spindles, and K complexes best seen in frontal and central derivations), there are serious limitations to adhering to this minimum recommended montage. Recording over only one hemisphere may result in inability to score sleep accurately if that hemisphere is affected by a pathological process (as in a patient with stroke or tumor) or in missing possible serious pathology in the contralateral hemisphere. Furthermore, the absence of a temporal lead may result in missing epileptiform activity which is most common in this region. Therefore, we use a montage that records over both hemispheres and includes the temporal regions (see Table 11.1), in addition to electrodes recommended by the AASM for the scoring of sleep. For patients in whom nocturnal seizures are suspected or likely to occur, a full seizure montage with parasagittal and temporal chains (not shown) is recommended [2].

Electro-oculography Eye movements are generally characteristic of the sleep stage in which they occur and are an essential part of scoring. Eye blinks, seen only in wakefulness, are conjugate vertical eye movements occurring at 0.5–2 hertz with the eyes open or closed. Rapid eye movements (conjugate, irregular, sharp eye movements with an initial deflection of less than half a second) occur in wakefulness along with high chin EMG tone, eye blinks, and a posterior dominant rhythm, and also occur in REM sleep, especially in phasic REM where they occur in bursts seen in all directions (horizontal, oblique, and vertical) and are accompanied by low to absent chin tone (interspersed with similar phasic bursting) and a desynchronized, amorphous EEG pattern. Slow lateral eye movements (SEMs or SLEMs) are seen in drowsiness and light sleep and are defined as conjugate, sinusoidal, regular eye movements with an initial

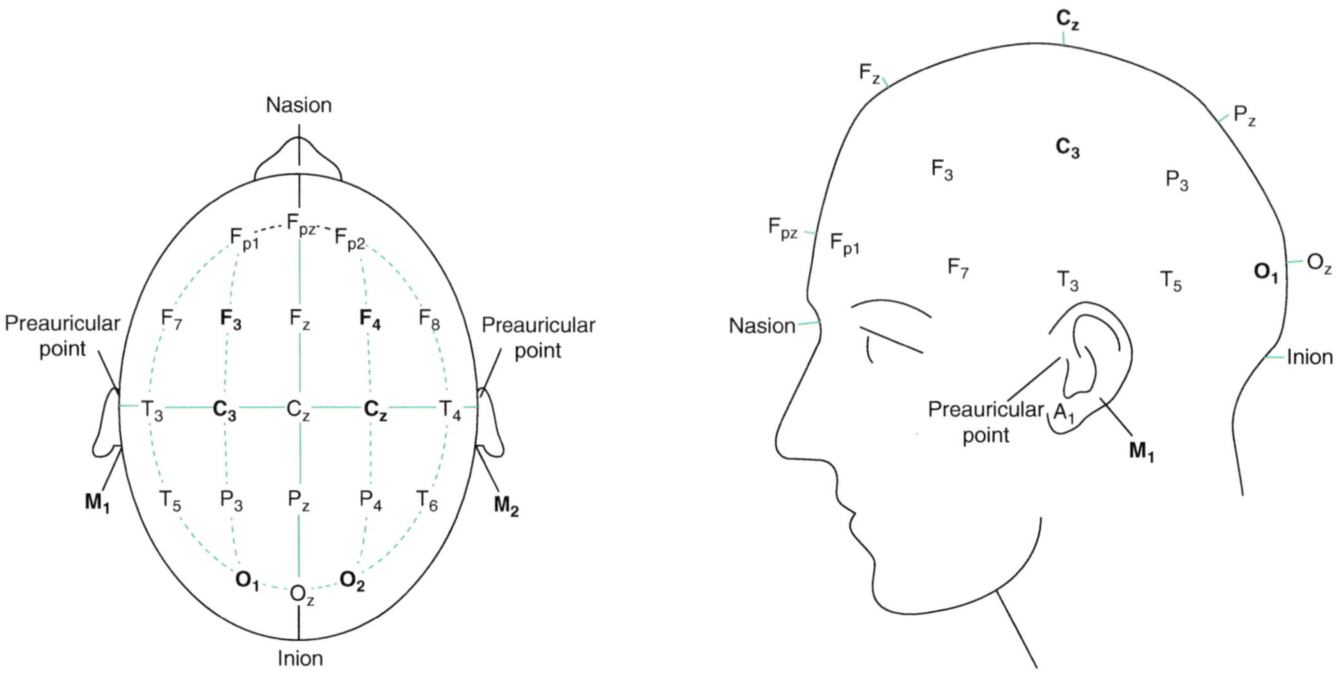

Fig. 11.2 The international 10–20 system of electrode placement, superior (*left*) and lateral (*right*) views. (From Butkov [6], with permission Synapse Media, Medford, Oregon)

deflection of greater than half a second. These eye movements are not under voluntary control and cannot be volitionally simulated. In approximately 10–15% of subjects who do not generate a posterior dominant rhythm, the appearance of SLEMs heralds stage N1 sleep. While they may persist into stage N2 during the early part of the night, they generally disappear in stage N3 and REM sleep (although there is no formal publication in this regard, but this information is derived from day-to-day routine PSG interpretation); the SLEMs may, however, may persist in deeper stages of sleep in patients on antidepressant medication).

Electromyography EMG channels provide important physiological characteristics that help determine sleep stage, as well as aiding in the diagnosis and classification of a variety of parasomnias. At a minimum, chin EMG channels recording activity from the mentalis and submental muscles (the mylohyoid and anterior belly of the digastric) and bilateral leg EMG channels recording activity from the tibialis anterior muscles should be included in PSG recordings.

Chin EMG tone aids in the staging of sleep. It follows a characteristic pattern as sleep progresses, decreasing with sleep onset and continuing to diminish through NREM sleep to a point where it is at its minimum and almost absent in REM sleep. Phasic bursts (myoclonic bursts) in the chin EMG (as well as limb EMG) are seen in phasic REM sleep.

Lower limb EMGs are generally recorded with electrodes placed over the tibialis anterior muscles 2–2.5 cm apart. The main utility of these channels is to detect periodic limb movements in sleep (PLMS) and are particularly useful when these movements occur as a result of respiratory events, as the correlation between these movements and the respiratory events can be easily appreciated on PSG. However, many patients with a history of abnormal movements or behavior in sleep require a more extended EMG montage (we call this a multiple muscle montage [MMM]) that includes extra channels recording from additional cranially innervated muscles (e.g., the sternocleidomastoideus, masseter, and mentalis), upper limb muscles (e.g., biceps, triceps, extensor digitorum communis, flexor digitorum Sublimis), lower limb muscles (e.g., quadriceps and gastrocnemius), and axial muscles (e.g., paraspinals, rectus abdominis, intercostals). The MMM is of particular utility in patients with suspected RBD, where REM without atonia may be missed if an adequate number of muscles is not sampled. While a standard montage for RBD has not yet been agreed upon, Fraucher et al. [8] found that simultaneous recording and quantitative analysis of the mentalis and flexor digitorum Sublimis in 3-s mini epochs was 100% specific for RBD, when activity was present in more than 31.9% of miniepochs. The heterogeneity of RBD appears to be expressed in the dissociated EMG findings in cranial as well as arm and the leg muscles, requiring recording from multiple muscles. The MMM recording may also be useful in patients with suspected restless legs syndrome (RLS or Willis-Ekbom disease) as PLMS may also occasionally occur in the arm muscles or, rarely, in the axial or cranially innervated muscles.

It is often helpful to also include external intercostal or diaphragmatic EMG (recording inspiratory muscle bursts) as well as rectus abdominis muscle (recording expiratory muscle activity). The intercostal EMG recorded from the seventh to ninth intercostal space with an active electrode on the anterior axillary line and the reference electrodes on the midaxillary line may also include some diaphragmatic muscle activity in addition to the intercostal activity. Diaphragmatic activity can be recorded by placing surface electrodes over the right or left side of the umbilicus or over the anterior costal margin, but these are contaminated by a mixture of intercostal activity and such noninvasive techniques are unreliable for quantitative assessment of diaphragmatic EMG. True diaphragmatic activity is typically recorded by intraesophageal recording. Intercostal or diaphragmatic EMG is useful in the differentiation between central and obstructive apneas, especially when the respiratory channels are unreliable; continued bursts of EMG activity in these channels would identify the event as obstructive while the absence of such bursts would indicate a central event.

Electrocardiography The PSG generally includes a single channel of EKG recorded by placing one electrode over the sternum and the other electrode at a lateral chest location. This recording detects bradytachyarrhythmias or other cardiac arrhythmias which may be seen in many patients with autonomic failure and OSA; a standard EKG should be later obtained to characterize the exact nature of the arrhythmia.

Recording of Respiratory Effort Intraesophageal pressure monitoring is the ideal method of detecting respiratory effort but is not routinely used in the usual sleep laboratory recording. The most commonly used channels measure respiratory effort by respiratory inductive plethysmography (RIP) belts, or by mercury-filled or piezoelectric strain gauges. Impedance pneumography and respiratory magnetometers are available but generally not used.

Respiratory Inductive Plethysmography (RIP) This measures changes in thoracoabdominal cross-sectional areas and the sum of these two components is proportional to airflow. Inductance refers to resistance to current flow. Transducers across the chest and abdomen detect changes in the cross-sectional areas of the thorax and abdomen during breathing. These belts are prone to dislodgement during the night by patient movement, causing inaccuracy in measurements of the respiratory effort.

Measurement of Airflow Airflow can be measured by oronasal thermal devices (thermistors or thermocouples) or nasal cannula–pressure transducers. Most standard PSGs use both types of devices due to limitations with using only one type.

Oronasal Temperature Monitoring An oronasal thermal device (thermistor or thermocouple) placed between the nose and mouth is commonly used to monitor airflow by detecting changes in temperature (cool air flows during inspiration and warm air flows during expiration). A thermistor consisting of wires records changes in electrical resistance, and thermocouples consisting of dissimilar metals (e.g., copper and constantan) register changes in voltage that result from this temperature variation. Thermal devices are not as sensitive as nasal pressure transducers for detecting airflow limitation and, hence, may miss hypopneas. For this reason, the nasal pressure technique to detect airflow (described below) should also be used in addition routinely during PSG recording. The thermistors, however, are used to score apneas.

The temperature of the thermal device must be below body temperature in order to sense the temperature difference between expired and inspired air. These devices must therefore not be in contact with the skin. Because of this, they are easily displaced, causing false changes in airflow.

Nasal Pressure Monitoring Nasal airway pressure decreases during inspiration and increases during expiration. In nasal pressure monitoring, a nasal cannula is connected to a pressure-sensitive transducer, which measures this pressure difference. This alternating decrement and increment of nasal pressure produce electrical signals, which indirectly register airflow.

Nasal pressure monitoring is more sensitive than the thermal devices in detecting airflow limitation and hypopneas. With increased upper airway resistance, the nasal pressure monitor will register a plateau indicating a flow limitation. A DC amplifier or an AC amplifier with a long time constant should be used. One disadvantage is that nasal pressure cannula cannot be used to measure airflow in mouth breathers and in patients with nasal obstruction. For this reason, nasal pressure transducers are not used to score apneas.

Oxygen Saturation Finger pulse oximetry is used to noninvasively measure oxygen saturation during sleep (SaO_2). It reflects the percentage of hemoglobin that is oxygenated (by measuring the difference in light absorption between oxyhemoglobin and deoxyhemoglobin), rather than the arterial partial pressure of oxygen. Continuous monitoring of SaO_2 is crucial because it provides important information about the severity of respiratory dysfunction. PSG reports mention the time the patient spent with an SaO_2 below 90%. Patients with OSA may have hyponea/apnea-related recurrent desaturations with a return of SaO_2 to baseline at the termination of the event ("respiratory event related hypoxemia").

Expired Carbon Dioxide Capnography or end-tidal CO_2 ($EtCO_2$) monitoring detects the expired carbon dioxide (CO_2) level, which closely approximates intra-alveolar CO_2. Capnography detects both airflow and the partial pressure of CO_2 in alveoli and is useful in evaluating OSA, sleep hypoventilation, and underlying pulmonary disease. An infrared analyzer over the nose and mouth detects CO_2 in the expired air, which qualitatively measures the airflow. This is the best noninvasive method to detect alveolar hypoventilation. The method is costly and therefore not used in most laboratories, but it should be used routinely in children with suspected OSA.

Home Sleep Apnea Testing (HSAT) In recent years, there has been a trend toward the increased use of portable monitoring devices for home sleep studies in preference to in-lab PSG. HSAT devices are classified into four types based on the number of characteristics they measure and the degree of attendance required. Type 1 devices are the traditional attended in-laboratory PSGs described above. Type 2 devices require a minimum of seven channels, including EEG/EOG, chin EMG, EKG, oximetry, and airflow and respiratory effort channels. Thus, they permit sleep scoring. Type 3 studies (also called "cardiopulmonary studies") have a minimum of four channels (airflow, respiratory effort, pulse oximetry, and EKG); these studies can be attended or unattended. Sleep scoring cannot be performed with these devices. An example for a type 4 device is overnight ambulatory pulse oximetry (a single-channel device recording a single physiological characteristic). Type 4 devices may also have a channel to measure airflow.

The advantages of HSAT include reduced cost; easier access to these devices for patients who are immobile, cannot travel, or who live far away from sleep laboratories; and quicker turnaround time for results. On the other hand, there are several disadvantages, including reduced sensitivity, especially with type 3 and 4 devices, which may miss mild or positional OSA, or may produce false negative results in patients who sleep poorly during the test. Additionally, type 3 and 4 devices cannot evaluate abnormal movements or seizures in sleep due to lack of EEG and EMG channels. A negative study in a patient in whom the clinical suspicion for sleep disordered breathing is high leads to an in-laboratory PSG anyway. In-lab PSG, rather than portable monitoring, should be used for the diagnosis of OSA in patients with significant cardiorespiratory disease (such as chronic obstructive pulmonary disease [COPD] or congestive heart failure [CHF]), potential respiratory muscle weakness due to neuromuscular condition, awake hypoventilation or suspicion of sleep-related hypoventilation, chronic opioid medication use, history of stroke, or severe insomnia.

Tests for Daytime Hypersomnolence

Although they are both tests for excessive daytime sleepiness, the MSLT and the MWT assess different functions. The MSLT unmasks physiologic sleepiness, which depends on both circadian and homeostatic factors; in contrast, the MWT is a reflection of the individual's capability to resist sleep and is influenced by physiologic sleepiness.

Multiple Sleep Latency Testing

The MSLT, developed by Carskadon and Dement in the late 1970s [9], is an objective test of hypersomnolence, which measures the rapidity with which a subject can fall asleep under standard conditions during the day. The MSLT has become the standard clinical method for objectively measuring excessive daytime sleepiness [10–12]. It is also used to document sleep-onset REM periods (SOREMPS), defined as the onset of REM sleep within 15 min of sleep initiation, one of the critical findings in narcolepsy. Therefore, the AASM has indicated that the MSLT should be used as part of an evaluation of suspected narcolepsy, which remains the single most important indication for performing the MSLT, and that it may be helpful in the evaluation of suspected idiopathic hypersomnia [13, 14]. The MSLT is not routinely recommended in patients with OSA, circadian rhythm disorders, or insomnia; however, those patients previously diagnosed with OSA, PLMS, or mood disorders who continue to have excessive sleepiness despite optimal treatment may require evaluation by the MSLT to exclude associated narcolepsy. Additionally, the MSLT is also often used to determine the efficacy of treatment in patients with narcolepsy. For patients with initially negative studies, following are the recommended indications for repeat MSLT: extraneous circumstances or inappropriate conditions affecting the initial MSLT, presence of ambiguous or uninterpretable finding, and initial MSLT without polygraphic confirmation in a patient suspected to have narcolepsy.

MSLT Guidelines

Guidelines for performing the MSLT have been standardized [15] and should be followed without deviation from protocol by all sleep laboratories. Where deviations are unavoidable, they should be justified by the technician and included in the final report. The sleep specialist must then make a determination with regard to whether the deviation from protocol invalidates the results.

The general procedures before the actual recording include keeping a sleep diary for 1–2 weeks before the test, which records information about usual bedtime, time of rising, napping, and any drug use. The test is mandatorily preceded by an overnight PSG, and the MSLT is scheduled about 2–3 h after the conclusion of the overnight PSG study. On the PSG, additional sleep disorders that may contribute to hypersomnolence (such as OSA) or insufficient sleep (less than 360 min) would invalidate any MSLT results, and the MSLT should be deferred until the underlying sleep disorders are addressed.

The actual test consists of four to five opportunities for napping at 2-h intervals and each recording session is scheduled to last for 20 min. Between tests, subjects must remain awake. The subjects must not smoke for 30 min before lights are turned off. The patient is instructed to relax and fall asleep, and the lights are turned off. The test must be conducted in a quiet, dark room. The specific recording includes a minimum of three channels of EEG (F3-A2, C3-A2, O1-A2, and C4-A1 are recommended to document alpha activity in relaxed wakefulness in adults and its disappearance at sleep onset), submental EMG to evaluate chin tone, and EOG recordings for detection of rapid eye movements. For each nap opportunity, the measurements recorded include sleep-onset latency (the time in minutes from lights out to the first epoch of any stage of sleep) and the presence of SOREMPs. If sleep is recorded, the test is run for an additional 15 min to provide an opportunity for a SOREMP to occur; if a SOREMP does occur, the nap is immediately terminated. If the technician is unclear about whether a SOREMP has occurred, then it is better to continue the test than to end it prematurely. If no sleep occurs, then the test is concluded 20 min after lights are turned off. A total of four to five nap opportunities is provided to the subject (only four need to be recorded if the patient develops two SOREMPs in those four naps or has a SOREMP on the preceding night PSG and at least one additional SOREMP on one of the first four naps) [16]. Mean sleep latency (MSL) is calculated as the average sleep latencies of each of the four or five individual naps.

MSLT Interpretation, Limitations, and Pitfalls

Based on AASM practice parameters, a mean sleep latency of 8 min or less indicates pathological hypersomnolence; a mean sleep latency of 10 min or more is considered normal and latencies between these two means are considered borderline pathologic [17]. The diagnosis of narcolepsy requires a mean sleep latency of 8 min or less and 2 SOREMPs; where insufficient SOREMPs are seen, the diagnosis of idiopathic hypersomnia may be made.

The sensitivity and specificity of the MSLT in detecting sleepiness have not been clearly determined. While the test-retest reliability of the MSLT has been documented to be high in normal subjects [18, 19], it was found to be poor in patients with diseases of central hypersomnolence [20]. In subjects with sleepiness caused by circadian rhythm sleep disorders, sleep deprivation, and ingestion of hypnotics and alcohol, pathologic sleepiness has been validated by MSLT [14]. However, there is poor correlation between the MSLT and subjective measures of sleepiness such as the Epworth Sleepiness Scale [21–23]. The patient's psychological and behavioral state also interferes with the MSLT results. If the patient suffers from severe anxiety or psychological disturbances causing behavioral stimulation, MSLT may not show sleepiness even in a patient complaining of EDS. Day-to-day variability in the degree of sleepiness and an inability to cooperate or understand instructions are other factors for unreliability. Use of centrally active stimulating medications (methylphenidate, amphetamines, modafinil, armodafinil, etc.) and REM suppressants (selective serotonin reuptake inhibitors, tricyclic antidepressants, monoamino oxidase inhibitors, etc.) may produce falsely increased sleep latencies or suppress SOREMPs. Furthermore, pathological sleepiness with two or more SOREMPS may occasionally be seen in other conditions (e.g., OSA, REM sleep dysregulation, circadian rhythm sleep disorders). In addition, the MSLT measures propensity to fall asleep in an environment (e.g., sleep laboratory) conducive to sleep but not in other conditions (e.g., work or driving). One should also be aware of false-positive and false-negative test results. Aldrich et al. [24] found that the sensitivity of the combination of two or more SOREMPs with a mean sleep latency of <5 min on an initial MSLT was 70% with a specificity of 97%, but 30% of all subjects with this combination of findings did not have narcolepsy. Repeat MSLT in those patients with narcolepsy with an initially negative study may yield positive findings in up to 20% of cases [25].

Maintenance of Wakefulness Testing

The MWT, which is performed less frequently than the MSLT, measures the ability of the subject to remain awake, and in contrast to MSLT, the instruction provided is to resist, rather than attempt, sleep [11, 12, 26]. The test protocol requires four trials ("wake opportunities") at 2-h intervals to test an individual's ability to stay awake. Based on studies published in the peer-reviewed literature, the Standards of Practice Committee of the AASM [13] recommends the MWT 40-min protocol. Unlike the MSLT, the MWT does not require prior overnight polysomnography. The test is performed about 1.5–3 h after the individual's usual wake-up time. The recording montage and patient calibrations are similar to those used for the MSLT. Prior to the beginning of the recording, subjects are asked to sit still in bed with a back and headrest and remain awake as long as possible. They are not allowed to read, use headphones to listen to music, use a mobile phone, watch television or use any digital device to read during each trial of 40 min. Sleep onset is defined as the time between lights off in the beginning of the recording and the onset of three consecutive epochs of stage 1 sleep or one epoch of any other stage of sleep. The trial should be terminated after sleep onset or after 40 min if no sleep occurs. A mean sleep latency (the arithmetic mean of the individual sleep latencies of four trials) of less than 8 min is considered abnormal as recommended by the standards of practice committee of the AASM [13]; values greater than this but less than 40 min are of uncertain significance.

The AASM Standards of Practice Committee recommended the following indications for the MWT [13]:

- Assessment of the individuals employed in occupations involving public transportation or safety for their ability to remain awake
- Assessment of response to treatment (e.g., response to stimulants in narcolepsy and CPAP titration in OSA patients)

Recently in an important study of MWT [27] concluded tha for driving impairment a sleep onset latency (SOL) of 0–19 minutes may be considered pathological(highl vulnerable) but those with a SOL of 20–33 minutes may also be vulneral but to a lesser extent whereas those with a SOL of 34–40 minutes are considered alert.

Techniques to Measure Body Movements/ Sleep-Wake Cycles

Actigraphy

An actigraph, also known as an actometer or actimeter, monitors body movements and other activities continuously for days, weeks, or even months, and thereby indirectly obtains information about sleep-wake cycles [12, 28, 29]. These devices can be worn on the wrist or alternatively on the ankle for recording arm, leg, and body movements. Actigraphs use piezoelectric sensors which function as accelerometers to record acceleration or deceleration of movements rather than the actual movements. The mechanical movements are converted into electrical signals, which are then sampled every tenth second over a predetermined time or epoch and then retrieved and analyzed in a computer. The principle of analysis is based on the fact that increased movements (*as indicated by black bars in the actigraph*) are seen during wakefulness in contrast to markedly decreased movements or no movements (*as indicated by the white area interrupting the black bars*) during sleep, although normal physiological body and limb movements and postural shifts during sleep will cause interruptions (*black bars of the white background*) (Fig. 11.3).

Actigraphy has been shown to compare favorably with PSG recordings in distinguishing sleep from wakefulness [30]. Compared to PSG, actigraphs have several advantages including easy accessibility, inexpensive recording over extended periods for days, weeks, or even months; recording of 24-h activities at all sites (home, work, or laboratories); usefulness in uncooperative and demented patients when laboratory PSG study is not possible; and ability to conduct longitudinal studies during therapeutic intervention (behavioral or pharmacological treatment) in patients with insomnia. However, actigraphy has several limitations compared to PSG: these include inability to diagnose sleep apnea and to clarify the etiology of insomnia; overestimation of sleep when some insomniacs may lie down in bed for prolonged periods without moving; and an inability to identify subjects who are feigning sleep problem and to discriminate types of movements such as PLMS from other body movements and provide any information about other physiological characteristics (e.g., EEG, EOG, respiration).

Consumer-Oriented Sleep Technology

In recent years, there has been an explosion of inexpensive, consumer-oriented, readily available technology that is meant to monitor, among other parameters, sleep quality and duration. Entries into this category include standalone wearable devices (e.g., FitBit, Jawbone) as well as smartphone-based software programs ("apps") [31, 32]. While they all essentially use accelerometry-based techniques, as does actigraphy, to score sleep or wake (and in some cases distinguish between "light" and "deep" sleep) based on body movement, in most cases, the exact technology is proprietary, which limits detailed evaluation. "No-contact" bedside devices that detect sleep through radio waves have recently become available [33]. Several smartphone apps that screen for OSA have also been marketed [34, 35]. Although the use of consumer-oriented sleep technology is undoubtedly likely to become more prevalent in the near future, its widespread clinical application is currently limited by the very little data validating it against established means of evaluating sleep [36]. Recently published studies do suggest that this technology, while showing variable correlation with PSG-based scoring, has a sensitivity and specificity for sleep-wake detection that may be comparable to actigraphy [37, 38]. However, the data are preliminary and much more research in the area is required. The AASM Position Statement on consumer-oriented sleep technology [39] recommends that, given the lack of validation and US Food and Drug Administration (FDA) clearance, this technology not be utilized for the diagnosis or treatment of sleep disorders currently.

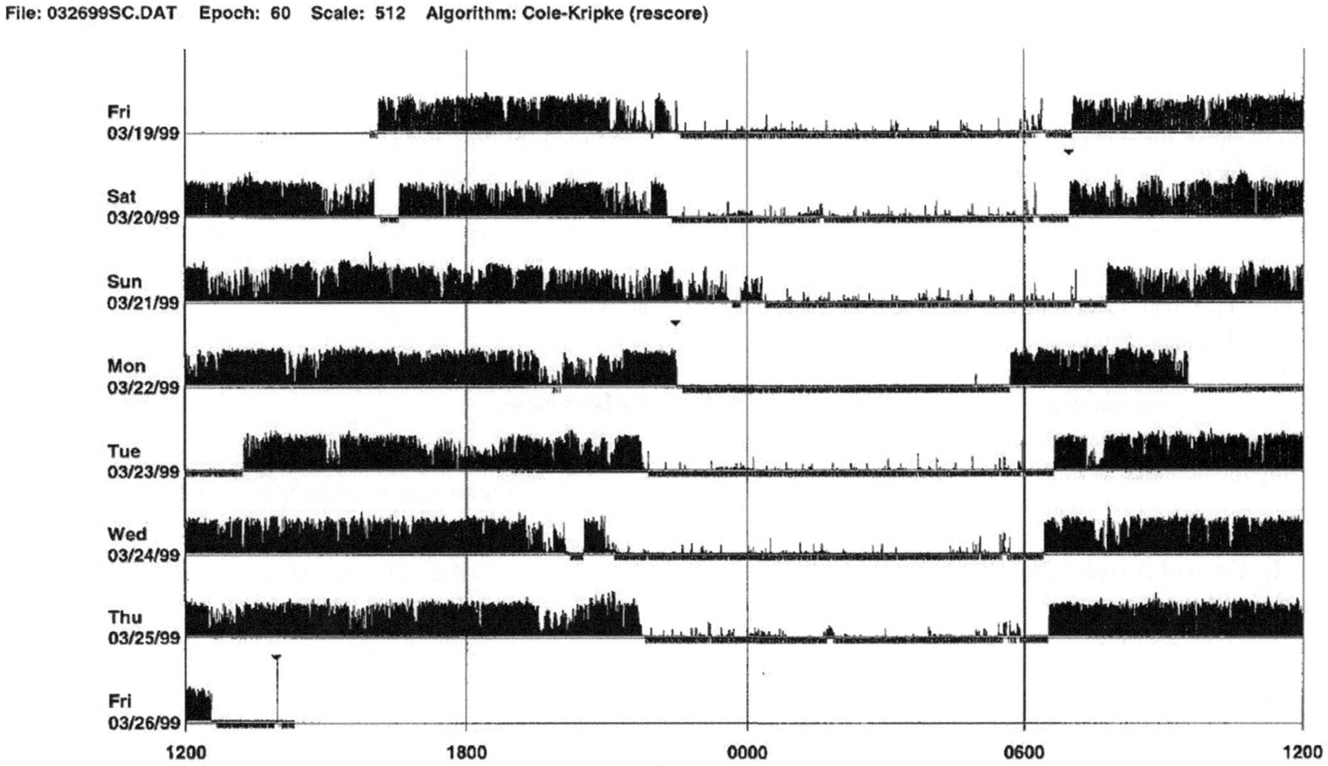

Fig. 11.3 Actigraphy showing normal sleep-wake schedule in a 55-year-old healthy woman without sleep complaints. This recording shows a fairly regular sleep-wake schedule except one weekend night (third from the top). She goes to bed between 10:30 PM and 11:00 PM and wakes up around 7:00 AM except on the third day. Physiological body shifts and movements during sleep are indicated by a few black bars in the white areas. The waking period is indicated by black bars. (From Chokroverty [12], with permission from Elsevier)

Brief Review of Sleep Laboratory Findings in Selected Cases of Autonomic Failure

Multiple System Atrophy (Formerly Known as the Shy-Drager Syndrome)

Sleep dysfunction is very common in MSA and PSG findings may include the following [40]: sleep onset and maintenance insomnia with repeated awakenings and sleep fragmentation; decreased sleep efficiency (SE); reduced slow wave sleep (SWS) and REM sleep; a variety of respiratory dysrhythmias (almost in 100% of cases in advanced stage of illness) consisting of OSA with oxygen desaturation; dysrhythmic breathing (irregular rate, rhythm, and amplitude of breathing becoming worse in sleep); Cheyne-Stokes breathing (CSB) and Cheyne-Stokes Variant breathing (hypopnea substituting apnea); prolonged period of central apneas accompanied by mild oxygen desaturation in relaxed wakefulness as if the respiratory center forgot to breathe; in occasional patients inspiratory gasps, apneustic breathing, and periodic breathing in the erect posture accompanied by postural fall of blood pressure; RBD (in 80–95% of cases characterized by violent behavior in about 80% of cases but non-violent in the remaining percentage as captured in the video-audio recordings which are part of the routine PSG recording in most of the laboratories); motor behavior accompanied by REM without atonia (RWA), which is the physiological signature of RBD; and nocturnal stridor which may be inspiratory, expiratory (due to an obstruction in the intrathoracic region), or both and gives rise to a striking noise likened to a "donkey braying." MSLT may show pathological excessive daytime sleepiness (EDS).

Postural Tachycardia Syndrome (POTS)

Sleep dysfunction is often an important component of this entity but has largely been neglected. PSG findings reflect heterogeneity (as is also noted in the spectrum of clinical presentation) and may include sleep onset and maintenance insomnia, PLMS, decreased or absent REM sleep, abnormal sweating in REM sleep, rarely OSA and CSA with ataxic breathing, and circadian dysrhythmia (e.g., delayed sleep phase syndrome). An important common presentation is fatigue, which may be difficult to differentiate from EDS.

Familial Dysautonomia (FD, Riley-Day Syndrome)

Approximately 85% of adults and 91% of pediatric patients with FD have some degree of SDB which, when untreated, is a risk factor for sudden unexpected death during sleep (SUDS), a leading cause of death in FD. Both CSA and OSA occur in about 50% of patients and hypoventilation is noted in 60% of cases without accompanying apnea in many of them [41]. Other PSG findings include increased arousals and awakenings, prolonged sleep onset, and reduced total REM sleep time as well as dysrhythmic breathing. MSLT may show hypersomnolence. In addition, one infant with FD was found to have periodic somnolence lasting for 4–15 h during the neonatal period.

Diabetic and Amyloidotic Polyneuropathies and Guillain-Barre Syndrome

Sleep and breathing disturbances characterized by PSG-documented obstructive and central apneas-hypopneas accompanied by oxygen desaturation and repeated awakenings have been described in some patients, particularly those with autonomic dysfunction.

Neurodegenerative Diseases (Synucleopathies, e.g., PD and DLBD)

Sleep dysfunction is present in 70–90% of cases of PD. PSG findings may include evidence of RBD (noted in about 40–50% of cases with dream-enacting behavior [DEB] which may precede, occur simultaneously, or after the onset of classic parkinsonian motor manifestations) accompanied by RWA (the physiological signature of RBD), insomnia and irregular sleep-wake schedule (circadian dysrhythmia) noted clearly in actigraphic study, as well as respiratory dysrhythmias in PSG characterized by OSA, hypoventilation, CSB and Cheyne-Stokes variant pattern of breathing, nocturnal stridor, and dysrhythmic breathing. Other breathing problems observed in PD during PSG recordings (video-audio) include laryngeal spasms associated with off-states as well as dystonic episodes and diaphragmatic dyskinesias related to the end-of-the dose and peak-dose levodopa medications. Additional PSG findings in PD may include PLMS, sleep onset blinking, REM onset blepharospasm, and intrusion of REMs into NREM sleep.

An important PSG finding in DLBD is RBD (REM motor dyscontrol with DEB and RWA) noted in 100% of cases and often preceding the onset of the illness. Other PSG findings include sleep apnea and insomnia. These patients may also have nocturnal visual hallucinations during PSG recording. MSLT may document hypersomnolence.

Fatal Familial Insomnia (FFI)

This is a rare autosomal dominant prion disease presenting with prominent sleep and autonomic dysfunction. The most prominent finding in the PSG is progressive decrease in the amount of NREM and REM sleep, eventually leading to patients having only brief episodes of REM sleep. PSG with video-audio recording shows oneiric episodes (RBD-like episodes with enactment of ordinary day-to-day activities).

References

1. Butkov N, Keenan SA. An overview of polysomnographic technique. In: Chokroverty S, editor. Sleep disorders medicine: basic science, technical considerations and clinical aspects. 4th ed. New York: Springer; 2017. p. 267–94.
2. Chokroverty S, Bhat S. Polysomnographic recording technique. In: Chokroverty S, Thomas RJ, editors. Atlas of sleep medicine. 2th ed. Philadelphia: Elsevier; 2014.
3. The American Academy of Sleep Medicine. The AASM manual for the scoring of sleep and associated events: rules, terminology, and technical specifications. Version 2.5. Darien: American Academy of Sleep Medicine; 2018.
4. Jasper HH. The ten twenty electrode system of the international federation. Report of the Committee on Methods of Clinical Examination in Electroencephalography. Electroencephalogr Clin Neurophysiol. 1958;10:371–5.
5. Bhat S, Chokroverty S. Electroencephalography, electromyography and electro-oculography: general principles and basic technology. In: Chokroverty S, editor. Sleep disorders medicine: basic science, technical considerations and clinical aspects. 4th ed. New York: Springer; 2017. p. 295–330.
6. Butkov N. Atlas of clinical polysomnography. 2nd ed. Medford: Synapse Media; 2010.
7. Chokroverty S, Radtke R, Mulligan J. Polysomnography: technical and clinical aspects. In: Schomer DL, Lopes Da Silva FH, editors. Niedermeyer's electroencephalography: basic principles, clinical applications, and related fields. 6th ed. Philadelphia: Lippincott, Williams and Wilkins; 2011. p. 817–64.
8. Frauscher B, Iranzo A, Gaig C, Gschliesser V, Guaita M, Raffelseder V, et al. Normative EMG values during REM sleep for the diagnosis of REM sleep behavior disorder. Sleep. 2012;35(6):835–47.
9. Carskadon MA, Dement W. The multiple sleep latency test: what does it measure? Sleep. 1982;5:567.
10. Roth T, Roehrs TA. Multiple sleep latency test. In: Chokroverty S, editor. Sleep disorders medicine: basic science, technical considerations and clinical aspects. 4th ed. New York: Springer; 2017. p. 392–8.
11. Chokroverty S. Sleep disturbances in general medical disorders. In: Chokroverty S, editor. Sleep disorders medicine: basic science, technical considerations and clinical aspects. 4th ed. New York: Springer; 2017. p. 997–1058.
12. Chokroverty S. Specialized techniques. In: Chokroverty S, Thomas RJ, editors. Atlas of sleep medicine. 2nd ed. Philadelphia: Elsevier; 2014.
13. Littner MR, Kushida C, Wise M, Davila DG, Morgenthaler T, Lee-Chong T, et al. Standards of Practice Committee of the American Academy of Sleep Medicine. Practice parameters for clinical use of the multiple sleep latency test and the maintenance of wakefulness test. Sleep. 2005;28(1):113–21.
14. Arand D, Bonnet M, Hurwitz T, Mitler M, Rosa R, Sangal RB. The clinical use of the MSLT and MWT. Sleep. 2004;8:123.

15. Carskadon MA, Dement WC, Mitler MM, Roth T, Westbrook PR, Keenan S. Guidelines for the multiple sleep latency test (MSLT): a standard measure of sleepiness. Sleep. 1986;9(4):519–24.
16. American Academy of Sleep Medicine. International classification of sleep disorders. 3rd ed. Darien: American Academy of Sleep Medicine; 2014.
17. Roehrs T, Zorick F, McLeaghan A, Sicklesteel J, Lamphere J, Wittig R, Roth T. Sleep and MSLT norms for middle age adults. Sleep Res. 1984;13:87.
18. Zwyghuizen-Doorenbos A, Roehrs T, Schaefer M, Roth T. Test-retest reliability of the MSLT. Sleep. 1998;11(5):562–5.
19. Seidel WF, Dement WC. The multiple sleep latency test: test-retest reliability. Sleep Res. 1981;10:105.
20. Trotti LM, Staab BA, Rye DB. Test-retest reliability of the multiple sleep latency test in narcolepsy without cataplexy and idiopathic hypersomnia. J Clin Sleep Med. 2013;9(8):789–95.
21. Aurora RN, Caffo B, Crainiceanu C, Punjabi NM. Correlating subjective and objective sleepiness: revisiting the association using survival analysis. Sleep. 2011;34(12):1707–14.
22. Chervin RD, Aldrich MS, Pickett R, Guilleminault C. Comparison of the results of the Epworth sleepiness scale and the multiple sleep latency test. J Psychosom Res. 1997;42(2):145–55.
23. Benbadis SR, Mascha E, Perry MC, Wolgamuth BR, Smolley LA, Dinner DS. Association between the Epworth sleepiness scale and the multiple sleep latency test in a clinical population. Ann Intern Med. 1999;130(4 Pt 1):289–92.
24. Aldrich MS, Chervin RD, Malow BA. Value of the multiple sleep latency test (MSLT) for the diagnosis of narcolepsy. Sleep. 1997;20(8):620–9.
25. Coelho FM, Georgsson H, Murray BJ. Benefit of repeat multiple sleep latency testing in confirming a possible narcolepsy diagnosis. J Clin Neurophysiol. 2011;28(4):412–4.
26. Goldstein C, Chervin R. Maintenance of wakefulness test. In: Chokroverty S, editor. Sleep disorders medicine: basic science, technical considerations and clinical aspects. 4th ed. New York: Springer; 2017. p. 399–404.
27. Phillip P, Chaufton C, Taillard J, et al. Maintenance of Wakefulness test scores and driving performance in sleep disorder patients. and controls. Int J Psychophysiol 2013;89:195–202
28. Sadeh A, Hauri PJ, Kripke DF, Lavie P. The role of actigraphy in the evaluation of sleep disorders. Sleep. 1995;18(4):288–302.
29. Walia HK, Mehra R. Practical aspects of actigraphy and approaches in clinical and research domains. Handb Clin Neurol. 2019;160:371–9.
30. Jean-Louis G, Kripke DF, Cole RJ, Assmus JD, Langer RD. Sleep detection with an accelerometer actigraph: comparisons with polysomnography. Physiol Behav. 2001;72(1–2):21–8.
31. Ko PT, Kientz JA, Choe EK, Kay M, Landis CA, Watson NF. Consumer sleep technologies: a review of the landscape. J Clin Sleep Med. 2015;11(12):1455–61.
32. Choi BH, Seo JW, Choi JM, Shin HB, Lee JY, Jeong DU, Park KS. Non-constraining sleep/wake monitoring system using bed actigraphy. Med Biol Eng Comput. 2007;45(1):107–14.
33. O'Hare E, Flanagan D, Penzel T, Garcia C, Frohberg D, Heneghan C. A comparison of radio-frequency biomotion sensors and actigraphy versus polysomnography for the assessment of sleep in normal subjects. Sleep Breath. 2015;19(1):91–8.
34. Nakano H, Hirayama K, Sadamitsu Y, Toshimitsu A, Fujita H, Shin S, Tanigawa T. Monitoring sound to quantify snoring and sleep apnea severity using a smartphone: proof of concept. J Clin Sleep Med. 2014;10(1):73–8.
35. Narayan S, Shivdare P, Niranjan T, Williams K, Freudman J, Sehra R. Noncontact identification of sleep-disturbed breathing from smartphone-recorded sounds validated by polysomnography. Sleep Breath. 2019;23(1):269–79.
36. Bianchi MT. Sleep devices: wearables and nearables, informational and interventional, consumer and clinical. Metabolism. 2018;84:99–108.
37. Bhat S, Ferraris A, Gupta D, Mozafarian M, DeBari VA, Gushway-Henry N, et al. Is there a clinical role for smartphone sleep apps? Comparison of sleep cycle detection by a smartphone application to polysomnography. J Clin Sleep Med. 2015;11(7):709–15.
38. Kolla BP, Mansukhani S, Mansukhani MP. Consumer sleep tracking devices: a review of mechanisms, validity and utility. Expert Rev Med Devices. 2016;13(5):497–506.
39. Khosla S, Deak MC, Gault D, Goldstein CA, Hwang D, Kwon Y, et al. American Academy of sleep medicine Board of Directors. Consumer sleep technology: an American Academy of sleep medicine position statement. J Clin Sleep Med. 2018;14(5):877–80.
40. Chokroverty S, Provini F. Sleep, breathing and neurologic disorders. In: Chokroverty S, editor. Sleep disorders medicine: basic science, technical considerations and clinical aspects. 4th ed. New York: Springer; 2017. p. 787–890.
41. Singh K, Palma JA, Kaufman H, Tkachenko N, Norcliffe-Kaufmann L, Spalink C, et al. Prevalence and characteristics of sleep disordered breathing in familial dysautonomia. Sleep Med. 2018;45:33–8.

Part III

Clinical Aspects

12 An Approach to a Patient with Suspected Autonomic and Sleep Dysfunction

Sudhansu Chokroverty

Introduction

An approach to an analysis of a patient's complaints must begin with a clear understanding of the evaluation process (see further on) when confronted with a patient suspected to have autonomic dysfunction (AD) or dysautonomia that could be defined as derangement of sympathetic, parasympathetic, or enteric nervous system function [1]. This may manifest more commonly as hypoactivity (autonomic failure, AF) more often rather than hyperactivity (autonomic dysreflexia or autonomic storms) of the autonomic nervous system (ANS). A correct diagnosis of AD is essential to design appropriate treatment, and to assess natural history and prognosis of the condition. Therefore, an approach must be formulated in a way to making an accurate diagnosis. For this purpose, it is essential to have a basic knowledge of the classification of AD and this is the first step. In this chapter, I shall outline the approach and evaluation in the subsections in the following order:

- **Classification of Dysautonomia**
- **General and Specific Clinical Manifestations of Autonomic Dysfunction and Physiology of Orthostatic Blood Pressure Control**
- **History and Physical Examination**
- **Clinical Scales and Questionnaires**
- **Autonomic Function and Other Laboratory Tests**
- **Brief Description of Some Important and Unusual Dysautonomic Entities**
- **Fits and Faints, Including Syncope and Other Mimics of Autonomic Dysfunction**
- **Clinical–Anatomical–Laboratory Correlations with Case Examples**
- **Principles of Therapy**

Classification of Dysautonomia

The ANS by innervating all body systems and organs controls major bodily functions to maintain internal homeostasis. The major functions include control of cardiovascular (CV), respiratory, gastrointestinal (GI), genitourinary (GU), endocrine and thermoregulatory systems as well as pupillary function and regulation of states of our existence (active wakefulness, relaxed wakefulness, nonrapid eye movement [NREM], and rapid-eye movement [REM] sleep [2–6]). History, therefore, should address possible dysautonomic symptoms affecting each of these systems and organs (see further on), and must include 24-h history.

Autonomic manifestations may be primary (idiopathic without any known cause) or secondary to (comorbid with) other conditions, for example, neurological, other medical or primary sleep disorders and iatrogenic (medication-related or surgically induced) cases that could be generalized (Box 12.1) and localized (Box 12.2; e.g., Horner syndrome, Adie's pupil, gustatory facial sweating, and Chagas disease [caused by *Trypanosoma cruzi* affecting predominantly Central and South American population, and affecting localized autonomic plexus in the heart and gut]). AD may also be transient or paroxysmal (Box 12.3), for example, vasovagal syncope in the young, and carotid sinus hypersensitivity in the elderly individuals. Sometimes patients present with features of autonomic overactivity or so called autonomic "storms" or dysreflexia (Box 12.4). An example of sympathetic overactivity in patients with spinal cord injury, particularly above T5 level may be cited causing paroxysmal hypertension resulting from spinal reflex activity (dysreflexia) in those

S. Chokroverty (✉)
Hackensack Meridian Health, Neuroscience Institute at JFK, JFK University Medical Center, Edison, NJ, USA

Seton Hall University & Hackensack Meridian School of Medicine at Seton Hall, South Orange, NJ, USA

Rutgers Robert Wood Johnson Medical School, New Brunswick, NJ, USA
e-mail: Sudhansu.Chokroverty@hackenssackmeridian.org

S. Chokroverty, P. Cortelli (eds.), *Autonomic Nervous System and Sleep*, https://doi.org/10.1007/978-3-030-62263-3_12

with quadriplegia. Another example is excessive vagal activity causing bradycardia in vasovagal syncope (a neurally mediated syncope) in young person with prolonged standing in a crowded environment. AF could sometimes be related to medications taken (e.g., clonidine and L-dopa) for some medical or psychiatric (e.g., anxiolytics and antidepressants) conditions or may be caused by some street drugs (e.g., cocaine, amphetamine, "crack," and phencyclidine) taken by many young individuals. Another iatrogenic cause of AF is surgical sympathectomy. Two important examples of primary diffuse chronic AF include multiple system atrophy (MSA, formerly known as the Shy-Drager syndrome) and pure autonomic failure (PAF) (see Box 12.1 and section "Brief Description of Some Important and Unusual Dysautonomic Entities"). Secondary diffuse AF may be caused by a variety of medical disorders. For example, diabetic autonomic neuropathy affecting cardiovagal function, postganglionic sympathetic sudomotor (with proximal–distal gradient), and adrenergic systems. Another example is familial amyloidotic polyneuropathy (somatic and autonomic) causing diffuse degeneration with selective loss of pain and temperature sensation (small fiber neuropathy), orthostatic hypotension, weight loss, and amyloid infiltration in the biopsied rectal and nerve tissues. Certain neurological diseases may cause secondary diffuse chronic AF (e.g., neurodegenerative disorders like Parkinson's disease, diffuse Lewy body disease with dementia, hypothalamic and brain stem tumors, spinal cord injury, and many others (see Box 12.1)). An important category of neurological disorders causing AF is neurodevelopmental diseases, such as congenital central hypoventilation syndrome (CCHS), and congenital megacolon (Hirschsprung's disease) (see Box 12.1). Fatal familial insomnia (FFI), a prion disease described relatively recently, presents with a variety of dysautonomic manifestations in addition to insomnia, ataxia, myoclonus, and oneiric behavior pursuing a relentlessly progressive course and ending in death in course of 1–2 years [7]. Most of the major entities listed in this section are described in separate chapters throughout this book.

Box 12.1 Classification of Generalized Autonomic Failure

A. **Primary Dysautonomia**

1. Pure autonomic failure (PAF) without associated somatic neurological deficits (Bradbury–Eggleston syndrome)
2. Multiple system atrophy (MSA), a neurodegenerative disease with progressive autonomic failure associated with somatic neurological manifestations, characterized either by predominant cerebellar (MSA-C) or parkinsonian features (MSA-P) or both parkinsonian-cerebellar syndrome (MSA-PC). When dysautonomia is the initial dominant feature, the entity is also known as the Shy–Drager syndrome, which has recently been replaced by multiple system atrophy)
3. Acute or subacute pandysautonomia (idiopathic variety)
4. A subset of postural tachycardia syndrome (POTS; idiopathic type)
5. Riley–Day syndrome (familial dysautonomia [FD])

B. **Secondary (Comorbid) Dysautonomia (Associated with Known Diseases or Iatrogenic)**

I. Neurological diseases

(a) Intracranial lesions
1. Hypothalamic, pituitary and brain stem tumors
2. Encephalitis and encephalopathies
3. Wernicke encephalopathy
4. Multiple encephalomalacia
5. Demyelinating diseases (including multiple sclerosis)
6. Neurodegenerative diseases (e.g., Parkinson's disease, dementia with Lewy body disease)
7. Oher brain stem lesions (e.g., trauma, stroke)
8. Epilepsy including diencephalic autonomic seizure

(b) Spinal cord dysfunction
1. Spinal cord injuries
2. Spinal cord tumors
3. Syringomyelia
4. Hematomyelia
5. Tabes dorsalis

(c) Neurodevelopmental or congenital disorders
1. Hirschsprung's disease (also known as aganglionic colon or megacolon), a developmental disorder due to absence or sparse enteric ganglia affecting most commonly the rectum or the distal sigmoid colon
2. Rett syndrome
3. Ehlers–Danlos syndrome
4. Congenital insensitivity to pain with anhidrosis (CIPA)
5. Congenital sensory neuropathy (HSAN Type II)
6. Dopamine beta-hydroxylase deficiency
7. Congenital central hypoventilation syndrome (CCHS)

(d) Peripheral neuropathies associated with Autonomic neuropathy
1. Diabetic neuropathies
2. Acute inflammatory demyelinating polyradiculoneuropathy (AIDP) [Landry–Guillain–Barré–Strohl syndrome]
3. Alcoholic neuropathy
4. Amyloidotic neuropathy
5. Hereditary sensory neuropathies
6. Acute pandysautonomia (secondary variety)
7. Acute or subacute immune mediated neuropathy
8. Toxic autonomic neuropathy (e.g., arsenic and thallium); Vacor, mercury, organic solvents (in some workers), *n*-hexane inhalation (industrial exposure), etc.

(e) Neuromuscular Junctional Disorders Comorbid with Autonomic Dysfunction:
1. Myasthenia gravis
2. Myasthenic syndrome (Lambert–Eaton syndrome)
3. Botulism

II. Nonneurological (general medical disorders):
1. Diabetes mellitus
2. Addison disease
3. Panhypopituitarism
4. Acute intermittent porphyria
5. Chronic fatigue syndrome
6. Collagen vascular disease (e.g., systemic lupus erythematosus [SLE] and Sjogren's syndrome)

III. Iatrogenic (surgically or drug induced):
1. Surgical sympathectomy (localized autonomic dysfunction)
2. Cordotomy (spinal cord surgery for intractable pain)
3. Drug induced
(i) Antidepressants
(ii) Tranquillizers
(iii) Hypotensive drugs
(iv) Other drugs (e.g., L-dopa, vincristine, amiodarone, cis-platinum)
(v) Anticholinergic (e.g., tricyclic antidepressants [amitriptyline] and antihistamines [Benadryl])
(vi) Diuretics

IV. Dysautonomia (hypo- or hyperactivity) in primary sleep disorders
1. Obstructive sleep apnea syndrome
2. Narcolepsy–cataplexy
3. Restless legs syndrome—periodic limb movements in sleep
4. Fatal familial insomnia (FFI)
5. Parasomnias (NREM and REMs)

V. Miscellaneous
1. Paraneoplastic autonomic neuropathy
2. Hyperbradykininism
3. Baroreflex Failure
4. Postural tachycardia syndrome (POTS) secondary to hypovolemia, deconditioning, selective autonomic neuropathy

Box 12.2 Localized Autonomic Dysfunction
1. Horner syndrome
2. Holmes–Adie syndrome
3. Argyll Robertson pupil
4. Ross syndrome
5. Harlequin syndrome
6. Gustatory sweating (auriculotemporal syndrome of Frey)
7. Crocodile tears (Bogorad syndrome)
8. Complex regional pain syndrome type I and type II
9. Chagas disease (caused by *Trypanosoma cruzi*, predominately in Central and South America)
10. Idiopathic palmar or axillary hyperhidrosis

Box 12.3 Transient or intermittent (episodic or paroxysmal) dysautonomia
- Episodic autonomic dysfunction reflexly induced (includes neurally mediated syncope):
  - Vasovagal, cough and micturition syncope
  - Carotid sinus hypersensitivity
  - Glossopharyngeal neuralgia
- Cardiac syncope (related to structural cardiac disease)
- Epileptic autonomic discharges in generalized or focal seizures and diencephalic autonomic seizure
- Subarachnoid hemorrhage
- Cerebral or brain stem transient ischemic episodes
- Paroxysmal hyperhidrosis
- Raynaud's phenomenon
- Erythromelalgia
- Shapiro syndrome (Agenesis of corpus callosum, hypothermia and hyperhidrosis)

Box 12.4 Autonomic Hyperactivity (Autonomic "Storms") or Autonomic "Dysreflexia"

A. Sympathetic hyperactivity (typically seen in complete spinal cord transection above the T5 segmental level interrupting the descending input to the spinal sympathetic preganglionic neurons. As a result of this interruption there is excessive sympathetic activity [autonomic dysreflexia]):
   1. Hyperhidrosis
   2. Altered thermal regulation
   3. High blood pressure
   4. Palpitation and tachycardia
   5. Pupillary dilation (*mydriasis*)
B. Parasympathetic hyperactivity
   1. Excessive salivation and lacrimation
   2. Hypotension
   3. Bradycardia
   4. Pupillary constriction (miosis)

Box 12.5 Clinical Manifestations of Autonomic Failure

A. The four most common presenting features
   1. Orthostatic intolerance symptoms related to orthostatic hypotension
   2. Urinary bladder dysfunction
   3. Anhidrosis or hypohidrosis
   4. Erectile dysfunction in men
B. Additional manifestations related to dysfunction of the peripheral or central autonomic neurons:
   1. Horner syndrome
   2. Impairment of pupillary response to light and accommodation
   3. Diminished lacrimation and dryness of the mouth
   4. Persistent tachycardia (palpitations) or in some cases, cardiac arrhythmias
   5. Difficulty in swallowing or vomiting
   6. Chronic constipation (persistent or intermittent) and often nocturnal diarrhea
   7. Fecal incontinence
   8. Respiratory dysrhythmias, which are observed particularly in multiple system atrophy

General and Specific Clinical Manifestations of Autonomic Dysfunction and Physiology of Orthostatic Blood Pressure Control

I. **The history and physical examination findings of a patient** referred for possible dysautonomia must be critically analyzed by the autonomic physician and she/he should be aware of symptoms resulting from a dysfunction of the ANS. Patients may present with a set of positive or negative dysautonomic symptoms [2, 3]. Moreover, certain symptoms and signs may suggest a specific dysfunction of a particular division of the ANS or may direct one's attention to a particular body system responsible for such manifestations.

   A. **General features**: The four most common presenting features in a patient with dysautonomia (Box 12.5) include [8] (i) orthostatic intolerance (OI) symptoms such as presyncope (e.g., dizziness, blurring of vision, nausea, sensation of abdominal bloating, and fullness) or syncope (transient loss of consciousness), and orthostatic hypotension (OH) in the upright posture (as a result of cerebral hypoperfusion) relieved by changing from erect to supine position; (ii) symptoms of urinary dysfunction (e.g., enuresis and frequency of micturition), which are often attributed to diseases of the prostate gland in men delaying the diagnosis; (iii) anhidrosis or hypohydrosis; and (iv) erectile dysfunction in men (this symptom frequently precedes other major manifestations by many years).

   Additional manifestations that may be presenting features in some patients are also listed in Box 12.5 [2, 3, 9].

   B. **Positive dysautonomic phenomena** that are infrequently the presenting features include the following:
      1. Autonomic dysreflexia or autonomic "storms" (e.g., after spinal cord transection usually above T5 level; see Box 12.4)
      2. Compensatory autonomic hyperactivity in normally innervated areas (e.g., facial hyperhidrosis in diabetic autonomic cranial neuropathy patients and segmental hyperhidrosis in partial peripheral nerve injuries)
      3. Hyperhidrosis seen in tetanus accompanied by hypertension and tachycardia

   C. **Negative autonomic phenomena:** These are more common (compared with positive features) presentation of dysautonomic patients:
      1. Faint feeling and dizziness (cerebral hypoperfusion) due to orthostatic hypotension
      2. Heat intolerance or heat stroke
      3. Accidental hypothermia, particularly in the older individuals
      4. Anhidrosis or hypohidrosis in parts of the body
      5. Sphincter dysfunction (incontinence of urine and feces)

D. **Specific features indicating parasympathetic failure:**
   1. Dry mouth
   2. Dry eyes (keratoconjunctivitis sicca) as a result of absent or decreased tear production (alacrima): very common along with dry mouth in Sjogren syndrome
   3. Sexual dysfunction
   4. Urinary bladder problem (retention or enuresis)
   5. Impaired pupillary light reflex (dilated poorly responsive pupils)
   6. Persistent tachycardia or fixed heart rate (HR) in all body positions
   7. Reduced heart rate variability (HRV) or altered low frequency/high frequency (LF/HF) ratio in HR frequency domain analysis
   8. Widespread anhidrosis or hypohidrosis (anatomically sympathetic but functionally cholinergic failure)

E. **Following symptoms or signs point to sympathetic failure:**
   1. Orthostatic hypotension
   2. Diffuse anhidrosis or hypohidrosis

F. **Features suggesting failure of the enteric nervous system (ENS):**

   Gastrointestinal dysmotility (e.g., achalasia, gastroparesis, intestinal pseudo-obstruction, and colonic atonia) manifested by the following symptoms: (i) anorexia, (ii) swallowing difficulty, (iii) early satiety, (iv) postprandial abdominal pain, (v) vomiting, (vi) constipation, (vii) diarrhea, often nocturnal, (viii) abdominal distension, and (ix) symptoms of intestinal pseudo-obstruction (intestinal obstruction without any structural lesion in the lumen), such as abdominal pain and distension, nausea, vomiting, dysphagia, diarrhea, and constipation depending on the GI part affected by dysmotility [10].

G. **Specific features pointing to an involvement of a particular body system and organ:**

   These features provide clues as to the possible cause for secondary dysautonomia. During history taking and physical examination, particular attention should be paid to symptoms and signs for uncovering specific system related involvement as listed below [11]:

1. Postural (orthostatic) hypotension in the head-up position (HUP; vertical) accompanied by OI symptoms normalized on lying supine (see above "A"). Of note, in the head-down position (HDP) BP and HR may increase above the baseline values in the supine position. The history must include inquiry into the following:
   (a) Triggering (or aggravating) factors for OH, such as exercise, prolonged bed rest, ingestion of food, environment (hot stuffy surrounding), hot bath, and time of the day (e.g., worse in the morning).
   (b) Sweat glands and sweating: see above "C", "D," and "E."
   (c) Cardiovascular system: see above "A" and "E."
   (d) Gastrointestinal system: see above "D' and "F."
   (e) Genitourinary system: see above "A", "C," and "D". Other symptoms may include recurrent urinary tract infection.
   (f) Neurological system: in addition to symptoms related to possible involvement of extrapyramidal system (e.g., stooped posture, rest tremor, rigidity, gait problem, postural instability, slowness of body and mind), unsteadiness and ataxic gait (cerebellar dysfunction), symptoms related to memory and cognitive impairment; other features related to neurological involvement may include droopy eyelids (ptosis), dryness of eyes (alacrimia), blurriness of vision, abnormal movements, particularly at night (may suggest rapid eye movement sleep behavior disorder [RBD]).
   (g) Respiratory system: this may have a variety of breathing problems, specifically during sleep (very common in multiple system atrophy), shortness of breath (dyspnea), and an unusual noise during sleep (e.g., stridor, which is very common in MSA).

II. **Physiology of orthostatic blood pressure control**

   Orthostatic hypotension is a cardinal sign of AF and orthostatic intolerance. In order to understand its pathophysiology, it is essential to have at least a basic knowledge about the physiological changes in BP and other hemodynamic aspects when a normal individual changes from a supine to erect position [12–15]. When humans became Homo sapiens, they made an enemy of gravity [16]. Chapter 3 outlines pathophysiological mechanism of control of BP and other hemodynamic characteristics in the erect posture. Chapter 3 also critically discusses how a breakdown of such mechanisms may adversely affect an individual.

History and Physical Examination

History is the most important initial step in the evaluation of a patient presenting with symptoms suggestive of dysautonomia [2, 3, 17]. It is important to have a high index of suspicion about AD based on the patient's complaints. One must be vigilant about classification (see section "Classification of Dysautonomia") and essential features (both general and specific, see section "General and Specific Clinical Manifestations of Autonomic Dysfunction and Physiology of Orthostatic Blood Pressure Control") of dysautonomia. History should be followed by physical examination of each body system including neurological, cardiovascular, respiratory, and GI systems. History must include 24 h information including sleep history (e.g., bedtime, wake-up time, awakenings and abnormal movements during sleep at night, and any daytime sleepiness or impairment of daytime function). Many with dysautonomia have sleep disturbance and conversely, many primary sleep disorders (e.g., obstructive sleep apnea [OSA], REM behavior disorder [RBD], narcolepsy, and some NREM parasomnias) may have autonomia dysfunction (see Box 12.1). There is clear evidence that the brain stem respiratory and autonomic premotor neurons share common rhythms. Furthermore, the coupling of the central autonomic network and sleep–wake generating neurons plays an important role in controlling cardiovascular and respiratory regulation during sleep and wakefulness [18, 19]. Sleep-related physiological alterations in the ANS may cause profound changes in breathing in some cases of AF (e.g., MSA), and likewise breathing disturbance in sleep (e.g., OSA and central sleep apnea [CSA] may cause impaired ANS function) [20].

Step 1. History

An important initial step in the history is to seek answers to the following questions based on a critical analysis of symptoms and signs.

- Q1. Does the patient have dysautonomia?
- Q2. Is the patient's AD significant? (Of note, many patients with mild AD remain asymptomatic requiring no treatment but may progress later to develop significant dysautonomia delaying the diagnosis.). Some autonomic scale scores (e.g., CASS, see further on) may determine severity and significance.
- Q3. If the patient has AD, is it primary or secondary, localized or generalized, transient, or persistent (see Box 12.1, 12.2, 12.3) or is it autonomic dysreflexia (see Box 12.4)?
- Q4. Does AD impair patient's quality of life? This can certainly be improved by symptomatic treatment. Identifying the type of dysautonomia and differentiating it from mimics (e.g., neurally mediated versus cardiac or other types of syncope and other causes of "fits and faints" [see section "Fits and Faints, Including Syncope and Other Mimics of Autonomic Dysfunction"]) may help in making a final diagnosis, ascertaining prognosis, and preventing life-threatening complications (e.g., cardiac arrhythmias and sudden cardiac death) as well as in designing appropriate treatment.

It is notable that certain symptoms may strongly suggest presence of AD, for example, OI symptoms with or without orthostatic hypotension; sudomotor dysfunction (hypo- or anhidrosis or rarely localized or generalized hyperhidrosis); genitourinary dysfunction (erectile and ejaculatory difficulties in men, and nocturnal enuresis); and temperature dysregulation (hypothermia or hyperthermia of unknown cause), including coldness and discoloration of the hands and feet (intermittent or persistent) [11].

History must also include inquiry into the onset of symptoms (sudden or insidious), progression, and triggering (aggravating) factors. The onset of dysautonomia is in general insidious but sometimes could be sudden (e.g., acute pandysautonomia, acute inflammatory demyelinating polyneuropathy [Guillain–Barré syndrome], acute paraneoplastic or immune-mediated autonomic neuropathy). AD usually presents with diffuse or generalized manifestations (e.g., multiple system atrophy, pure autonomic failure, generalized hypo- [or rarely] hyperhidrosis, hypo-or hyperthermia, and OI symptoms). AD could sometimes be localized (see Box 12.2) or transient (see Box 12.3) and rarely may present with hyperactivity (see Box 12.4).

It is also important to inquire about family history (some dysautonomia can be familial, for example, CCHS, familial dysautonomia [FD], FFI [see Box 12.1]), past illnesses, psychiatric, and drug-alcohol histories as well as social history that are all important in understanding etiology and pathophysiological mechanisms of AD.

Step 2. Physical Examination

This must include specific autonomic examination [21] directed at uncovering signs pointing to a possible dysautonomia in addition to general physical examination and attention to neurological, cardiovascular, respiratory, GI, and genitourinary systems for possible cause (secondary) of AD.

Autonomic Examination

(a) Record BP and HR in supine and standing positions. Significant fall of BP (>20 mm Hg fall of systolic and >10 mm Hg fall of diastolic BP) without any reflex tachycardia suggests neurally mediated OH. In contrast, reflex rise of HR (at least 30 beats more than the supine baseline reading in adults and 40 beats more in adolescents of 14–19 years in the erect position without significant fall of BP accompanied by OI symptoms [see section "General and Specific Clinical Manifestations of Autonomic Dysfunction and Physiology of Orthostatic Blood Pressure Control"]) suggests postural tachycardia syndrome (POTS) caused by hypovolemia, deconditioning, or restricted autonomic neuropathy.
(b) Measure core body temperature to document hypo- or hyperthermia.
(c) Inspect the skin for acrocyanosis (bluish discoloration of the hands or feet or tip of the nose) and pallor indicating vasospastic AD, and red-hot body parts, especially distally suggesting erythromelalgia.

(d) Look for impaired sweating by inspection or palpation of the skin (dryness of the skin) or by the "spoon test" (gliding the convex side of the spoon should be smooth and uninterrupted over the anhidrotic skin but the flow is interrupted and sticky over the sweaty skin [22]. In AD, there may be localized or generalized hypo- or anhidrosis and rarely hyperhidrosis. A proximal–distal grading pattern of sweating impairment (e.g., the presence of sweating in the forehead and axilla but absent sweating distally) may be found in peripheral neuropathy with autonomic fibers involvement.
(e) Examine the patient for allodynia (pain triggered by non-noxious stimuli), hyperalgesia (excessive perception of pain to minimally painful stimuli) or hyperpathia (excessive feeling of pain following application of minimally noxious stimuli after a latency of a few seconds). These are all dysautonomic symptoms resulting from a dysfunction of central or peripheral ANS.
(f) Inspect and feel for trophic sign (e.g., brittle nails, dry, scaly, or atrophic skin) or Charcot joints (disorganized joints with excessive range of motion), and alopecia.
(g) Pupillary examination for size, shape or inequality of pupils, light reflex and convergence reaction for dysautonomia (e.g., Argyll Robertson pupil in tabes dorsalis, Adie's pupil).
(h) Look for dry eyes and dry mouth suggesting parasympathetic dysfunction.

Step 3. General Physical Examination

This should include vital signs, appearance of skin including its color (see above) or cyanosis, ankle edema, general appearance of the patient, and peripheral arterial pulsation for peripheral atherosclerosis. General physical examination should also include otolaryngological examination, and measurement of neck circumference (risk factor for sleep apnea).

Step 4. Special Examination of Each System

This must include complete neurological examination, as well as inspection, palpation and auscultation of the heart and lungs, abdominal examination for tenderness, peristalsis, presence or absence of bowel sounds for gut atonia, urinary bladder distension (suggesting urinary retention), physical evidence of endocrinopathies (e.g., slow pulse rate, nonpitting ankle edema, and hung-up muscle stretch reflexes seen in hypothyroidism) that might suggest a secondary cause for AD. Neurological examination may uncover signs of extrapyramidal dysfunction (e.g., masked facies, slow shuffling gait, rigidity, postural, and gait problems as well as resting tremor suggesting Parkinson's disease) and cerebellar dysfunction (e.g., ataxic gait, intention tremor), which may indicate that the patient's dysautonomia may be due to MSA. Other neurological conditions (see Box 12.1) may be causing dysautonomia and may have abnormal neurological findings indicating involvement of a particular system in the CNS. Neurological findings may also provide evidence of peripheral neuropathy (e.g., muscle weakness, decreased or absent muscle stretch reflexes, decreased sensation in the stocking, and glove distribution).

After history and physical examination, the purpose after Step 4 is to strengthen the clinical suspicion by using autonomic questionnaires and scales (see section "Clinical Scales and Questionnaires") and assess severity.

The next step is to order a set of basic screening tests including scales, questionnaires (section "Clinical Scales and Questionnaires"), and autonomic functions (section "Autonomic Function and Other Laboratory Tests") to confirm the clinical diagnosis (see section "Autonomic Function and Other Laboratory Tests"). Box 12.6 lists some logical steps in an orderly manner for diagnostic evaluation of dysautonomia.

Box 12.6 Logical and Relevant Steps for Diagnostic Evaluation of Dysautonomia

- **Step 1:** Detailed history from the patient and caregiver
  (a) Think about relevant questions (see section "History and Physical Examination")
  (b) Be aware of general and specific dysautonomic symptoms (see section "General and Specific Clinical Manifestations of Autonomic Dysfunction and Physiology of Orthostatic Blood Pressure Control")
  (c) Be knowledgeable about classification of dysautonomia (see section "Classification of Dysautonomia")
- **Step 2:**
  (a) Physical examination with particular attention to general and autonomic examination findings and measurement of BP and HR in the supine and upright positions for 3–5 min (section "History and Physical Examination")
  (b) Specific physical examination findings in every body system to get some clues for the cause of orthostatic intolerance symptoms and orthostatic hypotension (section "History and Physical Examination")
- **Step 3:** Use relevant questionnaires and scales (see section "Clinical Scales and Questionnaires") to

assess autonomic function and severity of its dysfunction

- **Step 4:** Formulate a provisional diagnosis and differentiate from mimics (section "Fits and Faints, Including Syncope and Other Mimics of Autonomic Dysfunction")
- **Step 5:** Order a set of basic simple bedside screening tests to confirm the diagnosis of AD (section "Autonomic Function and Other Laboratory Tests")
- **Step 6:** If needed, order more sophisticated and complex laboratory investigations for arriving at an etiological diagnosis (section "Autonomic Function and Other Laboratory Tests")
- **Step 7:** Design appropriate treatment and arrange for follow-up evaluation and monitoring.

Clinical Scales and Questionnaires

Certain scales and questionnaires may help in supporting and strengthening the clinical impression of dysautonomia. There are, however, only a limited number of scales and questionnaires (e.g., ASP, COMPASS, SCOPA-AUT [see below]) available for evaluating dysautonomic symptoms [23–25].

The autonomic symptom profile (ASP) containing 169 questions ("domain of autonomic function was initially described by Suarez et al. [23]). There are too many questions and so the Composite Autonomic System Scale (COMPASS) was developed containing 84 questions derived from the ASP. Later COMPASS-31 containing 31 questions was developed that demonstrated high sensitivity but moderate specificity. The COMAPSS-31 [24] scores correlated reasonably well with the Composite Autonomic Scores Scale (CASS) derived from autonomic function test results. Many problems were noted with the COMPASS over the years including an overall weak correlation with symptoms of diabetic autonomic neuropathies [25, 26]. Another scale, the SCOPA-AUT [27], was originally developed to screen and assess autonomic function in PD as well as in MSA. This scale contains 25 items covering six domains (gastrointestinal, urinary, cardiovascular, thermoregulatory, pupillomotor, and sexual functions) [27]. The latest validated questionnaire from the University of Maryland with high sensitivity and specificity is the Survey of the Autonomic Symptoms (SAS) consisting of 11 questions for women and 12 for men to diagnose early and mild diabetic autonomic neuropathy [26]. This one is easy to administer and is comparable to other validated questionnaires. There are two other questionnaires for a specific disorder of the ANS, for example, "the United Multiple System Atrophy Rating Scale (UMSARS)" to assess severity of motor and autonomic symptoms as well as to monitor progress of the disease in MSA [28]. Another example is an "Orthostatic Hypotension Questionnaire" (OHQ) used to assess the severity of symptoms and impact on day-to-day function in OH (a 10-item scale) [29].

Autonomic Function and Other Laboratory Tests

For more detail, see also Chap. 9.

A. The purpose of autonomic function tests (AFTs) in patients suspected to have AD (hypo- or hyperactivity, positive, or negative symptoms) can be summarized as follows [2–4, 8, 9, 30, 31]:
   1. To confirm or exclude significant AD in a patient suspected to have dysautonomia from clinical evaluation (see above)
   2. To determine the severity and for confirmation of autonomic impairment as evident from clinical evaluation (see above) and the clinical scale scores (e.g., the COMPASS-31 and others; see section "Clinical Scales and Questionnaires")
   3. To assess if the AD is affecting predominantly one or both the major subdivisions (sympathetic or parasympathetic) of the ANS
   4. To further localize the lesion responsible for AF to a particular part of the baroreflex pathway (e.g., afferent, efferent, central regions, or diffusely affecting)
   5. To confirm if AD is localized or generalized (i.e., distribution of dysautonomia)
   6. To evaluate if the AD is minimal requiring no intervention (many of the patients with minimal dysfunction remain functionally asymptomatic) or moderate to severe (determined by autonomic function severity scale (COMPASS-31 and CASS) [24, 25]) requiring treatment to improve symptoms and quality of life
   7. To find a cause for the autonomic symptoms (e.g., evaluation of the ANS involvement in sensorimotor peripheral neuropathies [autonomic involvement in distal small fiber neuropathy, DSFN [32] or autoimmune or paraneoplastic syndrome]; etiological evaluation in POTS or OI syndrome; to evaluate the role of the sympathetic nervous system in maintaining pain in some painful conditions, and in contributing to dysesthetic symptoms in RLS)
   8. To monitor patient's response to drug therapy
   9. To ascertain progression and prognosis of the disease, and, finally
   10. To design appropriate treatment

B. I shall briefly summarize the autonomic function tests, which can be performed to achieve the objectives as outlined above (for further details, the readers are referred to Chap. 9). The tests for ANS assessment can be grouped into noninvasive and invasive tests and those that can be used during sleep as well as in wakefulness.

I. **Noninvasive ANS Function Tests**

(All these tests are age specific and must be compared with age-matched normal controls) [2, 3, 7, 8, 30, 31].

1. Orthostatic stress testing (BP and HR responses to standing form a supine position and head-up tilt [HUT] to 70°. Normal changes in HR and BP on standing for 3–5 min may include a fall of systolic BP of ≤20 mm Hg and diastolic BP of ≤10 mm Hg or an increase of HR to 15 beats/min or no significant changes in BP.
2. Valsalva ratio (VR): obtain a continuous electrocardiographic (ECG) monitoring during forced expiration for 10–15 s against a closed glottis maintaining a pressure of 35–40 mm Hg; the VR measures the ratio of longest R-R interval to the shortest R-R interval. Normal value for VR ≥ 1.21; (10–60 yrs. ≥1.45–1.50; >60 yrs. ≥1.35).
3. Response to HR after deep breathing (HRDB): instruct the subject to breathe deeply at six breaths per minute (5 s for inspiration and 5 s for expiration in each breath) and determine mean HR (continuous one channel of EKG monitoring is needed) or pulse rate change (note that the HR increases on inspiration and decreases on expiration) during inspiration and expiration; also determine expiratory–inspiratory (E–I) ratio. Normative values: difference in HR increase: ≥15 beats/min; abnormal: ≤10.
4. 30:15 Ratio: determine response to HR at 30 and 15 s after standing from a supine to upright position. Normative values: ≥1.04 (abnormal: 1.00 or less).
5. Handgrip: BP and HR responses to handgrip: Normative value: Increase of diastolic BP ≥ 16 (abnormal: ≤10).
6. Mental arithmetic (cognitive load) test (MAT): BP and HR response during simple mathematical calculation.
7. Cold pressor test (CPT): BP and HR response on dipping the hand in ice-cold water (4 °C): both latencies to threshold (first perception of painful sensation) and tolerance (too painful to keep hand dipped in ice-cold water).
8. Cold face test (CFT): (diving reflex): BP and HR response to submerging face in cold water.
9. Noninvasive pharmacologic tests: determination of plasma levels of renin and norepinephrine in supine and upright positions.
10. Sudomotor function tests: for cholinergic sympathetic integrity and for an early diagnosis of small fiber neuropathy [30, 31, 33].
    (a) Thermoregulatory sweating of the entire body using quinizarin dye.
    (b) Sympathetic skin response (SSR) [33]: This can be performed in the standard electromyographic (EMG) laboratory using an EMG machine and surface electrodes over the dorsum and palm of the hand or the dorsum and sole of the foot. This test is nonspecific and gives variable results.

II. **Invasive Tests**

1. Invasive Valsalva maneuver (VM): intra-arterial recording of continuous BP and HR during four stages of VM; it is particularly important to see BP and HR responses during stage 4 of VM (note "overshoot" of BP and relative bradycardia in normal subjects) [14, 30, 31].
2. Pharmacological tests after intravenous (IV) infusion:
    (a) IV phenylephrine and norepinephrine infusion tests to determine denervation (postganglionic) supersensitivity to alpha receptors
    (b) IV isoproterenol infusion (a test for beta-receptor supersensitivity)
    (c) Baroreflex sensitivity (BRS) testing (expressed as a change in the slope of HR per mm Hg increase in BP after IV infusion or mechanical challenge (e.g., neck suction) [34].
3. A cardiac MIBG scintigraphy (single photon emission tomographic [SPECT] scans) to determine uptake of metaiodobenzylguanidine (MIBG), a scintigraphic test for cardiac sympathetic innervation [35].
4. Sudomotor test: the quantitative sudomotor axon reflex test (QSART) measures postganglionic sweat gland innervation for sweating after acetylcholine iontophoresis [36]. It is a very useful test to evaluate for dysautonomia in small fiber neuropathy.

All the above autonomic function tests (AFTs) can be performed to assess ANS function during wakefulness.

III. **The Following Tests Are Useful for Assessing ANS Function During Sleep**

(see also Chap. 9)

1. Heart rate and heart period (HR [reciprocal of HR]): HR and HP can help in linear assessment of

cardiac ANS tone (average ANS activity) throughout the night as well as transient variation (beat-to-beat) of HR. HP is related in a linear fashion to the frequency of cardiac sympathetic and parasympathetic activities.

2. Heart rate variability (HRV) [37–39]: This is a quantitative measure of spectral power of HR broken down into low (0.04–0.15 Hz) and high (0.15–0.40 Hz) frequencies as well as measuring beat-to-beat variability of HR (i.e., time intervals between subsequent R-waves on the EKG). Low frequency (LF) reflects both sympathetic and vagal activities whereas high frequency (HF) reflects respiratory sinus arrhythmias and as such is an important measure of cardiac vagal modulation. LF/HF ratio is thought to reflect sympathovagal balance; although this has been challenged recently [40, 41]. HRV can be measured in "time domain" and "frequency domain" (see also Chap. 10).
3. Beat-to-beat BP monitoring by ambulatory BP recording to assess normal "dippers" or "extreme" and "reverse" dippers as well as individuals who are "nondippers." People in the latter three categories (extreme, reverse, and nondippers) are "at risk" for cardiovascular catastrophes [42].
4. Microneurography: Uses tungsten microelectrodes to obtain multiunit recordings from cutaneous and muscle vessel nerve endings (i.e., intraneural recording) to assess peripheral sympathetic nerve activity [43].
5. Photoplethysmography (PPG): Measures change in light absorption by skin vessels showing continuous changes in cutaneous blood perfusion. PPG can be obtained from pulse oximetry [44].
6. Impedance cardiography (ICG) [45].
7. Baroreflex sensitivity (see above).

IV. **The Initial Simple Screening Tests**

The AFTs must be reliable, simple (easy to perform), reproducible and noninvasive for using in day-to-day autonomic medical practice. The following five tests known as the Ewing [46] battery of tests are easy to perform as the first screening step in evaluation of patients after initial history and physical examination: (i) BP and HR response to standing for 3–5 min from the supine position, (ii) HRDB, (iii) VR, (iv) BP and HR response to handgrip, and (v) 30:15 ratio. These tests can be performed at the bedside or outpatient clinic using the following: (a) a sphygmomanometer, (b) an electrocardiogram (1–2 channels), (c) an aneroid manometer, (d) a handgrip dynamometer, and (e) a mouthpiece for forced expiration against a closed glottis during VM. Most commonly tests for cardiovagal function (e.g., the Ewing battery of tests) and sudomotor tests (particularly QSART) are used as the initial AFTs to confirm clinical diagnosis of dysautonomia. Of note, hand grip tests are often omitted and more than one AFTs should be performed to confirm dysautonomia in a patient.

V. **Other Laboratory Tests**

These may be needed in selected cases [2, 3, 5, 9, 11].

1. Hematological studies, biochemical, and urinary analyses to exclude systemic diseases, for example, anemia, amyloidosis, and collagen vascular disorders (e.g., systemic lupus erythematosus [SLE] and Sjogren syndrome).
2. Plasma volume measurement.
3. Twenty-four-hour urinary sodium estimation.
4. Autoantibody tests for suspected autoimmune disorders with AF and a paraneoplastic dysautonomia (see Chap. 25).
5. Gastrointestinal motility study including esophageal and anorectal manometry as well as gastric emptying and colonic transit time (see Chap. 30).
6. Tests to evaluate genitourinary systems in appropriate cases with dysautonomia.
7. Laser Doppler and thermography for vascular assessment (important in suspected complex regional pain syndromes [CRPS I and II] and erythromelalgia.
8. For suspected Sjogren syndrome, it will be useful to perform Schirmer's test (for tear production) as well as Rose Bengal stain and lip biopsy (to assess status of salivary glands).
9. Pharmacologic studies of the pupils in appropriate cases.
10. PSG and other recordings for sleep disorders (see Chaps. 9 and 11).
11. Specialized investigations like brain magnetic resonance imaging (MRI), single photon emission tomographic (SPECT), and positron emission tomographic (PET) scans of the brain as well as brain MRI spectroscopy may be needed in suspected neurological disorders causing dysautonomic symptoms (secondary dysautonomia). These tests may also be useful in differentiating MSA from PAF (see Chaps. 23 and 24).
12. Skin biopsy: This may be considered (although evidence is weak for diagnostic sensitivity and specificity) in a symptomatic patient to uncover the presence of small fiber sensory neuropathy with associated autonomic neuropathy [32, 47].
13. Urodynamic studies may be needed for evaluating possible neurogenic urinary bladder.
14. In patients with urinary and fecal incontinence, needle electromyography (an invasive test) of the

urethral and anal sphincters may be helpful [30, 31].

15. Catecholamine fluorescence in muscle biopsy samples [8, 48].

C. **Limitations and Pitfalls of Autonomic Function Tests**

Certain limitations and pitfalls in the AFTs must be kept in mind otherwise the interpretation of the AFTs results may be invalid [49].

(i) No single test is diagnostic of a significant AD. One must perform at least two tests from each category (sympathetic or parasympathetic function) for a valid interpretation.
(ii) Several AFTs (e.g., HRDB, 30:15 ratio, VR) vary with age and therefore control values must be obtained from age-matched subjects. In addition, comorbidities must be taken into consideration for interpretation of the findings.
(iii) All tests must be performed according to a valid scientifically recommended standardized manner; otherwise, the significance of the test results must remain questionable.
(iv) All tests may not have sufficient sensitivity and specificity and may give false positive or negative results (e.g., MAT, CPT, CFT, intravenous infusion test, and SSR).
(v) Some tests may be too complex to perform (e.g., certain invasive tests, such as invasive Valsalva maneuver, intravenous infusion, microneurography).
(vi) Each autonomic function laboratory may not be equipped with facilities to perform the recommended and complex tests (e.g., QSART, cardiac MIBG scan, and intravenous infusion tests).
(vii) There is not a single specific laboratory test to assess a lesion of the afferent limb of the baroreceptor reflex arc. Similarly, there is no single specific test to assess central component of the baroreceptor reflex arc.
(viii) Many AFTs are invasive and the patients may be reluctant to undergo those tests. The autonomic physician thus must depend only on noninvasive tests, which may not give a satisfactory answer to the question.
(ix) Emotional state of the patient (e.g., anxiety and agitation) may affect the AFT making interpretation and validity of the test unreliable.
(x) Certain medications may affect AFT results (e.g., anticholinergics and antidepressants).
(xi) Skin temperature must be measured and controlled to avoid interference with certain tests (e.g., QSART may give wrong result if skin temperature is not standardized; another example is a patient with complex regional pain syndrome type 1 or type 2 who also requires attention to skin temperature).
(xii) Patient's hydration states (by altering plasma volume) may affect BP and HR responses.
(xiii) For evaluating parasympathetic function patients must be in sinus rhythm; cardiac arrhythmia will invalidate the test results.
(xiv) Even after performing multiple AFTs, it may not be possible to locate the site of the lesion to the afferent, central, or efferent limbs of a reflex arc (e.g., baroreceptor reflex), and one may not be absolutely certain about affection of a particular division (sympathetic, parasympathetic, or localization to the preganglionic or postganglionic segments of the ANS). However, careful attention to the tests and their results may help the physician to localize the lesion (see further on).
(xv) Another limitation is an absence of standardized guidelines to perform minimum number of AFTs. Based on general consensus [49–51], there are certain suggestions for a minimum number of tests to evaluate autonomic function.

D. **Localization of the Lesion Based on Autonomic Function Tests**

In this segment, I shall list certain AFTs and their alteration that may suggest affection of either the sympathetic efferent (adrenergic dysfunction) or the parasympathetic (vagal) divisions of the ANS [8, 9, 17, 30, 31].

1. Abnormalities of the following tests will suggest involvement of the efferent sympathetic division of the ANS.
   (a) Head-Up Tilt (HUT) Table Test: OH without rise of HR or subnormal rise.
   (b) Valsalva maneuver (VM): Failure of rise of BP and HR in Phase 2 (during sustained strain) and failure of "Overshoot" in Phase 4 (release of strain).
   (c) Cold Pressor Test (CPT): Uses both sympathetic afferent and efferent pathways: Failure of rise of BP and HR.
   (d) Mental Arithmetic Test (MAT): Uses sympathetic efferent limb: Failure of rise of BP and HR.
   (e) Standing from supine position: Uses central and sympathetic efferent pathways: excessive fall of systolic BP by 20 mm Hg or more or diastolic BP by 10 mm Hg or more within 3–5 min of standing.
   (f) Sustained hand grip (about 30% of maximum voluntary contraction for several minutes); abnormal response: rise of diastolic BP to ≤10 mm Hg.
   (g) Noninvasive pharmacologic tests measuring plasma levels of norepinephrine and renin in

supine and erect positions: low levels of norepinephrine in the supine and failure of rise of renin and norepinephrine significantly or subnormal rise in the upright position signify efferent sympathetic (postganglionic) involvement.
   (h) Hypohidrosis or anhidrosis and impairment of sympathetic skin response.
2. Impairment of cardiovagal function: Abnormalities of the following tests will indicate impairment of efferent vagal (parasympathetic) function [2, 8, 52].
   (a) HRDB: Difference in HR between expiration and inspiration ≤ 10.
   (b) VM: Absence of reflex bradycardia in the fourth phase (release of strain).
   (c) VR: Abnormal value <1.21.
   (d) CFT (Diving reflex): Failure to show bradycardia.
   (e) 30:15 ratio: Abnormal value ≤ 1.00.
   (f) Neostigmine test: Failure to cause bradycardia after neostigmine injection.
   (g) Atropine test: Lack of tachycardia after intravenous atropine injection (provided sympathetic efferent is intact).
3. Localization of lesion to different components of the baroreceptor reflex arc in OH [8]:
   (a) Total baroreflex arc involvement
      (i) Abnormal HUT Test
      (ii) Abnormal VM
      (iii) Abnormal VR
   (b) Efferent arc: See above 1 and 2.
   (c) Central lesion: No single reliable test is available but a combination of tests may help. There were two papers, one published in 1960 in the journal *Lancet* by Sharpey-Schaffer and Taylor [53] and the other published by Sharpey-Schaffer earlier [54] suggesting vasomotor center (VMC) responsiveness in the medulla: Post hyperventilation (15 s) fall of BP and bradycardia imply intact central mechanism.
   (d) Afferent limb: Abnormal test of total reflex arc but normal efferent limb will suggest affection of either the afferent limb or the central component of the Baroreflex arc whereas presence of bradycardia after VM (phase 4) and intravenous norepinephrine infusion will imply intact (unaffected) afferent limb [8, 52].
4. There are also tests to localize to a preganglionic or postganglionic segment of the ANS as well as intraocular and other tests, which are beyond the scope of this chapter [2, 3, 30, 31].

Brief Description of Some Important and Unusual Dysautonomic Entities

(Details of most of the entities are available throughout this book)

I. **Generalized Primary ANS Failure**
   1. **Acute Pandysautonomia**

This is also known as autoimmune autonomic neuropathy (AAN) (see also Chap. 25). This condition must be differentiated from paraneoplastic autonomic neuropathy as well as drug-induced (e.g., heavy metals, such as inorganic mercury and arsenic poisoning, hexane inhalation [glue sniffing], acrylamide) autonomic neuropathies. The classic presentation of acute AAN is an acute onset of severe pandysautonomia (generalized sympathetic and parasympathetic failure) often preceded by a viral infection (e.g., flu-like or upper respiratory tract infection) and running a monophasic course with partial recovery in most cases (occasional complete recovery) [55, 56]. Evidence of an autoimmune mechanism is manifested by the presence of ganglionic nicotinic acetylcholine receptor (AChR) antibodies in high titers in serum in approximately 50% of cases. Most prominent clinical features include orthostatic hypotension with orthostatic intolerance symptoms, hypo- or anhidrosis, and in some cases also disturbances of gastrointestinal motility, urinary bladder and bowel dysfunction as well as dry mouth, dry eyes, and tonic pupils with impaired light reflex.

2. **Pure Autonomic Failure (Bradbury–Eggleston Syndrome)**

In 1925 Bradbury and Eggleston [57] described three patients presenting with pure autonomic failure (PAF) without any somatic manifestations presenting with orthostatic hypotension associated with orthostatic intolerance symptoms (see below) in the erect posture relieved by assuming supine position (see also Chap. 24). It is noteworthy that almost 100 years before this description the French physician Piorry in 1826 first recognized the importance of the gravitational force on the circulation in the upright position. Under the title of "Research on the Influence of Gravity on the Circulation of Blood: Diagnosis of Syncope and Apoplexy; Cause and Treatment of Syncope," Piorry gave a clinical description of four patients who became unconscious in the sitting and upright positions, but immediately regained consciousness when placed in the supine position [58]. Piorry concluded that the arterial, venous, and capillary circulation was under the influence of the law of gravity.

However, in the absence of documentation of postural variation of BP (sphygmomanometer was not invented at that time), considerable doubt remains as to whether Piorry's patients really had orthostatic hypotension. Nevertheless, Piorry was the first physician to realize the importance of the effect of gravity on circulation. Bradbury and Eggleston [57] from Cornell University Medical College, New York, however, were the first to define the syndrome of primary orthostatic hypotension (OH). Laubry and Doumer [59] first coined the term "orthostatic" in 1932 when they demonstrated the orthostatic nature of hypotension in a 41-year-old man. It is noteworthy that several publications with the description of Bradbury–Eggleston syndrome clearly showed phenoconversion of many PAF patients (≈10%) to a neurodegenerative disease (Shy–Drager syndrome, also known as multiple system atrophy [MSA] mostly and also as PD and DLBD) within an average interval of three to 5 years after onset [60] as exemplified by our case number one in section "Clinical–Anatomical–Laboratory Correlations with Case Examples". Risk factors (predictors) for such conversion include [61] the following (see also Chap. 24): subtle motor CNS signs (gait imbalance and subtle tremor) at presentation; CASS (see section "Autonomic Function and Other Laboratory Tests") score of <7; CASS vagal subscore of <2 (i.e., mild cardiovagal impairment); severe urinary bladder dysfunction; preganglionic pattern of sweat loss (e.g., impaired thermoregulatory sweating but preserved sweating in QSART [see section "Autonomic Function and Other Laboratory Tests"]); supine norepinephrine (NE) > 100 pg/ml; and orthostatic rise of NE > 65 pg/ml (in those converting to PD/DLBD).

3. **Multiple System Atrophy (Shy–Drager Syndrome)**

Since the description of PAF by Bradbury and Eggleston in 1925 [57], many reports of PAF appeared in the literature and some of these patients had diffuse CNS manifestations [62], but these were not emphasized and some even considered these as incidental features. However, in 1960, Shy and Drager gave a lucid clinical description of two patients with detailed postmortem findings on one of them, and for the first time suggested that a primary neurodegenerative disease may be one etiological factor in the so-called idiopathic orthostatic hypotension or PAF [63]. Subsequent reports [64] not only confirmed this suggestion but also changed the name of this neurodegenerative disease of the CNS to multiple system atrophy in 1969 by Graham and Oppenheimer and later researchers grouped this disease as one of the four synucleinopathies (e.g., Parkinson's disease [PD], MSA, diffuse Lewy body disease [DLBD], and PAF) [65, 66]. For further details about MSA and PAF, the readers are referred to Chaps. 23 and 24, respectively. The median survival of MSA is 9.8 years. The best known condition with AF in which sleep and respiratory disturbances have been reported and well described includes MSA presenting initially with prominent dysautonomic features progressing relentlessly with subsequent development of somatic neurological manifestations [2, 3, 7–9, 67] (e.g., parkinsonian-cerebellar or cerebellar-parkinsonian syndrome, upper motor neuron dysfunction, in occasional patient also degeneration of anterior horn cells, and cognitive impairment in the more advanced stage [usually significant impairment 5–6 years after onset in up to 31% of cases], generally with normal sensory findings) [68]. Sleep disturbance is very common in MSA and includes insomnia with sleep fragmentation, REM behavior disorder (RBD), and sleep-related respiratory dysrhythmias. Box 12.7 lists these respiratory disturbances in MSA [69].

Box 12.7 Respiratory Disturbances in Multiple System Atrophy

- Central sleep apneas
- Obstructive apneas–hypopneas
- The above were noted in both NREM and REM sleep associated with oxygen desaturation
- Dysrhythmic breathing (irregular rate, rhythm and amplitude of respiration becoming worse in sleep)
- Cheyne–Stokes breathing
- Cheyne–Stokes variant breathing (hypopnea substituting apnea)
- Prolonged periods of central apnea in relaxed wakefulness as if the respiratory center forgot to breathe
- Periodic breathing in the erect posture accompanied by postural fall of blood pressure
- Inspiratory gasps
- Apneustic breathing
- Nocturnal stridor due to posterior cricopharyngeal muscle denervation atrophy or laryngeal dystonia (stridor is mostly inspiratory but can be expiratory depending on the site of obstruction

4. **Neurogenic Orthostatic Hypotension**

Orthostatic hypotension (OH) may result from impairment of sympathetically mediated baroreflex mechanism [60, 61, 70]. The etiology and pathogenesis are multifactorial and include central and peripheral efferent mechanisms (e.g., MSA, PAF, other central neurodegenerative synucleinopathies, brain stem and spinal cord structural lesion, peripheral autonomic neuropathies [see also Box 12.1], drug-induced and iatrogenic causes as well as some rare conditions like dopamine-beta hydroxylase [DBH] deficiency, and hyperbradykininism).

Clinical features include orthostatic intolerance (OI) symptoms that include the following: postural dizziness, faint feelings, obscuration or blurring of vision, nausea, and bloating feeling in the abdomen. These symptoms (presyncope) occur in the erect posture before syncope (transient loss of consciousness) that may happen on prolonged standing when BP falls significantly with the relief of symptoms within 1 min after resuming the recumbent position. OI symptoms may worsen in the morning (time of day), after ingestion of food (postprandial), and after exercise. The presence of OI symptoms should direct attention to a possible generalized AF and the suspicion would be strengthened by documenting OH and abnormal autonomic function tests. Moreover, the fall of BP in the erect posture is accompanied by failure of rise or inadequate rise of HR. Elderly people are highly vulnerable that may be physiological and age-related impairment of baroreflex mechanism.

5. **Postural Tachycardia Syndrome (POTS;** See Also Chap. 20)

POTS is a heterogeneous syndrome (one subgroup is labeled "idiopathic") of selective autonomic failure characterized by an increase of HR by 30 or more beats/min within 10 min of standing (or on head-up-tilt, HUT) in adults but 40 or more beats/minute in adolescents (12–19 years) or absolute HR $\geq$ 120 beats/min unaccompanied by OH (defined as sustained drop of 20/10 mm Hg or more BP within 3 min of upright posture [71–73]). Clinical manifestations include OI symptoms for $\geq$6 months (e.g., symptoms of presyncope or syncope [cerebral hypoperfusion] as described above as well as non-OI symptoms [the two most common are fatigue and sleep dysfunction [74, 75] besides others]). Standard battery of laboratory ANS function tests is generally normal. Therapy includes both nonpharamacologic (e.g., increased sodium and fluid intake, compression garments, and cognitive behavioral therapy) and pharmacologic measures (e.g., volume expanders, vasoconstrictive agents, sympatholytics, or drugs to reduce HR) [71, 72, 74, 75].

6. **Hyperbradykininism**

This is also known as Streeten syndrome who along with his collaborators first described this rare entity as a new orthostatic syndrome in 1971 [76]. This is most commonly seen in young people (20–35 years) but may also occur in children and older persons. The clinical manifestations are characterized by OI symptoms (see above) accompanied by orthostatic tachycardia and excessive fall of pulse pressure due to a fall in systolic but a rise in diastolic BP in the erect posture. The other characteristic features include flushing of the face and upper trunk (anterior chest) in the recumbent position as well as ecchymoses and purple discoloration of the legs standing for 3–4 min. Plasma bradykinin, a vasodilator, is increased above the normal limits (mean normal is <1 ng/ml in supine fasting state) due to bradykininase-I deficiency. Patients respond very well to propranolol (a beta blocker), at least temporarily. They also respond to fludrocortisone, and cyproheptadine (a serotonin antagonist) [76, 77].

7. **Dopamine-Beta-Hydroxylase Deficiency**

Dopamine-beta-hydroxylase (DBH) is an enzyme converting dopamine into noradrenaline. A few cases of DBH deficiency (some of which have been familial) causing postural hypotension and OI symptoms have been described due to sympathetic adrenergic failure [78, 79]. This is a rare entity and the key laboratory finding consists of virtual absence of plasma levels of noradrenaline and adrenaline with elevated levels of dopamine, and undetectable DBH activity. These patients respond very well to the racemic mixture of both the dextrorotatory and levorotatory forms as in dihydroxyphenylserine (DL—DOPS) as well as the levorotatory form as in L-DOPS [80].

II. **Generalized Secondary Autonomic Failure**

1. **Polyradiculoneuropathies, AF, Sleep, and Respiratory Disturbances**

Diabetic, amyloidotic and paraneoplastic polyneuropathies with AF may cause a variety of sleep and respiratory disturbances. Mondini and Guilleminault [81], and Bottoni [82] and collaborators described central and upper airway obstructive sleep apneas-hypopneas in several diabetics with autonomic neuropathies. These sleep-respiratory disturbances have been observed in over 30% of nonobese patients independent of severity of their dysautonomia in Bottini's series. The most common subtype of Guillain-Barré-Strohl (GBS) syndrome is an acute inflammatory demyelinating polyradiculoneuropathy (AIDP). Mild autonomic dysfunction (AD) is common in most cases of GBS requiring no treatment. Some patients may have more severe AD that may be correlated with severe motor disability [83, 84] (although this has been contradicted by others). AD in GBS may involve both sympathetic and parasympathetic divisions. Cardiovascular autonomic neuropathy is common and potentially a serious complication of GBS [85].

2. **Neurodegenerative Synucleinopathies (other than MSA and PAF)**

Abnormal deposition of alpha-synuclein protein in the cytoplasm of neurons or glial cells constitutes a group of neurodegenerative diseases (e.g., PD and DLBD are two such additional synucleinopathies besides MSA and PAF) that may be associated with AF and sleep dysfunction.

A. **Parkinson's Disease**

Sleep dysfunction is a major nonmotor feature present in 70–90% of cases with progressive impairment concomitant with the progression of motor disability [86]. Sleep dysfunction includes sleep onset and maintenance insomnia, sleep fragmentation, and several nocturnal motor abnormalities, such as RBD (noted in 40–50% of cases) and PLMS. In addition, RLS, sleep-onset rapid blinking, REM-onset blepharospasm and intrusion of REMs into NREM sleep have been noted [86]. Respiratory dysrhythmias (e.g., obstructive and central apneas) are thought to be more common in PD than in age-matched controls, especially those with AF [87–89]. It is notable that Parkinson himself in his original description [90] alluded to sleep and respiratory problems in his patients and mentioned the following: "...but as the malady proceeds...in this state the sleep becomes much disturbed (pp. 6–7). ...and at the last, [advanced stage] constant sleepiness...announce the wish for release (p. 9)...some fetched their breath rather hard (p. 40)". The spectrum of respiratory dysrhythmias in PD includes sleep apnea–hypopnea, Cheyne–Stokes and Cheyne–Stokes variant pattern of breathing, nocturnal hypoventilation, dysrhythmic breathing, and nocturnal stridor [86]. Laryngeal spasm or stridor sometimes may be associated with off-states or dystonic episodes. Additionally, diaphragmatic dyskinesias as well as end-of-the-dose and peak-dose Levodopa-related respiratory dysrhythmias have been observed in some PD patients. Finally, many patients complain of daytime hypersomnolence and irresistible "sleep attacks" resembling narcolepsy phenotype that may be due to a combination of intrinsic disease process and dopaminergic medication [91].

AD in PD generally develops in more advanced stage of the illness affecting multiple systems, particularly cardiovascular, gastrointestinal and genitourinary systems as well as affecting sweating, thermoregulation, and saliva production. Some patients may have OH that may in part be related to Levodopa medication. Sometimes, AD may be present earlier in the course of the illness causing considerable difficulty in differentiating PD with AF from MSA. However, relentless progression of the disease, much shorter course of the natural history of the ailment compared with that in PD and absence of a dramatic response to Levodopa, at least initially may help in separating PD with AF from MSA (see also Chaps. 23 and 24).

B. **DLBD, Autonomic Failure, and Sleep**

The core diagnostic features of DLBD as listed by McKeith et al. [92] include fluctuating cognition, recurrent visual hallucinations and parkinsonian features (e.g., cogwheel rigidity, postural instability, and akinesia or bradykinesia) combined with other features such as repeated falls, sensitivity to neuroleptics, and RBD. OH and syncope occur in up to 30% of DLBD patients. Urogenital disturbance may be cited as additional dysautonomic feature. Sleep dysfunction in DLBD includes RBD (noted in 70–80% of cases and frequently precedes the onset of the illness), sleep apnea, nocturnal visual hallucinations, insomnia, and excessive daytime sleepiness [93].

3. **Narcolepsy–Cataplexy (Narcolepsy Type 1)**

Narcolepsy is classified in the international classification of sleep disorders (ICSD-3) [93] as a prominent and a chronic debilitating neurological disorder in the category of central hypersomnolence. This is divided into two subtypes: narcolepsy 1 (with cataplexy) and narcolepsy 2 (without cataplexy). Narcolepsy type 1 is characterized by excessive daytime sleepiness with irresistible and uncontrollable "sleep attacks" under inappropriate circumstances and in inappropriate places, cataplexy (sudden loss of muscle tone triggered mostly by emotional excitement) and characterized by head nodding, dropping of things from hands, knee buckling and falling to the ground, sleep paralysis (hypnagogic or hypnopompic), visual hallucinations (vivid, often fearful dreams), and sleep maintenance difficulties with repeated awakenings. Another important manifestation is automatic behavior (e.g., repeatedly doing the same thing, missing an exit on the highway as a result of microsleep). This disorder (narcolepsy) is associated with many comorbid conditions including RBD. Narcolepsy 1 is associated with 85–90% loss of hypocretin (orexin) neurons in the perifornical and lateral hypothalamic regions. Cerebrospinal fluid (CSF) hypocretin 1 deficiency (< 110 pg/ml) is noted in over 90% of cases of narcolepsy type 1. An important laboratory test is multiple sleep latency test (MSLT) preceded by an overnight PSG. A mean sleep latency of ≤8 min accompanied by two sleep-onset REM periods (SOREMs) out of 4–5 naps obtained after 20-min of recording every 2 h (one sleep onset REM obtained in the preceding overnight PSG may substitute one of two SOREMS in the MSLT) is strongly suggestive of a diagnosis of narcolepsy in context of appropriate clinical features (ICSD-3).

Hypocretins 1 and 2 (orexins A and B) are neuropeptides responsible for regulating circadian timing and sleep–wakefulness that also have multiple other physiologic functions such as feeding, energy homeostasis, arousal, as well as controlling thermoregulation, neuroendocrine, and cardiovascular functions via changes in the ANS [94–97]. Diffuse projections of hypocretins to rostral ventrolateral medulla (RVLM) [premotor sympathetic excitatory neurons in the so-called vasomotor center], caudal ventromedial medulla (RVMM), noradrenergic neurons in the locus coeruleus (LC), nucleus ambiguus, and dorsal motor nucleus of the vagus (parasympathetic premotor neurons) as well as nucleus tractus solitarius (NTS) [an important relay station for cardiovascular, pulmonary, and gastrointestinal afferents] may be responsible for ANS control by hypocretin neurons [98]. Orexin control of thermoregulation and metabolism remains controversial. However, experimental studies in animal models of narcolepsy–cataplexy point to an involvement of the orexin system in the sleep-state stabilization and arousal as well as in control of cardiovascular (CV) and respiratory functions (CO_2-induced breathing increase in orexin gene knockout mice while causing spontaneous apneas in both REM and NREM sleep) through the influence of orexin neurons on the ANS [95–97]. Controlled clinical studies in narcolepsy–cataplexy patients may provide further insight into the role of the hypocretin neurons in the ANS control, which will be clinically relevant because of increasing endeavor in finding orexin antagonist for treatment of obesity and insomnia, and for future drug development in CV disorders and narcolepsy.

Summary of ANS Dysfunction in Narcolepsy–Cataplexy

Several autonomic abnormalities have been observed in narcolepsy–cataplexy patients, which may be summarized as follows [99–101] (see also Chap. 17):

(a) Abnormal pupillary reaction in darkness (pupillometry study).
(b) Impaired REM-related penile tumescence in men.
(c) Impaired autonomic control of the CV system: the studies for assessing effect on CV functions have been inconsistent. But, overall, various studies suggest that orexin deficiency in narcolepsy may be associated with sympathetic cardiovascular withdrawal (deficiency) and may increase CV risks in these patients. A recent survey in general population confirmed these suggestions by showing an increased prevalence of cardiometabolic diseases (e.g., hypertension, diabetes and heart disease) in narcolepsy–cataplexy patients contrasted with matched controls. In a previous study [97], an enhanced sympathetic activity (using heart rate variability [HRV] study at rest and during orthostatic stress compared with controls) was noted but found no abnormalities in CV reflex tests in the narcoleptic patients. Grimaldi et al. [101] published their observations in 2012 on the 24-h-circadian rhythms including state-dependent changes in BP and HR in narcoleptic patients (on no medications) compared to controls. The pertinent findings in a recent study by Grimaldi et al. [97] include the following: (a) nondipping of nocturnal BP, (b) higher systolic BP during REM sleep, and (c) increased sleep fragmentation and arousal index including PLMS-related arousals.

4. **Idiopathic Hypersomnia and AF**

The entity of idiopathic hypersomnia (IH), included in the ICSD-3 [93] in the central hypersomnolence category, remains controversial and is often mistaken with and difficult to differentiate from narcolepsy type 2. In the past, there was cursory mention of autonomic dysfunction in IH (e.g., OH, Raynaud's phenomenon, tension headache, and migraine) but the symptoms were thought to be nonspecific but no formal autonomic function studies were available. Sforza and colleagues [102] found a significant rise of HF power during sleep and wakefulness and concluded that in IH there is an enhancement of vagal tone during wake and sleep that may explain some of the vegetative symptoms experienced by the IH patients (see also Chap. 17). These findings are in contrast to those noted in narcoleptic patients (see above).

III. **Generalized ANS Hyperactivity**

1. **Sleep, Autonomic Hyperactivity, Cardiac Arrhythmia, and Sudden Cardiac Death**

In normal young individuals, the most frequent cardiac dysrhythmia is sinus arrhythmia, many of whom (about 30%) had sinus pauses of 1.8–2 s and in about 6% episodes of atrioventricular block were noted [103]; in addition, sinus arrest lasting up to 9 s during REM sleep without associated apnea–hypopnea or oxygen desaturation was noted in some young healthy adults. There was a case report of several episodes of atrioventricular complete heart block lasting up to 7.8 s during phasic REM sleep associated with mild sleep apnea with minimal oxygen desaturation during both NREM and REM sleep but the episodes of block persisted despite normalization of apnea–hypopnea index and oxygen saturation following upper airway pressurization [104]. There are several reports of ventricular arrhythmia during arousal from sleep [105]. Nocturnal EKG changes (T wave inversion and ST segment elevation or depression) have been reported in patients with ischemic heart disease.

Muller et al. in 1987 [106] published an important paper reporting a high incidence of sudden cardiac death among hospitalized inpatients between 7 am and 11 am similar to the high incidence of nonfatal myocardial infarction and ischemia at that time (most likely due to sympathetic hyperactivity in the morning). There are three other entities which may cause sudden unexpected cardiac death: (i) congenital long QT syndrome (CLQTS), (ii) Brugada syndrome, and (iii) sudden unexpected nocturnal death syndrome (SUNDS) in South-East Asian young individuals. Both autonomic dysfunction and genetic mutation have been suggested as possible causes [107, 108].

Samuels [109] provided evidence suggesting that a generalized "autonomic storm" (ANS dysreflexia or hyperactivity) related to life-threatening stressor may explain so-called "voodoo" death (a term originally coined by Walter B. Cannon in 1942 [110]) meaning sudden unexpected death (SUD) in adults that remains unexplained. SUD is also noted in neurological disorders, sudden infant death syndrome (SIDS), sudden death during asthmatic attacks, alcohol withdrawal, and cocaine–amphetamine-related SUD [109]. It is speculated that this may also be the explanation in some cases of sudden unexpected death in epilepsy (SUDEP). All of these conditions associated with SUD may be linked by stress and catecholamine surge.

2. **Baroreflex Failure**

Baroreflex failure, an important but an uncommon condition manifesting autonomic dysfunction, may result from injury to the carotid and aortic baroreceptors or their afferents in the sinus nerve of Hering (a branch of glossopharyngeal nerve) and the aortic nerve of Ludwig and Cyon (a branch of vagus nerve) as well as the central medullary relay station in the nucleus tractus solitarius (NTS) [111]. The causes for this injury may consist of neck surgery including carotid surgery, carotid dissection and tumors, radiation to the neck, brain stem stroke or trauma, and syringobulbia. The clinical manifestations often resemble pheochromocytoma (which needs to be excluded by appropriate tests) and consist of hypertensive crises (fluctuating hypertension, tachycardia, profuse sweating, palpitation and headache resembling autonomic hyperreflexia, and marked elevation of plasma norepinephrine levels during hypertensive crises, less commonly presenting with OH, orthostatic tachycardia, severe bradycardia, and syncope) [111, 112]. Clonidine (a central alpha-2 agonist blocking RVLM sympathoexcitatory neurons) is the treatment of choice.

3. **Neuroblastoma**

Neuroblastoma is an example of secondary autonomic hyperactivity. This tumor, most frequently found within or adjacent to the sympathetic ganglia and adrenal tissue [113], causes catecholaminergic hyperactivity (e.g., hypertension, tachycardia, and hyperhidrosis) associated with excessive synthesis of norepinephrine and dopamine [113]. An unusual feature is an acute cerebellar encephalopathy, which is most likely a paraneoplastic expression. Clinical manifestations include truncal and limb ataxias as well as opsoclonus–myoclonus syndrome (rapid, ataxic, and chaotic conjugate eye movements accompanied by diffuse myoclonus). The onset is commonly before the age of 3 years. Most often the tumor is highly anaplastic and aggressive. Prognosis depends on the age of onset as survival varies inversely with age.

4. **Diencephalic Autonomic Seizure (DAS)**

This is an example of paroxysmal autonomic hyperactivity, first described by Penfield in 1929 [114]. The lesion is thought to be in the hypothalamus or related to lesions causing pressure on this structure. Clinical manifestations include paroxysmal episodes (occurring several times a day and each time lasting 30–60 s) of bifrontal headache, hypertension, restlessness, flushing, lacrimation, salivation, excessive sweating, tachycardia, pupillary dilation or constriction, periodic hypothermia, and periodic breathing of Cheyne–Stokes type. The episodes are often preceded by stereotypic symptoms of olfactory hallucination characterized by strange smell and abdominal sensation with nausea and retention of awareness but associated with increased surge of plasma catecholamines (about double the basal value) during these episodes with subsequent falls to normal levels after the spells are over [115]. EEG in most reports showed no epileptiform discharges. DAS should be differentiated from paroxysmal autonomic dysfunction, sometimes noted in epilepsy, especially temporal lobe epilepsy (TLE) as a result of excessive sympathetic discharge. Electroencephalogram (EEG) in TLE is generally positive showing epileptiform spikes or sharp waves in the temporal region. Some cases of SUDEP may be related to this autonomic hyperactivity.

5. **Fatal Familial Insomnia (FFI)** (See Chap. 18)

IV. **Localized ANS Dysfunction**

1. **Holmes–Adie Syndrome**

The other name is Adie's pupil or "Tonic pupil" with light-near dissociation [9, 116]. In 80% of cases, patients present with unilateral dilated pupil (larger than the unaffected eye). It is more commonly present in women than in men. The characteristic finding is impaired light reflex and slow but exaggerated response to convergence, and the pupil in the affected eye becomes smaller than that in the unaffected eye; then it dilates slowly. Another characteristic finding in most cases (90%) is absent (or markedly attenuated) muscle stretch reflexes [117], the cause of which remains disputed (one plausible suggestion is degeneration of spinal dorsal root ganglia). The site of lesion for the tonic dilated pupil is thought to be located in the postganglionic parasympathetic fibers in the ciliary ganglion; the cause is most likely degeneration of the fibers as was also documented by denervation supersensitivity (exaggerated response with marked constriction of the affected pupil to instillation of 2.5% mecholyl or dilute solution of pilocarpine [1%] which has no appreciable effect in normal pupils). There have been occasional reports of associated OH or impaired sweating response casting doubt on the concept of localized ANS dysfunction.

2. **Argyll Robertson Pupil** [9, 118, 119]

Both the pupils (in bilateral cases) are irregular, small with absent light reflexes but preserved convergence reaction (accommodation). The site of lesion is thought to be in the dorsal midbrain region interrupting the light reflex pathway. This was originally described in Tabes Dorsalis but Argyll Robertson-like pupil may be seen in diabetes mellitus.

3. **Ross Syndrome**

This is another rare entity with localized ANS dysfunction of unknown cause and a variant of Holmes–Adie syndrome. In addition to tonic pupil and areflexia, there is progressive segmental hypohydrosis [120].

4. **Harlequin Syndrome**

A rare condition with localized ANS dysfunction of the pre- and postganglionic cervical sympathetic fibers with normal ocular sympathetic innervation manifested by the loss of thermoregulatory sweating on one side of the face [121].

5. **Horner Syndrome**

The triad of Horner syndrome consists of miosis, mild ptosis, and ipsilateral (if unilateral) facial anhidrosis or hypohydrosis as a result of pre- or postganglionic cervical sympathetic dysfunction [9, 118]. Pharmacologic study with local instillation of eye drops shows evidence of sympathetic denervation supersensitivity in case of postganglionic dysfunction [9, 119].

6. **Unilateral Gustatory Sweating (Auriculotemporal Syndrome of Frey)**

Abnormal unilateral gustatory facial sweating during eating may occur most commonly after lesions including surgery of the parotid gland as a result of damage and subsequent regeneration of the parasympathetic fibers innervating salivary glands that are then misdirected to the postganglionic cervical sympathetic sudomotor pathways [2, 3, 5, 9]. The name auriculotemporal syndrome is derived from the fact that there is affection of the cervical sympathetic sudomotor fibers distributed along the auriculotemporal branch of the trigeminal nerve. This has also been described in diabetes mellitus and after upper thoracic sympathectomy [2, 3, 5, 9].

7. **Crocodile Tears (Bogorad Syndrome)**

Most commonly this has been described after a lower motor neuron facial nerve palsy (e.g., Bell's palsy) as a result of regenerating parasympathetic fibers (destined originally for submandibular glands) aberrantly coursing along the parasympathetic fibers to the lacrimal glands [2, 3, 9, 122]. Whenever there is salivation (e.g., eating or even thinking of food), there is tearing of the eye on the affected side. In most of the cases, it is not sufficiently distressing requiring treatment.

8. **Hirschsprung's Disease**

This is a congenital developmental condition, also known as *megacolon,* presenting in children and adolescents with the complaint of severe constipation since birth [10].The symptom results from obstruction of distal bowel showing radiographically as a spastic segment of the distal bowel with proximal dilation: the condition is due to congenital absence of intestinal ganglion cells (aganglionic segment) in the myenteric (Auerbach) and submucosal (Meissner) plexus due to arrest of embryonic development. Anorectal manometry reveals absence of internal anal sphincter relaxation. Resection biopsy has shown characteristic histopathological findings.

9. **Achalasia**

This is a rare disorder of the esophagus [2, 3, 10] due to incomplete relaxation of the lower esophageal sphincter (also known as cardiospasm) due to postganglionic denervation of the smooth muscles in the lower esophageal sphincter (degeneration of the myenteric [Auerbach] plexus of the enteric nervous system [ENS] division of the ANS). The cause is mostly undetermined (may be an autoimmune disease) but sometimes it is due to Chagas disease caused by *Trypanosoma cruzi,* mostly noted in Central and South America. Clinical manifestations of this GI dysautonomic disease include dysphagia, regurgitation, chest pain, aspiration pneumonia, and weight loss.

10. **Gastroparesis**

This is another manifestation of autonomic neuropathy due to dysfunction of the ENS division of the ANS [10]. A common cause is uncontrollable diabetes mellitus. Clinical features include epigastric discomfort, nausea, abdominal bloating, vomiting (may be projectile), weight loss, and anorexia. The condition may be a localized AD but often is part of a generalized autonomic failure. The gold standard test for gastroparesis is radiolabeled scintigraphy to quantify the emptying of a physiologic meal and evaluate stomach's motor function (gastric atonia) [123].

Fits and Faints, Including Syncope and Other Mimics of Autonomic Dysfunction

Orthostatic hypotension and syncope are two cardinal manifestations of autonomic dysfunction. This section briefly addresses syncope and various other conditions that may mimic and be mistaken for conditions causing AD. Box 12.8 lists these conditions (mimics), and Box 12.9 includes different types of syncope. All these entities must be kept in mind when approaching a patient with symptoms suggestive of dysautonomia [15, 124, 125].

Syncope, the most frequent cause of transient loss of consciousness (TLOC) as a result of transient cerebral hypoperfusion, may result from diverse lesions [15, 124, 125] (see Box 12.9). The list in Box 12.8 includes "common faint" (reflex syncope or vasodepressor syncope), cardiac arrhythmia and structural lesions ("cardiac syncope"), autonomic failure (specifically, OH [see section "Brief Description of Some Important and Unusual Dysautonomic Entities"]), epileptic seizure and nonepileptic or psychogenic seizure (NES), pseudo-syncope (PS), "drop attack" (e.g., frequently due to vertebrobasilar insufficiency or transient ischemic attacks [TIA], and other mimics (e.g., narcoleptic "sleep attacks", cataplectic episodes and posttraumatic concussion). All these should be differentiated from syncope and orthostatic intolerance (OI) symptoms associated with OH, particularly when a patient with OH has anoxic seizure. Reflex syncope could be vasovagal syncope including cough, swallow, and micturition syncope as well as carotid sinus hypersensitivity [15, 124, 125]. History will provide clues most of the time based on the presenting complaints and direct attention to a particular condition and etiology.

One must remember that consciousness has two components: *Awareness* (e.g., aware of the surrounding environment) and *arousal* (e.g., an ability to respond to a stimulus). In epileptic seizures, TIAs and TLOC associated with syncope (except "focal aware seizures") there is no awareness whereas in cataplexy, NES or PS there should be awareness but these subjects may not be arousable unless vigorous stimuli are applied.

In true epileptic seizures (generalized and focal impaired awareness seizure ["partial complex seizure" of old termi-

Box 12.8 Fits, faints, and mimics mistaken for autonomic dysfunction (differential diagnosis)

- Syncope
  - Reflex (as listed in Box 12.9)
  - Cardiac
  - Autonomic Failure with orthostatic hypotension related syncope
  - Pseudosyncope
- Seizure
  - Generalized (especially atonic and akinetic seizures)
  - Focal impaired awareness seizure (formerly partial complex seizure)
- Psychogenic or nonepileptic seizure (NES)
- Postural tachycardia syndrome
- "Drop attacks"
- Vertebrobasilar ischemia (transient ischemic-attack [TIA])
- Narcoleptic sleep attacks
- Cataplexy (as in narcolepsy type 1)
- Psychiatric disorders (e.g., generalized anxiety disorder [GAD], major depression)
- Hypovolemia (e.g., related to internal bleeding, dehydration and ingestion of diuretics)
- Deconditioning
  - Prolonged immobilization
  - Space flight
- Posttraumatic concussion

Box 12.9 Types of Syncope [124, 127]

1. Cardiac syncope.
2. Reflex syncope
   - (i) Vasovagal or vasodepressor syncope (neurally mediated or neurocardiogenic syncope)
   - (ii) Situational syncope
     - (a) Cough syncope (pulmonary syncope)
     - (b) Swallow syncope (esophageal syncope)
     - (c) Micturition and defecation syncope (pelvic syncope)
     - (d) Exercise-induced syncope
     - (e) Valsalva-like maneuver syncope
     - (f) Trumpet player's syncope
     - (g) Postprandial syncope
   - (iii) Carotid sinus supersensitive syncope
3. Convulsive syncope
4. Autonomic failure (primary or secondary): syncope associated with orthostatic hypotension
5. "Drop attacks" (cerebral syncope)
6. Hyperventilation syncope
7. Drug-induced syncope
8. Postural tachycardia syndrome (POTS) associated with orthostatic intolerance symptoms (presyncope-posture-related)
9. Breath-holding syncope
10. Overdrive pacemaker related syncope
11. Syncope with deafness and sudden death (Romano–Ward syndrome)

nology]), there is evidence of postictal confusion but not in other conditions listed above [124–126].

Tongue biting (particularly lateral side of the tongue) is commonly seen in generalized (primary or secondary generalization) and focal impaired awareness seizures; however, some patients with syncope rarely may have tongue biting (usually seen in the tip of the tongue).

In "drop attacks" due to vertebrobasilar TIAs besides TLOC, there may be other neighboring signs of brain stem dysfunction.

In generalized true seizure, any motor phenomena are usually synchronous (in phase) and symmetrical whereas in NES any movements (e.g., clonic versus myoclonic) are in general asynchronous or out of phase.

Vasovagal syncope (VVS) often occurs under circumstances of prolonged standing or straining in an overcrowded stuffy environment [15, 124, 125, 127]. OH is often associated with OI symptoms including presyncope or prodromal features (e.g., faint feeling, lightheadedness, dizziness, blurry vision, nausea, abdominal bloating feelings). Figure 12.1 schematically outlines suggested mechanism for VVS [127]. History should include the events in the preictal, ictal, postictal, and interictal periods for differentiating various conditions causing TLOC including syncope and seizures. Recording of BP and HR in supine and standing positions is important for diagnosis of OH and others causing syncope.

Most important items for diagnosis consist of the following: (i) history including that from the witness and family members; (ii) physical examination, particularly of the heart and nervous system; (iii) electrocardiography (ECG), and (iv) electroencephalography (EEG).

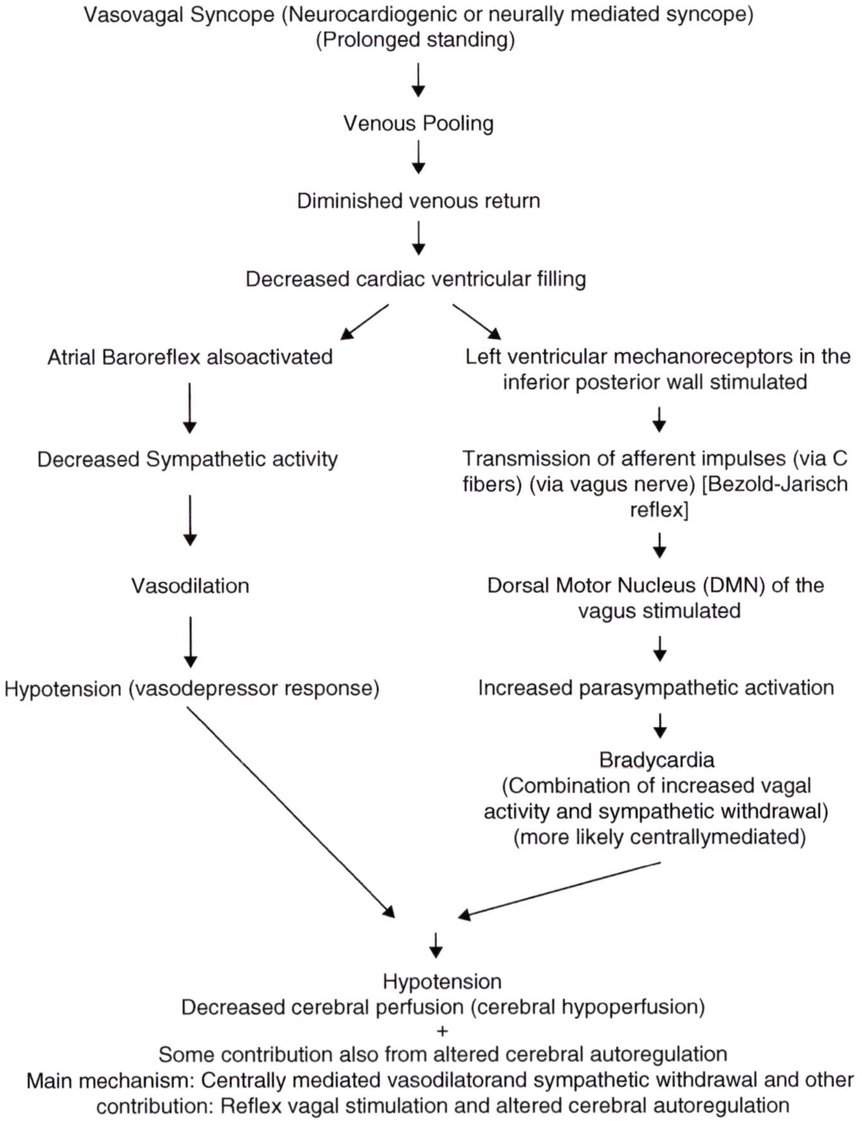

Fig. 12.1 Schematically shown the mechanism of vasovagal syncope [127]

Types of Syncope (see Box 12.9) [15, 124, 125, 127]

A. Cardiac syncope (see further on and Box 12.10)
B. Reflex syncope
   (i) Vasovagal (common faint): Neurally mediated or neurocardiogenic syncope in the elderly (vasodepressor syncope)
   (ii) Situational syncope
   (iii) Carotid sinus hypersensitivity syndrome with syncope
C. Others (see Box 12.9) [124]
D. Cardiac syncope (Box 12.10) [127]

Box 12.10 Points in favor of a diagnosis of cardiac syncope [127]

- Age of onset of syncope: 35 years or more
- Gender: Male
- A previous history of atrial fibrillation/flutter or other cardiac arrhythmias (e.g., sinus arrest, sinoatrial block, atrioventricular heart block, paroxysmal supraventricular arrhythmia or brady–tachy arrhythmia syndrome [sick sinus syndrome], pacemaker malfunction, and congenital deficit in cardiac conduction including congenital prolonged Q-T syndrome)
- Known history of hypertension and structural heart disease including cardiomyopathy, congestive heart failure, ischemic and congenital heart disease, and cardiac valvular disease
- Cyanosis witnessed during the episode of syncope
- Chest discomfort or dyspnea before transient loss of consciousness (TLOC)
- Abnormal cardiac examination
- Palpitation before TLOC
- Abnormal EKG
- Evaluation of Guidelines in Syncope Study (EGSYS) score of 3 points or more; (palpitation [4 points]; abnormal ECG/heart disease [3 points]; effort syncope [3 points]; syncope in supine position [2 points]; neurovegetative prodromes [−1 point]; predisposing and precipitory factors [−1 point])
- Vasovagal score (VVS): Less than −2
- Family history of sudden cardiac death, syncope or drowning
- History of two or fewer syncope episodes

A small percentage of patients presenting with syncope result from structural lesions of the heart or cardiac arrhythmias that should be differentiated form the common faint (vasovagal syncope) and other conditions listed in Box 12.9 as cardiac syncope carries high morbidity and mortality [127]. A careful clinical history and physical examination can identify patients with cardiac syncope most of the time but may require ECG, Holter monitoring, and other laboratory tests for confirmation in challenging situation [127]. Box 12.10 lists the pertinent features favoring a diagnosis of cardiac syncope [127].

Drop Attacks

The term was introduced by Kremer in 1958 [128, 129]. The condition is common in women and in up to 65% of cases no cause is found. Most likely cause (if found) is cardiovascular (evidence of heart disease; needs EKG and Holter monitoring) or cerebrovascular disease (history and neurological examination to detect other signs of brainstem ischemia; may require magnetic resonance imaging of the brain and magnetic resonance angiography (MRI-MRA) for investigation). Other causes may include narcoleptic "drop attack" (related to emotionally triggered cataplectic episodes or irresistible narcoleptic "sleep attacks" [93] and rarely "drop attacks" may be caused by psychogenic or true seizure (e.g., atonic or akinetic seizure). Most of the neurologists consider brain stem ischemia due to vertebrobasilar insufficiency (transient ischemic attacks-TIA) as a frequent cause of so-called "drop attacks."

Carotid Sinus Supersensivity Syncope

This is a type of reflex syncope similar to VVS but is due to hypersensitivity of carotid sinus in certain individuals as manifested by syncope triggered by carotid sinus massage (extreme caution is needed as this may trigger cardiac asystole) [15, 124, 127].

Miscellaneous: Four entities (e.g., glossopharyngeal neuralgia, postprandial syncope and hypotension, esophageal or swallow syncope, and pelvic syncope [see Box 12.9]) may all be due to similar reflex mechanism as in VVS and carotid sinus supersensitivity syndrome causing syncope.

Mastocytosis-Related Syncope

This is a rare condition [124]. There is overproduction of mast cells (normally found in connective tissue) in multiple organs releasing histamine as well as an overproduction of prostaglandin D2 (PGD2) causing diffuse allergic reactions. Women outnumber men (4:1) and the onset is most commonly around 45 years. Clinical features include flushing, palpitation, syncope, fatigue, and shortness of breath without any wheeze. A prominent cutaneous finding is urticaria pigmentosa, present in 99% of cases and is a useful diagnostic sign of mastocytosis. Narcotic analgesics, nonsteroidal anti-inflammatory agents as well as beta-receptor antagonists, alpha receptor and cholinergic agonists, and aspirin should be avoided as these may activate mast cells. The most effective medications are epinephrine, chlorpheniramine, and cimetidine.

Breath-holding Spells

In the very young (infants and children), special types of syncopal episodes have been described [124]. Breath-holding spells (two forms: cyanotic type [the most common type] related to a combination of apneic hypoxemia and forceful Valsalva-like maneuver and pallid type like a vasovagal spell related to sudden unexpected pain).

Other rare types in infants and children

Other rare types in infants and young children include syncope associated with prolonged Q-T interval, familial deafness, and sudden death (Jervell–Lange–Nielsen syndrome), Romano–Ward syndrome (a similar syndrome as above but without deafness and associated with syncope and sudden death in an infant), overdrive pacing causing syncope and faster HR with prolonged Q-T interval as well as syncope in children with multiple extrasystoles, and ventricular fibrillation.

Clinical–Anatomical–Laboratory Correlations with Case Examples

From an account of the functional neuroanatomy of the ANS as described in Chap. 3 as well as AFTs (section "Autonomic Function and Other Laboratory Tests") and brief clinical entities (section "Brief Description of Some Important and Unusual Dysautonomic Entities") described above, it will now be easy to understand the various clinical manifestations resulting from autonomic deficits.

The following three cases serve to illustrate clinical–anatomical correlations in three different types of autonomic disorders [52].

Case 1 A 57-year-old patient was admitted with a history of urinary frequency and incontinence, and impotence for 5 years. He also had been having syncopal episodes in assuming the upright posture. These fainting spells in the upright posture became very disabling. Neurological examination revealed that syncopal attacks were associated with severe postural hypotension. There was no evidence of somatic neurologic dysfunction. The patient denied any history of diabetes mellitus.

His BP in the supine position was 120/70 and the pulse rate was 80 per minute. Tilt-table examination showed that on tilting the table to 60° the BP fell rapidly to 40/0 but the pulse rate remained fixed at 80 per minute. The patient felt faint. Simultaneous EEG recording during the tilt-table test showed diffuse slowing of the background rhythm. Valsalva test showed reduced Valsalva ratio. Cystometrogram revealed an atonic urinary bladder. Intravenous norepinephrine infusion test revealed a supersensitive BP response but no reflex bradycardia. Intramuscular atropine did not produce any change in the pulse rate or the BP. Supine fasting plasma norepinephrine level was reduced and showed no further rise in the upright position. Plasma renin activity did not change significantly from the supine to the erect position. Cold pressor and mental arithmetic tests did not raise the BP or the HR. Thermal sweating was impaired over the abdomen and the legs. Conjunctival instillation of dilute (0.062%) pilocarpine solution produced pupillary constriction and 1:1000 adrenaline produced pupillary dilatation.

Comments This patient's symptoms of fainting spells accompanied by orthostatic hypotension, urinary incontinence, and impotence suggest autonomic deficits that are not associated with any somatic neurological dysfunction. The postural hypotension was confirmed by tilt-table test accompanied by slowing of the EEG background suggesting critical cerebral hypoperfusion. These findings in association with a fixed HR suggest an impairment of the ANS function affecting the heart as well as the resistance and the capacitance vessels. A supersensitive BP response after norepinephrine infusion and a supersensitive pupillary response to dilute (1:1000) adrenaline suggest peripheral sympathetic fiber denervation. Impairment of thermal sweating, abnormal cold pressor, and mental arithmetic tests in conjunction with other findings suggest widespread impairment of sympathetic efferent fibers. Absence of bradycardia despite supersensitive BP response to norepinephrine infusion, impotence, atonic urinary bladder and failure of pulse rate, and BP change after atropine injection as well as pupillary constriction after dilute pilocarpine solution (denervation super sensitivity) indicate that the parasympathetic system is also involved. Reduced fasting plasma norepinephrine and its failure to rise in the erect posture suggest postganglionic sympathetic dysfunction. Failure of plasma renin to rise in the upright position also suggests depletion of the sympathetic neurotransmitter at the renal sympathetic nerve endings. In summary, the clinical features and the AFTs suggest that this patient has been suffering from pure AF and fulfill the criteria of Bradbury–Eggleston syndrome [57].

Approximately 3 years after initial presentation neurological examination showed that he was developing parkinsonian-cerebellar syndrome consistent with conversion to MSA phenotype [14].

Case 2 A 52-year-old man was admitted for investigation of episodes of syncope in the upright position, urinary incontinence and frequency of 5 years duration, and impotence for 8 years. Recently, he noticed progressive difficulty in walking due to incoordination. His BP in the supine position was 140/90 mm Hg and the HR was 80 per minute. In the upright position, the BP fell rapidly to unrecordable level accompanied by faint feelings but the pulse rate remained fixed. Neurological examination showed evidence of cerebellar dysfunction in the upper and lower extremities including ataxia of gait. These findings continued to progress and later he developed mild cogwheel rigidity in both hands, stooped posture, and bradykinesia. The plantar responses were bilaterally extensor. Sensory examination and mental functions (no formal testing was performed) were normal. In the terminal stage, he developed dysrhythmic breathing and sleep apnea on PSG recording.

Cystometrogram showed an atonic bladder. A barium swallow and cineradiography of the esophagus showed evidence of mild impairment of the peristaltic waves. Thermal sweating was severely impaired over the trunk and the lower extremities. Valsalva test showed no "overshoot" of the BP. Cold pressor and mental arithmetic tests did not show any changes in the BP or the HR. Plasma renin activity remained unchanged in the erect position. Norepinephrine infusion test revealed small rise of BP and HR. Conjunctival instillation of dilute pilocarpine solution (0.062%) and 1:1000 adrenaline solution did not produce any alterations in pupillary size.

Three years after onset of the somatic neurological dysfunction, the patient died of pneumonia and respiratory failure. Postmortem examination disclosed significant structural alterations in the brain stem, cerebellum, basal ganglia, and spinal cord.

Comments The clinical manifestations of fainting spells in the upright position accompanied by orthostatic fall of BP and fixed HR, urinary incontinence and impotence suggest autonomic deficits. The initial presentation of these autonomic manifestations followed later by cerebellar-parkinsonian syndrome fulfills the criteria for the diagnosis of MSA with progressive AF (the Shy–Drager syndrome). The AFTs showing marked reduction of BP in the erect posture, relatively fixed HR in all body positions, absence of "overshoot" after Valsalva maneuver, no rise of BP and HR after cold pressor and mental arithmetic tests, failure of rise of plasma renin and norepinephrine in the erect posture all suggest evidence of sympathetic denervation. Absence of a supersensitive BP response after intravenous norepinephrine infusion and a lack of supersensitivity of the pupillary response to intraocular dilute adrenaline solutions suggest a central lesion and not a lesion of the postganglionic sympathetic fibers.

Absence of a rise of HR after atropine injection, absence of bradycardia after Valsalva maneuver, reduced Valsalva ratio, cystometric finding of an atonic bladder, impairment of respiratory beat-to-beat variation of HR, impairment of the peristaltic waves on cineradiography, and barium swallow examination of the esophagus as well as a lack of super sensitivity of the pupillary response to intraocular dilute pilocarpine solution all suggest evidence of parasympathetic denervation in this patient. Therefore, the clinical and AFTs provide evidence of central autonomic deficits accompanied by somatic neurological dysfunction, particularly involving extrapyramidal and cerebellar pathways. These findings are characteristic of those noted in the Shy–Drager syndrome (MSA).

The pathological findings [2, 3, 8, 14, 63, 67, 130] of olivopontocerebellar atrophy as well as degeneration and gliosis in the corpus striatum, substantia nigra, and locus ceruleus correlate anatomically with the cerebellar-parkinsonian syndrome in this patient. Intermediolateral neuronal cell loss in the spinal cord (also noted in every case of the Shy–Drager syndrome) and lesions around the NTS and ventral medulla explain severe sympathetic denervation including profound OH in this patient. Lesions of the nucleus tractus solitarius and nucleus ambiguus likely are responsible for respiratory dysrhythmia while involvement of the dorsal motor nucleus of the vagus and nucleus ambiguus explain GI motility disturbances and cardiac parasympathetic denervation. Lesions of the sacral spinal cord including Onuf's nuclei are responsible for the urinary and sexual dysfunction. Pyramidal tract degeneration correlates with extensor plantar responses. Loss of neurons in the sympathetic ganglia, anterior horn cells of the spinal cord, and the oculomotor nucleus are consistent with those noted in MSA.

Case 3 A 45-year-old patient has suffered from insulin-dependent diabetes mellitus for 15 years. He now complains of tingling and numbness in both feet and the hands, and mild weakness of the legs for the last 1 year. Recently, he has been having episodes of fainting spells in the upright position, urinary incontinence, and impotence. He has also noted lack of sweating in his feet. In addition, he has intermittent diarrhea, particularly nocturnal diarrhea. Occasionally, he has some difficulty in swallowing both solids and liquids.

On neurological examination, he has evidence of mild sensory-motor polyneuropathy in the legs. The feet and legs are dry and are relatively hairless. Supine BP is 150/95 and the pulse rate is 78 per minute. On standing for a minute the BP fell to 50/0 and the pulse rate increased to 80 per minute. Cold pressor and mental arithmetic tests show no change in BP or the HR. Valsalva test shows reduced VR and absence of "overshoot" of BP and a lack of reflex bradycardia. There is impairment of respiratory HR variation. Nerve conduction study shows evidence of sensory-motor axonal polyneuropathy. Sympathetic skin responses are absent in the palms and soles. Barium swallow with cineradiography shows impairment of the peristaltic waves. Thermal sweating is severely impaired in the trunk and legs. Supine fasting plasma norepinephrine level is markedly reduced and there is no rise on standing up. Intramuscular injection of atropine does not change the HR or the BP. Intravenous norepinephrine infusion test shows supersensitive BP response. Pupillary constriction after pilocarpine (0.062%) and pupillary dilation after 1:1000 adrenaline eye drops suggest postganglionic autonomic denervation.

Comments This patient with longstanding insulin dependent diabetes mellitus developed an axonal type of somatic polyneuropathy, which later was accompanied by evidence of autonomic neuropathy as is obvious from the clinical, nerve conduction, and the autonomic function tests. The abnormalities in the AFTs suggest evidence of affection of both sympathetic and parasympathetic fibers in the postganglionic regions.

The characteristic pathological changes (not obtained from this patient) as reported in the literature in diabetic autonomic neuropathy [131, 132] consist of involvement of the sympathetic and parasympathetic postganglionic neurons associated with lymphocytic infiltration, vacuolation, and poor Nissl staining. Additional findings include depletion of myelinated fibers in the vagus and greater splanchnic nerves, and the white rami communicantes [124, 125]. Thus, there is good clinical–physiological–anatomical correlation in diabetic autonomic neuropathy.

Principles of Therapy

In this last section, I shall briefly allude to principles of therapy in autonomic dysfunction but the details are beyond the scope of this chapter and are addressed in various chapters throughout this book.

Treatment should ideally include nonpharmacologic and drug treatment [2, 3, 5, 9]. Those with mild or minimal AD who are asymptomatic require no treatment. Those with mild AD and are symptomatic should benefit from nonpharmacologic therapy that includes avoidance of triggering factors and adherence to nonpharmacologic measures that may consist of use of compression stockings and other physical countermeasures for OH as well as drinking of plenty of fluids, especially in the morning and adequate intake of sodium chloride (salt) for POTS. Other nondrug therapy includes exercise, specifically designed for a particular type of AD. For specific sleep dysfunction appropriate measures include common sense sleep hygiene practice for all, cognitive behavioral therapy for chronic insomnia (CBT-I), as well as upper airway pressurization for OSA and other ventilatory measures for sleep-hypoventilation or central sleep apnea.

Secondary AD requires treatment of primary disorder supplemented by drug to control dysautonomic symptom for debilitating and symptomatic patients along with appropriate measures for sleep disorders. The pharmacologic treatment for OH (which is a cardinal and severely debilitating feature in many patients with dysautonomia) and orthostatic intolerance symptoms may include the following in a particular patient (treatment needs to be individualized): (i) volume expanders, (ii) medications to reduce heart rate (particularly in POTS), (iii) vasoconstrictive agents, and (iv) sympatholytics, especially in POTS.

Non-orthostatic and other systemic symptoms may benefit from melatonin (especially, circadian rhythm disorder), wake-promoting agents for fatigue, immunosuppressants for autoimmune AD, SSRIs for comorbid anxiety and depression, appropriate measures for GI motility and genitourinary disorders, and analgesics for comorbid painful conditions and headache.

In conclusion, an approach whether at the bedside or in the clinics should consist of pursuing the diagnostic steps in a logical and systematic manner as outlined above (see also Box 12.6) for optimal care of patients. Most important first step is clinical history and physical examination including specific autonomic examination before ordering laboratory tests in a haphazard manner otherwise the physician may run into a state of confusion in terms of correct diagnosis and appropriate treatment.

References

1. Goldstein DS, Holmes C, Cannon RO 3rd, Eisenhofer G, Kopin IJ. Sympathetic cardioneuropathy in dysautonomias. N Engl J Med. 1997;336(10):696–702.
2. Low PA, editor. Clinical autonomic disorders. 2nd ed. Philadelphia: Lippincott-Raven; 1997.
3. Mathias CJ, Bannister R, editors. Autonomic failure: a textbook of clinical disorders of the autonomic nervous system. 5th ed. Oxford: Oxford University Press; 2013.
4. Benarroch EE. Central autonomic network: functional organization and clinical correlations. Armonk: Futura Publishing; 1997.
5. Appenzeller O. The autonomic nervous system. Part I. Normal functions. Part II. Dysfunctions. In: Vinken PJ, Bruyn GW, editors. Handbook of clinical neurology, Vols. 74 and 75. Amsterdam: Elsevier; 1999 and 2000.
6. Robertson D, editor. Primer on the autonomic nervous system. 3rd ed. Amsterdam: Elsevier; 2012.
7. Montagna P, Chokroverty S, editors. Sleep disorders. Parts I and II. In: Aminoff MJ, Boller F, Swaab DF, series editors. Handbook of clinical neurology, Vols. 98 and 99. Amsterdam: Elsevier; 2010.
8. Chokroverty S. Autonomic dysfunction in olivopontocerebellar atrophy. In: Duvoisin RC, Plaitakis A, editors. The olivopontocerebellar atrophies. Advances in neurology, vol. 41. New York: Raven Press; 1984. p. 105–41.
9. Johnson RA, Lambie DG, Spalding JMK. The autonomic nervous system. In: Baker AB, Joynt NT, editors. Clinical neurology. Philadelphia: Harper and Row; 1986. p. 1–94.
10. Quigley EMM, Pfeiffer RF, editors. Neurogastroenterology. Philadelphia: Elsevier/ Butterworth-Heinemann; 2004.
11. Struhal W, Lahrmann H, Faneiulli A, Wenning GK, editors. Bedside approach to autonomic disorders: A clinical tutor. Cham: Springer International; 2017.
12. Best CH, Taylor NB. Physiological basis of medical practice. Baltimore: Williams & Wilkins; 1966.
13. Burton AC. Physiology and biophysics of the circulation. Chicago: Yearbook Medical; 1965.
14. Chokroverty S, Barron KD, Katz FH, Del Greco F, Sharp JT. The syndrome of primary orthostatic hypotension. Brain. 1969;92(4):743–68.
15. Grubb BP, Olshansky B, editors. Syncope: mechanisms and management. 2nd ed. Malden: Blackwell Publishing; 2005.
16. Jones JA. Effect of posture work on health of children. Am J Dis Child. 1933;46(1):148–54.
17. Mathias CJ. Autonomic disorders and their recognition: an editorial. N Engl J Med. 1997;336(10):721–4.
18. Parmeggiani PL. The autonomic nervous system in sleep. In: Kryger MH, Roth T, Dement WC, editors. Principles and practice of sleep medicine. Philadelphia: Saunders; 1994. p. 194–203.
19. Parmeggiani PL. Systemic homeostasis and poikilostasis in sleep. London: Imperial College Press; 2011.
20. Loewy AD, Spyer KM, editors. Central regulation of autonomic functions. New York: Oxford University Press; 1990.
21. Low PA. Clinical autonomic disorders: classification and clinical education. In: Low PA, editor. Clinical autonomic disorders. 2nd ed. Philadelphia: Lippincott/Raven; 1997. p. 3–13.
22. Tsementzis SA, Hitchcock ER. The spoon test: a simple bedside test for assessing sudomotor autonomic failure. J Neurol Neurosurg Psychiatry. 1985;48(4):378–80.
23. Suarez GA, Opfer-Gehrking TL, Offord KP, Atkinson EJ, O'Brien PC, Low PA. The autonomic symptom profile: a new instrument to assess autonomic symptoms. Neurology. 1999;52(3):523–8.
24. Sletten DM, Suarez GA, Low PA, Mandrekar J, Singer W. COMPASS 31: a refined and abbreviated composite autonomic symptom score. Mayo Clin Proc. 2012;87(12):1196–201.
25. Low PA, Benrud-Larson LM, Sletten DM, Opfer-Gehrking TL, Weigand SD, O'Brien PC, et al. Autonomic symptoms and diabetic neuropathy: a population-based study. Diabetes Care. 2004;27(12):2942–7.
26. Zilliox L, Peltier AC, Wren PA, Anderson A, Smith AG, Singleton JR, et al. Assessing autonomic dysfunction in early diabetic neuropathy: the survey of autonomic symptoms. Neurology. 2011;76(12):1099–105.
27. Visser M, Marinus J, Stiggelbout AM, Van Hilten JJ. Assessment of autonomic dysfunction in Parkinson's disease: the SCOPA-AUT. Mov Disord. 2004;19(11):1306–12.
28. Wenning GK, Tison F, Seppi K, Sampaio C, Diem A, Yekhlef F, et al. Multiple System Atrophy Study Group. Development and validation of the Unified Multiple System Atrophy Rating Scale (UMSARS). Mov Disord. 2004;19(12):1391–402.
29. Kaufmann H, Malamut R, Norcliffe-Kaufmann L, Rosa K, Freeman R. The Orthostatic Hypotension Questionnaire (OHQ): validation of a novel symptom assessment scale. Clin Auton Res. 2012;22(2):79–90.
30. Low PA. Laboratory evaluation of autonomic function. In: Low PA, editor. Clinical autonomic failure. 2nd ed. Philadelphia: Lippincott/Raven; 1997. p. 179–208.
31. Mathias CJ, Low DA, Iodice V, Bannister B. Investigation of autonomic disorders. In: Mathias CJ, Bannister R, editors. Autonomic failure. Oxford: Oxford University Press; 2013. p. 259–89.
32. England JD, Gronseth GS, Franklin G, Carter GT, Kinsella LJ, Cohen JA, et al. American Academy of Neurology. Practice parameter: evaluation of distal symmetric polyneuropathy: role of autonomic testing, nerve biopsy, and skin biopsy (an evidence-based review). Report of the American Academy of Neurology, American Association of Neuromuscular and Electrodiagnostic Medicine, and American Academy of Physical Medicine and Rehabilitation. Neurology. 2009;72(2):177–84.
33. Gutrecht JA. Sympathetic skin response. J Clin Neurophysiol. 1994;11(5):519–24.
34. Parati G, Di Rienzo M, Mancia G. How to measure baroreflex sensitivity: from the cardiovascular laboratory to daily life. J Hypertens. 2000;18(1):7–19.
35. Miyamoto T, Miyamoto M, Suzuki K, Nishibayashi M, Iwanami M, Hirata K. ^{123}I-MIBG cardiac scintigraphy provides clues to the underlying neurodegenerative disorder in idiopathic REM sleep behavior disorder. Sleep. 2008;31(5):717–23.
36. Low PA, Caskey PE, Tuck RR, Fealey RD, Dyck PJ. Quantitative sudomotor axon reflex test in normal and neuropathic subjects. Ann Neurol. 1983;14(5):573–80.
37. Heart rate variability: standards of measurement, physiological interpretation and clinical use. Task Force of the European Society of Cardiology and the North American Society of Pacing and Electrophysiology. Circulation. 1996;93(5):1043–65.
38. Stein PK, Pu Y. Heart rate variability, sleep and sleep disorders. Sleep Med Rev. 2012;16(1):47–66.
39. Tobaldini E, Nobili L, Strada S, Casali KR, Braghiroli A, Montano N. Heart rate variability in normal and pathological sleep. Front Physiol. 2013;4:294.
40. Billman GE. The LF/HF ratio does not accurately measure cardiac sympatho-vagal balance. Front Physiol. 2013;4:26.
41. Reyes del Paso GA, Langewitz W, Mulder LJ, van Roon A, Duschek S. The utility of low frequency heart rate variability as an index of sympathetic cardiac tone: a review with emphasis on a reanalysis of previous studies. Psychophysiology. 2013;50(5):477–87.
42. White WB. Ambulatory blood pressure monitoring: dippers compared with non-dippers. Blood Press Monit. 2000;5(Suppl 1):517–23.
43. Somers V, Dyken ME, Mark AL, Abboud FM. Sympathetic nerve activity during sleep in normal subjects. N Engl J Med. 1993;328:303–7.

44. Chan G, Cooper R, Hosanee M, Welykholowa K, Kyriacou PA, Zheng D, et al. Multi-site photoplethysmography technology for blood pressure assessment: challenges and recommendations. J Clin Med. 2019;8(11):1827.
45. Sherwood A, Allen MT, Fahrenberg J, Kelsey RM, Lovallo WR, van Doornen LJ. Methodological guidelines for impedance cardiography. Psychophysiology. 1990;27(1):1–23.
46. Ewing DJ, Clarke BF. Diagnosis and management of diabetic autonomic neuropathy. Br Med J (Clin Res Ed). 1982;285(6346):916–8.
47. Donadio V, Incensi A, Giannoccaro MP, Cortelli P, Di Stasi V, Pizza F, et al. Peripheral autonomic neuropathy: diagnostic contribution of skin biopsy. J Neuropathol Exp Neurol. 2012;71(11):1000–8.
48. Falck B, Hillarp NA, Thieme G, Torp A. Fluorescence of catechol amines and related compounds condensed with formaldehyde. Brain Res Bull. 1982;9(1–6):xi–v.
49. Low PA. Pitfalls in autonomic testing. In: Low PA, editor. Clinical autonomic disorders. 2nd ed. Philadelphia: Lippincott/Raven; 1997. p. 391–401.
50. Consensus statement: Report and recommendations of the San Antonio conference on diabetic neuropathy. American Diabetes Association American Academy of Neurology. Diabetes Care 1988;11(7):592–597.
51. Assessment. Clinical autonomic testing report of the Therapeutics and Technology Assessment Subcommittee of the American Academy of Neurology. Neurology. 1996;46(3):873–80.
52. Chokroverty S. Functional anatomy of the autonomic nervous system correlated with symptomatology of neurologic disease, American Academy of Neurology Course No. 246. San Diego: American Academy of Neurology; 1992. p. 49.
53. Sharpey-Schafer EP, Taylor PJ. Absent circulatory reflexes in diabetic neuritis. Lancet. 1960;1(7124):559–62.
54. Sharpey-Schafer EP. Circulatory reflexes in chronic disease of the afferent nervous system. J Physiol. 1956;134(1):1–10.
55. Young RR, Asbury AK, Corbett JL, Adams RD. Pure pandysautonomia with recovery. Description and discussion of diagnostic criteria. Brain. 1975;98(4):613–36.
56. Klein CM, Vernino S, Lennon VA, Sandroni P, Fealey RD, Benrud-Larson L, et al. The spectrum of autoimmune autonomic neuropathies. Ann Neurol. 2003;53(6):752–8.
57. Bradbury S, Eggleston C. Postural hypotension: a report of 3 cases. Am Heart J. 1925;1:73–86.
58. Piorry PA. Researches sur l'influence de la pesanteur sur le cours du sang: diagnostic de la syncope et de l'apoplexie; cause et traitement de la syncope. Arch Generales de Med. 1826;12:527–44.
59. Laubry C, Doumer E. L'hypotension orthostatique. Presse Med. 1932;40:17.
60. Coon EA, Singer W, Low PA. Pure autonomic failure. Mayo Clin Proc. 2019;94(10):2087–98.
61. Singer W, Berini SE, Sandroni P, Fealey RD, Coon EA, Suarez MD, et al. Pure autonomic failure: predictors of conversion to clinical CNS involvement. Neurology. 2017;88(12):1129–36.
62. Wagner HN Jr. Orthostatic hypotension. Bull Johns Hopkins Hosp. 1959;105:322–59.
63. Shy GM, Drager GA. A neurological syndrome associated with orthostatic hypotension: a clinical-pathologic study. Arch Neurol. 1960;2:511–27.
64. Graham JG, Oppenheimer DR. Orthostatic hypotension and nicotine sensitivity in a case of multiple system atrophy. J Neurol Neurosurg Psychiatry. 1969;32(1):28–34.
65. Brás IC, Dominguez-Meijide A, Gerhardt E, Koss D, Lázaro DF, Santos PI, et al. Synucleinopathies: where we are and where we need to go. J Neurochem. 2020. https://doi.org/10.1111/jnc.14965. Epub ahead of print.
66. Mendoza-Velásquez JJ, Flores-Vázquez JF, Barrón-Velázquez E, Sosa-Ortiz AL, Illigens BW, Siepmann T. Autonomic dysfunction in α-Synucleinopathies. Front Neurol. 2019;10:363.
67. Wenning GK, Fanciulli A. Multiple system atrophy. Vienna: Springer-Verlag; 2014.
68. Stankovic I, Krismer F, Jesic A, Antonini A, Benke T, Brown RG, et al. Movement Disorders Society MSA (MODIMSA) Study Group. Cognitive impairment in multiple system atrophy: a position statement by the Neuropsychology Task Force of the MDS Multiple System Atrophy (MODIMSA) study group. Mov Disord. 2014;29(7):857–67.
69. Chokroverty S, Provini F. Sleep, breathing, and neurological disorders. In: Chokroverty S, editor. Sleep disorders medicine: basic science, technical considerations and clinical aspects. 4th ed. New York: Springer; 2017. p. 787–890.
70. Freeman R. Clinical practice. Neurogenic orthostatic hypotension. N Engl J Med. 2008;358(6):615–24.
71. Benarroch EE. Postural tachycardia syndrome: a heterogeneous and multifactorial disorder. Mayo Clin Proc. 2012;87(12):1214–25.
72. Mathias CJ, Low DA, Iodice V, Owens AP, Kirbis M, Grahame R. Postural tachycardia syndrome – current experience and concepts. Nat Rev Neurol. 2011;8(1):22–34.
73. Jarjour IT. Postural tachycardia syndrome in children and adolescents. Semin Pediatr Neurol. 2013;20(1):18–26.
74. Miglis MG, Barwick F. Sleep disorders in patients with postural tachycardia syndrome: a review of the literature and guide for clinicians. Auton Neurosci. 2018;215:62–9.
75. Mallien J, Isenmann S, Mrazek A, Haensch CA. Sleep disturbances and autonomic dysfunction in patients with postural orthostatic tachycardia syndrome. Front Neurol. 2014;5:118.
76. Streeten DH, Kerr CB, Kerr LP, Prior JC, Dalakos TG. Hyperbradykininism: a new orthostatic syndrome. Lancet. 1972;2(7786):1048–53.
77. Garcia Leme J, Rocha E, Silva M. Competitive and noncompetitive inhibition of bradykinin on the Guinea-pig ileum. Br J Pharmacol Chemother. 1965;25(1):50–8.
78. Biaggioni I, Goldstein DS, Atkinson T, Robertson D. Dopamine-beta-hydroxylase deficiency in humans. Neurology. 1990;40(2):370–3.
79. Cheshire WP Jr, Dickson DW, Nahm KF, Kaufmann HC, Benarroch EE. Dopamine beta-hydroxylase deficiency involves the central autonomic network. Acta Neuropathol. 2006;112(2):227–9.
80. Mathias CJ, Bannister R. Dopamine beta-hydroxylase deficiency – with a note on other genetically determined causes of autonomic failure. In: Mathias CJ, Bannister R, editors. Autonomic failure: a textbook of clinical disorders of the autonomic nervous system. 5th ed. Oxford: Oxford University Press; 2013. p. 597–612.
81. Mondini S, Guilleminault C. Abnormal breathing patterns during sleep in diabetes. Ann Neurol. 1985;17(4):391–5.
82. Bottini P, Dottorini ML, Cristina Cordoni M, Casucci G, Tantucci C. Sleep-disordered breathing in nonobese diabetic subjects with autonomic neuropathy. Eur Respir J. 2003;22(4):654–60.
83. Zochodne DW. Autonomic involvement in Guillain-Barré syndrome: a review. Muscle Nerve. 1994;17(10):1145–55.
84. Flachenecker P, Wermuth P, Hartung HP, Reiners K. Quantitative assessment of cardiovascular autonomic function in Guillain-Barre syndrome. Ann Neurol. 1997;42(2):171–9.
85. Dalos NP, Borel C, Hanley DF. Cardiovascular autonomic dysfunction in Guillain-Barré syndrome. Therapeutic implications of Swan-Ganz monitoring. Arch Neurol. 1988;45(1):115–7.
86. Chokroverty S, Bhat S, Allen RP. Motor control and dyscontrol in sleep. In: Chokroverty S, editor. Sleep disorders medicine: basic science, technical considerations and clinical aspects. 4th ed. New York: Springer; 2017. p. 713–57.

87. Valko PO, Hauser S, Sommerauer M, Werth E, Baumann CR. Observations on sleep-disordered breathing in idiopathic Parkinson's disease. PLoS One. 2014;9(6):e100828.
88. Cochen De Cock V, Benard-Serre N, Driss V, Granier M, Charif M, et al. Supine sleep and obstructive sleep apnea syndrome in Parkinson's disease. Sleep Med. 2015;16(12):1497–501.
89. Apps MC, Sheaff PC, Ingram DA, Kennard C, Empey DW. Respiration and sleep in Parkinson's disease. J Neurol Neurosurg Psychiatry. 1985;48(12):1240–5.
90. Parkinson J. An essay on the shaking palsy. London: Whittingham & Rowland; 1817. p. 1–60.
91. Frucht S, Rogers JD, Greene PE, Gordon MF, Fahn S. Falling asleep at the wheel: motor vehicle mishaps in persons taking pramipexole and ropinirole. Neurology. 1999;52(9):1908–10.
92. McKeith IG, Galasko D, Kosaka K, Perry EK, Dickson DW, Hansen LA, et al. Consensus guidelines for the clinical and pathologic diagnosis of dementia with Lewy bodies (DLB): report of the consortium on DLB international workshop. Neurology. 1996;47(5):1113–24.
93. American Academy of Sleep Medicine. International classification of sleep disorders. 3rd ed. Darien: American Academy of Sleep Medicine; 2014.
94. Korczynski W, Ceregrzyn M, Matyjek R, et al. Central and local (enteric) action of orexins. J Physiol Pharmacol. 2006;57(Suppl 6):17–42.
95. Inutsuka A, Yamanaka A. The physiological role of orexin/hypocretin neurons in the regulation of sleep/wakefulness and neuroendocrine functions. Front Endocrinol (Lausanne). 2013;4:18.
96. Nattie E, Li A. Respiration and autonomic regulation and orexin. Prog Brain Res. 2012;198:25–46.
97. Grimaldi D, Silvani A, Benarroch EE, Cortelli P. Orexin/hypocretin system and autonomic control: new insights and clinical correlations. Neurology. 2014;82(3):271–8.
98. Peyron C, Tighe DK, van den Pol AN, de Lecea L, Heller HC, Sutcliffe JG, Kilduff TS. Neurons containing hypocretin (orexin) project to multiple neuronal systems. J Neurosci. 1998;18(23):9996–10015.
99. Calandra- Buonaura G, Cortelli P. Autonomic dysfunction and sleep disorders. In: Chokroverty S, Ferini-Strambi L, editors. Oxford textbook of sleep disorders. Oxford: Oxford University Press; 2017. p. 291–300.
100. Plazzi G, Moghadam KK, Maggi LS, Donadio V, Vetrugno R, Liguori R, et al. Autonomic disturbances in narcolepsy. Sleep Med Rev. 2011;15(3):187–96.
101. Grimaldi D, Calandra-Buonaura G, Provini F, Agati P, Pierangeli G, Franceschini C, et al. Abnormal sleep-cardiovascular system interaction in narcolepsy with cataplexy: effects of hypocretin deficiency in humans. Sleep. 2012;35(4):519–28.
102. Sforza E, Roche F, Barthélémy JC, Pichot V. Diurnal and nocturnal cardiovascular variability and heart rate arousal response in idiopathic hypersomnia. Sleep Med. 2016;24:131–6.
103. Parish JM, Shepard JW Jr. Cardiovascular effects of sleep disorders. Chest. 1990;97(5):1220–6.
104. Osuna E, Patiño G. REM sleep-related complete heart block: is it a specific sleep-related disorder? Sleep Med. 2006;7(4):387–8.
105. Verrier RL, Kirby DA. Sleep and cardiac arrhythmias. Ann N Y Acad Sci. 1988;533:238–51.
106. Muller JE, Stone PH, Turi ZG, Rutherford JD, Czeisler CA, Parker C, et al. Circadian variation in the frequency of onset of acute myocardial infarction. N Engl J Med. 1985;313(21):1315–22.
107. Antzelevitch C. Brugada syndrome. Pacing Clin Electrophysiol. 2006;29(10):1130–59.
108. Vatta M, Dumaine R, Varghese G, Richard TA, Shimizu W, Aihara N, et al. Genetic and biophysical basis of sudden unexplained nocturnal death syndrome (SUNDS), a disease allelic to Brugada syndrome. Hum Mol Genet. 2002;11(3):337–45.
109. Samuels M. Introduction to neurocardiology. In: Mathias CJ, Bannister R, editors. Autonomic failure. 5th ed. Oxford: Oxford University Press; 2013. p. 669–76.
110. Cannon WB. "Voodoo" death. Am Anthropol. 1942;44(new series):169–181. Am J Public Health. 2002;92(10):1593–6; discussion 1594–5.
111. Robertson D, Hollister AS, Biaggioni I, Netterville JL, Mosqueda-Garcia R, Robertson RM. The diagnosis and treatment of baroreflex failure. N Engl J Med. 1993;329(20):1449–55.
112. Benarroch EE. Baroreflex failure. In: Benarroch EE, editor. Central autonomic network: functional organization and clinical correlations. Armonk: Futura Publishing; 1997. p. 482–4.
113. Moskowitz MA. Diseases of the autonomic nervous system. Clin Endocrinol Metab. 1977;6(3):745–68.
114. Penfield W. Diencephalic autonomic epilepsy. Arch Neurol Psychiatr. 1929;22:358–74.
115. Metz SA, Halter JB, Porte D Jr, Robertson RP. Autonomic epilepsy: clonidine blockade of paroxysmal catecholamine release and flushing. Ann Intern Med. 1978;88(2):189–93.
116. Adie WJ. Tonic pupils and absent tendon reflexes: a benign disorder sui generis; its complete and incomplete forms. Brain. 1932;55(1):98–113.
117. Hardin WB Jr, Gay AJ. The phenomenon of benign areflexia. Review of the holmes-adie syndrome with case reports and a study of the achilles reflex. Neurology. 1965;15:613–21.
118. Dichter SL, Shubert GS. Argyll Robertson upil. In: StatPearls [Internet]. Treasure Island: StatPearls Publishing. p. 2020.
119. Wilhelm H. Disorders of the pupil. In: Kennard C, Leigh RJ, editors. Neuro-ophthalmology. Handbook of clinical neurology, vol. 102. Amsterdam: Elsevier; 2011. p. 428–66.
120. Ross AT. Progressive selective sudomotor denervation; a case with coexisting Adie's syndrome. Neurology. 1958;8(11):809–17.
121. Lance JW, Drummond PD, Gandevia SC, Morris JG. Harlequin syndrome: the sudden onset of unilateral flushing and sweating. J Neurol Neurosurg Psychiatry. 1988;51(5):635–42.
122. Modi P, Arsiwalla T. Crocodile tear syndrome. In: StatPearls [Internet]. Treasure Island: StatPearls Publishing. p. 2020.
123. Abell TL, Camilleri M, Donohoe K, Hasler WL, Lin HC, Maurer AH, et al. American Neurogastroenterology and Motility Society and the Society of Nuclear Medicine. Consensus recommendations for gastric emptying scintigraphy: a joint report of the American Neurogastroenterology and Motility Society and the Society of Nuclear Medicine. Am J Gastroenterol. 2008;103(3):753–63.
124. Ross RT. Syncope. Philadelphia: Elsevier/Saunders; 1988. p. 1–160.
125. van Dijk JG. Transient loss of consciousness. In: Mathias CJ, Bannister R, editors. Autonomic failure. 5th ed. Oxford: Oxford University Press; 2013. p. 677–89.
126. Fisher RS, Cross JH, D'Souza C, French JA, Haut SR, Higurashi N, et al. Instruction manual for the ILAE 2017 operational classification of seizure types. Epilepsia. 2017;58(4):531–42.
127. Albassam OT, Redelmeier RJ, Shadowitz S, Husain AM, Simel D, Etchells EE. Did this patient have cardiac syncope?: the rational clinical examination systematic review. JAMA. 2019;321(24):2448–57.
128. Kremer M. Sitting, standing, and walking. Br Med J. 1958;2(5088):63–8.
129. Kremer M. Sitting, standing, and walking. Br Med J. 1958;2(5089):121–6.
130. Jellinger KA. Neuropathology of multiple system atrophy: new thoughts about pathogenesis. Mov Disord. 2014;29(14):1720–41.
131. Dunchen LW. Neuropathology of the autonomic nervous system in diabetes. In: Bannister R, editor. Autonomic failure. Oxford: Oxford University Press; 1983. p. 437–52.
132. Low PA, Walsh JC, Huang CY, McLeod JG. The sympathetic nervous system in diabetic neuropathy. A clinical and pathological study. Brain. 1975;98(3):341–56.

13 Obstructive Sleep Apnea in Adults and the Autonomic Nervous System

Jose-Alberto Palma and Horacio Kaufmann

Introduction

Obstructive sleep apnea (OSA) is characterized by episodic collapse of the upper airway during sleep, resulting in periodic reductions or pauses in ventilation, resulting in hypoxia, hypercapnia, or arousals from sleep. OSA is frequent in the general population with an estimated prevalence of 3% among women and 10% among men aged 30–49 years and 9% among women and 17% among men aged 50–70 years [1].

Risk factors for OSA comprise factors that reduce the side of the pharynx at rest or increase the collapsibility of the airway and include obesity and increased adipose tissue within the tongue and pharynx. Male sex is a risk factor, although the reasons for this remain unknown. Additional risk factors include hypothyroidism, acromegaly, and craniofacial abnormalities such as retrognathia [2].

The diagnosis of OSA requires an overnight polysomnography to document the frequency of breathing events, apneas and hypopneas, during sleep. Obstructive apnea is defined as a near-complete or complete (>90%) cessation in airflow for more than 10 seconds in sleep despite ventilatory effort. Hypopneas are generally defined as a reduction in airflow of at least 30% accompanied by reductions in oxygen saturation of at least 3% or arousal from sleep. The number of apneas and hypopneas per hour of sleep is referred to as apnea-hypopnea index (AHI). OSA is defined as an AHI of at least 5 events per hour. Traditionally, the AHI can be classified according to the number of events per hour. Mild AHI is defined by 5–15 events per hour, moderate AHI is defined by 16–30 evens per hour, and severe AHI is defined by more than 30 evens per hour [3]. The AHI is typically worse during rapid eye movement (REM) sleep and in the supine position. Home sleep studies may be used instead of polysomnography in selected cases [4].

J.-A. Palma (✉) · H. Kaufmann
Dysautonomia Center, Department of Neurology, New York University School of Medicine, New York, NY, USA
e-mail: JoseAlberto.PalmaCarazo@nyulangone.org

Comorbidities Associated with OSA

An AHI of 15 or more events per hour is associated with a reduction in psychomotor speed equivalent to 5 years of aging. Also, the higher the AHI, the lower the subjective quality of life. Untreated OSA is associated with tripled risk of motor vehicle accidents compared to the general population [5].

Importantly, OSA is associated with increased risk of cardiovascular disease, specifically hypertension, stroke, coronary artery disease, and heart failure, even after adjustment for BMI and other risk factors. Patients with OSA are also at increased risk for cardiac arrhythmias, namely sinus bradycardia, atrioventricular block, and ventricular tachycardia [6–9] (Fig. 13.1).

An AHI of 20 or more events per hour is associated with increased risk of stroke by a factor of four in men and a factor of two in women [10]. In addition, OSA is associated with neuroendocrine abnormalities resulting in an increased risk of diabetes and glucose dysregulation, independent of obesity [11], as well as increased levels of total cholesterol, low-density lipoprotein cholesterol, and triglycerides [12]. Cancer mortality and all-cause mortality were significantly higher among men 40–70 years of age with an AHI of more than 30 events per hour [13].

The Autonomic Nervous System in OSA

In healthy individuals, hypoxia (i.e., reduction in oxygen levels with arterial pO_2 less than ~60 mmHg) causes chemoreceptor activation and triggers tachycardia and moderate increases in blood pressure. Hypoxia and hypercapnia promote both hyperventilation (resulting in enhanced oxygen delivery to blood), and increased sympathetic efferent activity resulting in vasoconstriction to redistribute oxygenated blood flow [14–16]. Baroreflex activation normally abolishes the increase in sympathetic activity induced by hypoxia,

S. Chokroverty, P. Cortelli (eds.), *Autonomic Nervous System and Sleep*, https://doi.org/10.1007/978-3-030-62263-3_13

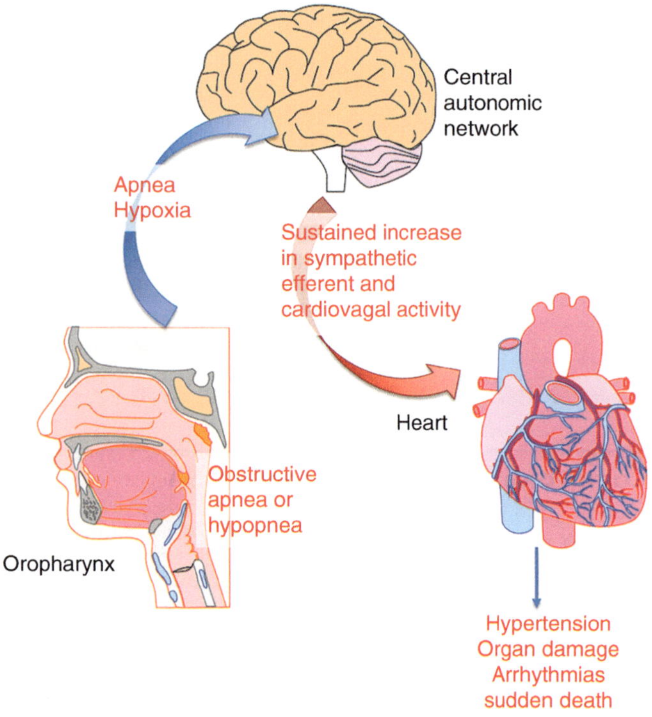

Fig. 13.1 Apnea-autonomic interactions. Sustained increased sympathetic efferent activity and cardiovagal tone promote cardiovascular disease and arrhythmias in patients with obstructive sleep apnea

which can result in vagal activation and bradycardia [17–19]. Apnea unbridles an intense cardiovascular response in order to maintain oxygen delivery, reduce cardiac oxygen demand, and ensure survival. This is similar to the diving reflex that occurs in humans during facial immersion and apnea [20].

Converging evidence obtained from studies with muscle sympathetic nerve activity, plasma catecholamine levels, and heart rate variability analysis indicates that in patients with OSA, hypoxia and apnea trigger a cascade of stimuli that elicit acute increases in efferent sympathetic activity during sleep that, when sustained over time, induce chronic sustained elevation of the setting point for central sympathetic outflow during wakefulness [21–26], resulting in higher risk of chronic hypertension, coronary artery disease, and stroke. Conversely, excessive sympathetic outflow results in baroreflex-mediated excessive cardiovagal efferent activity and bradycardia, atrioventricular block, and ventricular tachycardia, potentially resulting in sudden cardiac death [8, 9, 27]. Arousal at the termination of the obstructive event is associated with sleep fragmentation and further sympathetic efferent activity, leading to peripheral vasoconstriction and an abrupt increase in systolic and diastolic blood pressures and heart rate [28].

Intrathoracic Pressure Changes

The collapse of the upper airway during sleep resulting in obstructive apnea causes intrathoracic pressure swings resulting in myocardial stretch of the heart chambers and changes in transmural pressure gradients, particularly affecting the thin-walled atria. This may also contribute to atrial fibrillation and other arrhythmias [29, 30].

Additional Mechanisms

In addition to hypoxia and apnea, there might be other mechanisms contributing to the excessive sympathetic efferent activity that develops in patients with OSA. Obesity could not only mechanically obstruct the airway to cause OSA but also increase sympathetic efferent activity via leptin, insulin, angiotensin, and cytokine mechanisms [31]; on the other hand, many patients with OSA are not obese. Carotid body chemoreceptor hypersensitivity due to intermittent hypoxia has been confirmed in animal models and might contribute to the pathogenesis of OSA in humans [32]. Excessive activation of CNS nuclei induces neural changes that increase the excitatory drive to the rostral ventrolateral medulla and sustains a high sympathetic tone independently of the peripheral sensory signals [33].

The immune system contributes to cardiovascular diseases, including arrhythmias, hypertension, atherosclerosis, and heart failure. While it is well documented that patients with OSA have increased levels of serum inflammatory markers [34], it is unknown whether anti-inflammatory treatments can reduce or reverse OSA-associated sustained sympathetic drive and delay or prevent organ damage [35, 36].

Treatment of OSA

Treatment of OSA is recommended in patients with an AHI of 15 or more events per hour, as well as for patients with an AHI of 5–14 events per hour with significant symptoms (e.g., diurnal sleepiness and impaired cognition) or comorbid conditions (e.g., hypertension, history of stroke, or ischemic heart disease). Patients with an AHI of less than 5 must be treated if they are at high risk for sudden death during sleep, as it is the case of familial dysautonomia [37].

The most effective therapy to reduce OSA is positive airway pressure (PAP) applied with a tight seal to the nose or mouth (or both) serving to stent open the upper airway. Continuous positive airway pressure (CPAP) provides a constant level of positive pressure across inspiration and expiration and is the most commonly used modality. Although CPAP is highly effective, adherence is challenging due to difficulties in identifying the most suitable mask, positioning the mask, keeping the mask in place during sleep, and maintaining the equipment and supplies. There are many strategies that could help overcome these limitations, such as mask desensitization (e.g., using the mask at progressively increasing lengths of times each night to get used to it), or using variable-pressure approaches to CPAP, including higher pressure during inspiration than during expiration, auto-adjusting pressure in response to breath-to-breath airflow changes throughout the night, and lowered pressure just at the beginning of the expiratory phase; however, such approaches have not been proven to improve adherence rates.

Other therapies that might be suitable for patients with mild OSA include oral appliance to advance the mandible, positional therapy (avoiding a supine sleep position) or surgery (uvulopharyngopalatoplasty and maxillomandibular advancement surgical procedures) [38, 39].

Weight loss should be recommended to all overweight or obese patients with OSA, including those using CPAP [40, 41]. Muscle relaxants and medications that suppress the respiratory drive (e.g., benzodiazepines, opioids, and alcohol) exacerbate OSA and should be avoided.

Cardiovascular Autonomic Consequences of Treating OSA

Multiple studies indicate that CPAP therapy induces reductions in sympathetic efferent activity or sympathetic tone during sleep, both in the short and long terms [42–50]. Indeed, withdrawal of CPAP therapy for 1 week in patients with moderate to severe OSA was associated with increased urine norepinephrine levels [51]. The reductions in sympathetic efferent activity or tone appear to extend also to the daytime, when patients are not using CPAP [52–55].

The effects of treating OSA on hypertension and cardiovascular events remain uncertain. The use of a mandibular advancement splint appears to reduce systolic pressure [56]. In some randomized trials, but not in others, CPAP reduced blood pressure in both hypertensive and normotensive patients with obstructive sleep apnea [57–61]. Interestingly, a clinical trial to determine if nocturnal CPAP treatment can reduce nighttime supine hypertension in patients with efferent baroreflex (i.e., autonomic) failure, regardless of the presence of OSA, is underway (ClinicalTrials.gov: NCT03312556).

Whether the reductions in efferent sympathetic activity have actual clinical consequences is unclear. It might well be that in patients who have suffered from long-term OSA-related sympathetic efferent hyperactivity, the resolution of the OSA may not be sufficient to reduce hypertension. In keeping with this, in a large randomized controlled trial of patients with both cardiovascular disease and moderate to severe OSA, the use of CPAP had no significant effect on the prevention of cardiovascular events, despite improving daytime sleepiness and quality of life [62]. A recent meta-analysis of randomized trials concluded that there is insufficient evidence to determine the effect of CPAP on cardiovascular outcomes [63]. No controlled studies on the effects of CPAP on atrial fibrillation or other arrhythmias in patients with OSA have been completed yet [64].

Other Clinical Outcomes of Treating OSA

A study comparing CPAP and placebo showed that CPAP reduced fatigue and daytime sleepiness in patients with OSA [65]. An observational study showed that CPAP treatment was associated with a reduction in the risk of motor vehicle accidents, as compared with rates before treatment initiation, to a level similar to that of drivers without known OSA [5]. CPAP may also improve cognition, but results are inconsistent. A large, randomized, trial comparing 6 months of CPAP with sham CPAP showed no meaningful difference across groups in executive function, although the average nightly use of a CPAP device was only 4 hours [66]. In an ensuing analysis, adherence to therapy predicted improved psychomotor function [67].

Conclusions

OSA is highly prevalent in the general population. The repetitive apneas and hypoxic events elicit acute increases in efferent sympathetic activity during sleep that, when sustained over time, induce a carryover chronic sustained elevation of the setting point for central sympathetic outflow during wakefulness. Chronic increased sympathetic activity is asymptomatic but increases the risk of hypertension, coronary artery disease, stroke, arrhythmias, and sudden death. Treatment of OSA with CPAP results in reductions in sympathetic efferent activity or sympathetic tone during sleep, both in the short and long terms. The reductions in sympathetic efferent activity appear to extend also to the daytime. CPAP appears to reduce blood pressure in both hypertensive and normotensive patients with OSA, although the evidence is conflicting. Currently, there is insufficient evidence to determine the effect of CPAP on cardiovascular events, stroke, arrhythmias or death, for which additional, controlled trials are required. OSA should be considered in the differential diagnosis of hypertensive patients, particularly in those who are refractory to medications. Novel therapeutic approaches are redefining the relationship between OSA and autonomic dysfunction. For instance, treatment with CPAP may be a potential therapeutic option for the treatment of supine hypertension in patients with autonomic failure, regardless of the presence of OSA.

Conflict of Interests The authors report no conflict of interests related to this chapter.

References

1. Veasey SC, Rosen IM. Obstructive sleep apnea in adults. N Engl J Med. 2019;380(15):1442–9.
2. Shah N, Roux F. The relationship of obesity and obstructive sleep apnea. Clin Chest Med. 2009;30(3):455–65. vii
3. Ruehland WR, Rochford PD, O'Donoghue FJ, Pierce RJ, Singh P, Thornton AT. The new AASM criteria for scoring hypopneas: impact on the apnea hypopnea index. Sleep. 2009;32(2):150–7.
4. Kapur VK, Auckley DH, Chowdhuri S, Kuhlmann DC, Mehra R, Ramar K, et al. Clinical practice guideline for diagnostic testing for adult obstructive sleep apnea: an American Academy of sleep medicine clinical practice guideline. J Clin Sleep Med. 2017;13(3):479–504.
5. George CF. Reduction in motor vehicle collisions following treatment of sleep apnoea with nasal CPAP. Thorax. 2001;56(7):508–12.
6. Somers VK, White DP, Amin R, Abraham WT, Costa F, Culebras A, et al. Sleep apnea and cardiovascular disease: an American Heart Association/American College Of Cardiology Foundation Scientific Statement from the American Heart Association Council for High Blood Pressure Research Professional Education Committee, Council on Clinical Cardiology, Stroke Council, and Council On Cardiovascular Nursing. In collaboration with the National Heart, Lung, and Blood Institute National Center on Sleep Disorders Research (National Institutes of Health). Circulation. 2008;118(10):1080–111.
7. Mehra R, Benjamin EJ, Shahar E, Gottlieb DJ, Nawabit R, Kirchner HL, et al. Association of nocturnal arrhythmias with sleep-disordered breathing: the sleep heart health study. Am J Respir Crit Care Med. 2006;173(8):910–6.
8. Somers VK, Dyken ME, Mark AL, Abboud FM. Parasympathetic hyperresponsiveness and bradyarrhythmias during apnoea in hypertension. Clin Auton Res. 1992;2(3):171–6.
9. Gami AS, Olson EJ, Shen WK, Wright RS, Ballman KV, Hodge DO, et al. Obstructive sleep apnea and the risk of sudden cardiac death: a longitudinal study of 10,701 adults. J Am Coll Cardiol. 2013;62(7):610–6.
10. Redline S, Yenokyan G, Gottlieb DJ, Shahar E, O'Connor GT, Resnick HE, et al. Obstructive sleep apnea-hypopnea and incident stroke: the sleep heart health study. Am J Respir Crit Care Med. 2010;182(2):269–77.
11. Tasali E, Ip MS. Obstructive sleep apnea and metabolic syndrome: alterations in glucose metabolism and inflammation. Proc Am Thorac Soc. 2008;5(2):207–17.
12. Nadeem R, Singh M, Nida M, Kwon S, Sajid H, Witkowski J, et al. Effect of CPAP treatment for obstructive sleep apnea hypopnea syndrome on lipid profile: a meta-regression analysis. J Clin Sleep Med. 2014;10(12):1295–302.
13. Young T, Finn L, Peppard PE, Szklo-Coxe M, Austin D, Nieto FJ, et al. Sleep disordered breathing and mortality: eighteen-year follow-up of the Wisconsin sleep cohort. Sleep. 2008;31(8):1071–8.
14. Yang CF, Feldman JL. Efferent projections of excitatory and inhibitory pre Botzinger complex neurons. J Comp Neurol. 2018;526(8):1389–402.
15. Revill AL, Vann NC, Akins VT, Kottick A, Gray PA, Del Negro CA, et al. Dbx1 precursor cells are a source of inspiratory XII premotoneurons. elife. 2015;4 https://doi.org/10.7554/eLife.12301.
16. Del Negro CA, Funk GD, Feldman JL. Breathing matters. Nat Rev Neurosci. 2018;19(6):351–67.
17. Somers VK, Mark AL, Zavala DC, Abboud FM. Contrasting effects of hypoxia and hypercapnia on ventilation and sympathetic activity in humans. J Appl Physiol (1985). 1989;67(5):2101–6.
18. Somers VK, Mark AL, Zavala DC, Abboud FM. Influence of ventilation and hypocapnia on sympathetic nerve responses to hypoxia in normal humans. J Appl Physiol (1985). 1989;67(5):2095–100.
19. Somers VK, Mark AL, Abboud FM. Interaction of baroreceptor and chemoreceptor reflex control of sympathetic nerve activity in normal humans. J Clin Invest. 1991;87(6):1953–7.
20. Heistad DD, Abbound FM, Eckstein JW. Vasoconstrictor response to simulated diving in man. J Appl Physiol. 1968;25(5):542–9.
21. Floras JS. Sympathetic nervous system in patients with sleep related breathing disorders. Curr Hypertens Rev. 2016;12(1):18–26.
22. Carlson JT, Hedner J, Elam M, Ejnell H, Sellgren J, Wallin BG. Augmented resting sympathetic activity in awake patients with obstructive sleep apnea. Chest. 1993;103(6):1763–8.
23. Somers VK, Dyken ME, Clary MP, Abboud FM. Sympathetic neural mechanisms in obstructive sleep apnea. J Clin Invest. 1995;96(4):1897–904.
24. Marrone O, Riccobono L, Salvaggio A, Mirabella A, Bonanno A, Bonsignore MR. Catecholamines and blood pressure in obstructive sleep apnea syndrome. Chest. 1993;103(3):722–7.
25. Palma JA, Urrestarazu E, Lopez-Azcarate J, Alegre M, Fernandez S, Artieda J, et al. Increased sympathetic and decreased parasympathetic cardiac tone in patients with sleep related alveolar hypoventilation. Sleep. 2013;36(6):933–40.
26. Palma JA, Iriarte J, Fernandez S, Valencia M, Alegre M, Artieda J, et al. Characterizing the phenotypes of obstructive sleep apnea: clinical, sleep, and autonomic features of obstructive sleep apnea with and without hypoxia. Clin Neurophysiol. 2014;125(9):1783–91.
27. Xie J, Sert Kuniyoshi FH, Covassin N, Singh P, Gami AS, Wang S, et al. Nocturnal hypoxemia due to obstructive sleep apnea is an independent predictor of poor prognosis after myocardial infarction. J Am Heart Assoc. 2016;5(8):e003162.
28. Garpestad E, Katayama H, Parker JA, Ringler J, Lilly J, Yasuda T, et al. Stroke volume and cardiac output decrease at termination of obstructive apneas. J Appl Physiol (1985). 1992;73(5):1743–8.
29. Kasai T, Bradley TD. Obstructive sleep apnea and heart failure: pathophysiologic and therapeutic implications. J Am Coll Cardiol. 2011;57(2):119–27.
30. Linz D, Linz B, Hohl M, Bohm M. Atrial arrhythmogenesis in obstructive sleep apnea: therapeutic implications. Sleep Med Rev. 2016;26:87–94.
31. Gami AS, Hodge DO, Herges RM, Olson EJ, Nykodym J, Kara T, et al. Obstructive sleep apnea, obesity, and the risk of incident atrial fibrillation. J Am Coll Cardiol. 2007;49(5):565–71.
32. Prabhakar NR, Peng YJ, Kumar GK, Pawar A. Altered carotid body function by intermittent hypoxia in neonates and adults: relevance to recurrent apneas. Respir Physiol Neurobiol. 2007;157(1):148–53.
33. Guyenet PG. The sympathetic control of blood pressure. Nat Rev Neurosci. 2006;7(5):335–46.
34. Wang J, Yu W, Gao M, Zhang F, Gu C, Yu Y, et al. Impact of obstructive sleep apnea syndrome on endothelial function, arte-

rial stiffening, and serum inflammatory markers: an updated meta-analysis and metaregression of 18 studies. J Am Heart Assoc. 2015;4(11):e002454.
35. Zubcevic J, Waki H, Raizada MK, Paton JF. Autonomic-immune-vascular interaction: an emerging concept for neurogenic hypertension. Hypertension. 2011;57(6):1026–33.
36. Shi P, Diez-Freire C, Jun JY, Qi Y, Katovich MJ, Li Q, et al. Brain microglial cytokines in neurogenic hypertension. Hypertension. 2010;56(2):297–303.
37. Kazachkov M, Palma JA, Norcliffe-Kaufmann L, Bar-Aluma BE, Spalink CL, Barnes EP, et al. Respiratory care in familial dysautonomia: systematic review and expert consensus recommendations. Respir Med. 2018;141:37–46.
38. Caples SM, Rowley JA, Prinsell JR, Pallanch JF, Elamin MB, Katz SG, et al. Surgical modifications of the upper airway for obstructive sleep apnea in adults: a systematic review and meta-analysis. Sleep. 2010;33(10):1396–407.
39. Pliska BT, Nam H, Chen H, Lowe AA, Almeida FR. Obstructive sleep apnea and mandibular advancement splints: occlusal effects and progression of changes associated with a decade of treatment. J Clin Sleep Med. 2014;10(12):1285–91.
40. Chirinos JA, Gurubhagavatula I, Teff K, Rader DJ, Wadden TA, Townsend R, et al. CPAP, weight loss, or both for obstructive sleep apnea. N Engl J Med. 2014;370(24):2265–75.
41. Hudgel DW, Patel SR, Ahasic AM, Bartlett SJ, Bessesen DH, Coaker MA, et al. The role of weight management in the treatment of adult obstructive sleep apnea. An official American Thoracic Society Clinical Practice Guideline. Am J Respir Crit Care Med. 2018;198(6):e70–87.
42. Marrone O, Salvaggio A, Bue AL, Bonanno A, Riccobono L, Insalaco G, et al. Blood pressure changes after automatic and fixed CPAP in obstructive sleep apnea: relationship with nocturnal sympathetic activity. Clin Exp Hypertens. 2011;33(6):373–80.
43. Heitmann J, Ehlenz K, Penzel T, Becker HF, Grote L, Voigt KH, et al. Sympathetic activity is reduced by nCPAP in hypertensive obstructive sleep apnoea patients. Eur Respir J. 2004;23(2):255–62.
44. Hedner J, Darpo B, Ejnell H, Carlson J, Caidahl K. Reduction in sympathetic activity after long-term CPAP treatment in sleep apnoea: cardiovascular implications. Eur Respir J. 1995;8(2):222–9.
45. Veale D, Pepin JL, Wuyam B, Levy PA. Abnormal autonomic stress responses in obstructive sleep apnoea are reversed by nasal continuous positive airway pressure. Eur Respir J. 1996;9(10):2122–6.
46. Roche F, Court-Fortune I, Pichot V, Duverney D, Costes F, Emonot A, et al. Reduced cardiac sympathetic autonomic tone after long-term nasal continuous positive airway pressure in obstructive sleep apnoea syndrome. Clin Physiol. 1999;19(2):127–34.
47. Palma JA, Iriarte J, Fernandez S, Alegre M, Valencia M, Artieda J, et al. Long-term continuous positive airway pressure therapy improves cardiac autonomic tone during sleep in patients with obstructive sleep apnea. Clin Auton Res. 2015;25(4):225–32.
48. Narkiewicz K, Kato M, Phillips BG, Pesek CA, Davison DE, Somers VK. Nocturnal continuous positive airway pressure decreases daytime sympathetic traffic in obstructive sleep apnea. Circulation. 1999;100(23):2332–5.
49. Hall AB, Ziadi MC, Leech JA, Chen SY, Burwash IG, Renaud J, et al. Effects of short-term continuous positive airway pressure on myocardial sympathetic nerve function and energetics in patients with heart failure and obstructive sleep apnea: a randomized study. Circulation. 2014;130(11):892–901.
50. Kufoy E, Palma JA, Lopez J, Alegre M, Urrestarazu E, Artieda J, et al. Changes in the heart rate variability in patients with obstructive sleep apnea and its response to acute CPAP treatment. PLoS One. 2012;7(3):e33769.
51. Phillips CL, Yang Q, Williams A, Roth M, Yee BJ, Hedner JA, et al. The effect of short-term withdrawal from continuous positive airway pressure therapy on sympathetic activity and markers of vascular inflammation in subjects with obstructive sleep apnoea. J Sleep Res. 2007;16(2):217–25.
52. Ziegler MG, Mills PJ, Loredo JS, Ancoli-Israel S, Dimsdale JE. Effect of continuous positive airway pressure and placebo treatment on sympathetic nervous activity in patients with obstructive sleep apnea. Chest. 2001;120(3):887–93.
53. Usui K, Bradley TD, Spaak J, Ryan CM, Kubo T, Kaneko Y, et al. Inhibition of awake sympathetic nerve activity of heart failure patients with obstructive sleep apnea by nocturnal continuous positive airway pressure. J Am Coll Cardiol. 2005;45(12):2008–11.
54. Imadojemu VA, Mawji Z, Kunselman A, Gray KS, Hogeman CS, Leuenberger UA. Sympathetic chemoreflex responses in obstructive sleep apnea and effects of continuous positive airway pressure therapy. Chest. 2007;131(5):1406–13.
55. Henderson LA, Fatouleh RH, Lundblad LC, McKenzie DK, Macefield VG. Effects of 12 months continuous positive airway pressure on sympathetic activity related brainstem function and structure in obstructive sleep apnea. Front Neurosci. 2016;10:90.
56. Andren A, Hedberg P, Walker-Engstrom ML, Wahlen P, Tegelberg A. Effects of treatment with oral appliance on 24-h blood pressure in patients with obstructive sleep apnea and hypertension: a randomized clinical trial. Sleep Breath. 2013;17(2):705–12.
57. Pepperell JC, Ramdassingh-Dow S, Crosthwaite N, Mullins R, Jenkinson C, Stradling JR, et al. Ambulatory blood pressure after therapeutic and subtherapeutic nasal continuous positive airway pressure for obstructive sleep apnoea: a randomised parallel trial. Lancet. 2002;359(9302):204–10.
58. Becker HF, Jerrentrup A, Ploch T, Grote L, Penzel T, Sullivan CE, et al. Effect of nasal continuous positive airway pressure treatment on blood pressure in patients with obstructive sleep apnea. Circulation. 2003;107(1):68–73.
59. Dimsdale JE, Loredo JS, Profant J. Effect of continuous positive airway pressure on blood pressure: a placebo trial. Hypertension. 2000;35(1 Pt 1):144–7.
60. Engleman HM, Gough K, Martin SE, Kingshott RN, Padfield PL, Douglas NJ. Ambulatory blood pressure on and off continuous positive airway pressure therapy for the sleep apnea/hypopnea syndrome: effects in "non-dippers". Sleep. 1996;19(5):378–81.
61. Faccenda JF, Mackay TW, Boon NA, Douglas NJ. Randomized placebo-controlled trial of continuous positive airway pressure on blood pressure in the sleep apnea-hypopnea syndrome. Am J Respir Crit Care Med. 2001;163(2):344–8.
62. McEvoy RD, Antic NA, Heeley E, Luo Y, Ou Q, Zhang X, et al. CPAP for prevention of cardiovascular events in obstructive sleep apnea. N Engl J Med. 2016;375(10):919–31.
63. da Silva Paulitsch F, Zhang L. Continuous positive airway pressure for adults with obstructive sleep apnea and cardiovascular disease: a meta-analysis of randomized trials. Sleep Med. 2019;54:28–34.
64. Traaen GM, Aakeroy L, Hunt TE, Overland B, Lyseggen E, Aukrust P, et al. Treatment of sleep apnea in patients with paroxysmal atrial fibrillation: design and rationale of a randomized controlled trial. Scand Cardiovasc J. 2018;52(6):372–7.
65. Tomfohr LM, Ancoli-Israel S, Loredo JS, Dimsdale JE. Effects of continuous positive airway pressure on fatigue and sleepiness in patients with obstructive sleep apnea: data from a randomized controlled trial. Sleep. 2011;34(1):121–6.
66. Kushida CA, Nichols DA, Holmes TH, Quan SF, Walsh JK, Gottlieb DJ, et al. Effects of continuous positive airway pressure on neurocognitive function in obstructive sleep apnea patients: the Apnea Positive Pressure Long-term Efficacy Study (APPLES). Sleep. 2012;35(12):1593–602.
67. Holmes TH, Kushida CA. Adherence to continuous positive airway pressure improves attention/psychomotor function and sleepiness: a bias-reduction method with further assessment of APPLES. Sleep Med. 2017;37:130–4.

Primary Insomnia and Dysautonomia

14

Luigi Ferini-Strambi, Sara Marelli, and Maria Salsone

Introduction

Sleep disorders, including insomnia, are considered to be closely related to fatigue, decreased alertness, and concentration disturbances during daytime or impairment in family, social, vocational, academic, or other important areas of functioning [1]. Primary insomnia (PI) is commonly defined as sleep difficulties that affect daytime functioning. It is a chronic condition characterized by frequent and persistent sleep initiation or maintenance disorders, including difficulty in falling asleep. PI is considered an independent condition since it does not occur in the presence of another sleep disorder, mental disorder, or as a direct physiological effect of a substance or medical condition [1]. The clinical relevance of insomnia is strongly related to its prevalence. Indeed, insomnia is the most common sleep disorder and a public health concern considering that one-third of the general population presents insomnia symptoms and about 10% of the population meets the criteria for an insomnia diagnosis [2]. In this context, PI represents 10–15% of all chronic insomnias [3].

Although sleep has not traditionally been considered a phenomenon strictly regulated by the autonomic nervous system (ANS), there are overlapping areas in the central nervous system (CNS) that regulate both systems, resulting in relevant interactions impacting morbidity and mortality [4]. In addition, evidence from numerous experimental and epidemiological studies support the bidirectional nature of the relationship between sleep disorders and ANS dysfunctions. Indeed, patients with autonomic dysfunction may have sleep disorders and conversely patients with untreated sleep disorders may present features suggestive of autonomic dysfunction [5]. Thus, it is not surprising that a bidirectional relationship has been also proposed between insomnia and ANS dysregulation. In this view, the autonomic and cortical overactivations reported in insomnias patients might be considered a consequence of poor sleep quality [6]. On the other hand, autonomic hyperarousal state derived from the overactivations may predispose to poor sleep [7]. The exact chronopathological sequence of this bidirectional relationship remains to be determined.

In this chapter, we will give an overview of the relationship between primary insomnia and alterations of autonomic function emphasizing the crucial association between PI and cardiovascular disease (CVD) as well as clinical relevance of such relationship and therapeutic implications. We shall also briefly mention about the cardiovascular autonomic control in PI and insomnia phenotypes conferring increased risks to cardiovascular disorders most commonly reported in subjects with chronic insomnia. However, mechanisms linking adverse health consequences including those of cardiovascular health remain incomplete which should be the focus for future investigation.

Primary Insomnia and Cardiovascular Disease: The State of the Science

Over the past two decades, a growing scientific interest has focused on the association between insomnia and CVD. Yet, the existing literature has shown inconsistent findings. However, a considerable body of evidence has recently demonstrated that insomnia is associated with CVD and increased cardiovascular risk (particularly regarding hypertension or elevated resting heart rate) [8]. Moreover, in recent years,

L. Ferini-Strambi (✉) · S. Marelli
UO Neurology – Sleep Disorder Center, Department of Clinical Neurosciences, IRCCS San Raffaele Hospital, "Vita-Salute" San Raffaele University, Milan, Italy
e-mail: ferinistrambi.luigi@hsr.it

M. Salsone
UO Neurology – Sleep Disorder Center, Department of Clinical Neurosciences, IRCCS San Raffaele Hospital, "Vita-Salute" San Raffaele University, Milan, Italy

Institute of Molecular Bioimaging and Physiology, National Research Council (IBFM-CNR), Cantazaro, Italy

S. Chokroverty, P. Cortelli (eds.), *Autonomic Nervous System and Sleep*, https://doi.org/10.1007/978-3-030-62263-3_14

knowledge of the ANS's crucial role in cardiac control during sleep has emerged. To better clarify the nature of this association, however, some aspects should be taken into consideration. First, it is important to correctly measures and define subjective and objective sleep quality and its relation to insomnia. Furthermore, potential confounding variables (including hypnotic medication and caffeine intake as trigger of coronary events) should be also investigated. Despite advances in this field, certain questions remain. First, clarification is needed regarding which insomnia phenotypes have an increased risk of CVD. Second, identification of PI patients at increased risk for the opportunity of individualized therapeutic interventions should be emphasized.

Primary Insomnia and Cardiovascular Autonomic Control: The Neurophysiological Basis

PI is an established risk factor for the development of CVD. This connection is likely related to a dysregulation of ANS function (specifically, sympathetic overactivation). The increased cardiovascular sympathetic tone, in turn, plays a central role in the cardiovascular homeostasis with consequent increased risk of CVD. In this context, the association between PI and CVD raises two important questions: (1) What is the cause of the increased sympathetic activity that often occurs in patients with PI? (2) What is the link between this autonomic dysfunction and the development of cardiovascular damage?

Regarding the first question, the emerging hypothesis that could explain the phenomenon of sympathetic overactivation in patients with PI has centered on the concept of hyperarousal. Evidence from numerous pathophysiological models suggests that insomnia is characterized by an inappropriate physiological arousal resulting in a multisystem overactivation (including sympathetic hyperactivity), thus promoting wakefulness and blocking the occurrence of sleep at the desired time [9]. High-frequency electroencephalogram (EEG) activation, abnormal hormone secretion, and increased metabolic activation, as well as elevated heart rate and sympathetic nervous system activity during sleep, are the main consequences of the central and autonomic overactivation. Moreover, considering that this activation is chronic, this could really be responsible for elevated cardiovascular risk in insomnia patients. Of note, the concept of hyperarousal as a basis for insomnia offers several medical implications. Cardiac autonomic overactivation as biomarker of autonomic hyperarousal may be a potential pharmacological target. In this regard, the treatment of hyperarousal reducing the physiological activation and consequently the sympathetic activity may be a useful therapeutic strategy for the treatment of insomnia [9].

The second question is more complex than the first. The three proposed mechanisms related to sympathetic overactivation causing CVD in PI include the following: (1) impact of sympathetic hyperactivity on blood pressure and heart rate, (2) increased sympathoadrenal activity, and (3) an imbalance between the sympathetic and parasympathetic activities (Fig. 14.1).

Blood Pressure and Heart Rate

Blood pressure (BP) and heart rate (HR) are independently regulated by the circadian oscillations and sleep-related processes. While HR is widely regulated by the circadian system (e.g., the diurnal rhythm), BP seems to be influenced by sleep-state transitions [10]. Although the main determinant of the circadian influences of sleep on BP is physiological

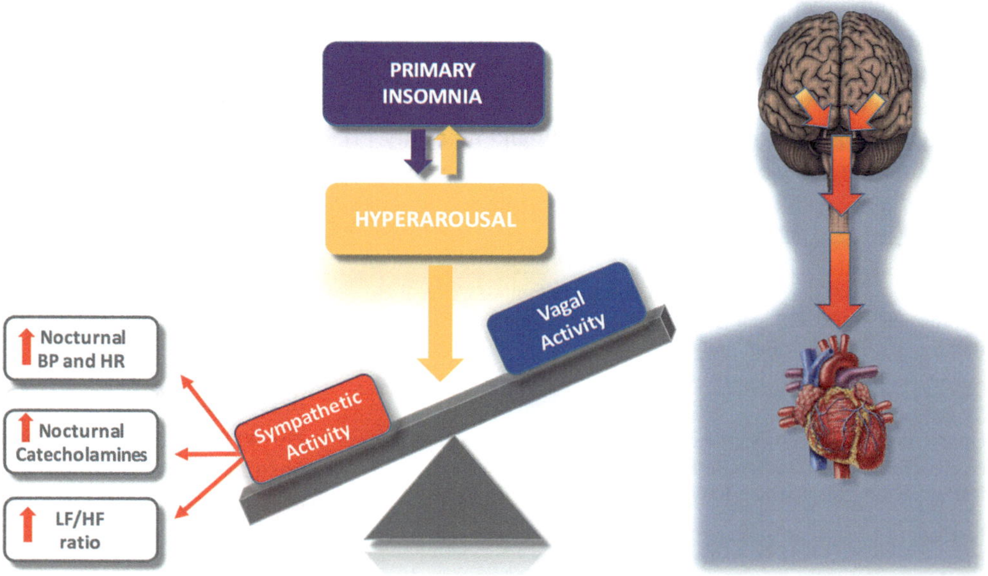

Fig. 14.1 Schematic representation of the pathophysiological mechanisms linking primary insomnia to cardiovascular disease. *BP* blood pressure, *HR* heart rate, *LF/HF ratio* low frequency/high frequency ratio

night time parasympathetic prevalence, many other mechanisms known to induce sleep or determine arousal play a crucial role in the mediation of sleep influences on BP. Alterations of one or more of such mechanisms may be reflected in altered circadian BP rhythms. Thus, it is possible to speculate that changes in the circadian BP rhythm may be strongly related to cardiovascular morbidity and mortality and represent strong prognostic indicators worthy of further investigation [11].

Over time, several pathophysiological models have analyzed BP and HR both separately and together (Table 14.1) [12–18]. Lanfranchi et al. [12] investigated the interaction between sleep and BP regulation. In order to provide daytime, night-time, and day-to-night BP changes, the authors performed a 24-hour BP recording in 13 normotensive subjects with PI and 13 sex- and age-matched good sleepers. An increase in nocturnal systolic BP and a reduction in systolic BP day-to-night dipping have been reported in insomniacs compared to the controls. The authors concluded suggesting this as a mechanism implicated in the development of cardiovascular morbidity and mortality in PI. Regarding HR, Stepanski et al. [13] assessed the physiological activity in 24 patients with chronic insomnia before sleep, during sleep, and in response to acute stress compared to 25 normal good sleepers. The authors found that HR was significantly higher in the insomniac group during the night. In accordance with these findings, a late spectral heart rate variability (HRV) analysis study [14] revealed significantly increased low-frequency power, suggestive of increased sympathetic nervous system activity in insomniacs versus controls across all stages of sleep thus supporting the hypothesis of nocturnal sympathetic hyperactivity. These data, however, have not been subsequently replicated by other authors reporting no difference in HR between insomnia patients and control subjects [15, 16, 19]. In a recent review of the literature, Dodds et al. [20] showed that 9 of their 12 included studies reported no statistically significant difference in HR values between insomnias and controls. Finally, Nilsson et al. [17] investigated blood sampling, BP, and pulse rate after 10 min supine rest in 22,444 men and 10,902 women, at baseline and after a follow-up period of several years in order to evaluate the impact of sleep disorders and resting HR on long-term mortality. They found that increased total mortality was shown in men reporting successively worse sleep problems (difficulty in initiating and maintaining sleep) and higher HR compared with men free from sleep problems and with normal HR, thus suggesting that sleep disorder is a risk factor for cardiovascular mortality [17].

Taken together, these findings suggest that despite the initial enthusiasm, evidence for elevated resting HR in patients with PI remains debatable. Conversely, nocturnal BP alterations occurring in PI patients may represent a starting point which warrants further research.

Table 14.1 Neurophysiological studies in insomnia patients

Studies	Participants	Methods	Findings
Lanfranchi et al. 2009 [12]	13 normotensive subjects with chronic primary insomnia and 13 sex- and age-matched good sleepers	24-h beat-to-beat BP	Altered BP profile in insomniacs could be one mechanism implicated in the link between insomnia and cardiovascular morbidity
Stepanski et al. 1994 [13]	24 patients with chronic insomnia before sleep, during sleep, and in response to acute stress compared to 25 normal good sleepers	HRV	HR was significantly higher in the insomniac group during the night
Bonnet et al. 1998 [14]	12 objectively defined insomniacs and age-, sex-, and weight-matched controls with normal sleep	HRV	Significantly increased low frequency power in insomniacs compared with the controls across all sleep stage
Jurysta et al. 2009 [15]	14 male patients with chronic primary insomnia matched with 14 healthy men	HRV and delta sleep determined at the EEG	Absence of modifications in HRV in patients with insomnia
Spiegelhalder et al. 2011 [16]	58 patients with primary insomnia and 46 healthy controls	HRV	Differences between groups in resting HR were not found
Nilsson et al. 2001 [17]	22,444 men and 10,902 women, a population-based health screening study	Examination of BP and pulse rate after 10 min supine resting	Increased total mortality was shown in men reporting successively worse sleep problems and higher HR
Irwin et al. 2003 [18]	17 subjects with primary insomnia and 14 patients with current major depression as compared to 31 controls	Sleep EEG, nocturnal sympathetic activity, and daytime measures of immune function	In insomnias patients, nocturnal increases of average levels of circulating norepinephrine and decreases of natural killer cell responses

BP blood pressure, *HRV* heart rate variability, *HR* heart rate, *EEG* electroencephalography

Sympathoadrenal Activity and Imbalance Between the Sympathetic and Parasympathetic Activities

There are limited studies with inconsistent results assessing the sympathoadrenal activity in PI. This is surprising, since norepinephrine is the main neurotransmitter released by the sympathetic terminal nerves, is easy to measure, and is considered to be a biomarker for sympathetic activity in humans. In order to investigate the sympathoadrenal activity, several studies measured the urinary levels of catecholamines, whereas there is only one report evaluating the plasma levels. The results on the catecholamine urinary levels in PI patients are not fully convergent and replicated. Nocturnal increases of average levels of circulating norepinephrine have been reported in PI compared to controls [18]. This evidence, although preliminary, suggests that insomnia may be associated with nocturnal sympathetic overactivation.

The correct balance between ANS sympathetic and parasympathetic activity is a crucial step in the chain of physiological responses mediated by the cardiovascular system. While parasympathetic regulation of the heart by the vagus nerve consists of an inhibition of the pacemaker activity with consequent reductions of heart rate, the opposite effect is produced by the sympathetic innervation by postganglionic neurons releasing norepinephrine [21]. One of the most promising quantitative markers of cardiac autonomic balance is HRV analysis, a simple and noninvasive measure of cardiac impulses. In the HRV spectral analysis, low-frequency (LF) components are conventionally considered to be influenced by the sympathetic system and high frequency (HF) influenced by the parasympathetic system. The LF/HF ratio expresses the physiological balance of sympathetic/parasympathetic activity. Despite the initial enthusiasm for the studies reporting a LF/HF ratio significantly higher in insomnia patients suggestive of an increase of sympathetic activity, recently, Dodds et al. [20] reviewed several observational studies finding no significant statistical differences in LF/HF between two groups. This review of existing literature seems not to support the hypothesis of the sympathetic hyperactivity in PI.

A significantly lower parasympathetic activity has been reported in PI patients with short sleep duration compared to the controls [16]. These results, however, have not been unambiguously replicated. Further HRV studies are needed to better elucidate whether an imbalance of sympathetic and parasympathetic activities is involved in the pathogenetic mechanism of PI.

In summary, there is a robust evidence demonstrating that PI is associated with CVD and increased cardiovascular risk. Our knowledge, however, on the mechanisms linking PI to cardiovascular risk remains incomplete.

Primary Insomnia and Cardiovascular Risk: The Experimental Data

During recent decades, identifying which insomnia phenotypes are at an elevated risk to develop CVD has been a primary goal of the clinical research. Therefore, quantifying the association between insomnia and poor sleep with objective short sleep duration and incident of CVD has important therapeutic implications. Furthermore, supporting evidence has demonstrated that objective measures of sleep quality as well as the severity of subjectively reported sleep are correlated with markers of increased autonomic activation. Moreover, it is necessary to determine which CVDs (e.g., hypertension, coronary heart disease, and heart failure) have a greater association with PI.

Insomnia Phenotypes and Cardiovascular Disease Risk

Insomnia with Short Sleep Duration

The finding on insomnia duration supports the hypothesis of the existence of two distinct phenotypes of insomnia (i.e., insomnia with and without objectively determined short sleep duration). Several epidemiological studies [22, 23] demonstrated that insomnia with objective short sleep is the most biologically severe phenotype of insomnia disorder. Indeed, it presents a greater clinical severity than phenotype characterized by insomnia symptoms without short sleep as well as short sleep without insomnia. The clinical importance to characterize the sleep phenotypes, however, is not exclusively related to severity of the symptoms but to a robust evidence suggesting that this phenotype is uniquely associated with higher cardiovascular risk [22, 24].

Notably, insomnia with objective short sleep duration is linked with a high risk for hypertension and type 2 diabetes [25]. In addition, in a large prospective population-based sample from central Pennsylvania, Vgontzas et al. examined the joint effects of chronic insomnia and objective sleep duration on mortality risk. Their study demonstrated that in men, chronic insomnia with objectively measured short sleep duration was associated with increased mortality, independent of comorbid conditions [26]. These findings suggest that (1) objective measures of sleep duration of insomnia might provide an index of the biological severity of the insomnia disorder and (2) the more severe form of insomnia is most likely associated with morbidity and possibly mortality [26]. The relationship between sleep phenotypes and cardiovascular risk yields two notable concepts: (1) a sex difference is observed in the vulnerability of cardiovascular risk and (2) insomnia with objective short sleep duration might represent a subtype of insomnia disorder responding differentially to the treatment.

While the relationship between insomnia with objective short sleep duration and increased mortality has been studied, the link between this sleep phenotype and major cardiovascular events (e.g., heart attack and stroke) remains unknown. Bertisch et al. were the first to quantify the association between insomnia or poor sleep with polysomnographically (PSG) measured short sleep duration and incident CVD. In their large prospective cohort study, the authors found that participants with insomnia or poor sleep and a PSG-defined sleep duration of less than 6 h. had a higher risk of incident CVD compared with participants without insomnia or poor sleep and sleep duration of at least 6 h. This evidence supports the need to characterize both objective sleep duration and insomnia symptoms in risk assessments [24].

Why insomnia with objective short sleep duration is the sleep phenotype more vulnerable to development of CVD remains to be investigated. However, physiological studies have demonstrated that the activation of the hypothalamic-pituitary-adrenal axis and hyperactivity of the sympathetic nervous system resulting in increased heart rate, 24-hour metabolic rate, and impaired HRV may occur in insomniacs who meet objective PSG criteria [26]. Several intermediate mechanisms have been also proposed in response to sympathetic hyperactivity (e.g., endothelial dysfunction, augmented inflammatory response, and alteration of coagulation system) (Fig. 14.2). These factors are of pivotal importance in the development of CVDs [27]. Thus, it is possible to speculate that insomnia with objective short sleep as well as acute or chronic sleep deprivation is associated with augmented sympathetic dysregulation and a pro-inflammatory response. Of note, various investigative methods evaluating the impact of short sleep duration in insomnia patients are heterogeneous leading to inconsistent and not replicable results.

Insomnia in Menopausal Transition State

Female sex is a strong risk factor for insomnia, with a female/male risk ratio of 1.41/1 [28]. Moreover, the prevalence of insomnia tends to vary as a function of a woman's reproductive state, being particularly evident during the menopausal transition, with 26% of women in the menopausal transition developing the disorder [29]. Therefore, it is not surprising that a growing scientific interest is focused on the potential impact of the menstrual cycle on the ANS in insomnia patients.

Recently, de Zambotti et al. [30] assessed the nocturnal BP and HR profiles in women with insomnia disorder in the menopausal transition period compared to the controls. Nocturnal systolic and diastolic BP patterns were increased in insomnia participants but remained low the in controls suggesting that altered regulatory control of BP during sleep may occur in these patients. However, the causes and consequences of this altered nocturnal BP profile remain to be determined. Currently, whether or how insomnia develops during the menopausal transition period and its impact on the cardiovascular system remains unknown. Yet, some answers may be found in another recent study from de Zambotti et al. [31] in which the authors aimed to determine whether the menopausal transition period subtype was characterized by autonomic hyperarousal similarly to the occurrence in insomnia patients not in a menopausal transition state. The question is legitimate since autonomic hyperarousal with consequent sympathetic activity plays a role in the etiology of insomnia disorder. HR was significantly elevated in insomnias compared to controls in both follicular and luteal phases and in all stages of the sleep. Moreover, in insomnia patients there is a trend of association between nocturnal increase of HR and lower nocturnal vagal activity, although the two did not show a statistically significant difference.

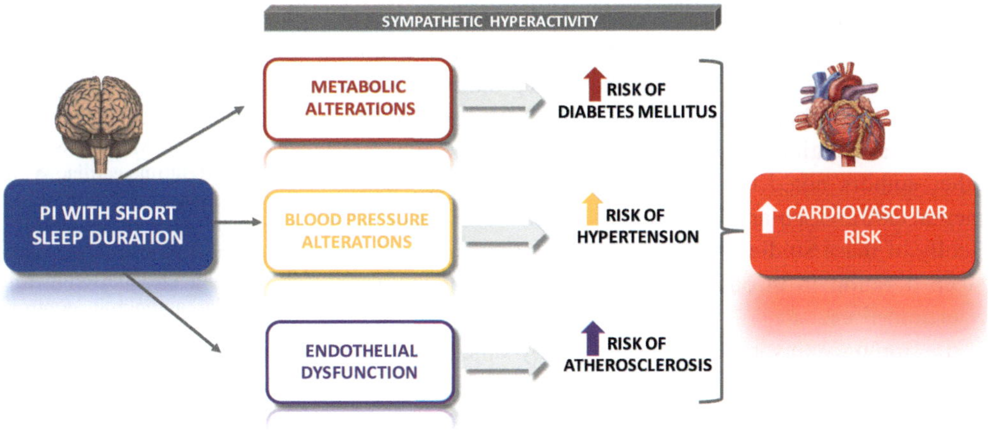

Fig. 14.2 Schematic representation of the pathophysiological mechanisms linking primary insomnia with short sleep duration to cardiovascular disease. *PI* primary insomnia

The authors concluded that insomnia in the menopausal transition may be characterized by nocturnal autonomic hyperarousal, which could be a factor in the etiology of menopausal transition insomnia (MTI) as well as a potential cardiovascular risk factor. Thus, whether insomnia patients in the menopausal transition state experience cardiac autonomic modulation during sleep differently from insomnia patients who are not, and consequently whether the MTI subtype is at a greater risk for CVD, remains to be determined.

Insomnia and Cardiovascular Diseases: The Link with Hypertension

Hypertension currently affects about 26.4% of adults worldwide. Given the clinical relevance, it is not surprising that its relationship with a very common sleep disorder (e.g., insomnia) has been documented in several cross-sectional observational and prospective adult cohort studies.

The most important research linking sleep phenotypes and hypertension risk has been conducted by Vgontzas and colleagues [26]. In a large prospective study (i.e., the Penn State Cohort), they used a sample of 1700 men and women from central Pennsylvania. After a 7-year follow-up, individuals having insomnia with short sleep duration had greater odds for hypertension incidence compared to normal sleepers. In contrast, neither individuals with chronic insomnia sleeping ≥6 h nor a control group of normal subjects showed elevated odds for either current or incident hypertension [22, 23, 26]. In addition, a recent meta-analysis of 17 prospective cohort studies assessing the relationship of sleep duration and insomnia to risk of hypertension incidence demonstrated that not only short sleep duration but also sleep continuity disturbance, early-morning awakening, and single/combined symptoms of insomnia were associated with an increased risk of hypertension incidence [32]. Finally, several factors including age, sex, smoking, obesity, and socioeconomic status seem to play a role in the relationship between insomnia with short sleep duration and higher risk of hypertension. Indeed, some authors found that short sleep duration was a significant risk factor for hypertension in younger subjects, with no association among older subjects [33, 34], whereas other authors noted that sleep deprivation produced detrimental cardiovascular effects among women. The major difficulty of these studies, however, is the assessment of short sleep duration in insomnia patients by using self-reported questionnaires.

In summary, insomnia characterized by objective PSG-short sleep duration is the most vulnerable phenotype of insomnia disorder associated with a higher risk of CVD. When insomnia disorder is present in the context of menopausal transition period, it could represent potential cardiovascular risk factor. Among CVDs, hypertension is commonly associated with this sleep phenotype.

Conclusion and Future Directions

The associations between PI and cardiovascular dysautonomia have been widely investigated by clinicians and researchers. The autonomic hyperarousal model has been proposed to explain the sympathetic hyperactivity occurring in patients with PI. Insomnia characterized by objective PSG-short sleep duration seems to be a unique phenotype of insomnia disorder associated with a higher risk of CVD. Given the clinical relevance and important therapeutic implications of the well-established PI-CVD association, we suggest that future research should be focused on (1) extending the pathogenetic mechanisms linking PI to cardiovascular risk in order to better characterize the etiology of this condition, (2) elucidating the mechanisms underlying increased cardiovascular risk in insomnia phenotype with objective short sleep duration, particularly the role of short sleep duration on the development of CVD, and (3) clarifying whether the phenotype of insomnia in menopausal transition state is at elevated risk more than insomnia patients who are not in this physiological state.

References

1. American Academy of Sleep Medicine. International classification of sleep disorders, third edition: diagnostic and coding manual. Darien: American Academy of Sleep Medicine; 2014.
2. Ohayon MM. Epidemiology of insomnia: what we know and what we still need to learn. Sleep Med Rev. 2002;6(2):97–111.
3. Becker PM. Insomnia: prevalence, impact, pathogenesis, differential diagnosis, and evaluation. Psychiatr Clin North Am. 2006;29(4):855–70.
4. Palma JA. Autonomic dysfunction in sleep disorders: introduction to the series. Clin Auton Res. 2018;28(6):507–8.
5. Miglis MG. Autonomic dysfunction in primary sleep disorders. Sleep Med. 2016;19:40–9.
6. Janackova S, Sforza E. Neurobiology of sleep fragmentation: cortical and autonomic markers of sleep disorders. Curr Pharm Des. 2008;14(32):3474–80.
7. de Zambotti M, Covassin N, Sarlo M, De Min Tona G, Trinder J, et al. Nighttime cardiac sympathetic hyper-activation in young primary insomniacs. Clin Auton Res. 2013;23(1):49–56.
8. Spiegelhalder K, Scholtes C, Riemann D. The association between insomnia and cardiovascular diseases. Nat Sci Sleep. 2010;2:71–8.
9. Grimaldi D, Goldsteinb MR, Carterc JR. Insomnia and cardiovascular autonomic control. Auton Neurosci. 2019;220:102551. Review.
10. Trinder J, Kleiman J, Carrington M, Smith S, Breen S, Tan N, Kim Y. Autonomic activity during human sleep as a function of time and sleep stage. J Sleep Res. 2001;10(4):253–64.
11. Smolensky MH, Hermida RC, Castriotta RJ, Portaluppi F. Role of sleep-wake cycle on blood pressure circadian rhythms and hypertension. Sleep Med. 2007;8(6):668–80.

12. Lanfranchi PA, Pennestri MH, Fradette L, Dumont M, Morin CM, Montplaisir J. Nighttime blood pressure in normotensive subjects with chronic insomnia: implications for cardiovascular risk. Sleep. 2009;32(6):760–6.
13. Stepanski EJ, Glinn M, Zorick F, Roehrs T, Roth T. Heart rate changes in chronic insomnia. Stress Med. 1994;10(4):261–6.
14. Bonnet MH, Arand DL. Heart rate variability in insomniacs and matched normal sleepers. Psychosom Med. 1998;60(5):610–5.
15. Jurysta F, Lanquart JP, Sputaels V, Dumont M, Migeotte PF, Leistedt S, et al. The impact of chronic primary insomnia on the heart rate-EEG variability link. Clin Neurophysiol. 2009;120(6):1054–60.
16. Spiegelhalder K, Fuchs L, Ladwig J, Kyle SD, Nissen C, Voderholzer U, et al. Heart rate and heart rate variability in subjectively reported insomnia. J Sleep Res. 2011;20(1 Pt 2):137–45.
17. Nilsson PM, Nilsson JA, Hedblad B, Berglund G. Sleep disturbance in association with elevated pulse rate for prediction of mortality consequences of mental strain? J Intern Med. 2001;250(6):521–9.
18. Irwin M, Clark C, Kennedy B, Gillin JC, Ziegler M. Nocturnal catecholamines and immune function in insomniacs, depressed patients, and control subjects. Brain Behav Immun. 2003;17(5):365–72.
19. Varkevisser M, Kerkhof GA. Chronic insomnia and performance in a 24-h constant routine study. J Sleep Res. 2005;14(1):49–59.
20. Dodds KL, Miller CB, Kyle SD, Marshall NS, Gordon CJ. Heart rate variability in insomnia patients: a critical review of the literature. Sleep Med Rev. 2017;33:88–100.
21. Benarroch EE. The central autonomic network: functional organization, dysfunction, and perspective. Mayo Clin Proc. 1993;68(10):988–1001.
22. Vgontzas AN, Fernandez-Mendoza J, Liao D, Bixler EO. Insomnia with objective short sleep duration: the most biologically severe phenotype of the disorder. Sleep Med Rev. 2013;17(4):241–54.
23. Fernandez-Mendoza J. The insomnia with short sleep duration phenotype: an update on its importance for health and prevention. Curr Opin Psychiatry. 2017;30(1):56–63.
24. Bertisch SM, Pollock BD, Mittleman MA, Buysse DJ, Bazzano LA, Gottlieb DJ, et al. Insomnia with objective short sleep duration and risk of incident cardiovascular disease and all-cause mortality: Sleep Heart Health Study. Sleep. 2018;41(6):zsy047.
25. Vgontzas AN, Liao D, Pejovic S, Calhoun S, Karataraki M, Bixler EO. Insomnia with objective short sleep duration is associated with type 2 diabetes: a population-based study. Diabetes Care. 2009;32(11):1980–5.
26. Vgontzas AN, Liao D, Pejovic S, Calhoun S, Karataraki M, Basta M, et al. Insomnia with short sleep duration and mortality: the Penn State cohort. Sleep. 2010;33(9):1159–64.
27. Tobaldini E, Fiorelli EM, Solbiati M, Costantino G, Nobili L, Montano N. Short sleep duration and cardiometabolic risk: from pathophysiology to clinical evidence. Nat Rev Cardiol. 2019;6(4):213–24.
28. Zhang B, Wing YK. Sex differences in insomnia: a meta-analysis. Sleep. 2006;29(1):85–93.
29. Ohayon MM. Severe hot flashes are associated with chronic insomnia. Arch Intern Med. 2006;166(12):1262–8.
30. de Zambotti M, Trinder J, Javitz H, Colrain IM, Baker FC. Altered nocturnal blood pressure profiles in women with insomnia disorder in the menopausal transition. Menopause. 2017;24(3):278–87.
31. de Zambotti M, Trinder J, Colrain IM, Baker FC. Menstrual cycle-related variation in autonomic nervous system functioning in women in the early menopausal transition with and without insomnia disorder. Psychoneuroendocrinology. 2017;75:44–51.
32. Meng L, Zheng Y, Hui R. The relationship of sleep duration and insomnia to risk of hypertension incidence: a meta-analysis of prospective cohort studies. Hypertens Res. 2013;36(11):985–95.
33. Wu X, Sun Y, Niu K, Yao W, Bian B, Yu X, et al. Association of self-reported sleep duration and hypertension: results of a Chinese prospective cohort study. Clin Exp Hypertens. 2016;38(6):514–9.
34. Kim J, Jo I. Age-dependent association between sleep duration and hypertension in the adult Korean population. Am J Hypertens. 2010;23(12):1286–91.

Restless Legs Syndrome, Periodic Limb Movements, and Dysautonomia

15

Marie-Hélène Pennestri, Rebecca Burdayron, and Alex Desautels

Restless Legs Syndrome: Description, Diagnosis, and Prevalence

Description

Restless legs syndrome (RLS) is a neurological sensorimotor disorder. Although its symptoms have been described for centuries, RLS was identified as a distinct clinical entity in 1945 by the neurologist Karl-Axel Ekbom [1]. More recently, it is also recognized as Willis-Ekbom disease. Patients with RLS report an urge to move the legs, which is usually associated with dysesthesia or unpleasant sensations. These sensations are particularly present when patients are at rest, with a worsening of the symptoms during the evening or night. In most patients, these sensations are described as uncomfortable or unpleasant. However, some patients describe painful sensations that are creepy-crawly, internally itchy, or shock-like. Up to 50% of RLS patients also have unpleasant sensations in the arms [2]. RLS is often associated with sleep complaints, especially with difficulty falling asleep at night because of the dysesthesia, as well as nighttime awakenings [3].

M.-H. Pennestri (✉) · R. Burdayron
Department of Educational and Counselling Psychology, McGill University, Montréal, QC, Canada

Hôpital en Santé Mentale Rivière-des-Prairies, CIUSSS du Nord-de-l'Ile-de-Montréal, Montréal, QC, Canada
e-mail: marie-helene.pennestri@mcgill.ca

A. Desautels
Department of Neurology, University of Montréal, Montréal, QC, Canada

Center for Advanced Research in Sleep Medicine, Sacré-Coeur Hospital, Montréal, QC, Canada

Diagnosis

No biological marker is available in order to diagnose RLS. Therefore, the diagnosis of RLS is based on a clinical evaluation where the clinician assesses the patient's subjective symptoms. The International RLS Study Group (IRLSSG) established five criteria required for a diagnosis of RLS: (1) an urge to move the legs, usually accompanied by uncomfortable and unpleasant sensations in the legs; (2) symptoms begin or worsen during periods of rest or inactivity, such as sitting or lying down; (3) symptoms are partially or totally removed by movement; (4) a worsening of the condition in the evening or at night; and (5) the occurrence of the symptoms is not solely accounted for as symptoms primary to another medical or behavioral condition such as myalgia, venous stasis, arthritis, or positional discomfort [4].

Moreover, there are common clinical features that can further support a diagnosis of RLS. Although they are not essential, they can be helpful in the case of diagnostic uncertainty. These features include the presence of periodic limb movements in sleep (PLMS), a clinical benefit of dopaminergic medications, a family history of RLS, and a lack of profound daytime sleepiness [4].

Prevalence

RLS is the most common movement disorder and one of the most common sleep disorders, with a prevalence between 5 and 10% in large epidemiologic surveys [5]. However, clinically significant cases account for about 2.7% [6]. While RLS symptoms usually begin around middle-age, some patients develop the disease at an earlier age. This is particularly true in familial cases of RLS, which usually have a slower disease progression [7, 8]. The prevalence is about twice as high in women than in men [9]. Unfortunately, RLS remains underdiagnosed and undertreated [10–12].

S. Chokroverty, P. Cortelli (eds.), *Autonomic Nervous System and Sleep*, https://doi.org/10.1007/978-3-030-62263-3_15

Periodic Limb Movements During Sleep and Wakefulness

Although not exclusively observed in RLS, PLMS are commonly associated with RLS. They can occur during sleep (PLMS) or wakefulness (PLMW) before sleep or during nighttime awakenings. They were first recorded in RLS patients by Coccagna and Lugaresi and were named nocturnal myoclonus [13]. They are described as a rhythmic extension of the big toe and dorsiflexion of the ankle, with occasional flexion of the knee and hip. Movements are considered as PLMS if they are part of a series of at least four consecutive leg movements, with each movement ranging between 0.5 and 10 seconds and an inter-movement interval between 10 and 90 seconds [14].

In RLS patients, the prevalence of PLMS is high, ranging between 80 and 90% [3, 15]. However, PLMS are not a distinct clinical entity and are also commonly observed in other sleep disorders, such as narcolepsy, REM sleep behavior disorder, obstructive sleep apnea, insomnia, and hypersomnia. Moreover, they are also found in healthy subjects without any sleep complaints and have been found to increase with age (Fig. 15.1) [16]. While they are less frequently observed in healthy children and adolescents, they are particularly prevalent in the elderly [16]. In adult populations, an index of more than 15 PLMS per hour of sleep is considered as clinically significant (ICSD-3) [17], with a prevalence ranging between 4.3 and 9.3% in the general population [18]. Whether PLMS have an impact on objective or subjective sleep quality in healthy and clinical populations remains unclear [19–21]. However, even though there are still controversies related to their functional significance, PLMS are commonly recorded and used to support a diagnosis of RLS.

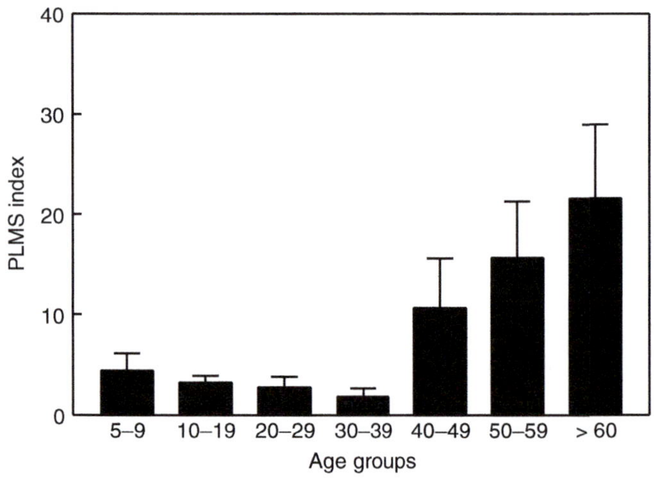

Fig. 15.1 Mean periodic leg movements during sleep (PLMS) index for healthy subjects according to seven age groups (5–9 y, 10–29 y, 20–29 y, 30–39 y, 40–49 y, 50–59 y, and 60 y and older). Vertical bars represent the SEM. (From Pennestri et al. [16] with permission)

Association Between RLS and Cardiovascular Disease

Epidemiological Cross-Sectional Studies

Other sleep disorders, such as sleep-related breathing disorders, have been studied extensively for their association with cardiovascular diseases (CVD). In contrast, the interest in the association between RLS and cardiovascular abnormalities is more recent. During the last few years, numerous cross-sectional studies have suggested positive associations between RLS and cardiovascular outcomes. In a mailed epidemiological survey, Ulfberg et al. [22] documented that in individuals fulfilling RLS criteria, the odds ratio of reporting heart problems was 2.5 (95% CI: 1.4–4.3). Ohayon and Roth also showed an OR of 1.41 (95% CI: 1.06–1.88) for the association between heart disease and RLS [15]. Winkelman and colleagues [23] evaluated the association between RLS and CVD with data from 2821 participants in the Wisconsin Sleep Cohort and found that daily symptoms of RLS were associated with 2.58 odds for CVD (95% CI: 1.38–4.84). In a second community-based, middle-aged, and elderly cohort of the Sleep Heart Health Study, Winkelman et al. [24] further found a 2.07 (95% CI: 1.43–3.00) odds for CVD in participants with RLS after adjustment for confounders. Notably, this association increased with RLS severity. For the most part, subsequent cross-sectional studies have reported similar associations [25]. Therefore, associations between RLS (defined as per IRLSSG criteria in most studies) and various manifestations of CVD (such as coronary artery disease (CAD), congestive heart failure, and myocardial infarction) have been described in several cohorts [9, 26–28].

However, some other cross-sectional studies did not find such an association [29–31]. For instance, the OR for overall CVD was 0.97 (95% CI 0.79–1.2) in a cohort of 22,786 men [32] and 0.98 (95% CI 0.74–1.29) in a cohort of 30,262 women [29]. In a recent case-control study of 487 patients with primary RLS and 354 controls, no association between RLS and CVD was found after adjusting for confounding variables [33].

Longitudinal Epidemiological Studies

A growing number of longitudinal studies have also evaluated associations between RLS and cardiovascular outcomes. While prospective studies can help determine causal relationships, these studies have yielded mixed results. In the Nurses' Health Study which accounted for RLS duration since diagnosis, women who reported having obtained a diagnosis of RLS at least three years prior were found to be at increased risk for CAD (HR = 1.72, 95% CI: 1.09–2.73) and fatal coronary heart disease (HR = 1.49, 95% CI: 0.55–4.04) [34]. In contrast, two large prospective cohort studies (Women's Health Study and Physicians' Health Study) by the same group reported no significant association between RLS and CVD in female (HR = 1.15, 95% CI: 0.88–1.50) and male (HR = 1.01, 95% CI: 0.81–1.25) health professionals with RLS [35].

Since RLS has been associated with other medical conditions (such as iron deficiency anemia and uremia), some authors have proposed to distinguish primary forms of RLS from secondary forms of RLS when the comorbid condition precedes the RLS manifestations. To that effect, Van Den Eeden et al. [36] prospectively examined the association between RLS and cardiovascular risk separately in primary and secondary RLS patients. They reported an increased risk for cardiovascular outcomes in patients with secondary RLS (HR = 1.33, 95% CI: 1.21–1.46), but not primary RLS (HR = 0.95, 95% CI: 0.86 – 1.04).

A recent meta-analysis of eight studies found no evidence for an increased risk of cerebrovascular or cardiovascular events in RLS patients after adjusting for putative confounders, despite a higher risk of all-cause mortality [37]. Another recent systematic review evaluated 18 cohorts (within 13 manuscripts) and also showed mixed findings regarding RLS as a prognostic factor for CVD [38]. The authors concluded that while the current state of the epidemiological literature on the association between RLS and cardiovascular risk is unclear, inconsistent outcomes may be attributed to differences in study populations, RLS diagnostic methods and criteria, presence of comorbidities, disease factors (e.g., severity and duration), and measured confounders, such as the presence of other sleep disorders or other cardiovascular risk factors.

In a recent study of 2823 community-based men, both RLS and PLMS were associated with myocardial infarction over eight years of average follow-up (although not to a composite of CVD outcomes). Of note, the association remained significant, even when considering both RLS and PLMS concurrently, suggesting that both of these entities potentially contribute independently to CVD risk [39]. Therefore, the presence of PLMS should also be considered when assessing the association between RLS and CVD.

Association Between PLMS and Cardiovascular Disease

While RLS and PLMS commonly co-occur, some authors have proposed that the presence of PLMS per se (i.e., not necessarily associated with RLS) could represent a specific cardiovascular risk factor and mortality risk [40–43]. To that effect, higher PLMS indexes have been observed in several types of CVD, such as in patients with congestive heart failure [44–46]. A higher PLMS index has also been shown to correlate with arteriolosclerosis, which is a known precursor to lacunar stroke [47]. Although PLMS indexes were not different in a group of patients with or without transient ischemic attack (TIA), PLMS indexes were higher in the TIA group after excluding obstructive sleep apnea syndrome [48].

In a large prospective study ($N = 2911$ elderly men), the frequency of PLMS was associated with increased cardiovascular events [41]. In a more recent population-based study of 2162 participants, a PLMS index greater than 15 per hour of sleep was associated with a higher prevalence of hypertension, diabetes, and metabolic syndrome. However, this difference was no longer present after adjusting for confounding factors [21]. In another retrospective study of 1163 participants with a PSG recording, no association was found between PLMS and daytime blood pressure [49].

Possible Mechanisms Linking RLS and PLMS with CVD

Several mechanisms have been proposed to explain the association between RLS, PLMS, and CVD. Three of these hypotheses will be discussed in this section: (1) sleep disruptions, (2) PLMS-related cardiovascular fluctuations, and (3) increased sympathetic activity in RLS.

Sleep Disruptions

In healthy subjects, we usually observe a significant decrease in blood pressure during the night (approximately 10%), a phenomenon called "nocturnal blood pressure dipping" [50]. However, indices of fragmented sleep, such as lower sleep efficiency and longer duration of wakefulness after sleep onset (WASO), are associated with an attenuation of this nocturnal blood pressure reduction in otherwise healthy subjects [51]. Moreover, in patients complaining of insomnia, increased heart rate variability (HRV), increased sympathetic tone, and the absence of this nocturnal dipping pattern were also documented [52–54]. Since a non-dipping pattern has been identified as a risk factor for cardiovascular morbidity and mortality [55–57] and that patients with RLS often complain of nocturnal sleep disruption [3, 6], this mechanism could at least partially contribute to the association between RLS and CVD. To further support this hypothesis, chronic sleep deprivation (sleeping less than 5 or 6 hours per night) and complaints of insomnia have both been associated with an increased risk of hypertension or CVD in large cohorts [58–61].

PLMS-Related Cardiovascular Changes

RLS patients not only suffer from sleep disruptions but they also often have high PLMS indexes. Therefore, another potential key mechanism linking RLS and CVD is PLMS-related cardiovascular fluctuations. It is now well known that every PLM is associated with a transient tachycardia, followed by a bradycardia [62, 63]. Furthermore, beat-to-beat recordings of blood pressure allowed for the observation of significant increases in systolic and diastolic blood pressure in association with PLMS [64–66]. On average, increases were about 22 mmHg for systolic blood pressure and 11 mmHg for diastolic blood pressure in RLS patients, but in some patients, increases could reach up to 29 mmHg for systolic blood pressure and 20 mmHg for diastolic blood pressure (Fig. 15.2) [64].

About one-third of PLMS are also associated with an EEG micro-arousal [62]. When PLMS occur in association with micro-arousals, the increases in heart rate and blood pressure are even more substantial [62–64, 66]. However, it is not clear whether the PLM provokes the micro-arousal or vice versa [67]. Notably, these two phenomena can be dissociated: dopaminergic agonists effectively decrease PLMS index but not arousals, as opposed to benzodiazepines, which reduce the presence of arousals but not PLMS [68, 69]. These results suggest that micro-arousals and PLMS are not necessarily the consequence of each other but are instead part of a global arousal mechanism.

These cardiovascular increases were also described to be higher when PLMS were bilateral [70] and when the inter-interval was shorter [71]. Although cardiovascular activations associated with PLMS have been reported to be of greater amplitude in RLS patients, they have also been observed in otherwise healthy non-RLS subjects with PLMS [72, 73]. It is well recognized that increased blood pressure variability is associated with both cerebrovascular and cardiovascular damages [74–76]. Considering that RLS patients often show very high indexes of PLMS, these repetitive increases of blood pressure occurring night after night during several years have the potential to contribute to the increased risk of CVD in RLS. Moreover, these repetitive blood pressure fluctuations during the night also have the potential to alter the nocturnal dipping and could explain the link between RLS and CVD.

Increased Sympathetic Activity

Alternatively, it has also been proposed that increased sympathetic activity in RLS patients could lead to a higher risk of CVD. In animal models of RLS, the hypodopaminergic state correlates with hypofunction of the A11 diecephalospinal descending pathway, which projects to the preganglionic sympathetic neurons located in the intermediolateral columns. Dysfunction in these spinal inhibitory projections may result in an increased sympathetic activation, hence predisposing to CVD [77–79].

Indeed, various indices of increased sympathetic activity have been described in RLS, such as an attenuated baroreflex gain [80] and lower levels of flow-mediated brachial artery dilation [81]. The odd of slow coronary flow was reported to be 3.11 times higher in patients with RLS compared to non-RLS healthy subjects (95% CI: 1.54–6.29) [82]. RLS has also been identified as an independent determinant for the non-dipping blood pressure pattern [83].

PLMS-related autonomic fluctuations could be one of these manifestations and represent one of the markers of this autonomic dysfunction. To that effect, HR and BP changes associated with PLMS have been described to precede the movement [62–64, 66, 72, 84] (see Fig. 15.2). Therefore, authors have proposed that PLMS could be part of a central periodic activation and that a central generator could periodically trigger cardiovascular changes, micro-arousals, PLMS, or other types of arousal responses that could follow a hierarchy of arousal [85–88].

Finally, some authors evaluated HRV in RLS patients. While some studies described a higher low frequency/high frequency (LF-HF) ratio in RLS patients (usually a marker of increased sympathetic activity), one needs to be careful in interpreting the significance of these findings [89, 90]. Indeed, PLMS typically have an inter-interval between 20 and 40 seconds, which corresponds explicitly to LF frequencies. Therefore, this temporal distribution likely explains this higher LF ratio [91], as opposed to an increase in sympathetic activity. When comparing HRV during wakefulness or sleep periods without PLMS, most studies did not find any difference between RLS and healthy subjects with or without PLMS [73, 92].

Conclusion

Although there are still controversies and some inconsistent findings, a growing body of literature shows cardiovascular abnormalities in RLS and PLMS, and a considerable number of epidemiological studies document such an association between RLS, PLMS, and CVD. However, a clear causal relationship remains to be clarified with prospective studies. Moreover, the frequent co-occurrence of RLS and PLMS contributes to the difficulty of disentangling the contribution of these two conditions on cardiovascular abnormalities. Since RLS and PLMS are prevalent, but under-recognized and undertreated conditions, a better understanding of their relationships with CVD is of major importance in clinical practice.

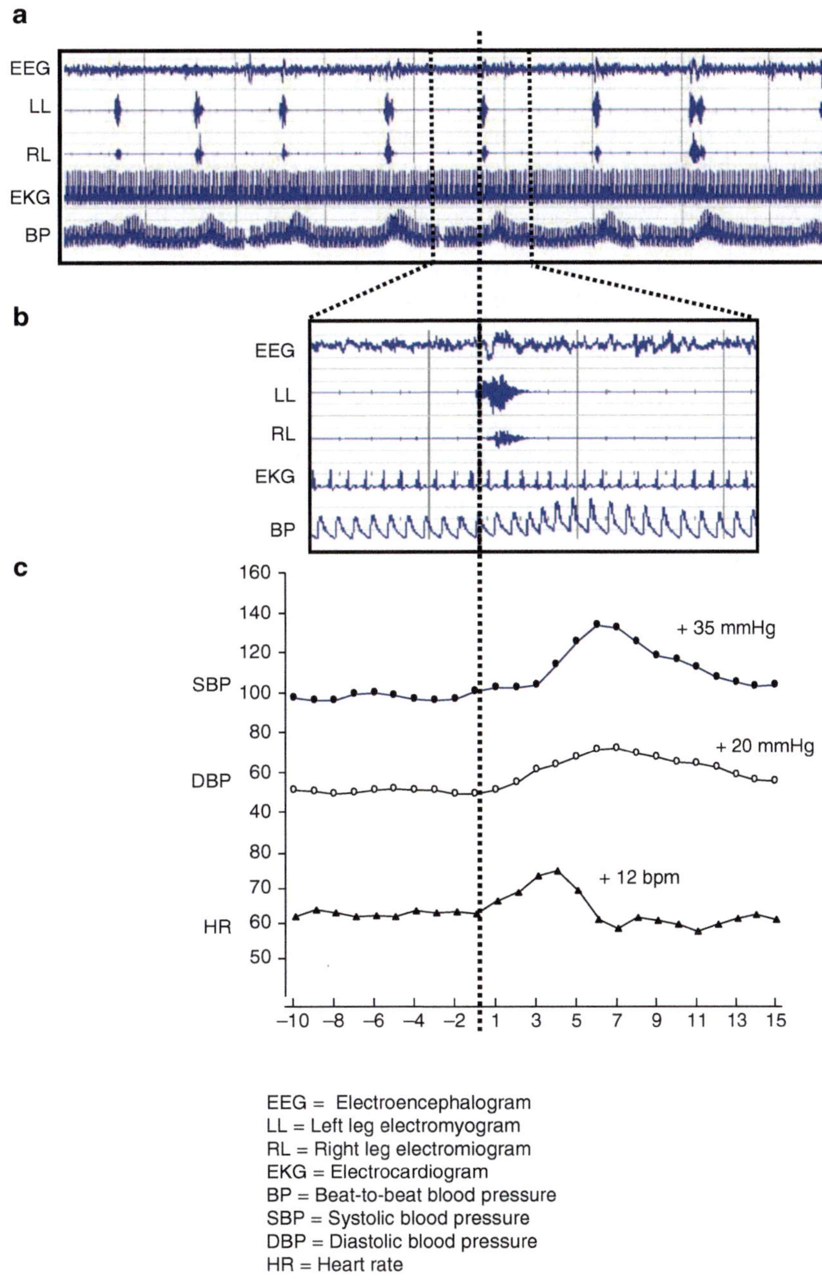

Fig. 15.2 Periodic leg movements during sleep-related beat-to-beat blood pressure, electrocardiogram, and EEG signals presented in a compact window (**a**) and wider temporal window (**b**). The portion of signals shown in (**b**) represents the temporal window used for the analyses. (**c**) The corresponding measurements of systolic blood pressure, diastolic blood pressure, and heart rate. (From Pennestri et al. [64] with permission)

References

1. Ekbom KA. Restless legs. Acta Med Scand. 1945;158(Suppl):1–123.
2. Michaud M, Chabli A, Lavigne G, Montplaisir J. Arm restlessness in patients with restless legs syndrome. Mov Disord. 2000;15(2):289–93.
3. Montplaisir J, Boucher S, Poirier G, Lavigne G, Lapierre O, Lespérance P. Clinical, polysomnographic, and genetic characteristics of restless legs syndrome: a study of 133 patients diagnosed with new standard criteria. Mov Disord. 1997;12(1):61–5.
4. Allen RP, Picchietti DL, Garcia-Borreguero D, Ondo WG, Walters AS, Winkelman JW, et al. Restless legs syndrome/Willis-Ekbom disease diagnostic criteria: updated International Restless Legs Syndrome Study Group (IRLSSG) consensus criteria – history, rationale, description, and significance. Sleep Med. 2014;15(8):860–73.
5. Allen RP, Earley CJ. Restless legs syndrome: a review of clinical and pathophysiologic features. J Clin Neurophysiol. 2001;18(2):128–47.
6. Allen RP, Walters AS, Montplaisir J, Hening W, Myers A, Bell TJ, et al. Restless legs syndrome prevalence and impact: REST general population study. Arch Intern Med. 2005;165(11):1286–92.
7. Whittom S, Dauvilliers Y, Pennestri MH, Vercauteren F, Molinari N, Petit D, et al. Age-at-onset in restless legs syndrome: a clinical and polysomnographic study. Sleep Med. 2007;9(1):54–9.
8. Winkelmann J, Muller-Myhsok B, Wittchen HU, Hock B, Prager M, Pfister H, et al. Complex segregation analysis of restless legs syndrome provides evidence for an autosomal dominant

mode of inheritance in early age at onset families. Ann Neurol. 2002;52(3):297–302.
9. Berger K, Luedemann J, Trenkwalder C, John U, Kessler C. Sex and the risk of restless legs syndrome in the general population. Arch Intern Med. 2004;164(2):196–202.
10. Einollahi B, Izadianmehr N. Restless leg syndrome: a neglected diagnosis. Nephro-urol Mon. 2014;6(5):e22009.
11. Innes KE, Selfe TK, Agarwal P. Prevalence of restless legs syndrome in North American and Western European populations: a systematic review. Sleep Med. 2011;12(7):623–34.
12. Högl B, Kiechl S, Willeit J, Saletu M, Frauscher B, Seppi K, et al. Restless legs syndrome: a community-based study of prevalence, severity, and risk factors. Neurology. 2005;64(11):1920–4.
13. Coccagna G, Lugaresi E. Restless legs syndrome and nocturnal myoclonus. Int. J Neurol. 1981;15(1-2):77–87.
14. Ferri R, Fulda S, Allen RP, Zucconi M, Bruni O, Chokroverty S, et al. World Association of Sleep Medicine (WASM) 2016 standards for recording and scoring leg movements in polysomnograms developed by a joint task force from the International and the European Restless Legs Syndrome Study Groups (IRLSSG and EURLSSG). Sleep Med. 2016;26:86–95.
15. Ohayon MM, Roth T. Prevalence of restless legs syndrome and periodic limb movement disorder in the general population. J Psychosom Res. 2002;53(1):547–54.
16. Pennestri MH, Whittom S, Adam B, Petit D, Carrier J, Montplaisir J. PLMS and PLMW in healthy subjects as a function of age: prevalence and interval distribution. Sleep. 2006;29(9):1183–7.
17. American Academy of Sleep Medicine. International classification of sleep disorders. 3rd ed. Darien: American Academy of Sleep Medicine; 2014.
18. Scofield H, Roth T, Drake C. Periodic limb movements during sleep: population prevalence, clinical correlates, and racial differences. Sleep. 2008;31(9):1221–7.
19. Hogl B. Periodic limb movements are associated with disturbed sleep. Pro J Clin Sleep Med. 2007;3(1):12–4.
20. Mahowald MW. Periodic limb movements are NOT associated with disturbed sleep. Con J Clin Sleep Med. 2007;3(1):15–7.
21. Haba-Rubio J, Marti-Soler H, Tobback N, Andries D, Marques-Vidal P, Vollenweider P, et al. Clinical significance of periodic limb movements during sleep: the HypnoLaus study. Sleep Med. 2018;41:45–50.
22. Ulfberg J, Nyström B, Carter N, Edling C. Prevalence of restless legs syndrome among men aged 18 to 64 years: an association with somatic disease and neuropsychiatric symptoms. Mov Disord. 2001;16(6):1159–63.
23. Winkelman JW, Finn L, Young T. Prevalence and correlates of restless legs syndrome symptoms in the Wisconsin Sleep Cohort. Sleep Med. 2006;7(7):545–52.
24. Winkelman JW, Shahar E, Sharief I, Gottlieb DJ. Association of restless legs syndrome and cardiovascular disease in the sleep heart health study. Neurology. 2008;70(1):35–42.
25. Innes KE, Selfe TK, Agarwal P. Restless legs syndrome and conditions associated with metabolic dysregulation, sympathoadrenal dysfunction, and cardiovascular disease risk: a systematic review. Sleep Med Rev. 2012;16(4):309–39.
26. Wesstrom J, Nilsson S, Sundstrom-Poromaa I, Ulfberg J. Restless legs syndrome among women: prevalence, co-morbidity and possible relationship to menopause. Climacteric. 2008;11(5):422–8.
27. Phillips B, Hening W, Britz P, Mannino D. Prevalence and correlates of restless legs syndrome: results from the 2005 National Sleep Foundation Poll. Chest. 2006;129(1):76–80.
28. Foley D, Ancoli-Israel S, Britz P, Walsh J. Sleep disturbances and chronic disease in older adults: results of the 2003 National Sleep Foundation Sleep in America Survey. J Psychosom Res. 2004;56(5):497–502.
29. Winter AC, Schurks M, Glynn RJ, Buring JE, Gaziano JM, Berger K, et al. Vascular risk factors, cardiovascular disease, and restless legs syndrome in women. Am J Med. 2013;126(3):220–7, 7.e1–2.
30. Cosentino FI, Arico D, Lanuzza B, Raggi A, Sciortino G, Tripodi M, et al. Absence of cardiovascular disease risk factors in restless legs syndrome. Acta Neurol Scand. 2012;125(5):319–25.
31. Lee HB, Hening WA, Allen RP, Earley CJ, Eaton WW, Lyketsos CG. Race and restless legs syndrome symptoms in an adult community sample in East Baltimore. Sleep Med. 2006;7(8):642–5.
32. Winter AC, Berger K, Glynn RJ, Buring JE, Gaziano JM, Schurks M, et al. Vascular risk factors, cardiovascular disease, and restless legs syndrome in men. Am J Med. 2013;126(3):228–35, 35.e1–2.
33. Cholley-Roulleau M, Chenini S, Béziat S, Guiraud L, Jaussent I, Dauvilliers Y. Restless legs syndrome and cardiovascular diseases: a case-control study. PLoS One. 2017;12(4):e0176552.
34. Li Y, Walters AS, Chiuve SE, Rimm EB, Winkelman JW, Gao X. Prospective study of restless legs syndrome and coronary heart disease among women. Circulation. 2012;126(14):1689–94.
35. Winter AC, Schürks M, Glynn RJ, Buring JE, Gaziano JM, Berger K, et al. Restless legs syndrome and risk of incident cardiovascular disease in women and men: prospective cohort study. BMJ Open. 2012;2(2):e000866.
36. Van Den Eeden SK, Albers KB, Davidson JE, Kushida CA, Leimpeter AD, Nelson LM, et al. Risk of cardiovascular disease associated with a restless legs syndrome diagnosis in a retrospective cohort study from Kaiser Permanente Northern California. Sleep. 2015;38(7):1009–15.
37. Katsanos A, Kosmidou M, Konitsiotis S, Tsivgoulis G, Fiolaki A, Kyritsis A, et al. Restless legs syndrome and cerebrovascular/cardiovascular events: systematic review and meta-analysis. Acta Neurol Scand. 2018;137(1):142–8.
38. Kendzerska T, Kamra M, Murray BJ, Boulos MI. Incident cardiovascular events and death in individuals with restless legs syndrome or periodic limb movements in sleep: a systematic review. Sleep. 2017;40(3)
39. Winkelman JW, Blackwell T, Stone K, Ancoli-Israel S, Redline S. Associations of incident cardiovascular events with restless legs syndrome and periodic leg movements of sleep in older men, for the outcomes of sleep disorders in older men study (MrOS sleep study). Sleep. 2017;40(4)
40. Alessandria M, Provini F. Periodic limb movements during sleep: a new sleep-related cardiovascular risk factor? Front Neurol. 2013;4:116.
41. Koo BB, Blackwell T, Ancoli-Israel S, Stone KL, Stefanick ML, Redline S. Association of incident cardiovascular disease with periodic limb movements during sleep in older men: outcomes of sleep disorders in older men (MrOS) study. Circulation. 2011;124(11):1223–31.
42. Yumino D, Wang H, Floras JS, Newton GE, Mak S, Ruttanaumpawan P, et al. Relation of periodic leg movements during sleep and mortality in patients with systolic heart failure. Am J Cardiol. 2011;107(3):447–51.
43. Benz RL, Pressman MR, Hovick ET, Peterson DD. Potential novel predictors of mortality in end-stage renal disease patients with sleep disorders. Am J Kidney Dis. 2000;35(6):1052–60.
44. Hanly PJ, Zuberi-Khokhar N. Periodic limb movements during sleep in patients with congestive heart failure. Chest. 1996;109(6):1497–502.
45. Javaheri S. Sleep disorders in systolic heart failure: a prospective study of 100 male patients. The final report. Int J Cardiol. 2006;106(1):21–8.
46. Skomro R, Silva R, Alves R, Figueiredo A, Lorenzi-Filho G. The prevalence and significance of periodic leg movements during sleep in patients with congestive heart failure. Sleep Breath. 2009;13(1):43–7.
47. Kang MK, Koo DL, Shin JH, Kwon HM, Nam H. Association between periodic limb movements during sleep and cerebral small vessel disease. Sleep Med. 2018;51:47–52.

48. Schipper MH, Jellema K, Alvarez-Estevez D, Verbraecken J, Rijsman RM. Sleep-related leg movements in patients with transient ischemic attack and controls. Eur Neurol. 2018;79(3-4):171–6.
49. Shin DS, Yang KI, Kim DE, Hwangbo Y, Koo BB, Cho YW. Periodic limb movements during sleep are not associated with hypertension in a clinical cohort of Korean adults. Am J Hypertens. 2018;31(11):1228–33.
50. Millar-Craig M, Bishop C, Raftery EB. Circadian variation of blood-pressure. Lancet. 1978;311(8068):795–7.
51. Loredo JS, Nelesen R, Ancoli-Israel S, Dimsdale JE. Sleep quality and blood pressure dipping in normal adults. Sleep. 2004;27(6):1097–103.
52. Irwin M, Clark C, Kennedy B, Christian Gillin J, Ziegler M. Nocturnal catecholamines and immune function in insomniacs, depressed patients, and control subjects. Brain Behav Immun. 2003;17(5):365–72.
53. Lanfranchi PA, Pennestri MH, Fradette L, Dumont M, Morin CM, Montplaisir J. Nighttime blood pressure in normotensive subjects with chronic insomnia: implications for cardiovascular risk. Sleep. 2009;32(6):760–6.
54. Vgontzas AN, Liao D, Bixler EO, Chrousos GP, Vela-Bueno A. Insomnia with objective short sleep duration is associated with a high risk for hypertension. Sleep. 2009;32(4):491–7.
55. Hansen TW, Li Y, Boggia J, Thijs L, Richart T, Staessen JA. Predictive role of the nighttime blood pressure. Hypertension. 2011;57(1):3–10.
56. Boggia J, Li Y, Thijs L, Hansen TW, Kikuya M, Bjorklund-Bodegard K, et al. Prognostic accuracy of day versus night ambulatory blood pressure: a cohort study. Lancet. 2007;370(9594):1219–29.
57. Verdecchia P, Porcellati C, Schillaci G, Borgioni C, Ciucci A, Battistelli M, et al. Ambulatory blood pressure. An independent predictor of prognosis in essential hypertension. Hypertension. 1994;24(6):793–801.
58. Laugsand LE, Strand LB, Platou C, Vatten LJ, Janszky I. Insomnia and the risk of incident heart failure: a population study. Eur Heart J. 2014;35(21):1382–93.
59. Fujikawa T, Tochikubo O, Kura N, Umemura S. Factors related to elevated 24-h blood pressure in young adults. Clin Exp Hypertens. 2009;31(8):705–12.
60. Gangwisch JE, Heymsfield SB, Boden-Albala B, Buijs RM, Kreier F, Pickering TG, et al. Short sleep duration as a risk factor for hypertension: analyses of the first National Health and Nutrition Examination Survey. Hypertension. 2006;47(5):833–9.
61. Hoevenaar-Blom MP, Spijkerman AM, Kromhout D, van den Berg JF, Verschuren WM. Sleep duration and sleep quality in relation to 12-year cardiovascular disease incidence: the MORGEN study. Sleep. 2011;34(11):1487–92.
62. Sforza E, Nicolas A, Lavigne G, RPGST AG, Petit D, Montplaisir J. EEG and cardiac activation during periodic leg movements in sleep support for a hierarchy of arousal responses. Neurology. 1999;52(4):786.
63. Winkelman JW. The evoked heart rate response to periodic leg movements of sleep. Sleep. 1999;22(5):575–80.
64. Pennestri MH, Montplaisir J, Colombo R, Lavigne G, Lanfranchi PA. Nocturnal blood pressure changes in patients with restless legs syndrome. Neurology. 2007;68(15):1213–8.
65. Cassel W, Kesper K, Bauer A, Grieger F, Schollmayer E, Joeres L, et al. Significant association between systolic and diastolic blood pressure elevations and periodic limb movements in patients with idiopathic restless legs syndrome. Sleep Med. 2016;17:109–20.
66. Siddiqui F, Strus J, Ming X, Lee IA, Chokroverty S, Walters AS. Rise of blood pressure with periodic limb movements in sleep and wakefulness. Clin Neurophysiol. 2007;118(9):1923–30.
67. Ferri R, Rundo F, Zucconi M, Manconi M, Bruni O, Ferini-Strambi L, et al. An evidence-based analysis of the association between periodic leg movements during sleep and arousals in restless legs syndrome. Sleep. 2015;38(6):919–24.
68. Manconi M, Ferri R, Zucconi M, Bassetti CL, Fulda S, Arico D, et al. Dissociation of periodic leg movements from arousals in restless legs syndrome. Ann Neurol. 2012;71(6):834–44.
69. Wu MN, Tseng PT, Chen TY, Chen YW, Liou LM, Lin PY, et al. The efficacy and tolerability of rotigotine on patients with periodic limb movement in sleep: a systematic review and meta-analysis. PLoS One. 2018;13(4):e0195473.
70. Ferri R, Zucconi M, Rundo F, Spruyt K, Manconi M, Ferini-Strambi L. Heart rate and spectral EEG changes accompanying periodic and non-periodic leg movements during sleep. Clin Neurophysiol. 2007;118(2):438–48.
71. Ferri R, Rundo F, Silvani A, Zucconi M, Arico D, Bruni O, et al. Short-interval leg movements during sleep entail greater cardiac activation than periodic leg movements during sleep in restless legs syndrome patients. J Sleep Res. 2017;26(5):602–5.
72. Pennestri MH, Montplaisir J, Fradette L, Lavigne G, Colombo R, Lanfranchi PA. Blood pressure changes associated with periodic leg movements during sleep in healthy subjects. Sleep Med. 2013;14(6):555–61.
73. Manconi M, Ferri R, Zucconi M, Clemens S, Rundo F, Oldani A, et al. Effects of acute dopamine-agonist treatment in restless legs syndrome on heart rate variability during sleep. Sleep Med. 2011;12(1):47–55.
74. Frattola A, Parati G, Cuspidi C, Albini F, Mancia G. Prognostic value of 24-hour blood pressure variability. J Hypertens. 1993;11(10):1133–7.
75. Zakopoulos NA, Tsivgoulis G, Barlas G, Papamichael C, Spengos K, Manios E, et al. Time rate of blood pressure variation is associated with increased common carotid artery intima-media thickness. Hypertension. 2005;45(4):505–12.
76. Roman MJ, Pickering TG, Schwartz JE, Pini R, Devereux RB. Relation of blood pressure variability to carotid atherosclerosis and carotid artery and left ventricular hypertrophy. Arterioscler Thromb Vasc Biol. 2001;21(9):1507–11.
77. Clemens S, Rye D, Hochman S. Restless legs syndrome: revisiting the dopamine hypothesis from the spinal cord perspective. Neurology. 2006;67(1):125–30.
78. Ferini-Strambi L, Walters AS, Sica D. The relationship among restless legs syndrome (Willis–Ekbom Disease), hypertension, cardiovascular disease, and cerebrovascular disease. J Neurol. 2014;261(6):1051–68.
79. Walters AS, Rye DB. Review of the relationship of restless legs syndrome and periodic limb movements in sleep to hypertension, heart disease, and stroke. Sleep. 2009;32(5):589–97.
80. Bertisch SM, Muresan C, Schoerning L, Winkelman JW, Taylor JA. Impact of restless legs syndrome on cardiovascular autonomic control. Sleep. 2016;39(3):565–71.
81. Koh SY, Kim MS, Lee SM, Hong JM, Yoon JH. Impaired vascular endothelial function in patients with restless legs syndrome: a new aspect of the vascular pathophysiology. J Neurol Sci. 2015;359(1-2):207–10.
82. Erden I, Cakcak Erden E, Durmus H, Tibilli H, Tabakci M, Kalkan ME, et al. Association between restless leg syndrom and slow coronary flow. Anadolu Kardiyol Derg. 2014;14(7):612–6.
83. Erden EC, Erden I, Türker Y, Sivri N, Dikici S, Ozsahin M. Incremental effects of restless legs syndrome on nocturnal blood pressure in hypertensive patients and normotensive individuals. Blood Press Monit. 2012;17(6):231–4.
84. Parrino L, Halasz P, Tassinari CA, Terzano MG. CAP, epilepsy and motor events during sleep: the unifying role of arousal. Sleep Med Rev. 2006;10(4):267–85.
85. Montplaisir J, Boucher S, Gosselin A, Poirier G, Lavigne G. Persistence of repetitive EEG arousals (K-alpha complexes) in RLS patients treated with L-DOPA. Sleep. 1996;19(3):196–9.

86. El-Ad B, Chervin RD. The case of a missing PLM. Sleep. 2000;23(4):450–1.
87. Sforza E, Jouny C, Ibanez V. Cardiac activation during arousal in humans: further evidence for hierarchy in the arousal response. Clin Neurophysiol. 2000;111(9):1611–9.
88. Ferrillo F, Beelke M, Canovaro P, Watanabe T, Arico D, Rizzo P, et al. Changes in cerebral and autonomic activity heralding periodic limb movements in sleep. Sleep Med. 2004;5(4):407–12.
89. Sforza E, Pichot V, Barthelemy JC, Haba-Rubio J, Roche F. Cardiovascular variability during periodic leg movements: a spectral analysis approach. Clin Neurophysiol. 2005;116(5):1096–104.
90. Guggisberg AG, Hess CW, Mathis J. The significance of the sympathetic nervous system in the pathophysiology of periodic leg movements in sleep. Sleep. 2007;30(6):755–66.
91. Walter LM, Foster AM, Patterson RR, Anderson V, Davey MJ, Nixon GM, et al. Cardiovascular variability during periodic leg movements in sleep in children. Sleep. 2009;32(8):1093–9.
92. Barone DA, Ebben MR, DeGrazia M, Mortara D, Krieger AC. Heart rate variability in restless legs syndrome and periodic limb movements of sleep. Sleep Sci. 2017;10(2):80–6.

NREM-Related Parasomnias and Dysautonomia

16

Federica Provini and Giuseppe Plazzi

Introduction

Parasomnias are defined as undesirable motor phenomena, behaviors, perceptions, or emotions that occur predominantly during the transition from wakefulness into sleep (and vice versa) or arise during arousals from sleep. According to the International Classification of Sleep Disorders (ICSD-3), there are three main categories of parasomnias: non-rapid eye movement (NREM), rapid eye movement (REM), and other parasomnias [1]. Parasomnias associated with NREM sleep consist of disorders of arousal (DoA) and sleep-related eating disorders.

This chapter focuses on DoA.

DoA are dissociated states in which awakening and sleeping features coexist, based on the fundamental hypothesis that sudden but incomplete arousals occur from slow wave sleep (SWS) because of disturbed or immature mechanisms of arousal [2–5]. During the episode (Fig. 16.1), the patient seems to be alert, but is sleeping, appearing confused, disoriented, and unresponsive to environmental stimuli [3]. Patients may exhibit a wide variety of behaviors, from inconsolable crying to complex actions such as dressing or playing an instrument, including an ability to interact with their environment, usually with relative unresponsiveness to external stimuli. In adults, the episodes could also involve the disinhibition of "basic drive states" such as feeding, aggression, and sex [6].

Traditionally, the manifestations of DoA can be considered along a spectrum with features of overlapping and increasing complexity from confusional arousal (CA) to sleep terror (ST) to sleepwalking (SW). Due to the large overlap, DoA share a number of common features. Symptoms usually arise during early childhood, with a tendency for spontaneous reduction to complete disappearance. Nevertheless, in some cases, episodes can persist beyond adolescence or can even emerge in adulthood. DoA episodes typically occur only once a night, in the first third of the night when the deepest stage of NREM sleep is predominant, usually within 1 to 2 hours after sleep onset. Since a positive family history is often reported, a common genetic background is also suspected. Sleep deprivation, sleep fragmentation (induced by sleep movements or sleep disordered breathing), fever, stress, some medications (thioridazine, lithium, perphenazine and desipramine), or alcohol consumption could enhance episodes or increase episodes frequency [7–9].Typically, patients have no recollection of the event the following morning, sometimes remembering only fragments, flashes, or vague impressions [10].

Current knowledge of DoA pathophysiology points to a dissociation between motor and mental arousal [2]. Clues supporting the above hypothesis come from studies showing a synchronous deactivation of the frontoparietal associative cortices and activation of the cingulate cortex without deactivation of thalamus, which is usually observed during NREM sleep [11–14].

Intense autonomic activation has commonly been reported in polysomnography of DoA. This is especially evident in ST, whose clinical definition includes autonomic signs (tachycardia, tachypnea, sweating, mydriasis, hyperventilation) [1]. However, detailed descriptions of autonomic activity in relationship with DoA episodes are lacking and the significance of the autonomic activation as a possible diagnostic marker is still debated, since relevant autonomic activation has also been observed in some forms of epileptic seizures [15] (Table 16.1).

The Role of Arousal

In 1968, Roger Broughton coined the term "disorder of arousal." Under this umbrella term, the author lumped parasomnias arising from slow wave sleep, like SW, ST, and CA

F. Provini (✉) · G. Plazzi
IRCCS Istituto delle Scienze Neurologiche, Bologna, Italy

Department of Biomedical and NeuroMotor Sciences (DIBINEM), University of Bologna, Bologna, Italy
e-mail: federica.provini@unibo.it

S. Chokroverty, P. Cortelli (eds.), *Autonomic Nervous System and Sleep*, https://doi.org/10.1007/978-3-030-62263-3_16

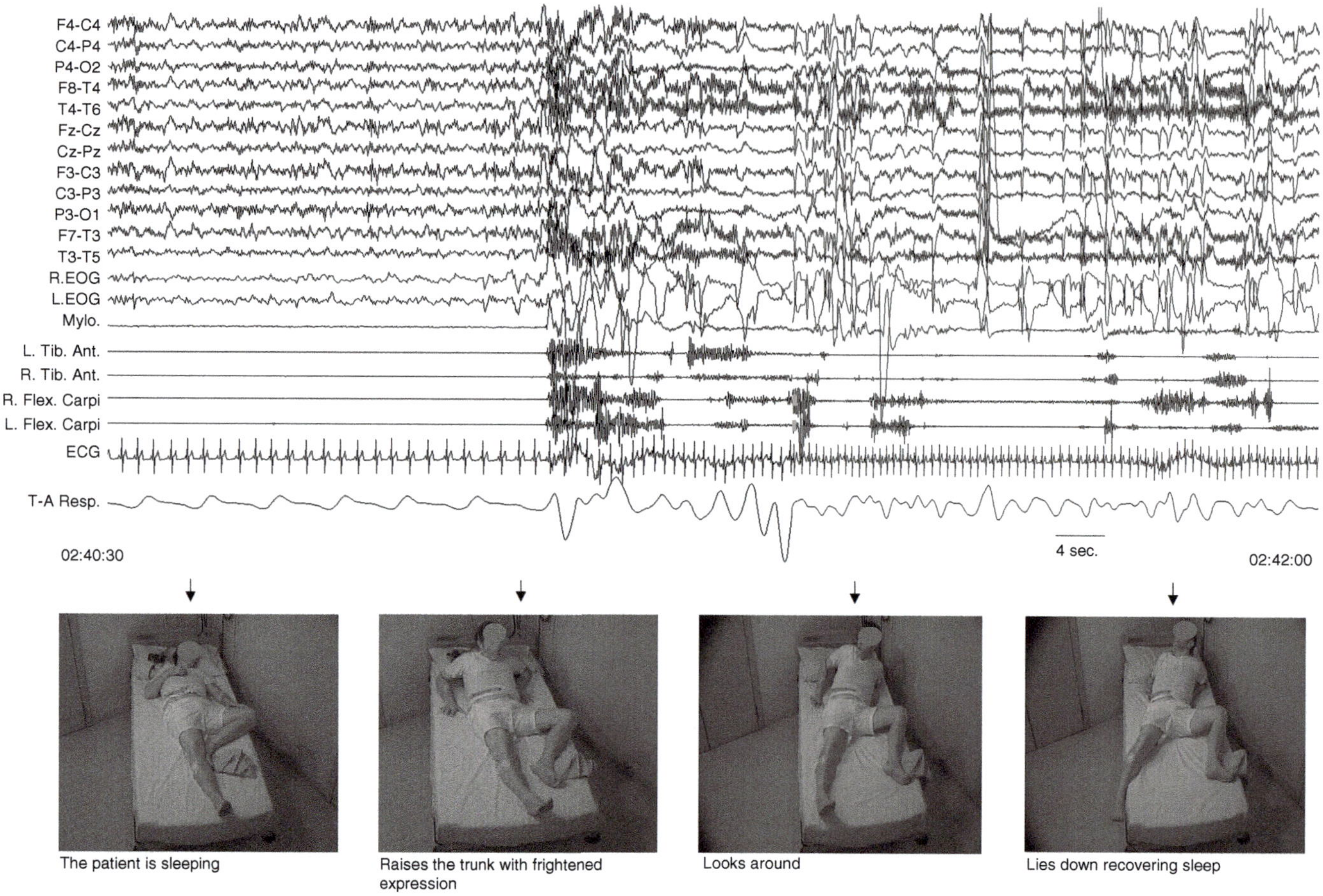

Fig. 16.1 A typical example of disorders of arousal (DoA) episode. Upper panel: Polysomnography (PSG) excerpt of the episode. The brief episode abruptly arises from non-rapid eye movement sleep (note the movement artifacts on electroencephalogram [EEG] tracing) and is associated with a marked increase in heart and breathing rate (*EOG* electro-oculogram, *Mylo.* mylohyoideus, *EKG* electrocardiogram, *Tib. Ant.* tibialis anterior muscle, *Flex* flexor, *R* right, *L* left, *T-A Resp.* thoraco-abdominal respirogram). Bottom panel: Photo-sequence of the CA episode

Table 16.1 Main features characterizing disorders of arousal

Features	Confusional arousals	Sleep terrors	Sleepwalking
Sitting on the bed and looking around as if confused	+++	++	++
Feeling of intense fear	–	+++	–/+
Frightening scream	–	+++	–
Sleeptalking	–	+	++
Ambulation	–	–	+++
Complex behaviors out of bed	–	–	++
Autonomic activation	+/–	+++	+/–
Inappropriate or no response to someone's attempts to intervene	+	+++	+++
Limited or no cognition	+	+	+
Partial or complete amnesia	+	+	+
Episode duration (min)	1–3	1–3	1–30

[16]. According to Broughton, "disorder of arousal" does not indicate the relationship between parasomnia episodes and arousal, but it indicates that the mechanism underlying the abnormal behaviors of parasomnia is an abnormal arousal process from SWS in DoA patients. In fact, in otherwise-normal subjects, a forced arousal does not precipitate an episode, while in DoA subjects, the attacks may be triggered experimentally by forced arousal. Guilleminault et al. and Gaudreau et al., observing a relevant increase in the relative power of slow delta rhythm just prior to the SW episodes, suggested that the cortical reaction to brain activation may avoid the interruption of sleep [17, 18]. Accordingly, an exaggeration of the antiarousal defense mechanisms, more evident in the first sleep cycle, may result in DoA.

Although the macrostructure of sleep does not show differences in the sleep parameters between DoA patients and age-matched controls, measures of sleep microstructure indicate an underlying increase in sleep instability and arousal oscillations in adults with SW and ST [19], as documented by an increased number of CAP cycles and a higher CAP rate (cyclic alternating pattern [CAP] scoring). This abnormal CAP sleep instability and arousal oscillation are markers of a sleep destabilizing process that plays a fundamental role for the onset of motor patterns, often already encoded in the brain (central pattern generators) [20, 21]. The isolated activation of these functional groups of motor neurons is associated not only with a relative paucity of activity in brain regions that control executive function but also memory. This accounts for the poor judgment and amnesia that characterize DoA.

Each physiological arousal induces an activation of the sympathetic system, whether these are associated with detectable modification of cortical activity or not, but more pronounced in the former case [22].

Sympathetic activation has been demonstrated to precede different stereotyped sleep-related movements such as periodic limb movements of sleep [23] and sleep bruxism [24] heralding the clear-cut EEG changes. Behavioral arousals are physiologically supported by the activation of autonomic functions. Autonomic activation, in particular an increase of heart rate, generally precedes all the other components of the behavioral arousals [22, 25].

Autonomic Activity

Autonomic nervous system activation appears differently in different DoA. Indeed, it has been described as intense in ST, low in CA, and low to moderate in SW. Nevertheless, these fluctuations have specifically been investigated in only a few studies [26].

In 1974, Fisher et al. analyzing cardiac and respiratory activity in SWS in ST in adults reported that the episodes typically arose from "physiological quiescence, with no gradual build-up" [27]. In fact, ST were associated with intense autonomic discharge, with rapid doubling or even tripling of the heart rate and a large increase in respiratory amplitude, along with a marked decrease in skin resistance.

In 1998, Schenck and Mahowald strongly supported the classification of SW/ST as disorders of arousals, performing a systematic electrophysiological analysis of 252 arousals from SWS in 38 SW/ST adults [28]. Assessing heart rate (HR) before and after behavioral and non-behavioral arousals, the authors found that HR acceleration emerged abruptly with SWS arousal, with significant changes in mean pre- versus post-arousal HR. The pre-arousal and post-arousal HR values were remarkably constant in both the parasomnia and non-parasomnia groups.

In 2005, Busek et al. conducted a spectral analysis of heart rate variability (HRV) during both sleep and wake in 10 sleepwalkers and 10 normal controls [29]. The authors found no differences between the groups of sleepwalkers and controls in the spectral analysis of HRV both during sleep and wake (horizontal position). Sleepwalkers showed a greater shift in the sympathovagal balance in favor of sympathetic activity, as a response to standing. In the authors' opinion, this autonomic nervous system reactivity was seen to be altered as a response to the orthostatic load in sleepwalkers, which could be the consequence of the instability of these patients' sleep.

Autonomic Activation in the Differential Diagnosis Between NREM Parasomnias and Epilepsy

Activation of the autonomic system is present not only in arousal reactions but also in many epileptic seizures [30]. Assuming different autonomic activation in DoA and in epileptic seizures, the analysis of autonomic reactivity could help to discriminate between these two clinical conditions. In addition, some authors suggest that autonomic activation may precede (or be asynchronous with) motor behaviors in epileptic seizures, especially in temporal lobe epilepsy and may be synchronized with cortical and motor activation in arousal disorders and physiological arousals [31].

Using wavelet analysis, Peter-Derex et al. [32] analyzed beat-to-beat RRI before and after the first motor manifestation in 50 patients during normal arousals, NREM parasomnia (CA and ST), nocturnal frontal lobe epilepsy (FLE), and temporal lobe epileptic patients (TLE). At least one nocturnal episode was recorded on video electroencephalography or video polysomnography. A significant decrease in RRI was observed at the onset of epileptic seizures, parasomniac behaviors, and physiological arousals with no significant differences between groups. The correlation analysis between the duration of the events and the autonomic responses did not show any relationship between the duration of the events and the mean RR, and between the duration of events and the LF/HF ratio. In temporal lobe epileptic patients, RRI modification started several seconds before motor manifestations and lasted longer suggesting that cardiac reactivity is not secondary to motor behavior or to arousal, rather depending on the direct activation of brain areas involved in autonomic control by the epileptic discharge. Analysis of the RRI slope showed faster and greater cardiac changes in ST and FLE than TLE and NA without any difference between ST and FLE. This result suggests that FLE and ST could trigger in a very fast and strong way the activation of the sympathetic system independent of the process that generates arousal. Similarly, Calandra-Buonaura et al. [33], assessing RRI variability by means of wavelet analysis, found that a similar autonomic activation preceded motor manifestations of FLE seizures and physiological arousal: they observed a shift of sympathetic/parasympathetic cardiac control toward sympathetic predominance in the 10 s immediately preceding seizure onset, while changes in HR were evident only 1 second before seizure onset. This sympathetic activation was not associated with a sleep-wake transition or changes in respiratory activity, both of which occurred concurrently with seizure onset. These findings challenge the idea that epileptic discharges could be responsible for autonomic activation in FLE and rather suggest that autonomic activation may represent a part of the arousal response that could be implicated in the occurrence of both seizure and arousal motor manifestations.

Conclusion

The activation of the autonomic system is an essential feature of arousal reactions. Autonomic nervous system activation is an essential feature of all DoA but especially of ST. Few studies specifically investigated the autonomic activation in DoA. Recent results indicate no differences between autonomic activation associated with DoA or physiological arousals or preceding sleep-related hyperkinetic seizures. Further studies are needed in this field, since DoA represent an ideal window to explore the functioning of the arousal circuits.

References

1. American Academy of Sleep Medicine. International classification of sleep disorders, third edition: diagnostic and coding manual. Darien: American Academy of Sleep Medicine; 2014.
2. Mahowald MW, Schenck CH. NREM sleep parasomnias. Neurol Clin. 1996;14(4):675–96.
3. Chokroverty S, Arousals C. In: Kushida CA, editor. Encyclopedia of sleep. Waltham: Academic Press; 2013. p. 199–201.
4. Stores G. Confusional arousals. In: Plazzi G, Thorpy MJ, editors. The parasomnias and other sleep-related movement disorders. Cambridge: Cambridge University Press; 2010. p. 99–108.
5. Zadra A, Desautels A, Petit D, Montplaisir J. Somnambulism: clinical aspects and pathophysiological hypotheses. Lancet Neurol. 2013;12(3):285–94.
6. Cicolin A, Tribolo A, Giordano A, Chiarot E, Peila E, Terreni A, et al. Sexual behaviors during sleep associated with polysomnographically confirmed parasomnia overlap disorder. Sleep Med. 2011;12(5):523–8.
7. Pilon M, Montplaisir J, Zadra A. Precipitating factors of somnambulism: impact of sleep deprivation and forced arousals. Neurology. 2008;70(24):2284–90.
8. Espa F, Dauvilliers Y, Ondze B, Billiard M, Besset A. Arousal reactions in sleepwalking and night terrors in adults: the role of respiratory events. Sleep. 2002;25(8):871–5.
9. Espa F, Ondze B, Deglise P, Billiard M, Besset A. Sleep architecture, slow wave activity, and sleep spindles in adult patients with sleepwalking and sleep terrors. Clin Neurophysiol. 2000;111(5):929–39.
10. Mason TB 2nd, Pack AI. Pediatric parasomnias. Sleep. 2007;30(2):141–51.
11. Bassetti C, Vella S, Donati F, Wielepp P, Weder B. SPECT during sleepwalking. Lancet. 2000;356(9228):484–5.
12. Terzaghi M, Sartori I, Tassi L, Didato G, Rustioni V, LoRusso G, et al. Evidence of dissociated arousal states during NREM parasomnia from an intracerebral neurophysiological study. Sleep. 2009;32(3):409–12.
13. Terzaghi M, Sartori I, Tassi L, Rustioni V, Proserpio P, Lorusso G, et al. Dissociated local arousal states underlying essential clinical features of non-rapid eye movement arousal parasomnia: an intracerebral stereo-electroencephalographic study. J Sleep Res. 2012;21(5):502–6.
14. Nobili L, Ferrara M, Moroni F, De Gennaro L, Russo GL, Campus C, et al. Dissociated wake-like and sleep-like electro-cortical activity during sleep. NeuroImage. 2011;58(2):612–9.
15. Zucconi M, Oldani A, Ferini-Strambi L, Smirne S. Arousal fluctuations in non-rapid eye movement parasomnias: the role of cyclic alternating pattern as a measure of sleep instability. J Clin Neurophysiol. 1995;12(2):147–54.
16. Broughton RJ. Sleep disorders: disorders of arousal? Enuresis, somnambulism, and nightmares occur in confusional states of arousal, not in "dreaming sleep". Science. 1968;159(3819):1070–8.
17. Guilleminault C, Poyares D, Aftab FA, Palombini L. Sleep and wakefulness in somnambulism: a spectral analysis study. J Psychosom Res. 2001;51(2):411–6.
18. Gaudreau H, Carrier J, Montplaisir J. Age-related modifications of NREM sleep EEG: from childhood to middle age. J Sleep Res. 2001;10(3):165–72.
19. Zucconi M, Manconi M, Bizzozero D, Rundo F, Stam CJ, Ferini-Strambi L, et al. EEG synchronisation during sleep-related epileptic seizures as a new tool to discriminate confusional arousals from paroxysmal arousals: preliminary findings. Neurol Sci. 2005;26(Suppl 3):S199–204.
20. Bruni O, Ferri R, Novelli L, Finotti E, Miano S, Guilleminault C. NREM sleep instability in children with sleep terrors: the role of slow wave activity interruptions. Clin Neurophysiol. 2008;119(5):985–92.
21. Tassinari CA, Rubboli G, Gardella E, Cantalupo G, Calandra-Buonaura G, Vedovello M, et al. Central pattern generators for a common semiology in fronto-limbic seizures and in parasomnias. A neuroethologic approach. Neurol Sci. 2005;26(Suppl 3):S225–32.
22. Sforza E, Jouny C, Ibanez V. Cardiac activation during arousal in humans: further evidence for hierarchy in the arousal response. Clin Neurophysiol. 2000;111(9):1611–9.
23. Guggisberg AG, Hess CW, Mathis J. The significance of the sympathetic nervous system in the pathophysiology of periodic leg movements in sleep. Sleep. 2007;30(6):755–66.
24. Lavigne GJ, Huynh N, Kato T, Okura K, Adachi K, Yao D, et al. Genesis of sleep bruxism: motor and autonomic-cardiac interactions. Arch Oral Biol. 2007;52(4):381–4.
25. Parrino L, Halasz P, Tassinari CA, Terzano MG. CAP, epilepsy and motor events during sleep: the unifying role of arousal. Sleep Med Rev. 2006;10(4):267–85.
26. Castelnovo A, Lopez R, Proserpio P, Nobili L, Dauvilliers Y. NREM sleep parasomnias as disorders of sleep-state dissociation. Nat Rev Neurol. 2018;14(8):470–81.
27. Fisher C, Kahn E, Edwards A, Davis DM, Fine J. A psychophysiological study of nightmares and night terrors. 3. Mental content and recall of stage 4 night terrors. J Nerv Ment Dis. 1974;158(3):174–88.

28. Schenck CH, Pareja JA, Patterson AL, Mahowald MW. Analysis of polysomnographic events surrounding 252 slow-wave sleep arousals in thirty-eight adults with injurious sleepwalking and sleep terrors. J Clin Neurophysiol. 1998;15(2):159–66.
29. Busek P, Vankova J, Opavsky J, Salinger J, Stepanova I, Nevsimalova S. Spectral analysis of the variations in heart rate and cardiac activation on waking up in sleepwalking. Rev Neurol. 2005;41(6):338–43.
30. Tinuper P, Provini F, Bisulli F, Vignatelli L, Plazzi G, Vetrugno R, et al. Movement disorders in sleep: guidelines for differentiating epileptic from non-epileptic motor phenomena arising from sleep. Sleep Med Rev. 2007;11(4):255–67.
31. Bruno E, Biondi A, Richardson MP, Consortium R-C. Pre-ictal heart rate changes: a systematic review and meta-analysis. Seizure. 2018;55:48–56.
32. Peter-Derex L, Catenoix H, Bastuji H, Chouchou F. Parasomnia versus epilepsy: an affair of the heart? Neurophysiol Clin. 2018;48(5):277–86.
33. Calandra-Buonaura G, Toschi N, Provini F, Corazza I, Bisulli F, Barletta G, et al. Physiologic autonomic arousal heralds motor manifestations of seizures in nocturnal frontal lobe epilepsy: implications for pathophysiology. Sleep Med. 2012;13(3):252–62.

Narcolepsy, Idiopathic Hypersomnia, and Dysautonomia

17

Lucie Barateau and Yves Dauvilliers

Introduction

Narcolepsy type 1 (NT1) and type 2 (NT2), idiopathic hypersomnia (IH), and Kleine-Levin syndrome (KLS) are central disorders of hypersomnolence [1]. NT1, formerly known as narcolepsy with cataplexy, is characterized by a pentad of symptoms: excessive daytime sleepiness, cataplexy, sleep paralysis and hypnagogic hallucinations, and disrupted nocturnal sleep [2]. NT2, formerly known as narcolepsy without cataplexy, shares most of the clinical features with NT1. IH patients also exhibit excessive daytime sleepiness and impaired daytime alertness, but with long and unrefreshing naps; their nocturnal sleep is prolonged and undisturbed, and they often report sleep inertia, a great difficulty in waking up after sleep [1]. KLS is characterized by relapsing-remitting episodes of severe hypersomnolence associated with behavioral and psychiatric disturbances, cognitive abnormalities, and hyperphagia or hypersexuality [3].

NT1 pathophysiology is well known; the disease is caused by the selective and irreversible destruction of a small population of neurons in the lateral hypothalamus that synthesizes hypocretin/orexin (ORX). A low level of ORX (<110 pg/ml on RIA assay) in the cerebrospinal fluid is very sensitive and specific for the diagnosis of NT1. On the other hand, NT2 and IH are still poorly understood disorders, probably heterogeneous, diagnosed on clinical and neurophysiological criteria only, with unspecific and unstable biomarkers and with some overlaps between these conditions [4, 5]. Some studies suggest recurrent primary hypothalamic dysfunction in KLS, but its pathophysiology also remains unclear.

L. Barateau (✉) · Y. Dauvilliers (✉)
Sleep-Wake Disorders Center, Department of Neurology, National Reference Network for Narcolepsy, Gui-de-Chauliac Hospital, CHU Montpellier, Montpellier, France

PSNREC, University Montpellier, INSERM 1061, Montpellier, France
e-mail: l-barateau@chu-montpellier.fr; y-dauvilliers@chu-montpellier.fr

NT1 is often associated with other sleep abnormalities (apnea, parasomnia, periodic leg movements, rapid eye movement (REM) sleep behavior disorder (RBD)), as well as with a wide range of comorbidities (e.g., neuropsychiatric disorders, obesity, and metabolic and autonomic disturbances). In particular, there is a higher frequency of cardiovascular diseases in human narcolepsy [6], and narcoleptic patients often report clinical autonomic impairment [7]. However, studies with objective markers of autonomic dysfunction in NT1 have so far yielded conflicting results, with some studies in favor of an increased and others in favor of a decreased sympathetic activity [8]. This autonomic imbalance in NT1 is probably directly related to the loss of ORX neurons. ORX neurons project widely through the brain (see further on).

In this chapter, we describe the pathophysiological mechanisms underlying dysautonomia in narcolepsy, related to ORX deficiency, with neuroanatomical bases and preclinical studies. The clinical aspects of autonomic impairment in narcolepsy are addressed in the second part, with a review of autonomic impairment and objective disturbances during wakefulness, sleep, and during a cataplectic episode. Literature about dysautonomia in other central disorders of hypersomnolence (NT2, IH, and KLS) is limited; however we will provide a general overview of the topic, its clinical implications and perspective for future research.

Dysautonomia in Narcolepsy Type I

Pathophysiological Aspects: Orexin and Autonomic Nervous System

Neuroanatomy

Orexin (ORX) neurons are a restricted group of 70–80,000 cells of the lateral hypothalamus, but they project widely to multiple neuronal systems and play a major role in various physiological functions such as the regulation of sleep-wake cycle, neuroendocrine and reward system, body temperature,

S. Chokroverty, P. Cortelli (eds.), *Autonomic Nervous System and Sleep*, https://doi.org/10.1007/978-3-030-62263-3_17

and metabolism [9]. In the central nervous system, autonomic nervous system (ANS) regulatory network is an interconnected set of brain structures, critical for the control of autonomic preganglionic neurons, and ORX neurons are a key component of this network [10] (Fig. 17.1). ORX neurons include pre-autonomic neurons directly targeting preganglionic sympathetic neurons in the intermediolateral column of the spinal cord and parasympathetic neurons in the dorsal motor nucleus of the vagus nerve. They also modulate the activity of other structures including pre-autonomic neurons, with projections to the rostral ventromedial medulla and caudal raphe nuclei, and rostral ventrolateral medulla and hypothalamic paraventricular nucleus. In addition, they project to and modulate the activity of neurons in the nucleus of the tractus solitarius in the medulla, receiving and relaying visceral afferent information, and in the dorsomedial nucleus of the hypothalamus and the extended amygdala. In rodents, ORX neurons innervate both parasympathetic and sympathetic regions of the ANS.

Pharmacological and Animal Studies

Several preclinical studies showed that ORX have a direct influence on autonomic functions such as heart rate (HR) and blood pressure (BP) regulation [11, 12], energy metabolism [13, 14], or gastrointestinal motility [15]. The injection of

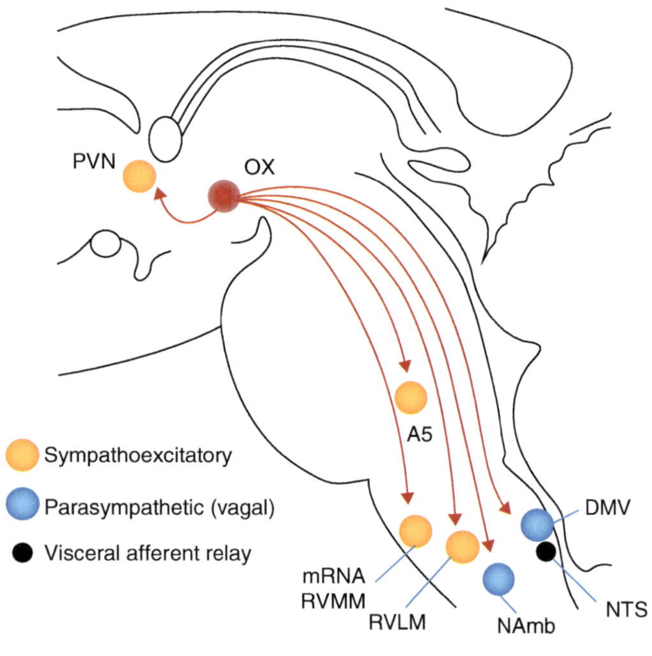

Fig. 17.1 Sagittal section of the human brainstem and diencephalon with the main projections from orexin neurons to areas of the central autonomic network. *A5* homonymous noradrenergic cell group of the pons, *DMV* dorsal motor nucleus of the vagus nerve, *mRN* medullary raphe nuclei, *Namb* nucleus ambiguous, *NTS* nucleus of the tractus solitarius, *OX* orexin neurons, *PVN* paraventricular nucleus of the hypothalamus, *RVLM* rostral ventrolateral medulla, *RVMM* rostral ventromedial medulla. (From Grimaldi et al. [10], with permission. © 2014 Wolters Kluwer Health)

ORX intrathecally or intracerebroventricularly in animals stimulates arousal and increases sympathetic drive, HR, oxygen consumption, body temperature, plasma catecholamine levels, and BP in a dose-dependent manner [11, 16–19]. A summary of all physiological responses to exogenously administered ORXs (via intravenous, intracerebroventricular, intraperitoneal, and in situ in different CNS areas) in rodents is provided in a review by Plazzi et al. [20]. Overall, the administration of ORX increases the sympathetic tone, but differences are sometimes observed, depending on the administration site. A lower sympathetic tone is a logical corollary of ORX deficiency, and lower HR and BP during wake were first reported in animal models of narcolepsy. However, further studies, and especially sleep studies, in transgenic and ORX knock-out (KO) mice have yielded contrasting results [21].

In physiological condition, arterial BP physiologically decreases from wakefulness to NREM sleep and rises again during REM sleep [22]. The blunted BP fall at night (called "non-dipping pattern") exists in animal models of narcolepsy [23], even though BP seems to be normal during sleep in narcoleptic mice [24]. A normal BP during wake but a relatively high BP in sleep, especially in REM sleep, was found in different animal models of the disease [23, 25]. Heart rate control is a subject of controversy. Similar HR was found in several narcoleptic animals compared with wild-type animals [23, 26–28]. However, a study reported higher HR in ORX-KO mice compared to control mice [23], and other authors found weaker HR responses to internal stimuli (defense reaction to psychological stressor) in animal models of narcolepsy [26, 28]. Subtle alterations of HR variability were also described in mouse models of narcolepsy [24, 25, 29]. Moreover, ORX/ataxin-3 transgenic mice are often obese that could increase sympathetic activity [30]. Overall, the complexity of these results could be due to the complex innervation and interaction between sympathetic and parasympathetic regions by ORX neurons. It has also been suggested that low doses of ORXs would increase parasympathetic tone through ORX-receptor 2, whereas high doses would increase sympathetic tone through ORX-receptor 1 [14].

Human Studies

Autonomic Symptoms

Fainting spells, erectile dysfunction, pupillary abnormalities, night sweats, gastric or digestive problems, hypotension, dry mouth, heart palpitations, and disturbed skin temperature profiles have all been described for decades in association with narcolepsy (for a comprehensive review of all clinical disturbances reported in narcolepsy, see Plazzi et al. [20]). However, the systematic assessment of autonomic symptoms has not been done until recently in a large cohort of well-characterized patients [7]. In this study, by using a reliable and valid instrument (the Scale for Outcomes in Parkinson Disease-Autonomic [SCOPA-AUT] self-questionnaire), a large spectrum of clinical autonomic dysfunction was reported in NT1, with impairment in every subdomain: gastrointestinal, urinary, cardiovascular, thermoregulatory, pupillomotor, and sexual. These symptoms were associated with older age, poorer quality of life, and more depressive symptoms. Narcolepsy management is nowadays only symptomatic, targeting sleepiness and cataplexy, and most drugs used (psychostimulants, sodium oxybate, antidepressant agents) may also interfere with the ANS functioning [31]. However, in this study, there was no significant effect of drugs for narcolepsy, suggesting that dysautonomia is more a trait than a state in ORX-deficient narcolepsy [7]. Besides these autonomic symptoms, objective findings of dysautonomia have been reported in NT1; an overview and synthesis of these studies published so far are provided in Table 17.1 [32–52].

Arterial Blood Pressure

The first study of the control of BP in patients with narcolepsy found normal values during wakefulness and sleep [32]. However, in line with animal models of narcolepsy, further studies with more patients included found a frequent occurrence of non-dipper BP profile in NT1 [38, 39, 46]. A normal BP in wake, but a relative higher BP in sleep, was also reported, especially in REM sleep [38, 42]. The beat-to-beat variability of BP within wake and each sleep stages has been studied little: it did not seem to vary during sleep in a small case-control study [40], but an increased variability was observed during wakefulness in another one [35]. A recent study failed to find a relationship between ORX levels and BP changes in NT1, but the sample was quite small [53]. The effect of medication for narcolepsy on BP was recently studied, and an increased diastolic BP and HR were found in NT1 patients treated by psychostimulants compared to untreated patients [47] (Fig. 17.2). To summarize, NT1 seems to be associated with a blunted fall of arterial BP from wakefulness to sleep, and particularly to REM sleep (Fig. 17.3, *double arrows*), coupled with a variable decrease in BP during wakefulness (see Fig. 17.3, *single arrow*) [12]. Further studies on the effect of different medications and related doses on BP and HR are warranted.

Heart Rate and Its Variability

Association between NT1 and HR control is subject to controversy. Some authors found similar HR in NT1 compared to controls, and similar HR regulation [34, 35, 39, 42], or subtle alterations of HR variability were described in NT1 patients [34, 35, 40]. Only one study showed lower HR during wakefulness in drug-naive patients [43]. Other studies reported higher HR than controls during sleep [38, 41, 45], and an increased LF/HF ratio [36, 38], suggesting an increased sympathetic tone. Blunted HR responses to arousals and leg movements (internal stimulus) were shown in narcolepsy [37, 41]. On the other hand, HR responses to emotional stimuli and acute administration of sodium oxybate seem normal in narcolepsy [44, 48].

Muscle Sympathetic Nerve Activity

A recording of muscle sympathetic nerve activity (MSNA) by microneurography was performed during sleep and wakefulness, being the first reports of the direct measure of sympathetic activity in NT1. A low sympathetic tone during wakefulness was demonstrated in a small sample of adult drug-naive patients (Fig. 17.4), in accordance with preclinical studies, and this reduction was correlated with ORX levels in the cerebrospinal fluid [43]. The recording during sleep was challenging and the sample was small [42]. The authors found a physiologic decrease of sympathetic activities from wake to NREM sleep, and an increase in REM sleep, comparable to controls. They also found unexpectedly a decrease of sympathetic activities during sleep-onset REM period (SOREMP), comparable to NREM sleep. Globally, the rarity of NT1, the cost of the material, the practical difficulty of execution of this technique, and especially the challenge to record MSNA during sleep in humans explain why these results have not been replicated. In this study, the authors also studied the skin sympathetic activity (SSA) that decreases in NREM sleep compared to wake but was similar during REM sleep and wakefulness in controls. In contrast, a progressive and significant decrease of SSA was found during SOREMP and NREM sleep in NT1, while an increase was found in REM sleep compared to wake [42].

Other Measures of Autonomic Disturbances

Orexin infusion in rodents increases peripheral and core body temperatures. In NT1, the circadian core body temperature cycle was initially reported to be preserved [54]; however, a more recent study reported an elevated distal skin temperature over the day in unmedicated NT1 patients [55]. This augmentation in distal temperature correlated with sleep propensity, and experimentally induced changes in core body and skin temperature could modify vigilance and sleepiness [56]. The authors attributed skin temperature alterations to a decreased sympathetic distal vasoconstrictor tone due to ORX deficiency.

A recent study used metaiodobenzylguanidine (MIBG) cardiac scintigraphy in NT1 patients and found an absence of cardiac sympathetic denervation compared to controls [51]. Five out of 56 NT1 patients, however, had low MIBG uptake associated with a threefold increase of phasic tonic REM sleep motor activities. In an old study, 24-h urinary and plasma catecholamine levels were reported to be normal in

Table 17.1 Summary of studies performed in human narcolepsy to assess objectively autonomic disturbances during wakefulness and sleep

Test/evaluation	Narcoleptic patients	Controls	Condition	Main results	ORX status	References
BP on ABPM	7 narcoleptic patients with cataplexy, adults, drug free	7, healthy	Sleep (2 or 3 nights)	Same mean BP and same nocturnal variations between patients and controls	–	Guilleminault et al. [32]
HR measured on ECG and BP measured by sphygmomanometer	22 narcoleptic patients with cataplexy, adults, drug free	–	Daytime W: at rest and after different doses of stimulants (orthostatic, deep breathing, Valsalva tests)	No abnormalities at baseline, dose-dependent rise in heart ration under medication	–	Hublin et al. [33]
Beat-to-beat HR calculated on ECG	10 narcoleptic patients (no mention of cataplexy), adults, drug naive	10, healthy	W and sleep (PSG)	Same mean HR during W, NREM and REM, increased LF/HF HRV during W before sleep for narcoleptics	–	Ferini-Strambi et al. [34]
BP continuously recorded by volume-clamp method (*Finometer*), beat-to-beat HR calculated on ECG	15 NT1, adults, drug free	15, healthy	Daytime W (20 min)	Increased variability of BP and HR in NT1, same mean HR	All ORX def	Fronczek et al. [35]
BP and HR continuously recorded by volume-clamp method (*Portapres*)	10 NT1 adults, drug free	18, healthy	Daytime W: at rest and during orthostatic stress (head-up tilt test, Valsalva, deep breathing and cold face tests)	Increased mean HR, increased LF/HF HRV, no increase during tilt test	9 LP/9 ORX def	Grimaldi et al. [36][a]
Beat-to-beat HR calculated on ECG	14 NT1, adults, drug free	14, healthy	Nocturnal sleep (PSG): responses to PLMS	Decreased HRV associated with PLMS	–	Dauvilliers et al. [37]
BP and HR continuously recorded by volume-clamp method (*Portapres*)	10 NT1, adults drug free	12, healthy	W and nocturnal sleep (PSG)	Non-dipping pattern in NT1, increased mean BP in REM, increased mean HR during W, NREM, and REM	9 LP/9 ORX def	Grimaldi et al. [38][a]
BP and HR on ABPM	36 NT1, adults, drug free	42, healthy	24-hour ambulatory measures	Non dipping pattern in 30% of patients, same mean HR during daytime and nighttime	17 LP / 17 ORX def	Dauvilliers et al. [39]
BP continuously recorded by volume-clamp method (*Portapres*), beat-to-beat HR calculated on ECG	9 NT1, adults, drug free	9, healthy	W and nocturnal sleep (PSG)	Similar variability of BP during W, NREM and REM sleep, increased mean HR during W, NREM, and REM	8 LP/8 ORX def	Silvani et al. [40][a]
Beat-to-beat HR calculated on ECG	67 narcoleptic patients (46 with cataplexy), adults, drug free	22, healthy	Nocturnal sleep (PSG): responses to arousals and PLMS	Decreased HRV associated with arousals, and with PLMS in narcoleptics vs controls, and in ORX-def condition vs ORX normal	61 LP/38 ORX def	Sorensen et al. [41]
BP and HR continuously recorded by volume-clamp method (*Finapres*), MSNA measured by microneurography, skin sympathetic activity by mean value of SVR and SSR	13 NT1, adults, drug naïve	5, healthy	Nocturnal sleep (PSG)	Physiologic decrease of SA from W to NREM, and increase in REM; non-dipping pattern; decrease of SA during SOREMP comparable to NREM1	All ORX def	Donadio et al. [42]

Table 17.1 (continued)

Test/evaluation	Narcoleptic patients	Controls	Condition	Main results	ORX status	References
BP and HR continuously recorded by volume-clamp method (*Finometer*), MSNA measured by microneurography	19 NT1, adults, drug naïve	19, healthy	Daytime W	Decreased MSNA, BP and HR mean values	All ORX def	Donadio et al. [43]
BP and HR continuously recorded by volume-clamp method (*Finapres*)	12 NT1, adults, drug naive	12, healthy	Daytime W: hemodynamic responses to emotional stimuli	No differences between patients and controls	All ORX def	De Zambotti et al. [44]
Beat-to-beat HR calculated on ECG	12 NT1, adults, drug naive	12, healthy	Nocturnal sleep (PSG)	Increased mean HR during W before sleep in NT1, NREM and REM; same HRV	All ORX def	van der Meijden et al. [45]
BP and HR on ABPM	8 NT1, adults, drug free	7 patients with insomnia	24-hour ambulatory measures	Non-dipping pattern in 7/8 patients, but no difference between narcoleptic and insomniac patients, and same mean HR	All ORX def	Sieminski et al. [46]
BP and HR on ABPM	160 NT1, adults (54 treated)	–	24-hour ambulatory measures	Higher diastolic BP and HR in treated than drug-free NT1; non-dipping pattern in 48% of untreated NT1, 44% treated	96 LP/94 ORX def	Bosco et al. [47]
Beat-to-beat HR calculated on ECG	12 NT1, children, drug naive	23, healthy children	Nocturnal sleep (PSG): baseline and response to sodium oxybate	Baseline: slightly higher HRV in all sleep stages; under sodium oxybate: tend to decreased HRV in REM	–	Antelmi et al. [48]
Activity of brown adipose tissue (BAT) measured by 123I-MIBG SPECT and 18-F-FDG PET	7 NT1, adults, no information on drug status	7, healthy	Daytime W, after 2 hours cold exposure	Same BAT activity in patients and controls	All ORX def	Enevoldsen et al. [49]
Cardiac sympathetic activity measured by 123-I-MIBG scintigraphy	34 NT1 with comorbid RBD, adults and adolescents (13 treated)	15 patients with idiopathic RBD, adults	Daytime W	MIBG cardiac uptake lower in iRBD than NT1	26 LP/26 ORX def	Barateau et al. [50][b]
Cardiac sympathetic activity measured by 123-I-MIBG scintigraphy	56 NT1, adults and children (16 treated)	91 adult controls from the general population without cardiac or neurologic disorder	Daytime W	Absence of cardiac sympathetic denervation in NT1 but association with REM motor deregulation	43 LP/43 ORX def	Barateau et al. [51][b]
Pulse transit time (PTT) based on ECG and pulse oximetry data, HR on ECG	27 NT1, children and adolescents, drug naive	19, clinical suspicion of hypersomnia, but no objective abnormalities	W and nocturnal sleep (PSG)	Same HR, but reduced lengthening of PTT during total sleep and REM compared to nocturnal W in NT1	26 LP/26 ORX def	Vandi et al. [52]

Studies are listed chronologically; studies during cataplectic episodes are not listed here; drug free means drug naive or withdrawal

ABPM ambulatory blood pressure monitoring, *BP* blood pressure, *ORX def* orexin deficient (CSF orexin levels <110 pg/mL), *ECG* electrocardiogram, *HR* heart rate, *HRV* heart rate variability, *LF/HF* low-frequency/high-frequency spectral power of HRV, *LP* lumbar puncture, *MSNA* muscle sympathetic nerve activity, *NT1* narcolepsy type 1, *NREM* non-rapid eye movement sleep, *ORX* orexin, *PLMS* periodic leg movements during sleep, *PSG* polysomnography, *RBD* REM sleep behavior disorder, *REM* rapid eye movement sleep, *SA* sympathetic activities, *SOREMP* sleep onset REM period, *SSR* skin sympathetic response, *SVR* skin vasomotor response, *W* wake

[a,b]These studies share narcoleptic patients

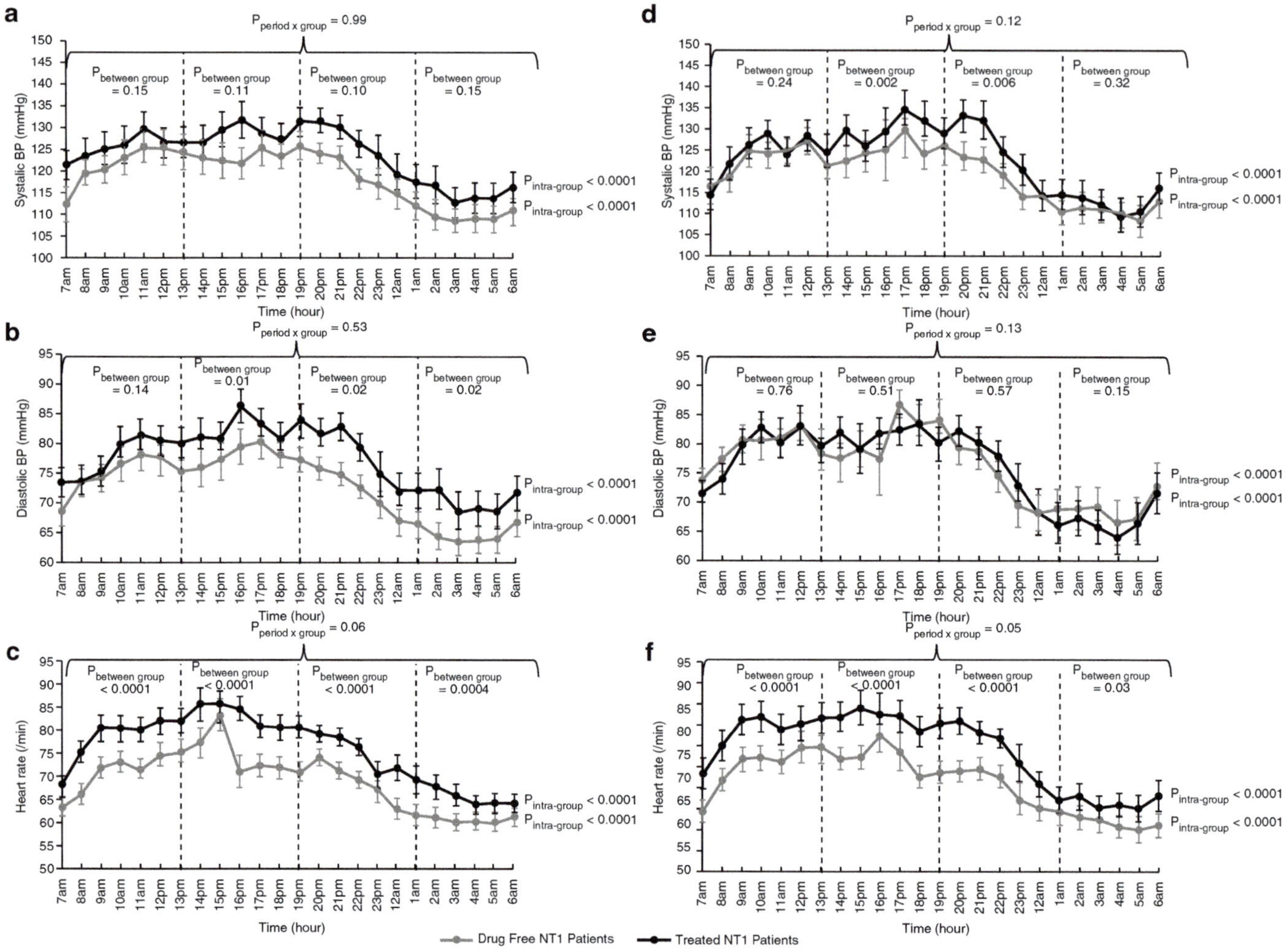

Fig. 17.2 Twenty-four-hour ambulatory blood pressure (BP) monitoring in NT1 patients. Twenty-four-hour ambulatory BP monitoring (divided into four periods: 7:00 AM–1:00 PM; 1:00 PM–7:00 PM; 7:00 PM–1:00 AM; and 1:00 AM–7:00 AM) in the independent sample (**a–c**) of untreated ($n = 68$) and treated ($n = 54$) patients with NT1 and in the dependent sample ($n = 38$) of patients with NT1 evaluated twice (drug-free and under treatment) (**d–f**). (**a, d**) systolic BP; (**b, e**) diastolic BP; (**c, f**) heart rate. P intragroup <0.0001 for all lines. Mixed models were used to analyze the 24-hour changes in systolic BP, diastolic BP, and HR. Between-group *p* values were calculated for each period. Variation over time within each group was examined over the whole period (intragroup *p* values). The difference in change over the 24 hours between the two groups is referred to as period × group *p* values. (From Bosco et al. [47], with permission. © 2018 Wolters Kluwer Health)

narcolepsy [57], but results have not been replicated. Finally, abnormal pupillary reaction during darkness [58] and impaired nocturnal penile tumescence [59] have been reported in narcolepsy.

Comorbid Disorders

Comorbid disorders are frequent in NT1, and of interest, most of them are also associated with autonomic dysfunction. Obesity is a condition known to be associated with increased sympathetic activity [60], and weight gain usually occurs at the onset of NT1, with more than 30% of patients becoming obese [13, 61]. Energy metabolism and basal metabolic rate have been investigated in NT1 but with inconsistent results. Rest energy expenditure, measured by indirect calorimetry, has been shown to be significantly lower in NT1 [62], but other studies found no difference with controls [35, 63]. As the ANS innervates white and brown adipose tissue (BAT) and induces catabolic processes through sympathetic inputs and anabolic processes through parasympathetic inputs [64], it has been suggested that the sympathetic tone reduction would explain the increased fat accumulation in NT1. A recent study evaluated the activity of BAT by ^{123}I-MIBG SPECT and ^{18}F-FDG PET in a small sample of NT1 patients versus control during wake and after 2 h of cold exposure but found no difference between the groups. Overall, the link between metabolic rate and sympathetic tone in narcolepsy remains to be explored as a function of obesity in NT1. Indeed, most previous studies did not focus on obese NT1 patients.

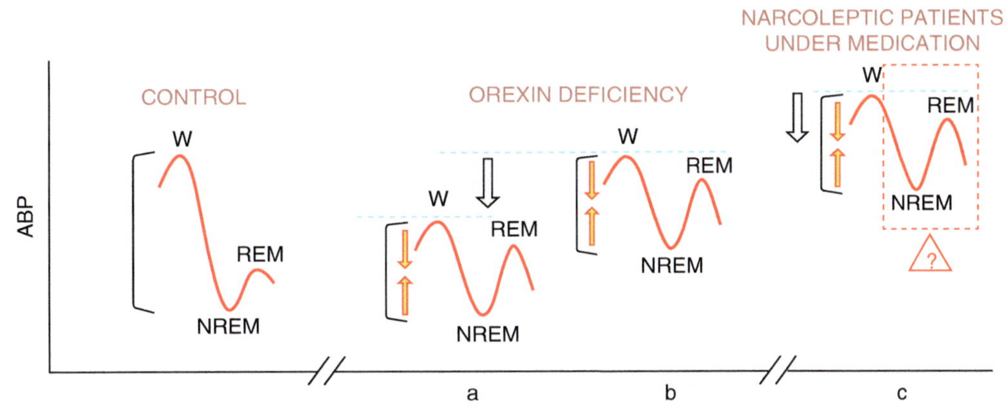

Fig. 17.3 Variations of arterial blood pressure (ABP) during wakefulness (W) and NREM and REM sleep in controls and in orexin deficiency condition. "Orexin deficiency may be associated with (**a**) ABP values lower than controls in W and APB values normal during sleep or (**b**) APB values normal in W, and ABP values higher than controls during sleep. ABP values are higher in treated than untreated narcoleptic patients (**c**), but variations of ABP during different stages of sleep in narcoleptic patients under medication have never been studied (*red box*, **c**). (Adapted with permission from Berteotti and Silvania [12]. © 2017 Springer Nature)

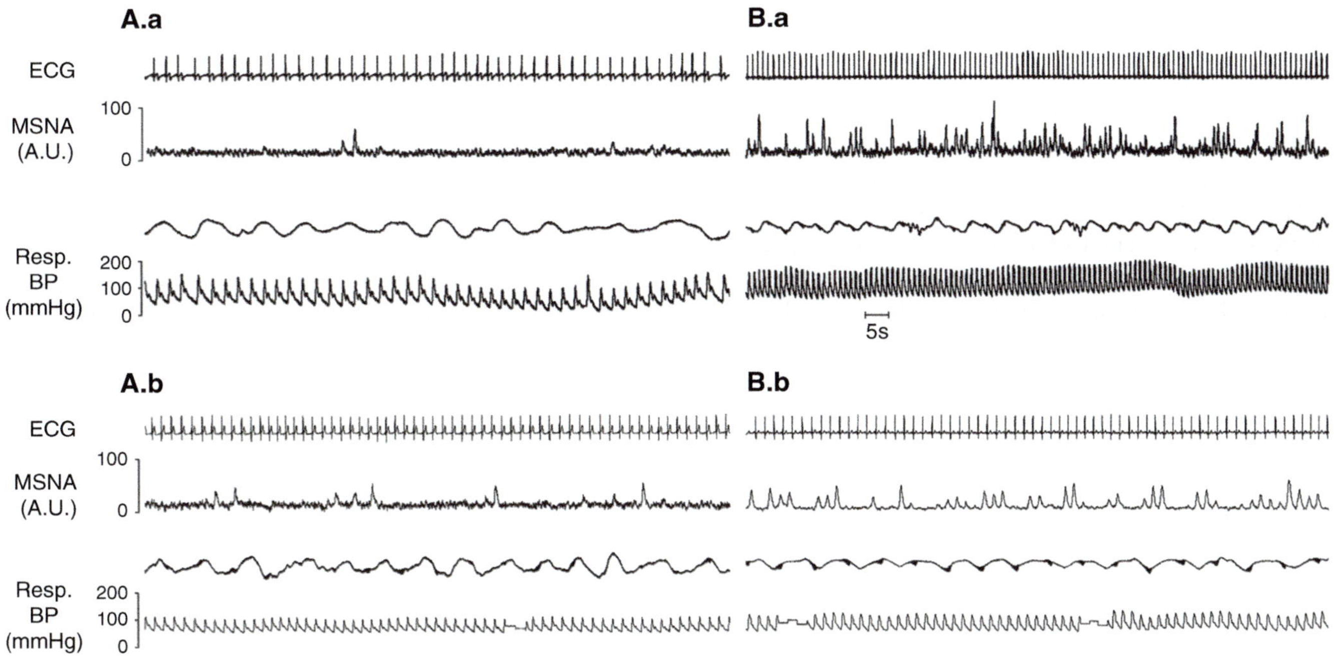

Fig. 17.4 Microneurographic recording and heart rate (HR) and blood pressure (BP) monitoring during wakefulness, in two patients with narcolepsy type 1 (**a.a**, **a.b**) and two matched healthy controls (**b.a**, **b.b**). Both patients displayed lower muscle sympathetic nerve activity (MSNA) compared to controls, with **a.a** showing lower HR and BP than **b.a**, and **a.b** showing similar HR and BP as **b.b**. (From Donadio et al. [43], with permission. © 2014 Wolters Kluwer Health)

Comorbid sleep disorders are also common in NT1. An estimated 25–30% of patients with narcolepsy may have sleep apnea syndrome, depending on age, body mass index (BMI) of the population, and apnea-hypopnea index (AHI) cutoff applied to diagnose obstructive sleep apnea syndrome [65], and this comorbidity may lead to increased sympathetic tone and diminished baroreceptor sensitivity, thus increasing the risk of hypertension and cardiovascular and cerebrovascular diseases. Sleep-maintenance insomnia and disrupted nocturnal sleep are common in NT1 [66], and this fragmented nocturnal sleep could also lead to an increased sympathetic drive. As many as 15% of narcoleptic patients have comorbid restless legs syndrome [67] and periodic leg movements in sleep (PLMS) are frequent in NT1 [68, 69]; these two conditions are associated with an increased sympathetic activity. PLMS can trigger a rapid rise in HR and BP, which is more pronounced if associated with a micro-arousal, but an impairment of this autonomic response to PLMS was shown in NT1 [37]. RBD is not only commonly associated with neurodegenerative disorders including parkinsonisms, but it is also reported in narcolepsy in up to 60% of patients [70]. Idiopathic RBD (iRBD) has been associated with reduced HR variability during sleep, and cardiac sympathetic denervation, but a recent study found that NT1 with comorbid RBD had a higher MIBG uptake on ^{123}I-MIBG cardiac scintigraphy than iRBD in the same range as controls [50]. However, in another study with the same technique, REM sleep without atonia in NT1 seemed related to cardiac sympathetic adrenergic nerve activity [51].

Dysautonomia During Cataplexy

Cataplexy is the pathognomonic symptom of NT1, a sudden involuntary loss of skeletal muscle tone while awake, typically triggered by positive emotions highly charged by autonomic changes [20, 71]. A cataplexy can be partial, with head drop, dysarthria, and jaw tremor, or limited to the upper or lower limbs. It can also be generalized, with a complete atonia resulting in a fall. The current pathophysiological hypothesis is a transient activation during wakefulness of the neural pathways that produce muscle atonia during REM sleep [72]. In ORX deficiency condition, the activation of the amygdala and medial prefrontal cortex induced by emotions decreases the excitation of noradrenergic neurons and hyperpolarizes motor neurons by GABA and glycine that are released by interneurons in the spinal cord and by long descending projections from the medial medulla [72, 73]. Behavioral and neurophysiological correlates of cataplexy, and especially autonomic changes, are challenging to study, because of the unpredictable nature of a cataplectic episode, a fluctuating and highly variable symptom in terms of frequency, duration, and intensity.

A study analyzed cataplectic episodes by video polygraphic study [74]. For 6 out of 11 attacks, an increase in HR several seconds before the episode was reported, followed by bradycardia starting at the onset of atonia, persisting throughout the cataplectic episode, and returning to baseline values 50–70 sec after the onset of the attack. Another study monitored muscle sympathetic nerve activity (MSNA), HR, respiratory movements, and arterial finger BP during 10 cataplectic episodes [75]. In contrast to the previous study, no significant autonomic changes were shown before cataplexy onset; however, cataplexy was associated with an increase in MSNA and systolic BP, while HR markedly decreased (Fig. 17.5) [42]. These data were further replicated in another study [76], suggesting a co-activation of sympathetic and parasympathetic autonomic systems during cataplexy.

Dysautonomia in Other Central Disorders of Hypersomnolence

In other central disorders of hypersomnolence (NT2, IH, and KLS), the literature on autonomic dysfunction is limited, and NT2 and IH (both characterized by normal ORX condition) are usually compared to NT1 patients. As mentioned previously, a study found a decreased HR variability associated with micro-arousals, with PLMS in narcoleptic patients (including NT2) versus controls, and in ORX-deficient condition versus ORX normal condition [41]. Another recent

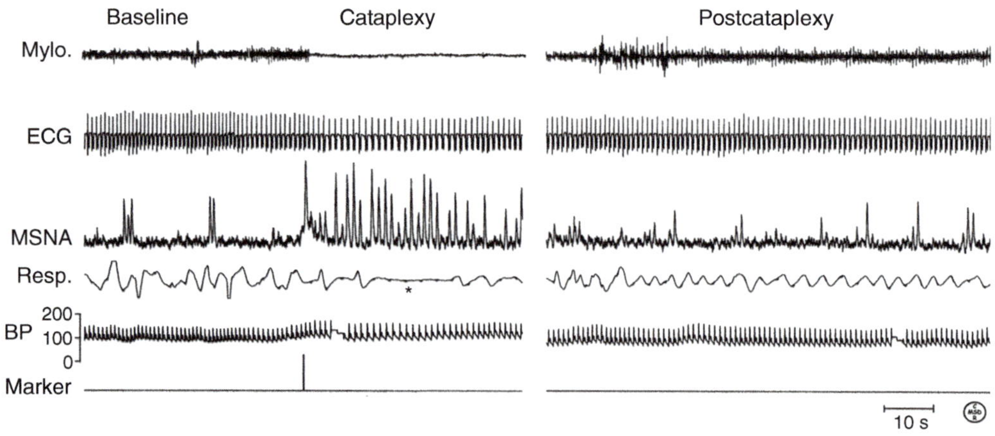

Fig. 17.5 Microneurographic recording before, during, and after a cataplectic episode, together with heart rate (HR), blood pressure (BP), and respiratory monitoring. The patient displayed a marked increase in incidence and amplitude of muscle sympathetic nerve activity (MSNA) and a decrease in HR, coinciding with muscle atonia (*Mylo* = mylohyoideus muscle). MSNA, BP, and HR returned to baseline after the episode. An irregular breathing pattern with apnea is also visible (*). The marker indicates speech arrest at cataplexy onset. (From Donadio et al. [42], with permission. © 2014 Elsevier)

study explored the HR variability in 11 patients with NT1, 20 patients with NT2, and 12 healthy controls [77]. The authors found a higher LF/HF ratio in patients than controls during NREM sleep, but a lower parasympathetic tone assessed by root mean square of successive RR interval differences in NT1 than NT2 during REM sleep. However, this study is retrospective, with a small number of patients, and ORX status was not available [77]. NT2 is probably an heterogeneous disease and sometimes an unstable condition, with some patients developing later cataplexy and becoming NT1 and some patients relapsing while others persisting into the NT2 phenotype. We may hypothesize that patients with NT2 who are prone to convert to NT1 would be more at risk to present with autonomic impairment, which is linked to a slow and progressive destruction of ORX neurons, but this remains speculative.

IH is a rare syndrome, with clinical heterogeneity suggesting a variable or multifactorial pathogenesis. Patients should be well characterized with standardized tests [4] before exploring a potential autonomic impairment. In IH, dysautonomia was reported in some case series [78], and a more recent case-control study found some functional equivalents (i.e., cold extremities and fainting), which is more frequent in patients than controls [79]. A large systematic assessment of dysautonomia in well-characterized patients is still lacking, and the mechanism underlying the occurrence of these symptoms remains unknown, but they could contribute to the burden of the disease. An older study reported lower BP in IH compared to narcoleptic patients, but the study lacked healthy controls [80]. Another study explored the HR variability in IH patients versus controls and found a dysfunction of the parasympathetic activity during wakefulness and sleep and an altered autonomic response to arousals [81]; however, patients were not diagnosed according to ICSD-3 criteria [2].

KLS is a very rare disorder of relapsing and remitting sleepiness, with ancillary features of cognitive impairment, apathy or disinhibition, hyperphagia, hypersexuality, derealization, and dysautonomia [3]. The underlying pathophysiology of this central disorder of hypersomnolence remains unclear, but a recurrent primary hypothalamic dysfunction mediated by immune mechanisms is suspected. Autonomic symptoms were never systematically assessed, but a recent study reported lower BP and HR, and lower ORX levels, associated with the symptomatic phase of the syndrome, compared to the remission phase, in a sample of 24 patients [82]. These noteworthy phenomena should be further studied.

When studying the cardiovascular tone in human disorders of hypersomnolence, a potential confounding factor would be the effects of sleep length and relative rest/inactivity linked to sleepiness, which might also result in a lowering of HR and BP. More detailed rest-activity profiles in central disorders of hypersomnolence might be informative.

Conclusion and Perspectives

The interactions between ANS and central disorders of hypersomnolence are complex. The recent integration of data from multiple approaches (including preclinical studies, animal models, and humans) has increased our understanding of these relationships and provided new insights into their physiology, as well as the morbidity and prognosis of ANS deregulation in these sleep disorders. Inconsistent results published so far on autonomic disturbances in narcolepsy might be explained by a lack of standardization; different populations involved; the use of different and often indirect methods to evaluate dysautonomia; and the various conditions tested during sleep, wakefulness, and at different moments of the day. The heterogeneity of age, gender, drug status (naive or withdrawal), and comorbidities (especially body weight, respiratory events during sleep, PLMS, and disturbed nocturnal sleep) as well as the small number of patients studied are elements that should also be taken into account when interpreting these findings. Many of these studies also lack data concerning cardiovascular risk factors such as dyslipidemia, hypertension, smoking status, physical activity, and associated cardiovascular treatments. In addition, even if NT1 starts in children/adolescent in most of the cases, narcoleptic children have been understudied in this regard. A recent study showed that adult NT1 patients with more severe autonomic disturbances had a poorer quality of life and more depressive symptoms [7], but the exact role of autonomic and metabolic impact on medical outcomes and lifetime expectancy in narcolepsy remains unknown. The non-dipping BP profile is a condition associated with greater cardiovascular risk, and narcoleptic patients seem to have greater cardiovascular morbidity [6]; however, further epidemiological studies are warranted to clarify the clinical importance of these complex autonomic changes. Narcolepsy is an active area for drug development with new wake-promoting agents developed over the past years, and very recently, non-peptide ORX receptor agonists [83–85]. The effect of medications should be further evaluated with new cardiovascular studies using state-dependent analysis and systematic monitoring of 24-hour BP and cardiac function in future clinical trials. A recent preclinical study demonstrated that reduced ORX signaling was associated with increased atherosclerosis burden in mouse models of NT1 and also unexpectedly in long-term sleep fragmentation [86]. Whether this observation is applicable in humans needs to be tested, especially in NT1 and disorders associated with severe sleep fragmentation. Overall, further research works are needed to fully understand the autonomic consequences of ORX-deficient narcolepsy (NT1), non-ORX-deficient narcolepsy (NT2) and IH, and their possible relation to cardiovascular risk, with large systematic assessment and careful follow-up of homogeneous groups of well-characterized patients with central disorders of hypersomnolence.

References

1. Dauvilliers Y, Barateau L. Narcolepsy and other central hypersomnias. Continuum (Minneap Minn). 2017;23(4, Sleep Neurology):989–1004.
2. American Academy of Sleep Medicine. International classification of sleep disorders, third edition: diagnostic and coding manual. Darien: American Academy of Sleep Medicine; 2014.
3. Arnulf I, Rico TJ, Mignot E. Diagnosis, disease course, and management of patients with Kleine-Levin syndrome. Lancet Neurol. 2012;11(10):918–28.
4. Evangelista E, Lopez R, Barateau L, Chenini S, Bosco A, Jaussent I, et al. Alternative diagnostic criteria for idiopathic hypersomnia: a 32-hour protocol. Ann Neurol. 2018;83(2):235–47.
5. Lopez R, Doukkali A, Barateau L, Evangelista E, Chenini S, Jaussent I, et al. Test–retest reliability of the multiple sleep latency test in central disorders of hypersomnolence. Sleep. 2017;40(12):zsx164.
6. Ohayon MM. Narcolepsy is complicated by high medical and psychiatric comorbidities: a comparison with the general population. Sleep Med. 2013;14(6):488–92.
7. Barateau L, Chenini S, Evangelista E, Jaussent I, Lopez R, Dauvilliers Y. Clinical autonomic dysfunction in narcolepsy type 1. Sleep. 2019;42(12):zsz187.
8. Miglis MG. Autonomic dysfunction in primary sleep disorders. Sleep Med. 2016;19:40–9.
9. Peyron C, Tighe DK, van den Pol AN, de Lecea L, Heller HC, Sutcliffe JG, et al. Neurons containing hypocretin (orexin) project to multiple neuronal systems. J Neurosci. 1998;18(23):9996–10015.
10. Grimaldi D, Silvani A, Benarroch EE, Cortelli P. Orexin/hypocretin system and autonomic control: new insights and clinical correlations. Neurology. 2014;82(3):271–8. https://doi.org/10.1212/WNL.0000000000000045.
11. Shirasaka T, Nakazato M, Matsukura S, Takasaki M, Kannan H. Sympathetic and cardiovascular actions of orexins in conscious rats. Am J Phys. 1999;277(6 Pt 2):R1780–5.
12. Berteotti C, Silvani A. The link between narcolepsy and autonomic cardiovascular dysfunction: a translational perspective. Clin Auton Res. 2018;28(6):545–55. https://doi.org/10.1007/s10286-017-0473-z.
13. Schuld A, Hebebrand J, Geller F, Pollmächer T. Increased body-mass index in patients with narcolepsy. Lancet. 2000;355(9211):1274–5.
14. Sakurai T. The role of orexin in motivated behaviours. Nat Rev Neurosci. 2014;15(11):719–31.
15. Okumura T, Nozu T. Role of brain orexin in the pathophysiology of functional gastrointestinal disorders. J Gastroenterol Hepatol. 2011;26(Suppl 3):61–6.
16. Samson WK, Gosnell B, Chang JK, Resch ZT, Murphy TC. Cardiovascular regulatory actions of the hypocretins in brain. Brain Res. 1999;831(1–2):248–53.
17. Shirasaka T, Kunitake T, Takasaki M, Kannan H. Neuronal effects of orexins: relevant to sympathetic and cardiovascular functions. Regul Pept. 2002;104(1–3):91–5.
18. Antunes VR, Brailoiu GC, Kwok EH, Scruggs P, Dun NJ. Orexins/hypocretins excite rat sympathetic preganglionic neurons in vivo and in vitro. Am J Physiol Regul Integr Comp Physiol. 2001;281(6):R1801–7.
19. Matsumura K, Tsuchihashi T, Abe I. Central orexin-A augments sympathoadrenal outflow in conscious rabbits. Hypertension. 2001;37(6):1382–7.
20. Plazzi G, Moghadam KK, Maggi LS, Donadio V, Vetrugno R, Liguori R, et al. Autonomic disturbances in narcolepsy. Sleep Med Rev. 2011;15(3):187–96.
21. Fronczek R, Thijs RD. Autonomic alterations in narcolepsy-contrasting results in mice and men. Sleep. 2013;36(1):9–10.
22. Pepin J-L, Borel A-L, Tamisier R, Baguet J-P, Levy P, Dauvilliers Y. Hypertension and sleep: overview of a tight relationship. Sleep Med Rev. 2014;18(6):509–19.
23. Bastianini S, Silvani A, Berteotti C, Elghozi J-L, Franzini C, Lenzi P, et al. Sleep related changes in blood pressure in hypocretin-deficient narcoleptic mice. Sleep. 2011;34(2):213–8.
24. Lo Martire V, Silvani A, Bastianini S, Berteotti C, Zoccoli G. Effects of ambient temperature on sleep and cardiovascular regulation in mice: the role of hypocretin/orexin neurons. PLoS One. 2012;7(10):e47032.
25. Silvani A, Bastianini S, Berteotti C, Cenacchi G, Leone O, Lo Martire V, et al. Sleep and cardiovascular phenotype in middle-aged hypocretin-deficient narcoleptic mice. J Sleep Res. 2014;23(1):98–106.
26. Kayaba Y, Nakamura A, Kasuya Y, Ohuchi T, Yanagisawa M, Komuro I, et al. Attenuated defense response and low basal blood pressure in orexin knockout mice. Am J Physiol Regul Integr Comp Physiol. 2003;285(3):R581–93.
27. Schwimmer H, Stauss HM, Abboud F, Nishino S, Mignot E, Zeitzer JM. Effects of sleep on the cardiovascular and thermoregulatory systems: a possible role for hypocretins. J Appl Physiol. 2010;109(4):1053–63.
28. Zhang W, Sakurai T, Fukuda Y, Kuwaki T. Orexin neuron-mediated skeletal muscle vasodilation and shift of baroreflex during defense response in mice. Am J Physiol Regul Integr Comp Physiol. 2006;290(6):R1654–63.
29. Silvani A, Bastianini S, Berteotti C, Lo Martire V, Zoccoli G. Control of cardiovascular variability during undisturbed wake-sleep behavior in hypocretin-deficient mice. Am J Physiol Regul Integr Comp Physiol. 2012;302(8):R958–64.
30. Hara J, Beuckmann CT, Nambu T, Willie JT, Chemelli RM, Sinton CM, et al. Genetic ablation of orexin neurons in mice results in narcolepsy, hypophagia, and obesity. Neuron. 2001;30(2):345–54.
31. Barateau L, Lopez R, Dauvilliers Y. Treatment options for narcolepsy. CNS Drugs. 2016;30(5):369–79.
32. Guilleminault C, Salva MA, Mancuso J, Hayes B. Narcolepsy, cataplexy, heart rate, and blood pressure. Sleep. 1986;9(1 Pt 2):222–6.
33. Hublin C, Matikainen E, Partinen M. Autonomic nervous system function in narcolepsy. J Sleep Res. 1994;3(3):131–7.
34. Ferini-Strambi L, Spera A, Oldani A, Zucconi M, Bianchi A, Cerutti S, et al. Autonomic function in narcolepsy: power spectrum analysis of heart rate variability. J Neurol. 1997;244(4):252–5.
35. Fronczek R, Overeem S, Reijntjes R, Lammers GJ, van Dijk JG, Pijl H. Increased heart rate variability but normal resting metabolic rate in hypocretin/orexin-deficient human narcolepsy. J Clin Sleep Med. 2008;4(3):248–54.
36. Grimaldi D, Pierangeli G, Barletta G, Terlizzi R, Plazzi G, Cevoli S, et al. Spectral analysis of heart rate variability reveals an enhanced sympathetic activity in narcolepsy with cataplexy. Clin Neurophysiol. 2010;121(7):1142–7.
37. Dauvilliers Y, Pennestri M-H, Whittom S, Lanfranchi PA, Montplaisir JY. Autonomic response to periodic leg movements during sleep in narcolepsy-cataplexy. Sleep. 2011;34(2):219–23.
38. Grimaldi D, Calandra-Buonaura G, Provini F, Agati P, Pierangeli G, Franceschini C, et al. Abnormal sleep-cardiovascular system interaction in narcolepsy with cataplexy: effects of hypocretin deficiency in humans. Sleep. 2012;35(4):519–28.
39. Dauvilliers Y, Jaussent I, Krams B, Scholz S, Lado S, Levy P, et al. Non-dipping blood pressure profile in narcolepsy with cataplexy. PLoS One. 2012;7(6):e38977.
40. Silvani A, Grimaldi D, Barletta G, Bastianini S, Vandi S, Pierangeli G, et al. Cardiovascular variability as a function of sleep-wake behaviour in narcolepsy with cataplexy. J Sleep Res. 2013;22(2):178–84.

41. Sorensen GL, Knudsen S, Petersen ER, Kempfner J, Gammeltoft S, Sorensen HBD, et al. Attenuated heart rate response is associated with hypocretin deficiency in patients with narcolepsy. Sleep. 2013;36(1):91–8.
42. Donadio V, Liguori R, Vandi S, Giannoccaro MP, Pizza F, Leta V, et al. Sympathetic and cardiovascular changes during sleep in narcolepsy with cataplexy patients. Sleep Med. 2014;15(3):315–21. https://doi.org/10.1016/j.sleep.2013.12.005.
43. Donadio V, Liguori R, Vandi S, Pizza F, Dauvilliers Y, Leta V, et al. Lower wake resting sympathetic and cardiovascular activities in narcolepsy with cataplexy. Neurology. 2014;83(12):1080–6. https://doi.org/10.1212/WNL.0000000000000793.
44. de Zambotti M, Pizza F, Covassin N, Vandi S, Cellini N, Stegagno L, et al. Facing emotions in narcolepsy with cataplexy: haemodynamic and behavioural responses during emotional stimulation. J Sleep Res. 2014;23(4):432–40.
45. van der Meijden WP, Fronczek R, Reijntjes RHAM, Corssmit EPM, Biermasz NR, Lammers GJ, et al. Time- and state-dependent analysis of autonomic control in narcolepsy: higher heart rate with normal heart rate variability independent of sleep fragmentation. J Sleep Res. 2015;24(2):206–14.
46. Sieminski M, Partinen M. "Non-dipping" is equally frequent in narcoleptic patients and in patients with insomnia. Sleep Biol Rhythms. 2016;14:31–6.
47. Bosco A, Lopez R, Barateau L, Chenini S, Pesenti C, Pépin J-L, et al. Effect of psychostimulants on blood pressure profile and endothelial function in narcolepsy. Neurology. 2018;90(6):e479–91. https://doi.org/10.1212/WNL.0000000000004911.
48. Antelmi E, Plazzi G, Pizza F, Vandi S, Aricò D, Ferri R. Impact of acute administration of sodium oxybate on heart rate variability in children with type 1 narcolepsy. Sleep Med. 2018;47:1–6.
49. Enevoldsen LH, Tindborg M, Hovmand NL, Christoffersen C, Ellingsgaard H, Suetta C, et al. Functional brown adipose tissue and sympathetic activity after cold exposure in humans with type 1 narcolepsy. Sleep. 2018;41(8) https://doi.org/10.1093/sleep/zsy092.
50. Barateau L, Jaussent I, Lopez R, Evangelista E, Chenini S, Benkiran M, et al. Cardiac sympathetic activity differentiates idiopathic and symptomatic rapid eye movement sleep behaviour disorder. Sci Rep. 2018;8(1):7304.
51. Barateau L, Lopez R, Chenini S, Evangelista E, Benkiran M, Mariano-Goulart D, et al. Exploration of cardiac sympathetic adrenergic nerve activity in narcolepsy. Clin Neurophysiol. 2019;130(3):412–8.
52. Vandi S, Rodolfi S, Pizza F, Moresco M, Antelmi E, Ferri R, et al. Cardiovascular autonomic dysfunction, altered sleep architecture, and muscle overactivity during nocturnal sleep in pediatric patients with narcolepsy type 1. Sleep. 2019;42(12):zsz169.
53. Sieminski M, Chwojnicki K, Sarkanen T, Partinen M. The relationship between orexin levels and blood pressure changes in patients with narcolepsy. PLoS One. 2017;12(10):e0185975.
54. Dantz B, Edgar DM, Dement WC. Circadian rhythms in narcolepsy: studies on a 90 minute day. Electroencephalogr Clin Neurophysiol. 1994;90(1):24–35.
55. Fronczek R, Overeem S, Lammers GJ, van Dijk JG, Van Someren EJW. Altered skin-temperature regulation in narcolepsy relates to sleep propensity. Sleep. 2006;29(11):1444–9.
56. Fronczek R, Raymann RJEM, Overeem S, Romeijn N, van Dijk JG, Lammers GJ, et al. Manipulation of skin temperature improves nocturnal sleep in narcolepsy. J Neurol Neurosurg Psychiatry. 2008;79(12):1354–7.
57. Clark RW, Boudoulas H, Schaal SF, Schmidt HS. Adrenergic hyperactivity and cardiac abnormality in primary disorders of sleep. Neurology. 1980;30(2):113–9.
58. Yoss RE, Moyer NJ, Ogle KN. The pupillogram and narcolepsy. A method to measure decreased levels of wakefulness. Neurology. 1969;19(10):921–8.
59. Karacan I. Erectile dysfunction in narcoleptic patients. Sleep. 1986;9(1 Pt 2):227–31.
60. Grassi G, Seravalle G, Cattaneo BM, Bolla GB, Lanfranchi A, Colombo M, et al. Sympathetic activation in obese normotensive subjects. Hypertension. 1995;25(4):560–3.
61. Kok SW, Overeem S, Visscher TLS, Lammers GJ, Seidell JC, Pijl H, et al. Hypocretin deficiency in narcoleptic humans is associated with abdominal obesity. Obes Res. 2003;11(9):1147–54.
62. Chabas D, Foulon C, Gonzalez J, Nasr M, Lyon-Caen O, Willer J-C, et al. Eating disorder and metabolism in narcoleptic patients. Sleep. 2007;30(10):1267–73.
63. Dahmen N, Tonn P, Messroghli L, Ghezel-Ahmadi D, Engel A. Basal metabolic rate in narcoleptic patients. Sleep. 2009;32(7):962–4.
64. Kreier F, Fliers E, Voshol PJ, Van Eden CG, Havekes LM, Kalsbeek A, et al. Selective parasympathetic innervation of subcutaneous and intra-abdominal fat--functional implications. J Clin Invest. 2002;110(9):1243–50.
65. Sansa G, Iranzo A, Santamaria J. Obstructive sleep apnea in narcolepsy. Sleep Med. 2010;11(1):93–5.
66. Roth T, Dauvilliers Y, Mignot E, Montplaisir J, Paul J, Swick T, et al. Disrupted nighttime sleep in narcolepsy. J Clin Sleep Med. 2013;9(9):955–65.
67. Plazzi G, Ferri R, Antelmi E, Bayard S, Franceschini C, Cosentino FII, et al. Restless legs syndrome is frequent in narcolepsy with cataplexy patients. Sleep. 2010;33(5):689–94.
68. Dauvilliers Y, Pennestri M-H, Petit D, Dang-Vu T, Lavigne G, Montplaisir J. Periodic leg movements during sleep and wakefulness in narcolepsy. J Sleep Res. 2007;16(3):333–9.
69. Plazzi G, Ferri R, Franceschini C, Vandi S, Detto S, Pizza F, et al. Periodic leg movements during sleep in narcoleptic patients with or without restless legs syndrome. J Sleep Res. 2012;21(2):155–62.
70. Dauvilliers Y, Jennum P, Plazzi G. Rapid eye movement sleep behavior disorder and rapid eye movement sleep without atonia in narcolepsy. Sleep Med. 2013;14(8):775–81.
71. Dauvilliers Y, Siegel JM, Lopez R, Torontali ZA, Peever JH. Cataplexy--clinical aspects, pathophysiology and management strategy. Nat Rev Neurol. 2014;10(7):386–95.
72. Luppi PH, Clément O, Sapin E, Gervasoni D, Peyron C, Léger L, et al. The neuronal network responsible for paradoxical sleep and its dysfunctions causing narcolepsy and rapid eye movement (REM) behavior disorder. Sleep Med Rev. 2011;15(3):153–63.
73. Barateau L, Pizza F, Lopez R, Antelmi E, Plazzi G, Dauvilliers Y. Persistence of deep-tendon reflexes during partial cataplexy. Sleep Med. 2018;45:80–2.
74. Rubboli G, d'Orsi G, Zaniboni A, Gardella E, Zamagni M, Rizzi R, et al. A video-polygraphic analysis of the cataplectic attack. Clin Neurophysiol. 2000;111(Suppl 2):S120–8.
75. Donadio V, Plazzi G, Vandi S, Franceschini C, Karlsson T, Montagna P, et al. Sympathetic and cardiovascular activity during cataplexy in narcolepsy. J Sleep Res. 2008;17(4):458–63.
76. Vetrugno R, D'Angelo R, Moghadam KK, Vandi S, Franceschini C, Mignot E, et al. Behavioural and neurophysiological correlates of human cataplexy: a video-polygraphic study. Clin Neurophysiol. 2010;121(2):153–62.
77. Aslan S, Erbil N, Tezer FI. Heart rate variability during nocturnal sleep and daytime naps in patients with narcolepsy type 1 and type 2. J Clin Neurophysiol. 2019;36(2):104–11.
78. Bassetti C, Aldrich MS. Idiopathic hypersomnia. A series of 42 patients. Brain. 1997;120(Pt 8):1423–35.
79. Vernet C, Leu-Semenescu S, Buzare M-A, Arnulf I. Subjective symptoms in idiopathic hypersomnia: beyond excessive sleepiness. J Sleep Res. 2010;19(4):525–34.
80. Baker TL, Guilleminault C, Nino-Murcia G, Dement WC. Comparative polysomnographic study of narcolepsy and idiopathic central nervous system hypersomnia. Sleep. 1986;9(1 Pt 2):232–42.

81. Sforza E, Roche F, Barthélémy JC, Pichot V. Diurnal and nocturnal cardiovascular variability and heart rate arousal response in idiopathic hypersomnia. Sleep Med. 2016;24:131–6.
82. Wang JY, Han F, Dong SX, Li J, An P, Zhang XZ, et al. Cerebrospinal fluid orexin a levels and autonomic function in Kleine-Levin syndrome. Sleep. 2016;39(4):855–60.
83. Dauvilliers Y, Bassetti C, Lammers GJ, Arnulf I, Mayer G, Rodenbeck A, et al. Pitolisant versus placebo or modafinil in patients with narcolepsy: a double-blind, randomised trial. Lancet Neurol. 2013;12(11):1068–75.
84. Irukayama-Tomobe Y, Ogawa Y, Tominaga H, Ishikawa Y, Hosokawa N, Ambai S, et al. Nonpeptide orexin type-2 receptor agonist ameliorates narcolepsy-cataplexy symptoms in mouse models. Proc Natl Acad Sci U S A. 2017;114(22):5731–6.
85. Thorpy MJ, Shapiro C, Mayer G, Corser BC, Emsellem H, Plazzi G, et al. A randomized study of solriamfetol for excessive sleepiness in narcolepsy. Ann Neurol. 2019;85(3):359–70.
86. McAlpine CS, Kiss MG, Rattik S, He S, Vassalli A, Valet C, et al. Sleep modulates haematopoiesis and protects against atherosclerosis. Nature. 2019;566(7744):383–7.

Fatal Familial Insomnia

18

Luca Baldelli, Giovanna Calandra-Buonaura,
Federica Provini, and Pietro Cortelli

Introduction

Fatal familial insomnia (FFI) was first described by Lugaresi et al. in 1986 [1] as a hereditary, autosomal dominant, and invariably fatal disease caused by a missense mutation at codon 178 of the prion protein gene (*PRNP*) cosegregating with methionine at methionine (M)–valine (V) polymorphic codon 129 on the mutated allele. The clinical hallmark of FFI is *agrypnia excitata* (AE), a syndrome characterized by a progressive and untreatable sleep loss with increasing difficulties in falling and remaining asleep both during the night and the day associated with 24-h motor and autonomic sympathetic overactivation and by a peculiar dream-like behavior known as oneiric stupor (OS) [2]. Pathologically, the thalamus, with severe but selective atrophy of its mediodorsal (MD) and anteroventral (AV) nuclei, appears to be the earliest and most severely affected brain structure in FFI [3]. Thalamic lesions cause the loss of slow wave sleep (SWS) and the disconnection of the limbic cortical areas and the cortical and subcortical regions that also regulate autonomic functions, resulting in an increase of autonomic activation [4].

Agrypnia excitata is not exclusive to FFI but it has been also described in Morvan syndrome (MS), an autoimmune limbic encephalopathy, and delirium tremens (DT), the well-known alcohol withdrawal syndrome [5, 6]. An anatomic (FFI) or functional (MS, DT) interruption of the thalamolimbic circuits regulating the sleep–wake cycle and the control of the autonomic nervous system (ANS) [7, 8] has been suggested as the pathogenetic mechanism for AF.

L. Baldelli
Department of Biomedical and NeuroMotor Sciences (DIBINEM), University of Bologna, Bologna, Italy

G. Calandra-Buonaura · F. Provini · P. Cortelli (✉)
IRCCS Istituto di Scienze Neurologiche, Bologna, Italy

Department of Biomedical and NeuroMotor Sciences (DIBINEM), University of Bologna, Bologna, Italy
e-mail: pietro.cortelli@unibo.it

Of major relevance is the role of the autonomic nervous system, permeating the clinical picture of FFI (and consequently of AE), a model disease for the investigation of the essential role of the thalamus for the central organization of body homeostasis integrating both sleep and autonomic function control [9, 10].

Fatal Familial Insomnia

Historical Notes

In 1986, Lugaresi et al. reported in detail an inherited condition named **fatal familial insomnia** (FFI) characterized by severe and progressive sleep impairment, dysautonomia, and motor hyperactivity associated with severe atrophy of the anterior and medial dorsal thalamic nuclei. The proband, a 53-year-old man, experienced a continuing inability to sleep associated with progressive dysfunction of the autonomic nervous system with pyrexia, diaphoresis, and urinary sphincter dysfunction over several months. Nocturnal sleep became disturbed by increasing movements and enacted dreams. Motor signs with tremor, dysarthria, clumsy gait, and myoclonus became more pronounced and memory deficit ensued [1].

The patient progressed into stupor, became comatose, and expired 9 months after clinical onset. Electroencephalographic (EEG) and polysomnographic (PSG) studies revealed loss of sleep, spindles, K complexes, and delta activity throughout 24 h. Autonomic tests disclosed sympathetic activation (increased heart rate, blood pressure, breathing rate, and core body levels temperature). Serial 24-h monitoring of hormonal and catecholamine levels revealed persistently elevated plasma concentrations of cortisol and especially norepinephrine (NE) levels and a lack of the physiological nocturnal rise of melatonin (MLT) secretion. No cognitive impairment was revealed on neuropsychological testing, even 7 months after disease onset.

S. Chokroverty, P. Cortelli (eds.), *Autonomic Nervous System and Sleep*, https://doi.org/10.1007/978-3-030-62263-3_18

Neuropathologic examination revealed 80–96% loss of large neurons in the anterior and medial dorsal thalamic nuclei with reactive astrogliosis associated with atrophy; these changes were also noted in the inferior olivary nucleus. In 1992, the mutation in FFI was associated with the substitution of aspartic acid for asparagine at codon 178 (D178N mutation) of the prion protein (PrP) gene *PRNP*. These findings conclusively established FFI as a new phenotype in familial human prion diseases [11, 12].

Demographics

FFI typically appears between the fourth and sixth decade of life, most often between the ages of 51 and 60 years [9], although early onset cases up to 17–18 years of age [13, 14] have also been reported [15–17]. The patients' genotype of the nonmutated allele of *PRNP* seems to influence both disease course and clinical presentation. FFI patients homozygous at codon 129 (codifying M also in the nonmutated allele at codon 129 of *PRNP*) have a more rapid evolution (11.6 ± 5.1 months) than FFI heterozygous patients (codifying V at position 129 of the nonmutated allele) who have a two- to threefold longer disease duration (21.8 ± 12.8 months) [18]. The reported shorter survival times in China and Japan (8.2 and 10.6 months, respectively) compared to Western countries, despite greater utilization of life-prolonging care, are likely to be related to the prevalence of the 129MM genotype in Asian countries [19–21]. The short-evolution cases (M-M patients homozygous at codon 129) present the most typical features of the disease [22], while the age at onset does not seem to be affected from prion protein (PrP) codon 129 genotype [23].

Up to date, more than 70 affected families have been identified all over the world and in every ethnic group, comprising more than 130 genetically or pathologically confirmed cases, with China presenting the absolute highest number (>25 kindreds), and Germany and Spain the highest prevalence in relation to their population [24].

Features

Symptoms and Signs The clinical picture of FFI can be divided into three categories including sleep disorders, autonomic and classic prion disease neurological symptoms such as disorders of ocular movements, pyramidal symptoms, myoclonus, gait disturbances, apraxia, and cognitive impairment [4, 24].

Changes in sleep with difficulties in falling asleep, early awakening, and inability to take usual naps is one of the earliest features of the disease. At the same time, patients appear drowsy (with head and eyelid drops) during daytime and apathetic, though social behavior is preserved. Hypertension, slight evening pyrexia, a tendency to perspire, lacrimate, and salivate, impotence in men and fluctuating diplopia accompany early insomnia in some cases. Sleep and autonomic alterations progressively get worse, and patients become increasingly taciturn and appear indifferent to their surroundings and even their fate. When left alone, patients lapse into a state of unresponsiveness showing peculiar motor behaviors during which they mimic daily-life activities, such as dressing, combing the hair, washing, and manipulating nonexistent objects. If questioned, patients link these gestures to an oneiric scene, justifying the term "oneiric stupor" [25, 26]. Disturbances of gait [27], disequilibrium, dysmetria, spontaneous and evoked myoclonus, and signs of upper motor neuron involvement such as hyperreflexia of muscle stretch reflexes and Babinski's sign progressively appear. Later stages are characterized by ever-increasing oneiric stupor, inability to stand and walk, increasing dysarthria and dysphagia. Death supervenes from cardiorespiratory failure or intercurrent respiratory or systemic infections [22].

Patients with 129MM genotype usually present sleep and vegetative disturbances as earliest symptoms, compared to 129MV who typically show visual symptoms and ataxia [18].Throughout the disease course, homozygotes tend to have more prominent insomnia, myoclonus, autonomic dysfunction, spatial disorientation, hallucinations, and weight loss, while heterozygotes are more likely to demonstrate ataxia with equilibrium impairment and latero-retropulsion, dysarthria, seizures, and bulbar symptoms [24, 27, 28].

Neurophysiological Features Longitudinal 24-h polysomnographic monitoring documents severe sleep fragmentation, reduction of total sleep time, and a sleep–wake cycle derangement with an early permanent and progressive reduction and consequent disappearance of sleep features (spindles and K complexes become impossible to generate even by pharmacologic means) and diminished deep sleep (delta sleep–slow wave sleep—SWS) [29, 30], more severe in the short disease course (Fig. 18.1) [31]. This derangement of physiological sleep, resulting from severe damage of the thalamic machinery, responsible for sleep generation, rules out the applicability of standard sleep scoring criteria [32].

Subwakefulness is the predominant nocturnal and diurnal EEG and behavioral pattern consisting of stage 1 NREM sleep. This stage can be interrupted by sudden onset of rapid-eye-movement (REM) sleep episodes with or without atonia lasting for a few seconds or minutes [2]. This condition represents the neurophysiological substrate of dream enactment behaviors characterizing oneiric stupor, which can emerge from any of these stages. Notably, quasiperiodic sharp wave

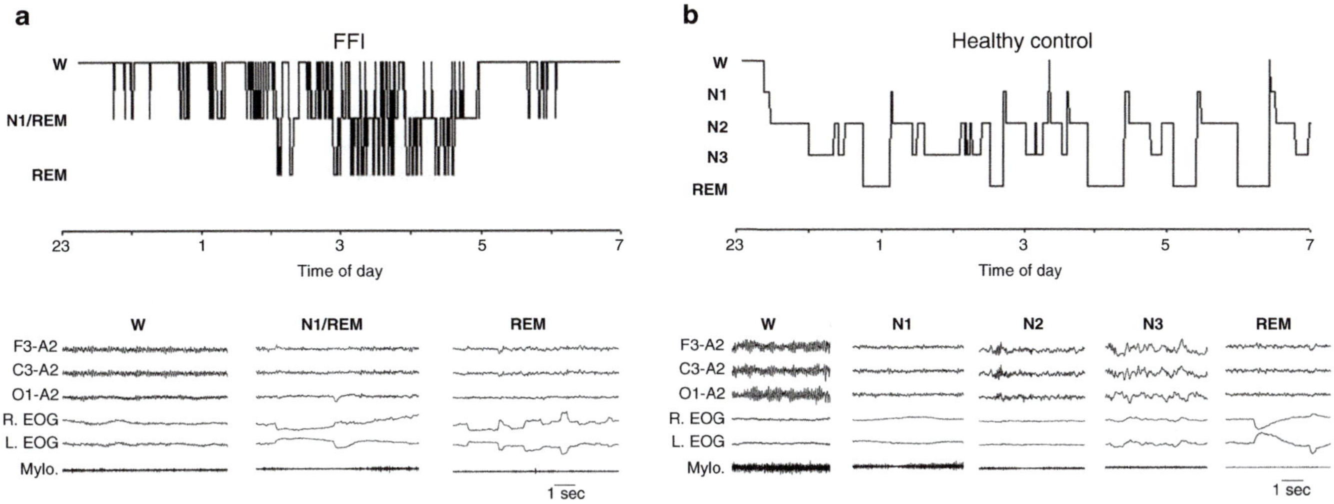

Fig. 18.1 Hypnogram (*upper graph*) and related excerpts of a polygraphic tracing (*lower graph*) in a patient with fatal familial insomnia (FFI) (**a**) and in an age-matched healthy control (**b**). In the FFI patient the hypnogram continuously fluctuates between wake and subwakefulness (N1/REM) with short intrusions of REM sleep; the polygraphic excerpts show abolishment of spindle and delta sleep. EEG (F3-A2; C3-A2; O1-A2); R, right; L, left; EOG, electrooculogram; Mylo, mylohyoideus muscle. (From Baldelli and Provini [31], © 2019 Elsevier with permission)

activity typical of Creutzfeldt–Jakob disease (CJD) is rarely recorded in short evolution patients but can occur in cases with long evolution just before death [9].

The loss of sleep is associated with a loss of 24-h circadian motor rhythmicity documented by long-term actigraphic monitoring [33]. Indirect calorimetry shows that energy expenditure is up to 60% more than in healthy controls [33], a feature associated with the severe metabolic exhaustion and cachexia in FFI patients [22].

Neuropsychological Features Serial neuropsychological examinations document an early progressive impairment of attention and vigilance (which varies within seconds from normal alertness to an oneiric status with enacted dreams), whereas intellectual function remains substantially intact until the advanced stages of disease, resembling more a disturbance of consciousness (confusional state) rather than true dementia [34].

Neuroimaging Computed tomography (CT) and magnetic resonance imaging (MRI) scans are unremarkable except for a mild cerebral and cerebellar atrophy in the most advanced disease stages. Serial positron emission tomography (PET) (18 fluorodeoxyglucose [FDG]–PET) scans invariably show an impaired thalamic metabolism from the early stages of the disease [35] or even several months before clinical disease onset in FFI mutation carriers [4]. Although hypometabolism is invariably more pronounced in the thalamus, it extends to the mesial areas of the frontal lobe as the disease progresses, affecting the entire cortex and basal ganglia in the most advanced disease stages of long-evolution cases. The metabolic impairment prevails in the mesial areas of the frontal lobe in both short- and long-evolution cases [35].

Pathology and Molecular Biology of Prion Protein Bilateral thalamic degeneration (with neuronal loss and astrogliosis) is the invariable finding of FFI. The MD and AV nuclei are the thalamic structures most consistently and most severely affected with neuronal loss often reaching 95–100% [3]. Other thalamic nuclei are variable and less severely involved. The inferior olives undergo similar atrophy in most cases. Other brain structures are usually unaffected, though minor and inconstant changes are represented by moderate astrogliosis of the hypothalamus and periaqueductal gray matter in the midbrain and basal ganglia [11, 36]. The involvement of the cerebral cortex is directly related to disease duration: mild spongiform degeneration confined to the orbitofrontal cortex and anterior cingulate gyrus is commonly seen in short duration cases, whereas the cortical spongiform degeneration is widespread in cases of long duration. However, in accordance with PET findings, the cortical involvement is always most prominent in the corticolimbic regions regardless of the disease duration [3, 24, 37].

Immunoblot analysis of the brain homogenates shows that, following deglycosylation, treatment with proteinase K (PK), the protease-resistant (PK-res) fragment of the abnormal, disease-related prion protein (PK-resPrP^{Sc}), displays electrophoretic mobility corresponding to a relative mass of 19 kilodalton a (kDa) in FFI which is different from the 21 kDa form described in familial Creutzfeldt–Jakob Disease (fCJD[178]) [38]. Amino-acid sequencing of the PK-resPrP^{Sc} fragments isolated in the two diseases shows that the fragment N-terminus is amino acid 97 in FFI and 82 in fCJD[178] [39]. These data show that the PrP^{Sc} species associated with FFI and fCJD[178], respectively, are cleaved by PK at distinct sites (97 and 82) generating fragments of different sizes. In turn the finding that PK cleaves PrP^{Sc} at distinct sites in FFI and fCJD[178] provides strong evidence that the conformation of PrP^{Sc} associated with these two diseases is different [23].

Dysfunction of the Autonomic Nervous System: Unbalanced Autonomic Control and Sympathetic Hyperactivation

The main autonomic features of FFI all point toward a dysregulated overactivation of ANS manifesting itself by means of: (1) the setting of BP, HR and temperature circadian rhythms to a higher level and their later disruption, (2) exaggerated NA and BP increase in response to physiologic stimuli (orthostatism and Valsalva, respectively), (3) increased mean level of resting awake muscle sympathetic nerve activity (MSNA), (4) absent BP rise after NA infusion, (5) abnormal HR increase after atropine infusion, (6) reduced effects of clonidine, (7) increased paroxysmal or persistent sweating, salivation and lacrimation, and (8) sphincteric dysregulation leading to complete insufficiency, point out the presence of an increased sympathetic tone, responsive (even if only partially) to stimuli at early stages and completely dysregulated and unhinged in later phases in FFI patients (Figs. 18.2 and 18.3). Hence, the sympathetic hyperactivation and the loss of its control, in terms of lack of any circadian rhythms and response to stimuli, are the two focal clinical points in FFI autonomic alterations. Illustrative of this condition are "autonomic storms," a possible event in FFI, characterized by a paroxysmal burst of sympathetic activity clinically translating into episodic hyperthermia, hypertension, and tachycardia associated with excessive sweating, salivation, and lacrimation which can precede short periods of SWS usually felt by patients as very restorative even if lasting only few minutes [40].

Unbalanced autonomic functions with a prevalent sympathetic activity are of utmost clinical relevance in FFI, not only for the above-mentioned signs and symptoms, but also for the related increased risk of mortality [41–45]. Described as dysautonomia in more than 80% of patients reported in literature, it could actually be a feature of all FFI patients, as some authors could not have specifically looked for it. In many cases, cardiovascular and neuroendocrine domains only studied in detail. Of note, among more than 120 patients, only in 5 of them the absence of dysautonomia was described [14, 46, 47].

Cardiovascular

Blood Pressure and Heart Rate

Cardiovascularsigns and symptoms, clinically expressing as increased heart rate (HR) or elevated arterial blood pressure (BP), are recorded or measured in about 35% of patients [48] (Fig. 18.4 and see also Fig. 18.2).

Nocturnal BP fall is the first component of BP circadian rhythm to be markedly reduced or completely lost in FFI patients (Fig. 18.4) [49]. However, at the early stage of the disease 24-h BP and HR profiles remain unchanged or mildly reduced in amplitude overall and patients are generally normotensive [49, 50]. As the disease progresses, the amplitude of circadian variations of BP and HR decreases further and patients develop full-blown and steady hypertension and tachycardia [49, 51], until complete obliteration of BP and HR rhythm profiles in the preterminal stage of the disease (Fig. 18.5a, *black line and dots*) [1, 49].

Hormonal and Catecholamine Circadian Rhythms

In FFI early stages, although hormonal circadian rhythms are maintained, cortisol levels are already persistently increased, positively modulating vascular response to catecholamines and increasing sympathetic activity (Figs. 18.4 and 18.5b, *gray shade*). In later stages, further elevation in cortisol with normal adrenocorticotropin (ACTH) has been documented in association with a pathological nocturnal peak of cortisol and ACTH. In addition, elevation of norepinephrine (noradrenaline—NA) and epinephrine (adrenaline—A) levels shows synchronism with the persistent tachycardia (Fig. 18.5a, b, *black line and dots*). Only the preterminal stage of the disease sees complete obliteration of the hormonal rhythms [49].The circadian secretory patterns of somatotropin and prolactin [52] are abnormal, negatively affecting menstrual cycle [53, 54]. Moreover, melatonin secretion is reduced, as most of the patients lack its physiological nocturnal peak, until the complete obliteration of its rhythm later on [55] (Fig. 18.5).A sympathetic overactivity in FFI patients is also supported by the responses to autonomic functions tests [1, 51, 54]. Already at early stage of the disease, although normotensive, patients usually present supine tachycardia and a high rise in NA at head-up tilt test. Later, with disease progression, patients can develop mainly systolic orthostatic hypotension, probably due to the deconditioning of patients, often bedridden at this stage, counterbalanced by a greater HR, plasma NA, and A increase in response to orthostatism excluding sympathetic failure. At Valsalva maneuver, a prompt rise in HR during the hypotension phase, which is sometimes excessively marked [51], is followed by a greater blood pressure overshoot with maintained compensatory bradycardia, which is maintained also during deep breathing test [54]. In other cases, BP is increased until no further change is seen during overshoot

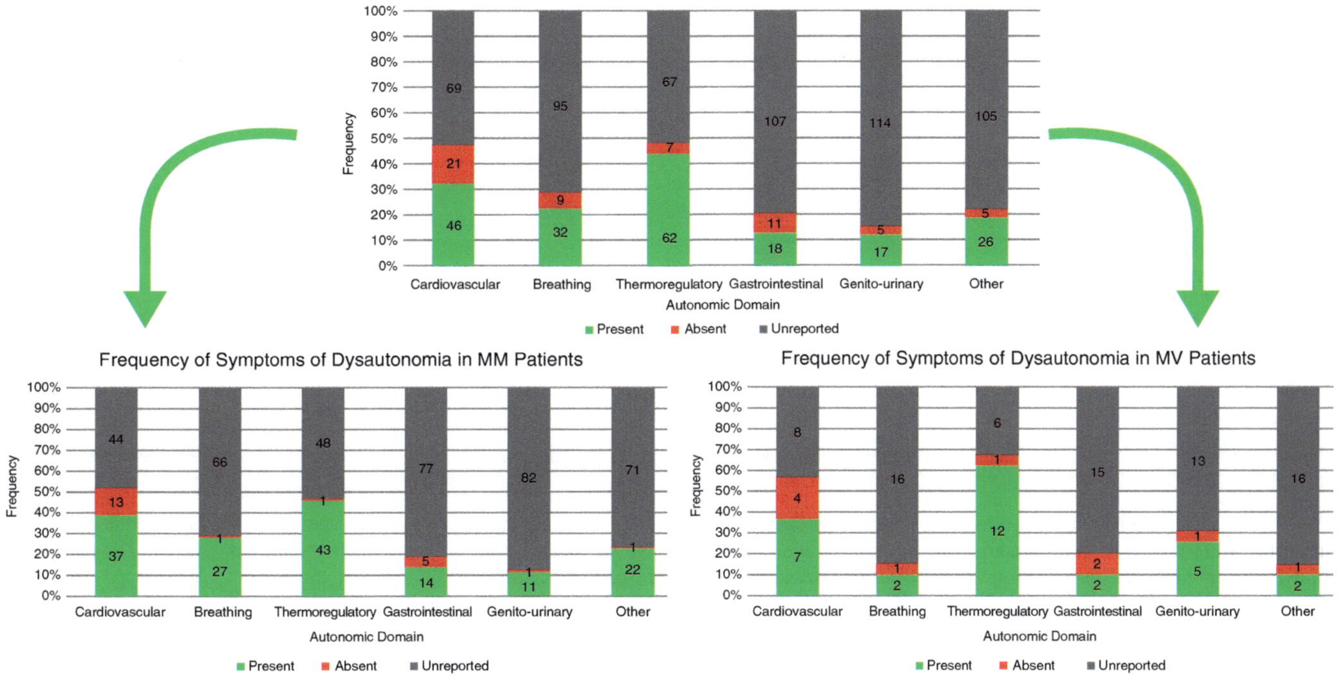

Fig. 18.2 Frequency of symptoms of dysautonomia throughout the disease course in published cases of confirmed (genetically and/or pathologically) fatal familial insomnia, homozygous (MM) and heterozygous (MV) at codon 129 as in Baldelli and Provini [31]. (*Other* = findings belonging to the salivary, lacrimal and pupillary domains. The number of described cases has been indicated inside each column's section)

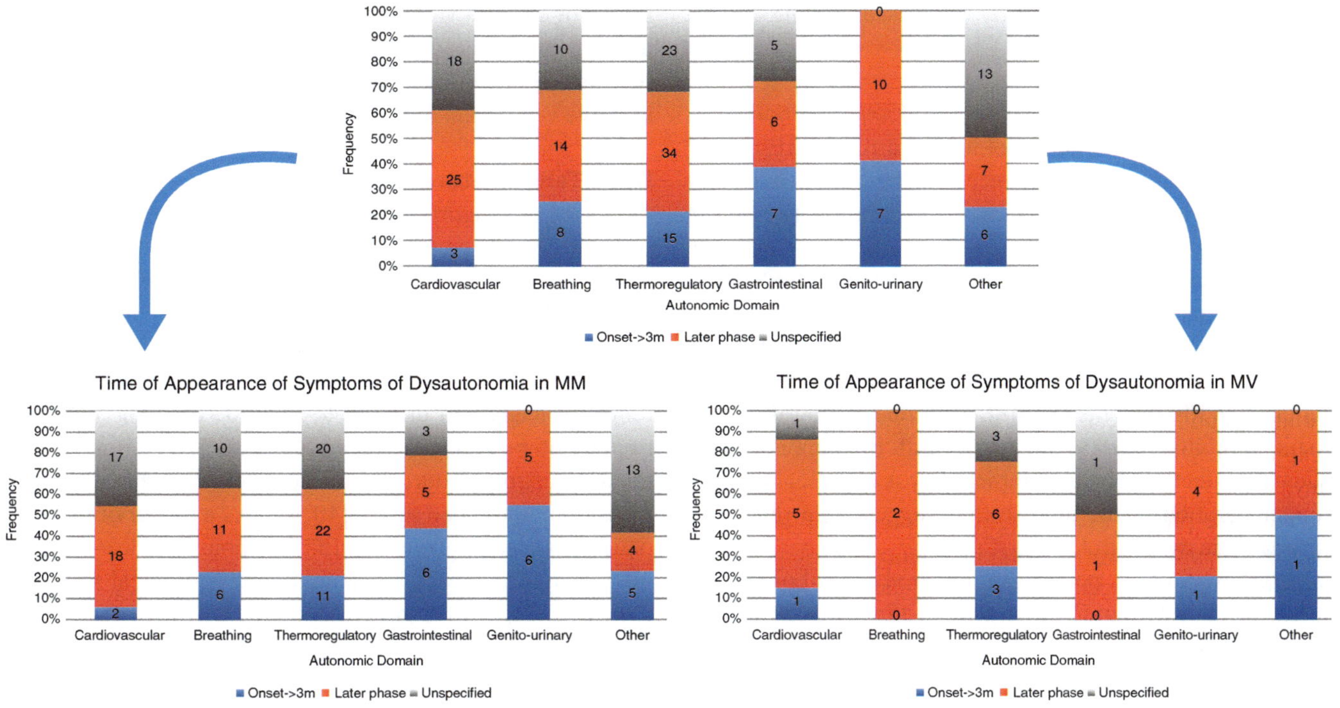

Fig. 18.3 Correlation between symptoms of dysautonomia and time of appearance during the disease course in published cases of confirmed (genetically and/or pathologically) fatal familial insomnia, homozygous (MM), and heterozygous (MV) at codon 129 as in Baldelli and Provini [31]. (*Other* = findings belonging to the salivary, lacrimal and pupillary domains. The number of described cases has been indicated inside each column's section)

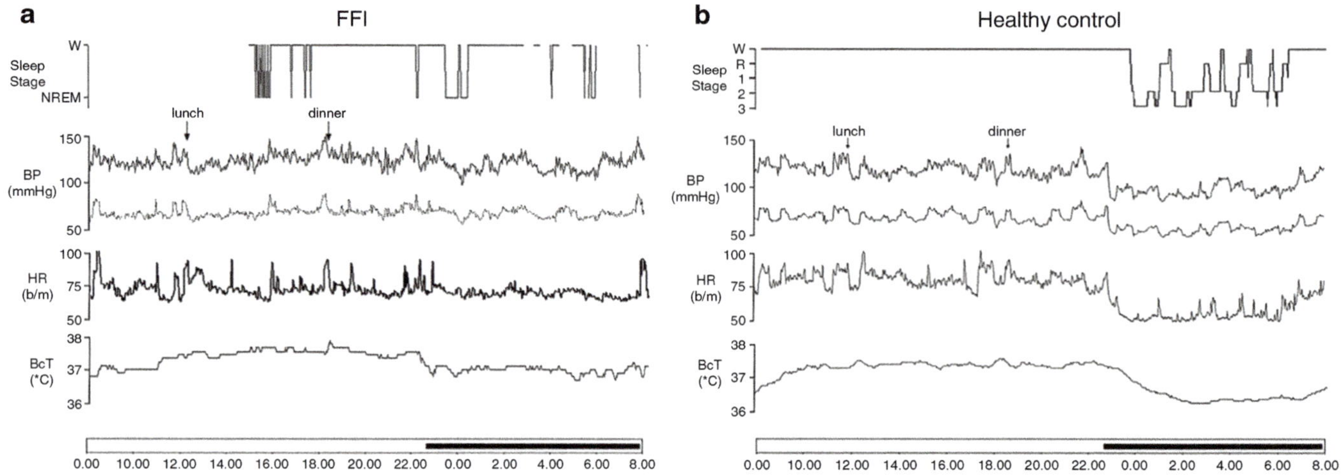

Fig. 18.4 Twenty-four-hour polygraphy in a patient with fatal familial insomnia (FFI) (**a**) and in an age-matched healthy control individual (**b**) showing (from top to bottom) hypnogram and circadian rhythms of systolic and diastolic blood pressure (BP), heart rate (HR), body core temperature (BcT). In comparison to the control, 24-h systolic and diastolic BP recordings lack the physiological nocturnal fall. The amplitude of HR circadian variation is markedly decreased; daytime HR peaks correspond to assumption of orthostatism. BcT nocturnal drop is impaired. (Image modified from Baldelli and Provini [31], © 2019 Elsevier with permission)

[1], suggesting that the response to sympathetic stimuli is not only increased but also not appropriately modulated [54], as it is also seen in cold pressure test where BP rise is conversely lower than normal rise [51]. Moreover, sympathetic overactivity is confirmed by abnormal diastolic BP rise at handgrip test [54] and by increased resting awake MSNA [56].

Pharmacological Tests Evaluating Autonomic Function

Infusing noradrenaline does not lead to a rise in BP, even if dosage is increased, in accordance with the already markedly increased levels of catecholamines, which probably result in the downregulation of adrenoreceptors. On the other hand, atropine induces an abnormal rise in HR [1, 54] highlighting that, when parasympathetic tone is artificially withdrawn, an unrestrained sympathetic activity is exposed. Finally, although arterial hypertension can be controlled with beta-blockers in FFI patients [57, 58], clonidine, a central sympathetic inhibitor, fails to obtain its full BP depressor and sedative effect, which is completely lost in patients with a longer duration of the disease [54] suggesting a refractory sympathetic dyscontrol.

All these findings point to an impaired control of the cardiovascular system in FFI characterized by a higher sympathetic activity with preserved parasympathetic activity.

Breathing

Autonomic dysfunction of breathing control is reported in about one-fifth of literature cases (see Fig. 18.2). Nocturnal breathing disorders have been described at onset or within 3 months in six patients, either as an irregular rhythm [59] or as respiratory pauses [42, 47] (see Fig. 18.3); in one case a respiratory noise functionally compatible with vocal cord adduction has also been clinically reported [60]. Later on, patients develop diurnal alterations of breathing such as persistent tachypnea at rest [40] and labored breathing. Terminal stages of FFI are variably characterized by respiratory failure, vocal cord adduction [61], or abnormal breathing rhythms (Biot's breathing) [43, 50], which often require non-invasive ventilation [44] or intubation [22, 43, 53, 62].

Body Temperature

Increased body temperature has been observed in more than one-third of FFI patients at early stages (see Fig. 18.3), presenting as mild forms of evening pyrexia [60] or as more structured intermittent fever spikes without inflammatory correlates [62, 63]. As the disease progresses, the patients can experience a stabilization of the hyperthermia, which remains steady and difficult to treat [1, 61]. The circadian rhythm of body core temperature (BCT) is progressively severely disrupted during the disease course with a full suppression in advanced stages [40, 43]. As a matter of fact, FFI patients present higher mean BCT without any clear-cut fluctuations during the 24-h lacking the physiological nocturnal reduction (Figs. 18.4 and 18.5).

Hyperstimulation of sweat glands leads to hyperhidrosis, described in about 40% of the patients in the literature (see Fig. 18.2). Frequently present at onset [64, 65], nocturnal or diurnal [46, 54, 66], intense sweating can be a steady condition or a part of an episodic "autonomic storm" [40]. Overall, dysfunction of the thermoregulatory control of ANS is the most frequently reported abnormality in about 45% of the patients.

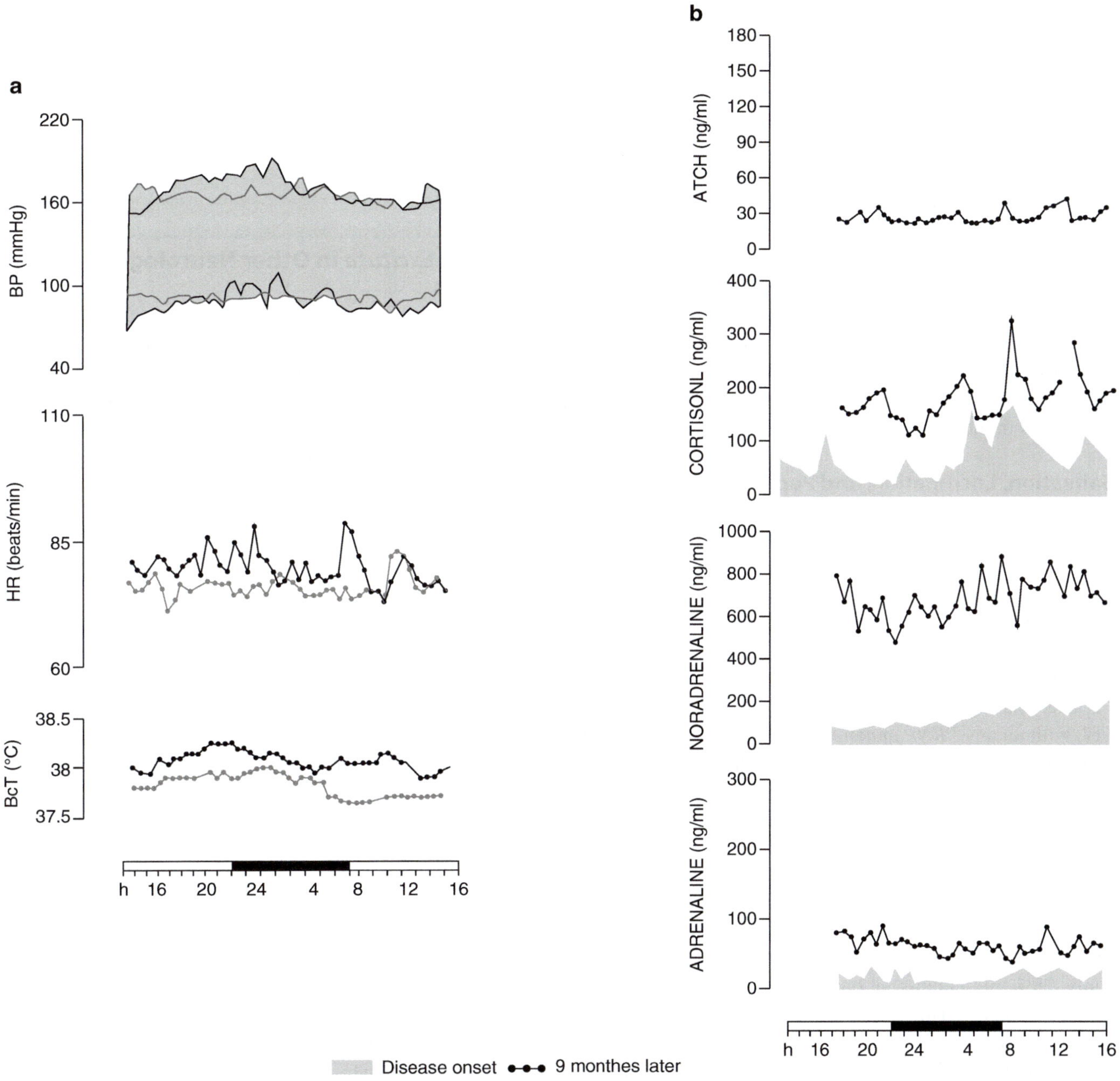

Fig. 18.5 Progressive disruption of 24-h rhythms of systolic and diastolic blood pressure (BP), heart rate (HR), and body core temperature (BcT) (**a**), adrenocorticotropin (ACTH), cortisol and catecholamines (**b**) during fatal familial insomnia disease course. The gray line and shade represent values at disease onset, black lines after 9 months of disease. BP, HR, BcT, catecholamines, and cortisol progressively set to higher levels. (From Baldelli and Provini [31], © 2019 Elsevier with permission)

Gastrointestinal

Decrease of gut motility due to sympathetic hyperactivity is probably the cause of constipation, generally reported among FFI patients, sometimes at onset [14, 41]. Gastrointestinal control impairment can manifest also as diarrhea [46] or bloating feeling (abnormal digestion) due to rapid accumulation of gas in the gastrointestinal tract [67]. When the disease reaches advanced phases, dysregulation of sphincter control, causing incontinence can appear [1, 54].

Genitourinary

Genitourinary dysautonomia is frequent in FFI patients, especially at onset, in 40% of the cases presenting these symptoms (see Fig. 18.3). When at onset, it often presents as impotence in men or loss of libido in both sexes [68–70], while urinary symptoms are less relevant at this stage, especially in short course MM patients.

In later stages, similarly to gastrointestinal alterations, the impairment of sphincter control affects also micturition leading to incontinence [1, 54, 65]. Few cases, however, report the association of constipation and urinary retention [71, 72]. This manifestation could suggest a dyssynergia of urinary sphincters rather than an insufficiency, probably related to a pathological adaptation to the underlying chronic sympathetic overactivity; however, urodynamic testing was never performed in these patients.

Salivation, Lacrimation, and Pupillary Tone

Excessive salivation and lacrimation can be found, either persistent [1, 73] or paroxysmal [40]. Pupillary tone alteration, miotic [47, 74] or mydriatic [53] and more frequently delayed or nonresponsive (to light stimuli) pupils [53, 75] have been described.

Sporadic Familial Insomnia

Patients sharing clinical and histopathologic features with FFI, without any *PRNP* mutation or any positive familial history, have been ascribed to the clinical definition of Sporadic Fatal Insomnia (sFI) [22, 76], often referred to as the thalamic form of sCJDMM2 [77–79].

The sFI clinical and histopathologic phenotype appears to be more variable than that of the FFI variant linked to the 129 homozygous genotype [9, 24]. Consequently, although many symptoms of sFI overlap with those observed in FFI, insomnia has not been a prominent symptom in many cases of sFI (only 29% of patients at onset) [80], unless specifically investigated [77]. This is true also for autonomic symptoms, reported only in half of the cases and in one-third of the recently reviewed European patients [76]. Impaired breathing control and genitourinary symptoms are the most frequent, while cardiovascular features resembling FFI are described in just one patient with hypertension. On the one hand, this outcome is predictable since the specific FFI mutation, D178N, is likely to impose more constraints on the initial spontaneous conversion to a prion-like conformation of the mutated PrP compared to the presumably idiopathic conversion [81, 82]. On the other, autonomic symptoms may not have been the main focus of these reports and therefore not searched in detail. Several cases have been generically described as "with dysautonomia," which probably, if specifically investigated, could have been more frequent in sFI patients [76].

Other symptoms overlap with those observed in FFI such as cognitive decline and/or ataxia (42%) at disease onset and cognitive impairment, ataxia, insomnia and myoclonus in the more advanced stages. Moreover, symptoms characterizing atypical parkinsonian syndromes, such as oculomotor symptoms, dyskinesia, and parkinsonism are often present in sFI at presentation [83, 84].

Agrypnia Excitata in Other Neurological Disorders

The clinical hallmark of FFI, AE is a definite clinico-neurophysiological condition characterized by (1) slow wave sleep loss with disruption of the physiological sleep–wake cycle, (2) a 24-h motor, sympathetic, and aminergic overactivity, and (3) peculiar episodes of oneiric stupor [2, 7, 8, 26, 85]. All these criteria must be fulfilled to make the diagnosis. Following are the three fundamental features of AE: (1) Disruption of the sleep–wake cycle consists of (a) disappearance of spindle-delta activities and failure of (b) REM sleep to stabilize, appearing only in short recurrent episodes or mixed with stage 1 NREM sleep [25]. (2) Twenty-four-hour diurnal and nocturnal (circadian) motor, sympathetic, and aminergic overactivity. Of particular interest is the steady higher secretion of NA during both day and night along with reduced MLT levels and the absence of its nocturnal peak. This inverse correlation between the circadian secretion of NE and MLT could constitute a biological marker of AE [2]. (3) Oneiric stupor (OSS), the third characteristic sign of AE, consists of the recurrence of stereotyped gestures mimicking daily-life activities (Fig. 18.6). OS should not be confused with REM Sleep Behavior Disorder (RBD), real enacted dreams, appearing during REM sleep without atonia. Moreover, while OS episodes are clinically reported by patients as a single oneiric scene, RBD is characterized by enactments of a true dream in which emotions and memories are transformed into a fantastic movie-like plot [86].

Outside FFI, AE has been observed in other diseases presenting different pathophysiological mechanisms, such as Morvan syndrome (MS) and delirium tremens (DT).

Morvan Syndrome

Diffuse muscle contractions (myokimias and cramps), associated with acute insomnia, anxiety and profuse perspiration characterize the syndrome first described by Morvan [87]. In most cases, MS resolves in a few weeks or months, but in others the progressive worsening of symptoms leads to a confusional-oneiric state preceding death by months or more

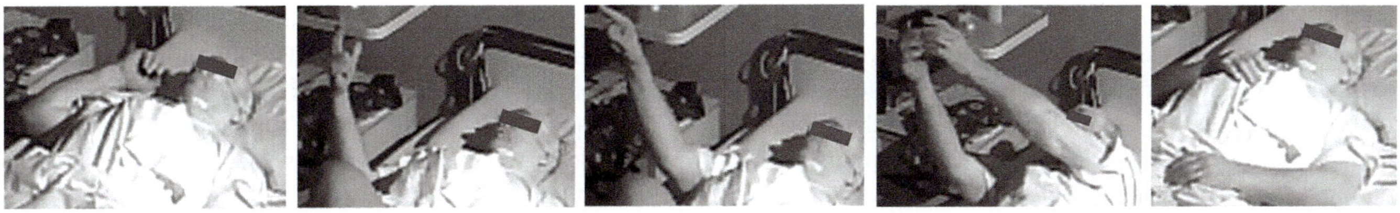

Fig. 18.6 Frame sequence of an oneiric stupor episode in a patient with fatal familial insomnia. The patient performs gestures such as pointing at something and manipulating an inexistent object, quietly mimicking usual daily life activities. (From Baldelli and Provini [31], © 2019 Elsevier with permission)

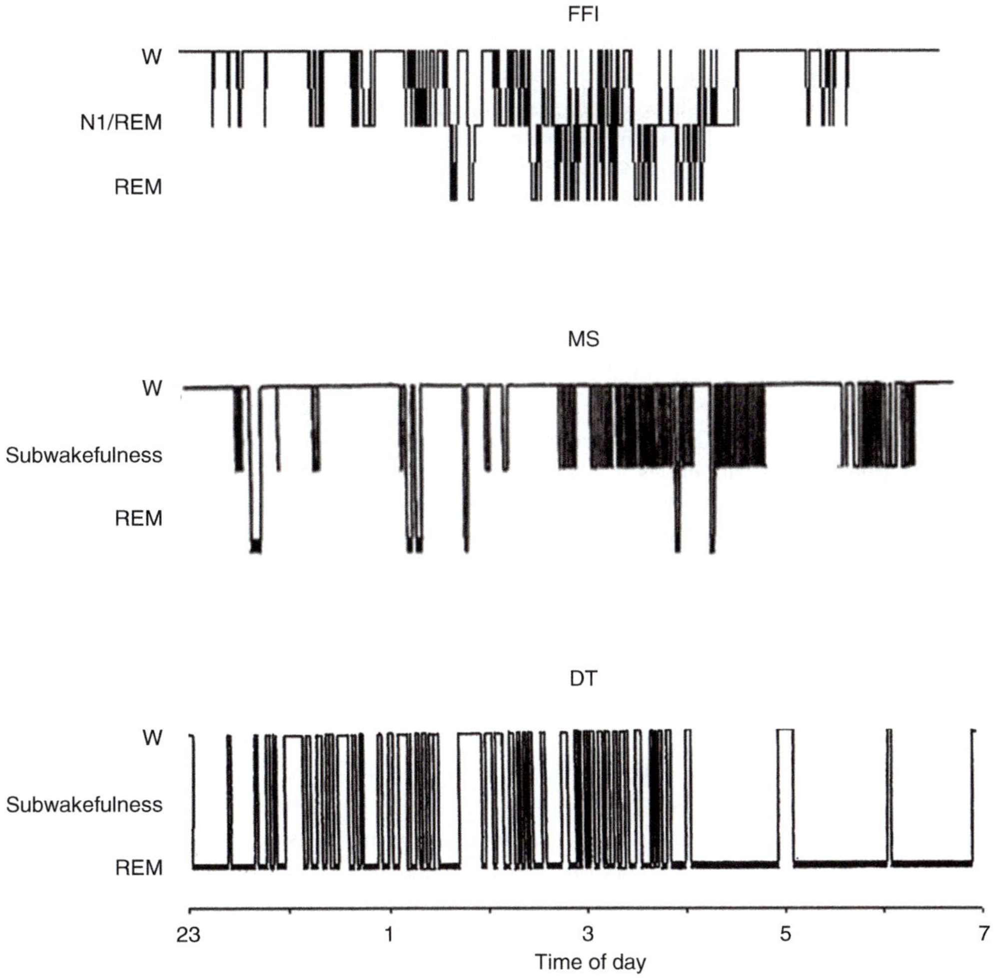

Fig. 18.7 Hypnograms in a patient with fatal familial insomnia (FFI, *upper graph*) and in patients with Morvan syndrome (MS, *middle graph*) and Delirium Tremens (DT, *lower graph*). Deep sleep is absent in all the three conditions; N1/REM-subwakefulness and REM sleep episodes are the only stages recorded. (From Baldelli and Provini [31], © 2019 Elsevier with permission)

seldom years, as described by Liguori et al. [5]. MS is usually an autoimmune disease presenting serum antibodies against voltage-gated K^+ channels (VGKC) and may have a paraneoplastic origin [5, 88]. Experimental laboratory data have shown that subfamilies of VGKCs are involved in wake–sleep cycle regulation [89–91]. Since Fisher-Perroudon's observations polysomnographic recordings in MS usually document a complete absence of spindles and delta activity with the predominance of a state intermediate between stage 1 (dominant theta activity and slow eye movements) and REM sleep (transient reduction of muscle tone or REM discharges), resembling the state of "subwakefulness" described in FFI patients, interspersed with intrusions of more definite REM epochs (Fig. 18.7, *middle graph*) [5, 92–94].

Hyperhidrosis, tachycardia, fluctuations in blood pressure with hypertensive crisis are common findings [95], while laboratory examinations reveal increased and disrupted hormonal rhythms and altered responses to physiological stimuli [5].

Twenty-four-hour plasma levels of NA can be up to twofold higher than in healthy controls, without any physiological nocturnal decrease [5] or even with an increased nychthemeral secretion [96]. Blood levels of ACTH and cortisol are reported to be slightly raised at night with preserved physiological early morning increases. Melatonin levels are lower than normal in the absence of any circadian rhythm. Prolactin and growth-hormone levels are negatively affected too [5].

Plasma NA, already increased at supine rest, presents an abnormal increase in erect posture; the appearance of numerous extrasystoles makes it almost impossible to measure HR response to further testing [5, 96]. After plasma exchange treatment, autonomic responses remain pathological, but to a lesser extent, allowing us to highlight the absence of HR adjustment during Valsalva maneuver and deep breathing test [5]. Moreover, MSNA showed that sympathetic activity was much more elevated than in controls during resting wakefulness in two MS patients [56].

Delirium Tremens

Alcohol withdrawal syndrome (AWS) generally arises within 48 h after the last drink in alcohol abusers. The signs and symptoms of AWS consist of tremors, nausea, excessive perspiration, anxiety, motor agitation, and insomnia. Unless prompt appropriate treatment is given, AWS may develop into a fluctuating disturbance of consciousness accompanied by hallucinations, delirium, and dream enactment with motor agitation and severe autonomic signs (profuse perspiration, tachycardia, and hyperventilation), an acute psychotic state commonly termed delirium tremens (DT) [97].

In a typical case of DT Plazzi et al. [6] described a confusional-oneiric state characterized behaviorally by episodes of oneiric stupor and polygraphically by a total disappearance of spindle and delta sleep during 24-h polysomnographic recordings.

As already described both in FFIs [22] and in seminal works on AWS by Japanese authors [98, 99] wake and subwake EEG features mixed with intrusion of REM sleep were the only polygraphic feature (Fig. 18.7, *lower graph*). Profuse perspiration, tachycardia, and hypertension are particularly common in patients with DT [6, 98, 99], who present also with increased cortisol and plasma catecholamines levels [8]. A dramatic change in gamma-aminobutyric acid (GABA) inhibitory synapses downregulated by the long-standing alcohol abuse, together with the upregulation of the *N*-methyl D-aspartate (NMDA) glutamatergic receptors [6, 100], is speculated to be the cause of DT [2].

Whipple Disease

Whipple disease (WD), an infection caused by *Tropheryma whippelii*, usually occurs with gastrointestinal and rheumatologic symptoms. Oculomasticatory myorhythmia (OMM), which is characterized by pendular vergence oscillations of the eyes at 1 Hz and synchronous with rhythmic contractions of masticatory muscles, is pathognomonic for WD. Hypothalamic dysfunction, supranuclear ophthalmoplegia, sleep–wake cycle, and movement disorders are also described [101–103].

In 2013, Calandra-Buonaura et al. reported the case of a 33-year-old man with WD [104] and features highly suggestive of AE as documented by a 24-h vPSG. A severe reduction of total sleep time and the absence of spindles, K-complexes, slow-wave, and REM sleep were documented with the presence of only wake and stage 1 NREM sleep. Behaviorally, the patient presented with OMM during both wake and sleep and a subcontinuous motor activity characterized by quasi-purposeful gestures mimicking daily life activity resembling oneiric stupor [25]. Diaphoresis, increased HR and a mean body core temperature 38.6 °C were also present.

FFI and Agrypnia: The Role of the Thalamus Not Only in Sleep–Wake Organization, But Also in Autonomic Control

Thalamus is fundamental to govern the sleep–wake cycle in terms of both wake promotion with thalamocortical loops [2] and slow-wave sleep onset and continuity by means of its MD nucleus allowing extra thalamic connections for the reticular nucleus [9, 105], original generator of sleep spindles [106]. Spindling and SWS invariably disappear in FFI and AE, independent of their etiology, as the thalamus is most severely impaired or damaged and thalamocortical and corticothalamic circuits are deeply involved by the pathological processes [2]. REM sleep, in contrast, continues to be present or even becomes overrepresented (as in DT) because its pontine generator is undamaged and transmission of the signal originating from the REM-on system to the forebrain follows extrathalamic pathways, as originally proposed by Jouvet [107] and since confirmed [108, 109]. Somnolence and stupor are the consequences of long-lasting and severe sleep deprivation. However, it cannot be excluded that the pathologic process affecting the thalamolimbic system may also have an impact on wake-promoting thalamocortical loops, as suggested by the fact that, in FFI, continuous somnolence and an inability to sleep appear together at disease onset [2].

Several nuclei of the thalamus have connections with areas of the central autonomic network (CAN): the paraventricular nucleus (PVT) projects to the medial prefrontal cortex and receives multimodal visceral and somatosensory inputs; the MD nucleus is connected with several limbic areas involved in autonomic control [10].

In FFI, postmortem examination [1, 11] and PET scan [4, 34, 110] indicate that the MD and the AV nuclei of the thalamus are selectively affected, with sparing of the hypothalamus and brainstem autonomic areas. Evidence of thalamic dysfunction is also present in AE as demonstrated in MS and DT [2]. While AV projects primarily to areas involved in learning and visuospatial memory (i.e., the "posterior" limbic circuit), the MD nucleus is the most likely candidate to be involved in the mechanisms of autonomic hyperactivation, and a general overactivation of homeostatic control [10].

From the autonomic point of view, the MD nucleus presents reciprocal connections with hypothalamus, amygdala, and prefrontal cortex [111]. Its medial region is connected with various limbic areas involved in the control of autonomic functions such as anterior cingulate gyrus and insular cortex, while its most central part, immediately adjacent to the PVT, receives inputs from the infralimbic area, amygdala, and lateral preoptic area, and to some extent, the dorsomedial nucleus of the hypothalamus [10]. Functionally, the MD nucleus serves as an integral relay between the inhibitory effect of the cortex, integrating instinctive, emotional and cognitive inputs, and the hypothalamus, organizing biologic rhythms, endocrine, and autonomic functions [10, 111]. Thus, disconnection caused by MD degeneration/dysfunction results in a functional imbalance of an unbridled and activated hypothalamus, leading to an increase of autonomic activation with tachycardia, tachypnea, systemic arterial hypertension, hyperthermia, and a rise in circulating catecholamine levels typical of AE [9, 112]. Indeed, the flattening of circadian rhythmicity is a consequence of autonomic hyperactivation, as in a system oscillating between two extremes, the amplitude of oscillations diminishes as the axis of equilibrium shifts toward one end [112]. Autonomic hyperactivity (increase in BP and tachycardia) can be reproduced in anesthetized and conscious rats by injections of GABA antagonist bicuculline into the medial portion of the MD nucleus of the thalamus [113]. In addition, thalamic neurons showing phasic neuronal activity related to systolic BP and thought to be involved in the integration of afferent baroreceptor information have been identified in humans. Their derangement may contribute to cardiovascular disturbances [114].

Conclusion: From Homeostasis to Allostatic Overload

We can hypothesize that thalamic lesions introduce a *diaschisis* (from the classical Greek διά—dia = throughout, and σχίζω—schizò = to separate—"separated throughout") between limbic regions involved in instinctive behavior and those cortical–subcortical areas (basal forebrain, hypothalamus, brainstem) that promote sleep, allowing for a functional imbalance to arise in the form of sympathergic and motor activation and loss of deep sleep [112].

FFI, caused by degeneration of medial thalamolimbic structures, mechanistically involved in deep sleep generation and autonomic balance, is a basic disorder of the control of body homeostasis, traditionally defined as a steady state in which all physiological parameters operate within normal values. In light of past and recent evidence, this condition can be better explained with the more dynamic process of allostasis, whereby an organism maintains physiological stability by changing parameters of its internal milieu by matching them appropriately to environmental demands [115–117].

Allostasis refers to multiple adaptive and survival-promoting systemic and neural processes that are activated by novel and potentially threatening experiences. By mediators, not only hormonal signaling such as cortisol and adrenalin is conceived, but also the parasympathetic nervous system and pro- and anti-inflammatory cytokines [116, 118, 119].

When repeated allostatic responses are activated (e.g., during stressful situations) and real or interpreted threats to homeostasis initiate consecutive activation of sympathetic drive and glucocorticoid secretion, the body starts to experience the "wear and tear" of allostatic load [120]. Allostatic load is sustained by the very same mediators, when they become overused and dysregulated among themselves (e.g., too much or too little cortisol or inflammation, not enough parasympathetic tone, or insulin resistance) [119], "allostatic states" arise, conditions of dysregulated activity in the brain and body which can occur during the development of an illness [121]. At its extremes, dysregulation of allostatic responses, often in response to chronic stressors, leads to the overtly pathologic condition of allostatic overload [122], where sympathetic and neuroendocrine overdrive, similarly to sympathetic hyperactivity of FFI, leads to a condition of disease. In light of this, FFI could represent also a natural model where patients experience a maximal allostatic overload of exclusive internal origin due to the maladaptive effect of thalamic lesions on the equilibrium of the central autonomic network regulation.

References

1. Lugaresi E, Medori R, Montagna P, Baruzzi A, Cortelli P, Lugaresi A, et al. Fatal familial insomnia and dysautonomia with selective degeneration of thalamic nuclei. N Engl J Med. 1986;315(16):997–1003.
2. Lugaresi E, Provini F, Cortelli P. Agrypnia excitata. Sleep Med. 2011;12(Suppl 2):S3–10.
3. Kong Q, Surewicz WK, Petersen RB, Zou W, Chen SG, Gambetti P, et al. Inherited prion diseases. In: Prusiner SB, editor. Prion biology and diseases. 2nd ed. New York: Cold Spring Harbor Laboratory Press; 2004. p. 673–775.
4. Cortelli P, Perani D, Montagna P, Gallassi R, Tinuper P, Provini F, et al. Pre-symptomatic diagnosis in fatal familial insomnia: serial neurophysiological and 18fdg-pet studies. Brain. 2006;129(Pt 3):668–75.

5. Liguori R, Vincent A, Clover L, Avoni P, Plazzi G, Cortelli P, et al. Morvan's syndrome: peripheral and central nervous system and cardiac involvement with antibodies to voltage-gated potassium channels. Brain. 2001;124(Pt 12):2417–26.
6. Plazzi G, Montagna P, Meletti S, Lugaresi E. Polysomnographic study of sleeplessness and oneiricisms in the alcohol withdrawal syndrome. Sleep Med. 2002;3(3):279–82.
7. Lugaresi E, Provini F. Agrypnia excitata: clinical features and pathophysiological implications. Sleep Med Rev. 2001;5(4):313–22.
8. Montagna P, Lugaresi E. Agrypnia excitata: a generalized overactivity syndrome and a useful concept in the neurophysiopathology of sleep. Clin Neurophysiol. 2002;113(4):552–60.
9. Montagna P. Fatal familial insomnia: a model disease in sleep physiopathology. Sleep Med Rev. 2005;9(5):339–53.
10. Benarroch EE, Stotz-Potter EH. Dysautonomia in fatal familial insomnia as an indicator of the potential role of the thalamus in autonomic control. Brain Pathol. 1998;8(3):527–30.
11. Manetto V, Medori R, Cortelli P, Montagna P, Tinuper P, Baruzzi A, et al. Fatal familial insomnia: clinical and pathologic study of five new cases. Neurology. 1992;42(2):312–9.
12. Medori R, Tritschler HJ, Leblanc A, Villare F, Manetto V, Chen HY, et al. Fatal familial insomnia, a prion disease with a mutation at codon 178 of the prion protein gene. N Engl J Med. 1992;326(7):444–9.
13. Dimitri D, Jehel L, Durr A, Levy-Soussan M, Andreux V, Laplanche JL, et al. Fatal familial insomnia presenting as psychosis in an 18-year-old man. Neurology. 2006;67(2):363–4.
14. He R, Hu Y, Yao L, Tian Y, Zhou Y, Yi F, et al. Clinical features and genetic characteristics of two Chinese pedigrees with fatal family insomnia. Prion. 2019;13(1):116–23.
15. Harder A, Gregor A, Wirth T, Kreuz F, Schulz-Schaeffer WJ, Windl O, et al. Early age of onset in fatal familial insomnia. Two novel cases and review of the literature. J Neurol. 2004;251(6):715–24.
16. Almer G, Hainfellner JA, Brucke T, Jellinger K, Kleinert R, Bayer G, et al. Fatal familial insomnia: a new Austrian family. Brain. 1999;122(Pt 1):5–16.
17. Rupprecht S, Grimm A, Schultze T, Zinke J, Karvouniari P, Axer H, et al. Does the clinical phenotype of fatal familial insomnia depend on *PRNP* codon 129 methionine-valine polymorphism? J Clin Sleep Med. 2013;9(12):1343–5.
18. Montagna P, Cortelli P, Avoni P, Tinuper P, Plazzi G, Gallassi R, et al. Clinical features of fatal familial insomnia: phenotypic variability in relation to a polymorphism at codon 129 of the prion protein gene. Brain Pathol. 1998;8(3):515–20.
19. Gao C, Shi Q, Tian C, Chen C, Han J, Zhou W, et al. The epidemiological, clinical, and laboratory features of Sporadic Creutzfeldt-Jakob disease patients in China: surveillance data from 2006 to 2010. PLoS One. 2011;6(8):E24231.
20. Nagoshi K, Sadakane A, Nakamura Y, Yamada M, Mizusawa H. Duration of prion disease is longer in Japan than in other countries. J Epidemiol. 2011;21(4):255–62.
21. Chen C, Wang J-C, Shi Q, Zhou W, Zhang XM, Zhang J, et al. Analyses of the survival time and the influencing factors of Chinese patients with prion diseases based on the surveillance data from 2008–2011. PLoS One. 2013;8(5):E62553.
22. Montagna P, Gambetti P, Cortelli P, Lugaresi E. Familial and sporadic fatal insomnia. Lancet Neurol. 2003;2(3):167–76.
23. Gambetti P, Kong Q, Zou W, Parchi P, Chen SG. Sporadic and familial CJD: classification and characterisation. Br Med Bull. 2003;66:213–39.
24. Cracco L, Appleby BS, Gambetti P. Fatal familial insomnia and sporadic fatal insomnia. Handb Clin Neurol. 2018;153:271–99.
25. Guaraldi P, Calandra-Buonaura G, Terlizzi R, Montagna P, Lugaresi E, Tinuper P, et al. Oneiric stupor: The peculiar behaviour of agrypnia excitata. Sleep Med. 2011;12(Suppl 2):S64–7.
26. Lugaresi E, Provini F. Fatal familial insomnia and agrypnia excitata. Rev Neurol Dis. 2007;4(3):145–52.
27. Cortelli P, Fabbri M, Calandra-Buonaura G, Capellari S, Tinuper P, Parchi P, et al. Gait disorders in fatal familial insomnia. Mov Disord. 2014;29(3):420–4.
28. Krasnianski A, Sanchez Juan P, Ponto C, Bartl M, Heinemann U, Varges D, et al. A proposal of new diagnostic pathway for fatal familial insomnia. J Neurol Neurosurg Psychiatry. 2014;85(6):654–9.
29. Sforza E, Montagna P, Tinuper P, Cortelli P, Avoni P, Ferrillo F, et al. Sleep-wake cycle abnormalities in fatal familial insomnia. Evidence of the role of the thalamus in sleep regulation. Electroencephalogr Clin Neurophysiol. 1995;94(6):398–405.
30. Tinuper P, Montagna P, Medori R, Cortelli P, Zucconi M, Baruzzi A, et al. The thalamus participates in the regulation of the sleep-waking cycle. A clinico-pathological study in fatal familial thalamic degeneration. Electroencephalogr Clin Neurophysiol. 1989;73(2):117–23.
31. Baldelli L, Provini F. Fatal familial insomnia and agrypnia excitata: autonomic dysfunctions and pathophysiological implications. Auton Neurosci. 2019;218:68–86. https://doi.org/10.1016/j.autneu.2019.02.007.
32. Berry RB, Brooks R, Gamaldo CE, Harding SM, Lloyd RM, Quan SF, et al. American Academy of Sleep Medicine. The AASM manual for the scoring of sleep and associated events: rules, terminology and technical specifications. Version 2.4. Darien: American Academy of Sleep Medicine; 2017.
33. Plazzi G, Schutz Y, Cortelli P, Provini F, Avoni P, Heikkila E, et al. Motor overactivity and loss of motor circadian rhythm in fatal familial insomnia: an actigraphic study. Sleep. 1997;20(9):739–42.
34. Gallassi R, Morreale A, Montagna P, Cortelli P, Avoni P, Castellani R, et al. Fatal familial insomnia: behavioral and cognitive features. Neurology. 1996;46(4):935–9.
35. Cortelli P, Perani D, Parchi P, Grassi F, Montagna P, De Martin M, et al. Cerebral metabolism in fatal familial insomnia: relation to duration, neuropathology, and distribution of protease-resistant prion protein. Neurology. 1997;49(1):126–33.
36. Gambetti P, Parchi P, Petersen RB, Chen SG, Lugaresi E. Fatal familial insomnia and familial Creutzfeldt-Jakob disease: clinical, pathological and molecular features. Brain Pathol. 1995;5(1):43–51.
37. Parchi P, Petersen RZ, Chen SG, Autilio-Gambetti L, Capellari S, Monari L, et al. Molecular pathology of fatal familial insomnia. Brain Pathol. 1998;8(3):539–48.
38. Monari L, Chen SG, Brown P, Parchi P, Petersen RB, Mikol J, et al. Fatal familial insomnia and familial creutzfeldt-jakob disease: different prion proteins determined by a DNA polymorphism. Proc Natl Acad Sci U S A. 1994;91(7):2839–42.
39. Parchi P, Zou W, Wang W, Brown P, Capellari S, Ghetti B, et al. Genetic influence on the structural variations of the abnormal prion protein. Proc Natl Acad Sci U S A. 2000;97(18):10168–72.
40. Lugaresi A, Baruzzi A, Cacciari E, Cortelli P, Medori R, Montagna P, et al. Lack of vegetative and endocrine circadian rhythms in fatal familial thalamic degeneration. Clin Endocrinol. 1987;26(5):573–80.
41. Peng B, Zhang S, Dong H, Lu Z. Clinical, histopathological and genetic studies in a case of fatal familial insomnia with review of the literature. Int J Clin Exp Pathol. 2015;8(9):10171–7.
42. Sun C, Xia W, Liu Y, Jia G, Wang C, Yan C, et al. Agrypnia excitata and obstructive apnea in a patient with fatal familial insomnia from China: a case report. Medicine (Baltimore). 2017;96(49):E8951.
43. Montagna P, Cortelli P, Tinuper P. Fatal familial insomnia: a disease that emphasizes the role of the thalamus in the regulation of sleep and vegetarive functions. In: Guilleminault C, Lugaresi E, Montagna P, Gambetti P, editors. Fatal familial insomnia: inher-

ited prion diseases, sleep, and the thalamus. New York: Raven Press; 1994. p. 1–14.
44. Casas-Mendez LF, Lujan M, Vigil L, Sansa G. Biot's breathing in a woman with fatal familial insomnia: is there a role for noninvasive ventilation? J Clin Sleep Med. 2011;7(1):89–91.
45. Dauvilliers Y, Cervena K, Carlander B, Espa F, Bassetti C, Claustrat B, et al. Dissociation in circadian rhythms in a pseudohypersomnia form of fatal familial insomnia. Neurology. 2004;63(12):2416–8.
46. Mclean CA, Storey E, Gardner RJ, Tannenberg AE, Cervenakova L, Brown P. The D178n (cis-129m) "fatal familial insomnia" mutation associated with diverse clinicopathologic phenotypes in an australian kindred. Neurology. 1997;49(2):552–8.
47. Julien J, Vital C, Deleplanque B, Lagueny A, Ferrer X. [Subacute familial thalamic atrophy. memory disorders and complete insomnia]. Rev Neurol (Paris). 1990;146(3):173–178. [*Article in French*].
48. Calandra-Buonaura G, Provini F, Guaraldi P, Plazzi G, Cortelli P. Cardiovascular autonomic dysfunctions and sleep disorders. Sleep Med Rev. 2016;26:43–56.
49. Portaluppi F, Cortelli P, Avoni P, Vergnani L, Contin M, Maltoni P, et al. Diurnal blood pressure variation and hormonal correlates in fatal familial insomnia. Hypertension. 1994;23(5):569–76.
50. Cortelli P, Gambetti P, Montagna P, Lugaresi E. Fatal familial insomnia: clinical features and molecular genetics. J Sleep Res. 1999;8(Suppl 1):23–9.
51. Colombier C, Geraud G, Delisle MB, Laplanche JL, Pavy Le Traon A, Alize P, et al. [Fatal familial insomnia: phenotypic changes determined by polymorphism of the codon 129]. Rev Neurol (Paris). 1997;153(4):239–243.
52. Portaluppi F, Cortelli P, Avoni P, Vergnani L, Maltoni P, Pavani A, et al. Dissociated 24-hour patterns of somatotropin and prolactin in fatal familial insomnia. Neuroendocrinology. 1995;61(6):731–7.
53. Tabernero C, Polo JM, Sevillano MD, Munoz R, Berciano J, Cabello A, et al. Fatal familial insomnia: clinical, neuropathological, and genetic description of a Spanish family. J Neurol Neurosurg Psychiatry. 2000;68(6):774–7.
54. Cortelli P, Parchi P, Contin M, Pierangeli G, Avoni P, Tinuper P, et al. Cardiovascular dysautonomia in fatal familial insomnia. Clin Auton Res. 1991;1(1):15–21.
55. Portaluppi F, Cortelli P, Avoni P, Vergnani L, Maltoni P, Pavani A, et al. Progressive disruption of the circadian rhythm of melatonin in fatal familial insomnia. J Clin Endocrinol Metab. 1994;78(5):1075–8.
56. Donadio V, Montagna P, Pennisi M, Rinaldi R, Di Stasi V, Avoni P, et al. Agrypnia excitata: a microneurographic study of muscle sympathetic nerve activity. Clin Neurophysiol. 2009;120(6):1139–42.
57. Bar KJ, Hager F, Nenadic I, Opfermann T, Brodhun M, Tauber RF, et al. Serial positron emission tomographic findings in an atypical presentation of fatal familial insomnia. Arch Neurol. 2002;59(11):1815–8.
58. Synofzik M, Bauer P, Schols L. Prion mutation D178N with highly variable disease onset and phenotype. J Neurol Neurosurg Psychiatry. 2009;80(3):345–6.
59. Lee MJ, Shin J, Chung EJ, Kim SJ, Kwon S, Kim JH, et al. Midbrain hypometabolism in fatal familial insomnia: a case report and a statistical parametric mapping analysis of a Korean family. Case Rep Neurol. 2014;6(3):243–50.
60. Shi XH, Han J, Zhang J, Shi Q, Chen JM, Xia SL, et al. Clinical, histopathological and genetic studies in a family with fatal familial insomnia. Infect Genet Evol. 2010;10(2):292–7.
61. Reder AT, Mednick AS, Brown P, Spire JP, Van Cauter E, Wollmann RL, et al. Clinical and genetic studies of fatal familial insomnia. Neurology. 1995;45(6):1068–75.
62. Fukuoka T, Nakazato Y, Yamamoto M, Miyake A, Mitsufuji T, Yamamoto T. Fatal familial insomnia initially developing parkinsonism mimicking dementia with Lewy bodies. Intern Med. 2018;57(18):2719–22.
63. Silburn P, Cervenakova L, Varghese P, Tannenberg A, Brown P, Boyle R. Fatal familial insomnia: a seventh family. Neurology. 1996;47(5):1326–8.
64. Bosque PJ, Vnencak-Jones CL, Johnson MD, Whitlock JA, Mclean MJ. A Prp gene codon 178 base substitution and a 24-bp interstitial deletion in familial Creutzfeldt-Jakob disease. Neurology. 1992;42(10):1864–70.
65. Harder A, Jendroska K, Kreuz F, Wirth T, Schafranka C, Karnatz N, et al. Novel twelve-generation kindred of fatal familial insomnia from Germany representing the entire spectrum of disease expression. Am J Med Genet. 1999;87(4):311–6.
66. Frobose T, Slawik H, Schreiner R, Vesely Z, Wiegand M, Bauml J, et al. Agomelatine improves sleep in a patient with fatal familial insomnia. Pharmacopsychiatry. 2012;45(1):34–6.
67. Zerr I, Giese A, Windl O, Kropp S, Schulz-Schaeffer W, Riedemann C, et al. Phenotypic variability in fatal familial insomnia (d178n-129m) genotype. Neurology. 1998;51(5):1398–405.
68. Saitoh Y, Ogawa M, Naito Y, Komatsuzaki Y, Tagaya H, Arima K, et al. Discordant clinicopathologic phenotypes in a Japanese kindred of fatal familial insomnia. Neurology. 2010;74(1):86–9.
69. Rossi G, Macchi G, Porro M, Giaccone G, Bugiani M, Scarpini E, et al. Fatal familial insomnia: genetic, neuropathologic, and biochemical study of a patient from a new Italian kindred. Neurology. 1998;50(3):688–92.
70. Friedrich M, Korte R, Portero C, Arzberger T, Kretzschmar HA, Zerr I, et al. [Fatal familial insomnia – a rare differential diagnosis in dementia]. Fortschr Neurol Psychiatr. 2008;76(1):36–40. (*Article in German*).
71. Lu T, Pan Y, Peng L, Qin F, Sun X, Lu Z, et al. Fatal familial insomnia with abnormal signals on routine MRI: a case report and literature review. BMC Neurol. 2017;17(1):104.
72. Spacey SD, Pastore M, Mcgillivray B, Fleming J, Gambetti P, Feldman H. Fatal familial insomnia: the first account in a family of Chinese descent. Arch Neurol. 2004;61(1):122–5.
73. Shi Q, Chen C, Gao C, Tian C, Zhou W, Zhang B, et al. Clinical and familial characteristics of ten Chinese patients with fatal family insomnia. Biomed Environ Sci. 2012;25(4):471–5.
74. Medori R, Montagna P, Tritschler HJ, Leblanc A, Cortelli P, Tinuper P, et al. Fatal familial insomnia: a second kindred with mutation of prion protein gene at codon 178. Neurology. 1992;42(3 Pt 1):669–70.
75. Haik S, Galanaud D, Linguraru MG, Peoc'h K, Privat N, Faucheux BA, et al. In vivo detection of thalamic gliosis: A pathoradiologic demonstration in familial fatal insomnia. Arch Neurol. 2008;65(4):545–9.
76. Abu-Rumeileh S, Redaelli V, Baiardi S, Mackenzie G, Windl O, Ritchie DL, et al. Sporadic fatal insomnia in europe: phenotypic features and diagnostic challenges. Ann Neurol. 2018;84(3):347–60.
77. Moda F, Suardi S, Di Fede G, Indaco A, Limido L, Vimercati C, et al. MM2-thalamic Creutzfeldt-Jakob disease: neuropathological, biochemical and transmission studies identify a distinctive prion strain. Brain Pathol. 2012;22(5):662–9.
78. Hayashi Y, Iwasaki Y, Yoshikura N, Asano T, Hatano T, Tatsumi S, et al. Decreased regional cerebral blood flow in the bilateral thalami and medulla oblongata determined by an easy Z-score (eZIS) analysis of (99m)Tc-ECD-SPECT images in a case of MM2-thalamic-type sporadic Creutzfeldt-Jakob disease. J Neurol Sci. 2015;358(1–2):447–52.
79. Iwasaki Y, Mori K, Ito M, Mimuro M, Kitamoto T, Yoshida M. An autopsied case of MM1 + MM2-cortical with thalamic-type sporadic Creutzfeldt-Jakob disease presenting with hyperintensities on diffusion-weighted MRI before clinical onset. Neuropathology. 2017;37(1):78–85.

80. Puoti G, Bizzi A, Forloni G, Safar JG, Tagliavini F, Gambetti P. Sporadic human prion diseases: molecular insights and diagnosis. Lancet Neurol. 2012;11(7):618–28.
81. Collinge J, Clarke AR. A general model of prion strains and their pathogenicity. Science. 2007;318(5852):930–6.
82. Imberdis T, Harris DA. Synthetic prions provide clues for understanding prion diseases. Am J Pathol. 2016;186(4):761–4.
83. Parchi P, Giese A, Capellari S, Brown P, Schulz-Schaeffer W, Windl O, et al. Classification of sporadic Creutzfeldt-Jakob disease based on molecular and phenotypic analysis of 300 subjects. Ann Neurol. 1999;46(2):224–33.
84. Cracco L, Notari S, Cali I, Sy MS, Chen SG, Cohen ML, et al. Novel strain properties distinguishing sporadic prion diseases sharing prion protein genotype and prion type. Sci Rep. 2017;7:38280.
85. Provini F. Agrypnia excitata. Curr Neurol Neurosci Rep. 2013;13(4):341.
86. Provini F, Tachibana N. Acute REM sleep behavior disorder. In: Schenck CH, Högl B, Videnovic A, editors. Rapid-eye-movement sleep behavior disorder. Cham: Springer Nature; 2019. p. 153–71.
87. Morvan A. [De la chorée fibrillaire]. Gaz Hebd Mèd Chir. 1890;27:173–200). (*Article in French*).
88. Vincent A, Buckley C, Schott JM, Baker I, Dewar BK, Detert N, et al. Potassium channel antibody-associated encephalopathy: a potentially immunotherapy-responsive form of limbic encephalitis. Brain. 2004;127(Pt 3):701–12.
89. Cirelli C, Bushey D, Hill S, Huber R, Kreber R, Ganetzky B, et al. Reduced sleep in drosophila shaker mutants. Nature. 2005;434(7037):1087–92.
90. Espinosa F, Marks G, Heintz N, Joho RH. Increased motor drive and sleep loss in mice lacking Kv3-type potassium channels. Genes Brain Behav. 2004;3(2):90–100.
91. Espinosa F, Torres-Vega MA, Marks GA, Joho RH. Ablation of Kv3.1 and Kv3.3 potassium channels disrupts thalamocortical oscillations in vitro and in vivo. J Neurosci. 2008;28(21):5570–81.
92. Cornelius JR, Pittock SJ, Mckeon A, Lennon VA, Aston PA, Josephs KA, et al. Sleep manifestations of voltage-gated potassium channel complex autoimmunity. Arch Neurol. 2011;68(6):733–8.
93. Murri L, Bonuccelli U, Iudice A, Simonetti C. [Sleep disturbances in a case of Morvan's Chorea (Author's Transl)]. Riv Patol Nerv Ment. 1976;97(6):350–356. (*Article in Italian*).
94. Fischer-Perroudon C, Trillet M, Mouret J, Tommasi M, Jouvet M, Schott B, et al. [Polygraphic and metabolic studies of persistent insomnia with hallucinations. apropos of an antomo-clinical study of a case of morvan's fibrillar chorea]. Rev Neurol (Paris). 1974;130(3–4):111–125. (*Article in French*).
95. Abou-Zeid E, Boursoulian LJ, Metzer WS, Gundogdu B. Morvan syndrome: Acase report and review of the literature. J Clin Neuromuscul Dis. 2012;13(4):214–27.
96. Spinazzi M, Argentiero V, Zuliani L, Palmieri A, Tavolato B, Vincent A. Immunotherapy-reversed compulsive, monoaminergic, circadian rhythm disorder in Morvan syndrome. Neurology. 2008;71(24):2008–10.
97. Provini F, Cortelli P, Montagna P, Gambetti P, Lugaresi E. Fatal insomnia and agrypnia excitata: sleep and the limbic system. Rev Neurol (Paris). 2008;164(8–9):692–700.
98. Tachibana M, Tanaka K, Hishikawa Y, Kaneko Z. A sleep study of acute psychotic states due to alcohol and meprobamate addiction. In: Weitzman E, editor. Advances in sleep research. New York: Spectrum; 1975. p. 177–203.
99. Kotorii T, Nakazawa Y, Yokoyama T, Kurauchi H, Sakurada H, Ohkawa T, et al. The sleep pattern of chronic alcoholics during the alcohol withdrawal period. Folia Psychiatr Neurol Jpn. 1980;34(2):89–95.
100. Mckeon A, Frye MA, Delanty N. The alcohol withdrawal syndrome. J Neurol Neurosurg Psychiatry. 2008;79(8):854–62.
101. Louis ED, Lynch T, Kaufmann P, Fahn S, Odel J. Diagnostic guidelines in central nervous system Whipple's disease. Ann Neurol. 1996;40(4):561–8.
102. Schwartz MA, Selhorst JB, Ochs AL, Beck RW, Campbell WW, Harris JK, et al. Oculomasticatory myorhythmia: a unique movement disorder occurring in Whipple's disease. Ann Neurol. 1986;20(6):677–83.
103. Voderholzer U, Riemann D, Gann H, Hornyak M, Juengling F, Schumacher M, et al. Transient total sleep loss in cerebral Whipple's disease: a longitudinal study. J Sleep Res. 2002;11(4):321–9.
104. Calandra-Buonaura G, Provini F, Guaraldi P, Pizza F, Cecere A, Barletta G, et al. Oculomasticatory myorhythmia and agrypnia excitata guide the diagnosis of Whipple disease. Sleep Med. 2013;14(12):1428–30.
105. Lugaresi E, Provini F, Montagna P. The neuroanatomy of sleep. Considerations on the role of the thalamus in sleep and a proposal for a caudorostral organization. Eur J Anat. 2004;8(2):85–93.
106. Steriade M, Mccormick DA, Sejnowski TJ. Thalamocortical oscillations in the sleeping and aroused brain. Science. 1993;262(5134):679–85.
107. Jouvet M. [Research on the neural structures and responsible mechanisms in different phases of physiological sleep]. Arch Ital Biol. 1962;100:125–206. (*Article in Italian*).
108. Lu J, Sherman D, Devor M, Saper CB. A putative flip-flop switch for control of REM sleep. Nature. 2006;441(7093):589–94.
109. Saper CB, Fuller PM, Pedersen NP, Lu J, Scammell TE. Sleep state switching. Neuron. 2010;68(6):1023–42.
110. Perani D, Cortelli P, Lucignani G, Montagna P, Tinuper P, Gallassi R, et al. [18f]FDG PET in fatal familial insomnia: the functional effects of thalamic lesions. Neurology. 1993;43(12):2565–9.
111. Benarroch EE. The central autonomic network: functional organization, dysfunction, and perspective. Mayo Clin Proc. 1993;68(10):988–1001.
112. Lugaresi E, Tobler I, Gambetti P, Montagna P. The pathophysiology of fatal familial insomnia. Brain Pathol. 1998;8(3):521–6.
113. Stotz-Potter E, Benarroch E. Removal of gabaergic inhibition in the mediodorsal nucleus of the rat thalamus leads to increases in heart rate and blood pressure. Neurosci Lett. 1998;247(2–3):127–30.
114. Oppenheimer SM, Kulshreshtha N, Lenz FA, Zhang Z, Rowland LH, Dougherty PM. Distribution of cardiovascular related cells within the human thalamus. Clin Auton Res. 1998;8(3):173–9.
115. Sterling P, Eyer J. Allostasis: a new paradigm to explain arousal pathology. In: Fisher S, Reason J, editors. Handbook of life stress, cognition and health. New York: John Wiley & Sons; 1988. p. 629–49.
116. McEwen BS. Stress, adaptation, and disease. Allostasis and allostatic load. Ann N Y Acad Sci. 1998;840:33–44.
117. McEwen BS. Allostasis and the epigenetics of brain and body health over the life course: the brain on stress. JAMA Psychiat. 2017;74(6):551–2.
118. McEwen BS, Gray JD, Nasca C. 60 years of neuroendocrinology: redefining neuroendocrinology: stress, sex and cognitive and emotional regulation. J Endocrinol. 2015;226(2):T67–83.
119. McEwen BS. Physiology and neurobiology of stress and adaptation: central role of the brain. Physiol Rev. 2007;87(3):873–904.
120. McEwen BS, Stellar E. Stress and the individual. Mechanisms leading to disease. Arch Intern Med. 1993;153(18):2093–101.
121. Koob GF, Le Moal M. Drug addiction, dysregulation of reward, and allostasis. neuropsychopharmacology. 2001;24(2):97–129.
122. Juster RP, Mcewen BS, Lupien SJ. Allostatic load biomarkers of chronic stress and impact on health and cognition. Neurosci Biobehav Rev. 2010;35(1):2–16.

Sleep-Related Epilepsy, Dysautonomia, and Sudden Nocturnal Death

19

Paola Proserpio, Thea Giacomini, Elio Clemente Agostoni, and Lino Nobili

Sleep-Related Epilepsy

The strong relationship between sleep and epilepsy has long been documented, but it is not completely understood because of the multiple aspects involved and the possible bidirectional influences. Sleep may favor seizure occurrence and in some epilepsy syndromes seizures occur mostly or exclusively during sleep or on awakening (sleep-related epilepsies [SRE]). Sleep deprivation aggravates epilepsy due to decreased seizure threshold; in addiction, different sleep disorders may represent relevant factors in seizure control. Conversely, epilepsy may alter sleep structure, both directly through seizures and epileptiform activity and indirectly through antiepileptic drug's (AED) side effects.

Evidence reported an alteration of cardiac autonomic control (CAC) in patients with epilepsy [1]. The study of the autonomic function in epilepsy is important for several reasons. For instance, the majority of patients with epilepsy display altered interictal heart rate variability (HRV) with a shift in the autonomic balance toward an increase of the sympathetic tone. Moreover, different types of seizures are associated with a rapid change in autonomic balance, probably depending on the activation of brain regions involved in the autonomic modulation. Finally, autonomic dysfunction has been identified as one of the major pathogenetic mechanisms of sudden unexpected death in epilepsy (SUDEP) [2]. Although it is well known that the autonomic balance oscillates during sleep, only few studies have examined HRV in sleep and wakefulness in epilepsy patients.

In this chapter, we present an overview of the clinical aspects of SRE, reporting the available data regarding the modification of the cardiac autonomic modulation in each type of SRE. Finally, we will update the new findings about SUDEP, focusing on the role of sleep and the autonomic nervous system (ANS) dysfunction in its pathogenesis.

Seizures Occurring Predominantly or Exclusively During Sleep Associated with ANS Dysfunction

Sleep-Related Hypermotor Epilepsy

Sleep-related hypermotor epilepsy (SHE)—formerly known as *nocturnal frontal lobe epilepsy*—was first described in 1981 by Lugaresi and Cirignotta in five patients with sleep-related stereotyped episodes characterized by bizarre movements or dystonic/tonic posturing of the limbs [3]. Considering the absence of electroencephalographic (EEG) abnormalities, the complex motor features of the manifestations and their sleep-related occurrence, the authors initially considered the episodes as "unusual motor disorder of sleep,", coining the term of "hypnogenic paroxysmal dystonia,", modified 5 years later to "nocturnal paroxysmal dystonia" (NPD) [4]. Clinicians debated for several years about the epileptic or nonepileptic nature of NPD. Subsequently, different studies conducted in patients with frontal lobe seizures undergoing neurosurgical treatment for drug-resistant epilepsy led to a better understanding of the physiopathological mechanism based on these manifestations, suggesting their epileptic origin. Therefore, the term "nocturnal frontal lobe epilepsy" was adopted [5–7].

In 2014, a consensus conference including experts in epilepsy and sleep medicine was convened in Bologna, with the aim of defining the electroclinical features and the diagnostic

P. Proserpio · E. C. Agostoni
Sleep Medicine Center, Department of Neuroscience, Grande Ospedale Metropolitano Niguarda, Milan, Italy

T. Giacomini · L. Nobili (✉)
Child Neuropsychiatry Unit, IRCCS Giannina Gaslini Institute, Genoa, Italy

Department of Neuroscience, Rehabilitation, Ophthalmology, Genetics and, Child and Maternal Health (DINOGMI), University of Genova, Genoa, Italy
e-mail: lino.nobili@unige.it

S. Chokroverty, P. Cortelli (eds.), *Autonomic Nervous System and Sleep*, https://doi.org/10.1007/978-3-030-62263-3_19

Table 19.1 Diagnostic criteria for sleep-related hypermotor epilepsy

Core clinical features
1. Brief (<2 min) seizures with stereotyped motor pattern within individuals and abrupt onset and offset
• Clustering is characteristic but not obligatory
2. The most common motor pattern consists of "hypermotor" events
• "Hypermotor" includes seizures with vigorous hyperkinetic features and seizures with asymmetric tonic or dystonic posturing
• Awareness of the episode does not exclude diagnosis
3. Seizures occur predominantly during sleep
• Episodes may occur occasionally in wakefulness
4. Diagnosis not excluded by:
(a) Intellectual disability, neuropsychiatric features
(b) The absence of clear interictal and ictal EEG correlates
(c) Extrafrontal origin
Three levels of certainty
1. Witnessed (possible):
• Core clinical features provided by eyewitness
2. Video-documented (clinical):
• Recording of at least one but preferably two stereotyped events (confirmed to be typical by eyewitness)
• High quality audio-video, including the onset and with clear visualization of the entire events, showing the evolution and offset of the attacks
• Minor motor events or PA excluded, making diagnosis unreliable
3. Video-EEG documented (confirmed):
• Recording of at least one but preferably two stereotyped events during a daytime sleep recording after sleep deprivation, or during a full night sleep recording, with at least 19 EEG channels (10–20 international system), ECG, oculogram, and chin EMG
• Clear-cut ictal epileptic discharge or interictal epileptiform abnormalities

EEG electroencephalography, *PA* paroxysmal arousals, *ECG* electrocardiography, *EMG* electromyography

criteria of the disorder [8] (for diagnostic criteria see Table 19.1). One of the major outcomes of the consensus conference was the need to change nomenclature; the proposed new name was "sleep-related hypermotor epilepsy," reflecting evidence that the attacks are associated with sleep rather than time of day, seizures can have an extrafrontal origin and the motor features of the seizures are specific to this entity.

Epidemiology

SHE is not a homogeneous disease as familial, idiopathic, sporadic, cryptogenetic or symptomatic forms exist [9–11]. The nonlesional cases of SHE seem to be predominant in the familial form [12]. This epileptic syndrome is characterized by onset during infancy or childhood with persistence in adulthood [13]. SHE is reported to be a rare disorder but epidemiologic data are scanty. In 1999, Provini et al. showed that SHE represented the diagnosis in 13% of patients referred to their tertiary center for a video-polysomnographic evaluation [10]. More recently, a population-based retrospective cohort study conducted in the northeast of Italy showed that SHE is a rare epileptic condition with a crude prevalence of 1.8 per 100,000 residents [12]. The majority of SHE patients show a positive response to antiepileptic drugs, especially carbamazepine. However, 30% of cases are resistant to carbamazepine and other antiepileptic drugs [10].

Genetic Forms of Sleep-Related Hypermotor Epilepsy

The first genetic form of SHE was described by Scheffer et al. in 1994 in a large Australian family with autosomal-dominant inherited SHE (ADSHE) associated with a mutation of the CHRNA4 (neuronal acetylcholine receptor subunit alpha-4) gene coding for the alpha4 subunit of the neuronal nicotinic acetylcholine receptor (nAChR) [9]. Subsequently, further mutations in genes (CHRNA2, neuronal acetylcholine receptor subunit alpha-2, and CHRNB2, neuronal acetylcholine receptor subunit beta-2) coding for other nAChR subunits (alpha2 and beta2) [14, 15] were found to be implicated in ADSHE with phenotype usually indistinguishable [16].

More recently, additional mutations in genes not coding for the cholinergic receptor were discovered in ADSHE. Specifically, mutations of the *KCNT1* gene (coding for a sodium-activated potassium channel subunit 1) have been associated with a severe form of ADSHE accompanying intellectual disabilities, regression, and behavioral and psychiatric symptoms [17]. Of note, the same gene has been found to be mutated also in a rare early infantile epileptic encephalopathy with poor prognosis, "epilepsy with migrating focal seizures of infancy" [18, 19].

In some families with ADSHE and in rare sporadic SHE cases mutations have been found in DEPDC5 (DEP domain containing 5) and NPRL (nitrogen permease regulator-like protein) 2 and 3, proteins coding for the mTORC1 (mammalian target of rapamycin complex 1)-regulating GATOR1 (Gap Activity TOward Rags 1) complex, implicated in the cell growth regulation [20–22]. Of note, DEPDC5 has been associated with a variety of familial epilepsies, including familial focal epilepsy with variable foci, familial temporal lobe epilepsy, epileptic spasms, and epilepsies associated with cortical dysplasia [23–25].

Recently, mutation in the *CABP4* gene, encoding the neuronal Ca^{2+}-binding protein 4 (CaBP4), was found in a Chinese family with 11 individuals diagnosed with ADSHE [26]. Finally, Peres et al. described a case of SHE with peri-ictal hypotension associated with syntaxin-1B gene mutation [27].

Symptomatic Forms

Studies conducted in patients with drug-resistant epilepsy showed that the most frequent etiological substrate of SHE is represented by type II focal cortical dysplasia (type II FCD) [28]. Notably, although type II FCD is more frequently located within the frontal lobe, evidence demonstrated that regardless of its anatomical localization, type II FCD (especially the type IIb) increases the risk of sleep-related epilepsy [29]. This correlation could be probably ascribed to the particular firing pattern of FCD IIb during non-REM sleep, characterized by the periodic occurrence of fast discharge frequently evolving into a seizure.

Clinical Features

From a clinical point of view, patients with familial forms of SHE do not show a clear distinction from sporadic NFLE cases, except for certain ADSHE mutations frequently associated with specific additional neurological or psychiatric symptoms. Seizure frequency is usually high and sometimes diminishes during adulthood. Almost 30–40% of SHE patients experience occasional seizures during wakefulness [10, 30]. Of note, subjective seizure manifestations, uncommon during the night, are more frequently reported by patients during diurnal events [10, 31].

SHE patients frequently exhibit different sleep-related motor manifestation of increasing complexity and duration during a single night [10, 11, 32, 33]. These include (a) *minor events*, consisting of short-lasting (2–4 s) stereotyped movements involving the limbs, the axial musculature, and/or the head; (b) *paroxysmal arousals* (PA), characterized by frequent and recurring abrupt brief arousals lasting about 5–10 s, accompanied by stereotyped movements (trunk and head elevation) often associated with vocalization and frightened expression; and (c) *major attacks*. Moreover, a minority of patients may show ictal ambulatory behavior (wandering behavior) often associated with frightened expression and fear, called "*epileptic nocturnal wanderings.*".

It has been postulated that the increasing complexity of the ictal motor manifestation is strictly related to a different duration and propagation of the epileptic discharge. This hypothesis was confirmed by studies conducted in drug resistant SHE patients with seizure arising from supplementary motor area, studied with intracerebral implanted electrodes during the presurgical evaluation [33, 34]. However, more recent evidence has demonstrated that minor motor events, whose occurrence is highly related to the presence of intracerebrally recorded epileptic discharges, may not be differentiated from physiological movements [35]. In fact, other studies by means of stereo-EEG investigations in drug-resistant SHE patients showed that periodic epileptic discharges, not detectable on scalp EEG, can increase arousal fluctuations and in turn increase and modulate the occurrence of physiological movements or different kinds of sleep disturbances such as periodic leg movements, sleep-talking, and bruxism [34, 36]. On the other hand, the resulting increased arousal instability might facilitate the production of epileptic discharges in a bi-directionally influenced system [37].

Considering major attacks, early studies focusing on seizure semiology in SHE have highlighted the heterogeneous features of the sleep-related manifestations [9, 10]. A recent retrospective study on 135 patients with drug-resistant SHE patients identified peculiar ictal semiologic patterns in this population of patients [31]. In particular, seizures were classified according to four semiology patterns (SPs): SP1, characterized mainly by *early elementary motor signs*, which included early clonic signs, asymmetric tonic postures or an asymmetric facial contraction; SP2, consisting of *unnatural hypermotor movements*, that is, nonintegrated or anarchic gestural hypermotor movements with axial tonic postures or symmetric facial contractions; SP3, characterized by *integrated hypermotor movements*, which included hyperkinetic behaviors (pedaling, kicking, rocking), distal stereotypies, or manipulation/utilization movements in the absence of a clear goal-directed purpose; and SP4, including *gestural behaviors with high emotional content*, such as integrated gestural behaviors of fear, fight or flight behavior, frightened facial expression or autonomic signs. Within the frontal lobe, the occurrence of a peculiar SP was strictly related to the location of the seizure onset zone (SOZ) with an anteroposterior distribution of the SOZ in relation to the SP: SP1 was mainly placed in the vicinity of the precentral sulcus (posterior mesial or posterior lateral surface of the frontal lobe) whereas SP4 was located predominantly near the frontopolar and orbitofrontal regions; SOZ in SP2 and SP3 was more scattered but followed the same anteroposterior tendency.

Sleep-Related Hypermotor Epilepsy: Always a Frontal Onset?

Hypermotor (hyperkinetic or dystonic) seizures, sleep-related or not, have been considered for a long time the hallmark of frontal lobe seizures (hence the name NFLE). However, over the past decade many case reports and case series have challenged this idea, demonstrating that other sites of seizure onset may trigger tonic/dystonic or hyperkinetic behaviors. Studies by means of Stereo-EEG investigations documented an extrafrontal origin in up to 30% of cases of drug-resistant SHE [28]. The majority of the described extrafrontal SHE cases displayed a temporal or an insular-opercular onset although cases of parietal lobe and even occipital lobe onset have been reported [31, 38–41]. Distinguishing a frontal from an extrafrontal form of SHE may be challenging. In the above-mentioned study [31], it has been shown that extrafrontal drug-resistant SHE exhibited the same SPs described for frontal SHE, but certain SPs were more likely or unlikely to occur in some extrafrontal SHE subgroups. In particular, seizures characterized by gestural behaviors with high emotional content (SP4) were frequently observed in temporal SHE, while they were absent in operculo-insular and parietal SHE, suggesting that the presence of SP4 in SHE could be strongly related to a SOZ involving a network between the ventromedial prefrontal cortex and the anterior temporal region. As far as the early nonmotor manifestations, the study [32] showed that some nonmotor features may provide useful localizing and/or lateralizing information. For instance, auditory and visual manifestations were observed only in extrafrontal SHE. As expected, visual symptoms were associated with posterior cortex SOZ while auditory symptoms were found in both temporal and operculoinsular SOZ. Conversely, cephalic symptoms were observed only in frontal SHE while a focal sensory onset was observed in both frontal and extrafrontal (parietal and operculoinsular) SHE. The characteristic of the sensory manifestation was sometimes very helpful to localize the SOZ. For example, insular patients frequently experienced pain or a choking sensation at the beginning of their seizures. Conversely, patients with parietal SOZ reported more often vertigo or falling sensation. Finally, epigastric and autonomic features were present in all but the posterior subgroup, while emotional manifestations were observed only in frontal and temporal SHE.

Another recent work on drug resistant SHE patients with different location of the SOZ found that the mean duration of electrographic seizures and clinically observable ictal manifestations were significantly shorter in frontal SHE compared to extrafrontal SHE. Moreover, the mean latency between the first video-detectable movement (e.g., eye opening or a minor motor event) and the onset of hypermotor manifestations was also shorter in frontal SHE [42].

Electroencephalographic Features

The interictal and ictal scalp electroencephalographic features of SHE patients are often uninformative, especially in cases in which SOZ is located in deep brain regions [9, 10, 43]. However, prolonged video-EEG recordings can sometimes be useful in characterizing the EEG abnormalities in selected subgroups of patients undergoing presurgical investigation. In the study of Gibbs et al. [32], it has been shown that the majority of drug resistant patients (82%) with both frontal or extrafrontal SHE exhibited interictal abnormalities during scalp EEG recordings (routine and video-EEG). However, this percentage decreased when the localizing value of EEG based on postoperative outcome was assessed (48%), except in temporal SHE where 93% of interictal abnormalities correctly localized to the epileptogenic temporal lobe [31].

Treatment

About two thirds of SHE/ADSHE patients benefit from carbamazepine administration [9, 10]. More recently, studies conducted in small population of SHE patients demonstrated the efficacy of other antiepileptic drugs administered as single or add-on therapy, such as oxcarbazepine, topiramate, acetazolamide, lacosamide, and fenofibrate [44]. Finally, different studies demonstrated the high efficacy of epilepsy surgery in selected patients with drug resistant SHE [45].

SHE and Autonomic System

Ictal and interictal abnormalities in autonomic control of cardiac frequency have been reported in different population of patients with focal and generalized epilepsies. For instance, faster interictal heart rates and reduced parasympathetic drive have been reported in patients with frontal lobe epilepsy [46]. However, studies analyzing modifications of cardiac autonomic control (CAC) specifically in patients with SHE are scant.

From a physiological point of view, sleep is characterized by oscillatory changes of CAC, with a predominant sympathetic modulation during REM sleep and, in contrast, a shift toward a vagal predominance during NREM sleep [47]. Furthermore, NREM sleep does not represent a stable phenomenon but it is punctuated by the occurrence of "arousals," consisting of transient episodes of cortical and autonomic activation. Notably, some studies demonstrated that autonomic modification can precede cortical/EEG activation during an arousal event [47]. Specifically, the physiological arousal response seems to follow a hierarchic pattern, starting with an early autonomic activation followed by different phasic EEG changes and ending in delayed cortical activation for stimuli of greater intensity [48].

As discussed above, a bidirectional association between arousal fluctuations and SHE has been observed [37], and higher level of arousal activity during NREM sleep has been described in SHE patients [49]. Calandra et al. [50] conducted a study to investigate whether signs of autonomic activation precede onset of seizure motor manifestations. Analysis of HRV showed a shift of sympathetic/parasympathetic cardiac control toward a sympathetic predominance in the 10 s immediately preceding seizure onset, while changes in HR were evident only 1 s before seizure onset. Moreover, to clarify the nature (epileptic or physiologic) of the CAC changes preceding the seizures, they also investigated time-dependent variations in HR and HRV related to physiological cortical arousals associated with motor activity (phases of transitory activation [PAT]). Notably, patterns of CAC variation before the motor onset of PAT reproduced the features of the autonomic activation observed before seizures. Therefore, authors hypothesized that the sympathetic activation observed before the onset of seizure motor manifestations may reflect the autonomic preparation that preceded the cortical and behavioral response to spontaneous arousal and not the direct effect of the discharge involving cortical areas of the CAC.

More recently, a study investigated interictal CAC modification in SHE patients. In particular, authors analyzed HRV modification during the cyclic alternating pattern (CAP) in patients with SHE with respect to controls [51]. SHE patients showed a significant increase in LF/HF (low frequency/high frequency) and LF (low frequency) power with respect to healthy subjects only around A1 phases. Conversely, the CAC control during A2 and A3 phases was similar in the two populations. This seems to suggest that A1 phases in SHE patients may be characterized by a shift in the sympathovagal balance toward a more sympathetically mediated control of heart rate. Authors hypothesized that this autonomic behavior could be related to a higher arousal activity described in SHE patients [49].

Benign Epilepsy with Centrotemporal Spikes (BECTS)

Benign epilepsy with centrotemporal spikes is the most frequent type of idiopathic age-dependent childhood epilepsy (8–20% of childhood epilepsy) [52]. The onset is usually between 3 and 13 years and remission is frequently before 16 years of age. Seizures are mainly characterized by hemi lateral clonic deviation of the mouth and tongue often associated with sialorrhea. Seizure frequency is usually low and up to 70% occur during NREM sleep, typically just after falling asleep or before awakening. EEG is characterized by the interictal presence of high-voltage centrotemporal spikes and sharp waves with amplitude and frequency increment during NREM sleep when they often become synchronous or asynchronous bilaterally. Even if this kind of epilepsy is often described as "benign" with good prognosis and no cognitive impairment, it is known that mild cognitive impairment may be present when associated with a marked increment of interictal discharges during sleep [53]. A recent systematic review and metanalysis comprising 1237 [off therapy) children with BECTS and 1137 healthy controls showed significantly lower scores predominantly in the cognitive domain, regarding long-term storage and retrieval [54]. Cognitive impairment both in language and academic performance has also been observed [55]. According to other studies, cognitive disturbances seem to be associated with the presence of bilateral discharges [56]. The observed cognitive dysfunction somehow fills the gap between the apparently benign BECTS and the atypical variants that can proceed to severe epileptic encephalopathies phenotypes as Landau–Kleffner syndrome and electrical status epilepticus in sleep (ESES), supporting the concept of a clinical spectrum of BECTS [52]. Genetic disposition has been observed; about one-fourth of patients present one or more relatives with seizures and recently, *GRIN2A*, *PRRT2*, *SRPXA*, and *ELP4* pathogenic variants were detected in some children with BECTS [57, 58]. Treatment (usually valproic acid, carbamazepine, levetiracetam, etc.) is indicated only when seizures are frequent or interfere significantly with daily life.

The analysis of HRV in 50 patients with BECTS compared with 50 controls revealed that during wakefulness BECTS patients exhibited an increased vagal and reduced sympathetic tone expressed by a higher HF and a lower LF/HF index than typically developing controls [59]. Thus, the study revealed a negative relationship between both seizure load as well as frequency of interictal sleep EEG abnormalities, and parasympathetic drive levels. Authors hypothesized that higher parasympathetic activation could be associated with a more effective seizure control and that failure of these adaptive processes might result in more difficult controlling seizures.

Panayiotopoulos Syndrome

Panayiotopoulos syndrome, also known as early onset childhood occipital epilepsy, is another common type of age-related focal epilepsy (estimated prevalence of 13% in children aged 3–6 years) [60]. Onset is usually between 1 and 11 years, frequently before 6 years of age. Remission occurs typically also without treatment within 1–2 years of the onset [60]. Seizures are generally characterized by nausea and vomiting often associated with a various combination of autonomic symptoms such as pallor, flushing, thermoregulatory alterations, mydriasis, urinary incontinence, and cardiorespiratory irregularities. Visual symptoms may be rarely present at onset and facial clonic manifestations, and loss of consciousness may follow. Evolution into secondary generalized seizures is common, and duration longer than 30 min may occur. Seizure frequency is usually extremely low, with a majority of patients reporting only one to five seizures in their lifetime [61]. About two-thirds of seizures occur during sleep, soon after falling asleep, or in the early hours of the morning [62, 63]. Interictal EEG is characterized by focal or multifocal spikes with variable localization, frequently involving occipital areas and with an increase during NREM sleep, even if less intense than in BECTS. A robust correlation of interictal epileptiform discharges (IEDs) with sleep spindles in this and other age-related epilepsies was specifically observed [64]. Occipital interictal spikes may be "fixation off" sensitive (meaning precipitated by the suppression of visual fixation) and brief diffuse discharges of small spikes and slow waves are occasionally observed [62]. Ictal EEG usually starts before clinical symptoms onset; it is usually characterized by theta waves mixed with small spikes and fast rhythms that may start variably (unilateral or bilateral) and spreading to other brain areas. Autonomic symptoms are not associated with a specific localization of ictal EEG abnormalities [65]. The genetic background is unknown. Rectal diazepam should be administered for prolonged seizures. Treatment should be prescribed only in patients with frequent and prolonged seizures; valproic acid and carbamazepine are the most frequently used drugs.

Juvenile Myoclonus Epilepsy

Juvenile myoclonus epilepsy (JME) is also known as Janz syndrome. The prevalence of JME has been estimated to be 5–10% of all epilepsies [66]. Onset is typical during adolescence, even if it can seldom occur before 10 years of age or in early adulthood. Seizures are characterized by the presence of brief, spontaneous, bilateral, arrhythmic, irregular, single, or repetitive myoclonic jerks repeatedly occurring on or shortly after awakening, without loss of consciousness. Myoclonic jerks usually present in brief clusters with upper limbs predominant involvement, and according to a consensus meeting in 2011 their presence is an obligatory requisite for JME diagnosis [67]. Sleep deprivation and forced awakening during sleep are known as triggers [68]. Generalized tonic-clonic seizures (GTCs), absences, perioral myoclonia, and praxis induced seizures may also occur. In particular, generalized tonic-clonic seizures are often subsequent to a cluster of myoclonic jerks, frequently intense and associated with prolonged postictal asthenia. Absences are rare (prevalence 10–38%), short, with partial consciousness impairment, and often are detected only during prolonged EEG recording [68]. Perioral and praxis-induced seizures are often precipitated by reading, speaking, and other neuropsychological activation [69]. Photosensitivity could be also present. Interictal EEG shows normal background activity and sleep pattern; widespread polyspikes and diffuse spike and waves at 2.3–3.5 Hz increased during sleep onset and awakening are typical. Myoclonic jerks usually are associated with rapid 5–20 polyspikes of increasing amplitude mainly localized in the frontal areas, followed or preceded by high amplitude slow waves [70]. Sleep disturbances have been often observed in JME patients, such as daytime sleepiness, disturbed night sleep, despite adequate medications and good seizure control [71]. A recent study observed the absence of expected apnea mediated HRV changes, including long-term HRV changes during sleep in JME patients compared with healthy controls, suggesting an impairment of reflex baroceptor activation and autonomic nervous system in these patients [72]. JME is not usually self-limiting, although the response to pharmacological treatment is satisfactory in most patients [61, 67]. Most used and efficacious drugs are valproic acid, topiramate, and levetiracetam. Lamotrigine may aggravate myoclonic jerks, carbamazepine, oxcarbazepine, gabapentin, phenytoin, and vigabatrin may worsen absences, GTCs (generalized tonic-clonic seizures), and myoclonic seizures and should be avoided [73].

West Syndrome

West syndrome is characterized by infantile spasms and hypsarrhythmia on EEG. Onset is usually between 3 and 12 months of life, even if earlier or later start is not uncommon. The estimated incidence is 2.5–10/10.000 newborns and the prevalence is around 1–2/10.000 children at the age of 10 years with onset within 1 year of age in 90% of cases [74]. The spasms usually manifest shortly before awakening as brief, synchronous flexor or extensor movement of head, trunk, and limbs and occur in clusters. Sometimes spasms may be very subtle presenting as a series of tonic contractions or focal jerks or even isolated eye deviation and facial grimacing. EEG is characterized by high amplitude pathognomonic hypsarrhythmic pattern, more prominent during early NREM sleep and in some cases occurring only during sleep [75, 76]. The etiology is the most important prognostic factor, but also the lack of physiological sleep patterns and the severity of hypsarrhythmia play a role for the developmental outcome [77, 78]. In particular, previous studies observed, similarly to ESES/CSWS, significant impairment of overnight slow wave sleep and alterations of NREM slow oscillations (with steeper slow waves] [79]. There is increasing evidence of NREM sleep slow wave activity playing an important role in synaptic homeostasis, synaptic plasticity regulation, and brain reorganization [80–82]. Slow wave sleep alteration may be a further causative factor for cognitive impairment in children with West syndrome. Possible etiologies are several including genetic, metabolic, hypoxic, ischemic, malformation, or other brain damages. Treatment should be started as soon as possible, and the effect frequently monitored by sleep EEG recordings. According to international recommendations, the most effective drugs are vigabatrin, adrenocorticotropic hormone (ACTH), and large doses of oral steroids (prednisolone) [83–85].

A few studies analyzed HRV in children with epileptic spasms. In particular, Moller et al. found an initial and transient reduction of HRV at the time of onset of West syndrome, probably related to the presence of hypsarrhythmia [86]. Moreover, while two studies reported a sympathetic dominance in patients with epileptic spasms [86, 87], one did not find significant differences other than lower heart rate in slow wave sleep [88]. A fourth study analyzing HRV during NREM sleep found an increased orthosympathetic component in patients with West syndrome with respect to control group [89]. Finally, ACTH treatment seems to induce a shift toward recovery of parasympathetic function [86, 87, 89].

Lennox–Gastaut Syndrome

Lennox–Gastaut syndrome is a severe developmental and epileptic encephalopathy characterized by the presence of drug-resistant tonic, tonic-clonic, myoclonic and atypical absence seizures and intellectual disability. It is a rare disorder, representing 1–5% of all epilepsies and 3–10% of childhood epilepsies with an annual estimated incidence of

0.2–2.8/10,000 births in European countries [90]. The typical age of onset is between 2 and 8 years, and it can appear as apparently cryptogenic or symptomatic of various etiologies such as pre- or perinatal ischemic or hypoxic brain damages, infections, tumors, and malformations. It is often preceded by a West syndrome or focal seizures [90]. Tonic seizures typically occur during sleep, although they can be subtle and detectable only with video-EEG polysomnographic recordings. Interictal EEG usually shows diffuse slow spike-wave complexes (<3 Hz) increasing during NREM sleep and fast rhythmic bursts (10 Hz) during sleep; ictal EEG typically presents diffuse fast 10–20/s activity often preceded by attenuation of the background activity [91]. The long-term outcome is poor and it is associated with high mortality and severe morbidity [92]. Several drugs are available for the treatment of Lennox–Gastaut syndrome and have been validated through randomized, controlled trials. However, at present, there is no evidence to suggest that any one drug is more efficacious than another [93]. Nonpharmacological treatment (e.g., ketogenic diet, epilepsy surgery or vagus nerve stimulation) has also been tried with variable results and may be considered after failure of two-to-three drugs [93].

Koenig et al. reported a case of a patient affected by Lennox–Gastaut syndrome with a severe impairment of HRV at baseline, which improved after implantation of a vagus nerve stimulator [94].

Electrical Status Epilepticus During Slow Sleep (ESES)

ESES, also known as *continuous spike-wave during slow wave sleep* (CSWS), is a developmental epileptic encephalopathy with seizure onset between 2 months and 12 years [95]. Seizures are frequent and types are various with focal motor or generalized seizures occurring during sleep, atypical absences, and atonic seizures during the awake state. Tonic seizures are not observed, allowing differential diagnosis with Lennox–Gastaut syndrome. EEG is characterized by continuous diffuse spike-waves during slow waves sleep, which is usually noted after seizure onset. Spike-waves index (SWI) is a parameter frequently used to assess ESES severity and it is usually ranged between 85% and 100% during all night NREM sleep stages [95, 96]. Global cognitive regression, either acute or insidious, is typical some months after seizure onset, generally associated with behavioral disturbances [97]. As in West syndrome, an impairment in physiological decrease of slow waves during sleep has been observed. The impairment is directly correlated with the amount of SWI during sleep. The evolution of seizures is usually benign, but neuropsychological disorders and behavioral disturbances may be pronounced, irrespective of previous cognitive functions and development [63]. The severity of neuropsychological impairment correlates with duration of CSWS EEG pattern and the topography of the spike-waves is associated with the type of cognitive deficit [98]. Half of the patients present brain malformation or lesions, in particular pre or perinatal thalamic lesions have been reported in these patients [97, 99]. Two epileptic syndromes, BECTS and Landau–Kleefner, show similar characteristic to ESES syndrome; both are characterized by a specific increase of spike-waves during sleep. These three syndromes have been indeed associated with the same genes pathogenic variants *GRIN2A, PRRT2, SRPXA*, and *ELP4* and the hypothesis is that they constitute an electro-clinical spectrum with a continuum between these disorders [100, 101]. Treatment options are various comprising steroids, benzodiazepines, levetiracetam, ethosuximide, valproic acid, ketogenic diet, but there are no controlled trials establishing the efficacy of different antiepileptic drugs and successful treatment is often difficult to achieve. The primary goal of treatment is to prevent cognitive deterioration or to improve neuropsychological impairment that are directly associated with CSWS duration and aggressive approach including steroid use should be considered [102].

Sudden Unexpected Death in Epilepsy (SUDEP)

Definitions

Epileptic patients have a higher probability to die prematurely with respect to the general population. Indeed, the risk of sudden unexpected death is considered to be 24–40 times higher in patients with epilepsy compared to people not affected [103]. Sudden unexpected death in epilepsy (SUDEP) has been defined as "sudden, unexpected, witnessed or unwitnessed, non-traumatic, and non-drowning death that occurs in benign circumstances in an individual with epilepsy, with or without evidence for a seizure, and excludes documented status epilepticus, in which postmortem examination does not reveal a cause of death" [104]. In the 1990s, two complementary definitions were published [105, 106] and since then, these two definitions have been used in most SUDEP studies, but often with variations. For this reason, in 2012 Nashef et al. proposed a unified SUDEP definition and classification to resolve current ambiguities and to retrieve cases that would not have been further studied if the previous definitions were used [104] (for details regarding the definitions see Table 19.2).

Epidemiology

Incidence of SUDEP varies depending on several factors, such as the modality of assessment of the causes of death, selection criteria, different definitions of SUDEP, and documentation requirements. In general, the risk of SUDEP is

Table 19.2 New SUDEP definition and classification according to Nashef et al. ([104], © 2012 John Wiley and Sons, with permission)

Definite SUDEP[a]	Sudden, unexpected, witnessed or unwitnessed, non-traumatic and non-drowning death, occurring in benign circumstances, in an individual with epilepsy, with or without evidence for a seizure and excluding documented status epilepticus (seizure duration ‡30 min or seizures without recovery in between), in which postmortem examination does not reveal a cause of death
Definite SUDEP plus[a]	Satisfying the definition of definite SUDEP, if a concomitant condition other than epilepsy is identified before or after death, if the death may have been due to the combined effect of both conditions, and if autopsy or direct observations/recordings of terminal event did not prove the concomitant condition to be the cause of death
Probable SUDEP/Probable SUDEP plus[a]	Same as definite SUDEP but without autopsy. The victim should have died unexpectedly while in a reasonable state of health, during normal activities, and in benign circumstances, without a known structural cause of death
Possible SUDEP[a]	A competing cause of death is present
Near-SUDEP/Near-SUDEP plus	A patient with epilepsy survives resuscitation for more than 1 h after a cardiorespiratory arrest that has no structural cause identified after investigation
Not SUDEP	A clear cause of death is known
Unclassified	Incomplete information available; not possible to classify

[a]If a death is witnessed, an arbitrary cutoff of death within 1 h from acute collapse is suggested

estimated in two types of studies: general community-based populations and clinical cohorts (for a review see Thurman et al. [107]). Considering community-based studies including all age groups, estimates ranged from 0.33 to 1.35 cases of SUDEP annually per 1000 people with epilepsy. Nine clinic-based studies, mainly representing people with treatment-resistant epilepsy, yielded higher estimates of SUDEP occurrence, ranging from 1.2 to 6.3 cases of SUDEP annually per 1000 individuals. In 2017, the American Academy of Neurology (AAN) and American Epilepsy Society (AES) published a clinical practice parameter guideline on SUDEP risk factors and incidence [108]. They found that the SUDEP risk in children with epilepsy is low (0.22/1000 patient-years) and increases in adults (1.2/1000 patient-years). However, this finding was challenged by two recent studies conducted with a more comprehensive study design employing multiple data sources to screen for SUDEP cases. In particular, Keller et al. [109] reported the overall incidence of pediatric SUDEP as 1.17 per 1000 person-years in the province of Ontario, Canada while Sveinsson et al. [110], using linked records from the Swedish National Patient Registry and National Cause of Death Registry, reported the incidence of SUDEP to be similar across all age groups: 1.1 per 1000 person-years in children <16 years and in adults 1.13 (age 16–50 years) and 1.29 (age > 50 years), respectively.

Studies analyzing the frequency of SUDEP in patients with sleep-related epilepsy are rare. In 2015, Mostacci et al. conducted a retrospective study showing an incidence of SUDEP in SHE patients similar to that observed in the general epilepsy population (0.36 per 1000 person-years) [13]. Authors hypothesized that the low prevalence of SUDEP could be probably related to the low occurrence of generalized tonic-clonic seizures in people with SHE. Considering that recent findings demonstrated that SOZ in SHE can be located also outside the frontal lobe, it is possible that SHE patients with an insular onset are at higher risk of SUDEP. Indeed, it has been shown that seizures originating from the insula may be accompanied by more evident autonomic dysfunctions.

Three boys with a diagnosis of BECTS were identified among 189 cases reported in the North American SUDEP Registry [111]. The three patients spanned the spectrum of BECTS severity: one had only a few seizures, one had more than 30 focal motor seizures, and one had four witnessed generalized tonic-clonic seizures and approximately 30 suspected generalized tonic-clonic seizures. None of the patients was prescribed antiseizure drugs, either owing to physician recommendation or mutual decision by the physician and parents. All three patients were found dead in circumstances typical of SUDEP.

A population study was conducted in Finland to analyze long-term survival and mortality among 207 patients treated for West syndrome in three tertiary care hospitals [112]. Etiology at onset was symptomatic in 87% patients and cryptogenic in 13%; six of the latter 26 patients later turned out to be symptomatic. During follow-up, 10 of 207 patients had died of SUDEP, representing the most common epilepsy-related cause of death. The mean age at SUDEP was 27.4 years. All but one of the SUDEP cases had intellectual disability and all but one had an underlying neurologic disorder.

Risk Factors for SUDEP

The identification of risk factors is essential to support clinicians to recognize individuals at risk and to identify how SUDEP risk can be mitigated and prevented, but also potentially help understand the underlying pathophysiology of SUDEP. Studies analyzing SUDEP risk factors are different with regard to the populations studied, methodology, and study design. The above cited AAN/AES guidelines [108] considered the presence and frequency of generalized tonic-clonic seizures (GTCs) as the most important risk factors for SUDEP (OR 10). Other factors associated with higher SUDEP risk were not being seizure free for 1–5 years (OR 4.7) and not adding an antiepileptic drug (AED) when patients are medically refractory (OR 6); the presence of nocturnal supervision was found to reduce SUDEP risk (OR 0.4), as did the use of a nocturnal listening device (OR 0.1).

Previous studies reported that specific AEDs (i.e., lamotrigine or carbamazepine) were associated with heightened SUDEP risk; however, these findings have been challenged from the results of recent studies. Therefore, the AAN/AES concluded that the evidence was low or low/conflicting for specific AED use and polytherapy, respectively, for SUDEP risk [108]. Conversely, optimization of AED therapy may reduce SUDEP risk: hence, in individuals with refractory epilepsy, the risk of SUDEP seems to be increased when an AED is not added to the treatment regimen.

Different scales are in development to help identify persons at risk. DeGiorgio et al. [113] reported the first SUDEP Inventory (the SUDEP-7), which was drawn from a single large cohort study [114]. The SUDEP-7 has been proposed to quantify SUDEP risk in living people with epilepsy based upon five factors: frequency of generalized tonic–clonic seizures, monthly seizure frequency, number of antiepileptic drugs in use, duration of epilepsy, and intellectual disability. Each risk factor is assigned a point score based on its respective odds ratio for SUDEP, with a possible score of 0–12. The revised SUDEP-7 (rSUDEP-7) combines generalized tonic-clonic seizures and seizure frequency measures to reduce score inflation [115] (Table 19.3).

Table 19.3 Comparing the SUDEP-7 to the revised SUDEP-7

Risk factors	SUDEP-7	Revised SUDEP-7
GCTS in the past 12 months	0 seizures → 0 points 1–3 seizures → 1 point ≥4 seizures → 3 points	0 seizures → 0 points 1–3 seizures → 1 point ≥4 seizures → 2 points
Any seizure, frequency per month in the past 12 months	0 seizures → 0 points 1–49 seizures → 1 point ≥50 seizures → 3 points	0 seizures → 0 points 1–49 seizures → 1 point ≥50 seizures → 2 points
Epilepsy duration	0–29 years → 0 points ≥30 years → 3 points	
Number of AEDs	0–2 drugs → 0 points ≥3 drugs → 1 point	
Cognitive impairment	IQ ≥ 70 → 0 points IQ < 70 → 2 points	
Total score	**12 points**	**10 points**

AED anti-epileptic drug, *GCTS* generalized tonic-clonic seizures, *IQ* intelligence quotient, *SUDEP-7* SUDEP Risk Inventory

Genetics of SUDEP

Recently, several pathogenic alterations in different genes have been reported to increase SUDEP risk through multiple pathophysiological mechanisms. Specific genetic and epilepsy syndromes are also associated with increased risk of SUDEP. Patients with Dravet syndrome (DS), a genetic epileptic encephalopathy in which a SCN1A loss-of-function mutation is found in 80% of cases, are at increased risk of SUDEP and premature mortality [116]. Analogously, individuals with mutations in SCN8A, associated with early-infantile encephalopathy, may also be at increased risk of SUDEP although a recent review of all-cause mortality in SCN8A did not confirm this association [117]. Moreover, patients with isodicentric chromosome 15 syndrome —especially those with severe neurological dysfunction —have higher risk of SUDEP. Several other genes have been found to be associated with SUDEP such as, SCN2A, SCN5A, KCNA1, KCNQ1, KCNH2, DEPDC5 (for a detailed review see [118]). Notably, some of these ion channel mutations are co-expressed in the brain and heart and predispose to both epileptic seizures and cardiac arrhythmias.

SUDEP and Sleep

Prince John the youngest child of King George V of England died having SUDEP during sleep. At that time, the royal doctor, Alan Reeve Manby wrote: "His Royal Highness Prince John, who has since infancy suffered from epileptic fits, which have lately become more frequent and severe, passed away in his sleep following an attack this afternoon at Sandringham." This is one of the first witnessed SUDEP case that happened during sleep. Subsequently, different studies demonstrated an association between SUDEP and night time or sleep [119, 120]. For instance, Lamberts et al. observed that 62% of SUDEP cases happened between midnight and noon and that 58% of SUDEP cases were sleep-related [121]. Similarly, a recent systematic review and meta-analysis [122] demonstrated that SUDEP is significantly associated with sleep as compared to wakefulness (69.3% of cases occurred during sleep and 30.7% occurred during wakefulness).

All these data suggest that sleep exert a fundamental role as a risk factor that can act in a particular circumstance with a peri-ictal coincidence of several precipitating factors. Moreover, other than the function of sleep as a possible precipitating factor for SUDEP, recent evidence suggests that sleep-epilepsy interaction could also exert a long-standing effect leading to an increase of SUDEP susceptibility. Different studies showed that ANS factors affecting cardiac or respiratory functions play a pivotal role in the SUDEP pathogenesis. However, evidence on how they might be related to one another or to an epileptic seizure, eventually leading to sudden death, especially during sleep, are not conclusive [2, 119].

Longstanding Effects of Sleep and Epilepsy Interaction: Implications for SUDEP

Different studies reported autonomic changes in epileptic patients, especially during sleep. Interictal HRV abnormalities have been described in various populations of both focal (especially temporal] and generalized epilepsy [1]. These HRV variations seem to be more pronounced during night time, suggesting that this period might be more vulnerable to impaired ANS heart control. Moreover, HRV modifications in epileptic patients improve after epilepsy surgery; in particular, patients with a poor surgical outcome show a more pronounced HRV impairment than those individuals with a good outcome [123]. These findings suggest that the ANS control could be mainly related to seizure reduction.

It is not completely clarified if HRV modifications reported in epileptic patients during sleep are related to a direct effect of interictal discharges or to their indirect effect on arousal instability. Indeed, as discussed above for SHE, periodic epileptic discharges can increase arousal fluctuations, inducing in turn a chronic sympathetic over activation. Moreover, among drug-resistant patients, a further vulnerability factor is represented by the repeated effects of seizures on the cardiovascular system that might also result in damage to the nervous network regulating excitation of the cardiac tissue. Indeed, sudden cardiac death (SCD) is more frequent in patients with underlying cardiac structural abnormalities. However, although several studies demonstrated postmortem myocardial injuries in SUDEP subjects [124], to date no evidence exists to support this possibility.

Some studies correlate specific AEDs use with greater degrees of autonomic dysfunction. For instance, carbamazepine can slow cardiac conduction, reduce HRV and, rarely, induce atrio-ventricular (AV) conduction block in elderly patients [125]. Moreover, the side effects of some AEDs such as weight gain or hyperhomocysteinemiae may in turn cause an indirect dysfunction of the cardiovascular system [119]. Different studies analyzed the effects of weaning AEDs in adults, including the rapid tapering that typically occurs during epilepsy monitoring unit admissions with conflicting results. While two studies demonstrated that rapid AEDs reduction led to acute decreases in HRV, the third study found instead no significant differences [1]. Another study in seizure-free outpatients with epilepsy on drug monotherapy demonstrated that slow withdrawal of AEDs appeared to improve HRV [126]. In summary, there is not enough evidence of a negative impact of AEDs on sleep-related autonomic changes; conversely, achieving complete seizure control represents one of the main tools to reduce SUDEP risk. Moreover, AEDs may show beneficial effects not only on the control of neuronal excitability but also on stabilization of sleep structure, with a consequent reduction of sleep arousals and in turn an indirect positive improvement of ANS functions.

Although different studies analyzed HRV in epileptic living patients, evaluating HRV parameters in relation to SUDEP risk factors and prospective data on HRV from SUDEP patients are scanty. In 2009, Surges et al. did not find significant differences in interictal HRV measures on seven patients with SUDEP with respect to a control group [127]. In a recent work, Myers et al. analyzed HRV data in wakefulness and sleep from 80 patients with drug-resistant epilepsy, half of whom had sodium channel mutations. They found that patients with sodium channel mutations who died due to SUDEP showed more extreme HRV derangements with low HRV in wakefulness and extremely high or very low values of sleep/awake HRV ratios [1].

Seizures During Sleep: Precipitating Factors for SUDEP

Studies evaluating the circumstances of death suggest that the most common scenario for SUDEP is a convulsive seizure occurring during sleep especially in prone position. The MORTEMUS study represents the largest study to date describing cardiorespiratory function at the time of death in epilepsy [128]. In this study, seven of the 10 cases for which sleep state could be determined occurred during sleep (one during REM, one during stage 1, two in stage 2, and three in sleep stages 3 or 4). Moreover, all SUDEP death happened after a convulsive seizure. In summary, the triggering seizure was followed by a short period of normal or increased heart and respiratory rates, after which a combination of central apnea, severe bradycardia, or transient asystole occurred concomitant with postictal generalized EEG suppression (PGES), typically after 1–3 min. This cardiorespiratory collapse was terminal in a third of patients. In the other patients, this was followed by transient restoration of cardiac function associated with abnormal and possibly ineffective respiration, probably aggravated by the prone position. Respiration then progressively worsened until terminal apnea, which occurred before terminal asystole in all cases. These data suggest that the highly abnormal cardiorespiratory patterns seen in all these cases could have been induced by a catastrophic autonomic dysfunction consequent to a severe brainstem problem.

Although a severe cardiorespiratory dysfunction induced by a GTCS represents the most common pathogenetic mechanism in SUDEP, rare cases of ventricular tachyarrhythmia in near-SUDEP or SUDEP patients were described. For instance, Espinosa et al. reported a case of near-SUDEP in a 51-year-old woman with refractory temporal lobe epilepsy. During video-EEG, a right temporal focal seizure occurred out of sleep, followed by a secondary generalization, which triggered ventricular tachycardia, requiring placement of an implantable cardiac defibrillator [129].

Studies conducted in animal models showed that both interictal and ictal epileptic activity may affect cardiac rhythm. Moreover, different kind of cardiac arrhythmias (i.e., severe tachyarrhtythmias, bradycardia, or asystole) have been shown not only in GTCS but also in focal seizures, especially originating from the temporal lobes, the insular cortex, or the limbic system. A study conducted with long-term ECG recording via implantable loop recorders in patients with refractory epilepsy reported the occurrence of at least one episode of ictal bradycardia or asystole in 21% of patients [130]. A retrospective analysis of multiday ECG data obtained during video-EEG recording in a population of drug resistant patients found that patients who subsequently died having SUDEP had greater increases in heart rate during seizures as compared with a clinically similar group of patients with refractory epilepsy. These changes in heart rate were particularly evident during sleep-onset seizures in the SUDEP group [131].

Different studies investigated the role of the respiratory system in the pathophysiology of SUDEP. Indeed, ictal respiratory impairment, often closely linked to cardiac dysfunction, is a prominent feature in witnessed SUDEP cases as demonstrated by the MORTEMUS study [128]. Since 1950s, Kaada and Jasper demonstrated that electrical stimulation of different brain regions such as human insular cortex, ventromedial prefrontal cortex, hippocampus, and amygdala produced an autonomic dysfunction which may cause respiratory arrest in rare cases [132]. It has been shown that ictal desaturations and ictal central apnea strongly correlate with temporal lobe epilepsy. In particular, intracerebral recordings in drug-resistant epileptic patients revealed that ictal apnea is related to the spread of a temporal onset seizure to the contralateral temporal lobe rather than the seizure onset itself [133]. More recently, another study with stereo EEG in patients with medically intractable epilepsy found that central apnea and O_2 desaturation occurred when seizures spread to the amygdala. Moreover, in the same patient localized electrical stimulation of the amygdala reproduced the same respiratory dysfunction [134]. Severe and prolonged increases in end-tidal CO_2 ($ETCO_2$) and modification of regional cerebral oxygen saturation are also reported to occur with seizures. Indeed, a study conducted with video-EEG telemetry with recording of respiratory data revealed that one-third of patients with focal epilepsy had seizures with $ETCO_2$ elevation above 50 mm Hg. Of note, ictal/postictal $ETCO_2$ increase above baseline was recorded for a mean duration of 424 s [133]. Moreover, studies by means of near-infrared spectroscopy reported decreased regional cerebral oxygenation with ictal onset [135].

In the majority of SUDEP cases, the victim is found in the prone position [136]. It is generally agreed that ending a convulsive seizure in the prone position may increase the risk of SUDEP. The most plausible explanation for this is that this position might increase the risk of an obstruction of the nose and mouth due to pressure against the bed clothing and alter ventilation by reducing vital capacity and tidal volume [137].

Serotonergic neurons seem to be implicated in the basic neurobiological mechanisms for SUDEP. Indeed, serotonergic neurotransmission modulates different brain functions, such as breathing, sleep-wake transitions and circadian rhythmicity. Serotonin levels are highest during wakefulness, reduced during NREM sleep, and almost absent during REM sleep [138]. Stable breathing requires serotonergic neurotransmission [139]. During sleep, increase in serotonergic neurotransmission is essential for the arousal response to inspired CO_2. An ictal epileptic discharge induces a suppression of serotonergic neurotransmission during both ictal and postictal period [140]. Therefore, a disruption of normal serotonergic arousal mechanisms may alter the normal arousal response to CO_2 in the postictal period during sleep, thus favoring death. In DBA/2 mice which lack several 5 HT receptor proteins in the brainstem, provoked audiogenic seizures leading to death due to respiratory arrest, which can be prevented with oxygenation. It is noteworthy that this seizure-related death is reduced by use of selective serotonin reuptake inhibitors (SSRI) [141]. An animal study conducted with kainic acid to induce recurring seizures, showed that seizure activity caused increased firing of the recurrent laryngeal nerve resulting in laryngospasm and airway occlusion, with a consequent obstructive apnea followed by ST segment elevation, bradycardia, and death [142].

An electrophysiological phenomenon which can be observed following seizures is PGES. This consists in the absence of detectable scalp EEG activity at <10 microvolts amplitude, typically following a primary or secondarily GTCS. In rare cases of SUDEP, a PGES started before the occurrence of any fatal cardiac or respiratory arrest [143]. A primary cause of this unclear phenomenon could be an alteration of cerebral blood flow autoregulation that induce a sudden drop of cerebral perfusion and a subsequent cessation of electrical activity. In epileptic patients, an overactivity of the sympathetic drive is reported to induce an impairment of interictal cerebrovascular autoregulation [144]. During NREM sleep, a reduction of cerebral blood flow and cerebrovascular response to hypercapnia and especially to hypoxia occurs, thus suggesting that during this sleep stage cerebral circulation may be particularly vulnerable [145].

Sleep Disorders Comorbidities in Epileptic Patients: Implications for SUDEP

Patients suffering from nocturnal epilepsy and, in general, from epilepsy can also suffer from primary sleep disorders. These can manifest themselves independently from epilepsy in the same patient but can negatively influence the epileptic disorder itself; conversely, the expression of sleep disorders can be negatively influenced by the epileptic condition. The most frequent sleep disorder in epilepsy patients is represented by obstructive sleep apnea (OSA). The frequency of comorbid OSA in various epilepsy cohorts has been estimated to range between approximately 10% and 30%. Recently, McCarter et al. demonstrated that drug resistant epilepsy patients are at an increased risk of sleep disordered breathing, particularly OSA [146]. Moreover, they also found a possible association between OSA and SUDEP risk. Indeed, OSA has been identified as an independent risk factor for sudden cardiac death [147]. The autonomic dysfunction and lower resting oxygen saturation observed in OSA patients might increase a patient's vulnerability to SUDEP. In particular, recurrent apnea/hypopnea episodes may lead to an increase in sympathetic tone and hypoxemia that, in turn, increase myocardial oxygen demand, resulting in cardiac ischemia and potentially fatal dysrhythmias. Moreover, OSA could further increase the QTc interval in vulnerable refractory epilepsy patients who may already have underlying prolonged QTc due to seizures or AEDs side effects [148]. Finally, OSA could induce a further impairment of HRV, worsening a poor pre-existing underlying autonomic function in patients with epilepsy that, in turn, could favor the development of tachydysrhythmias and sudden death [149]. The increased SUDEP risk in epileptic patients with OSA may be also mediated by a respiratory dysfunction. A chronic hypercapnia with a decreased ventilatory response to higher carbon dioxide levels has been described in patients with OSA [150]. Therefore, the above-mentioned dysfunctional serotonin transmission induced by seizures together with the blunted respiratory response to hypercapnia caused by chronic OSA may further reduce the respiratory drive following postictal apnea, increasing the risk of SUDEP. Finally, OSA could induce a sleep fragmentation and a consequent sleep deprivation [151], lowering the seizure threshold, and increasing the risk for refractory seizures and, in turn, the susceptibility for SUDEP.

Prevention of SUDEP

The primary purpose of understanding the incidence, risk factors, and biomarkers for SUDEP is to help identify individuals at risk and to determine how risk can be mitigated and SUDEP prevented. As discussed above, the most important risk factor for SUDEP is the presence of GTCS. The American Academy of Neurology and American Epilepsy Society recommend that clinicians inform their patients about the SUDEP risk [108]. Different survey studies revealed that epilepsy patients and family members prefer to know about the risk factors of SUDEP during the early phase of management [152]. However, recent evidence showed that only a small minority of neurologists counsel all of their patients about SUDEP [153]. A meta-analysis conducted by Ryvlin et al. found that an adjunctive AED treatment might reduce the SUDEP risk by seven times in drug resistant epilepsy patients [154]. In case of refractory epilepsy, other treatments should be evaluated, such as epilepsy surgery, vagal nerve stimulation (VNS), responsive neurostimulation, and the ketogenic diet.

Considering the role of sleep as risk factor for SUDEP, nocturnal supervision and nocturnal listening devices have been proposed as preventive measures for SUDEP. In accordance with the AAN/AES guideline, "for persons with frequent GTCS and nocturnal seizures, clinicians may advise selected patients and families, if permitted by their individualized epilepsy type and psychosocial circumstances, to use nocturnal supervision or other nocturnal precautions, such as the use of a remote listening device, to reduce SUDEP risk" [108].

Moreover, a growing number of automated devices to help detect seizures are now available in the market. There are two categories of devices: EEG-based systems (i.e., video EEG, ambulatory EEG, neurostimulation devices, VNS) and non-EEG systems, which employ several different technologies, such as accelerometry, electrodermal activity or skin resistance/conductance, near-infrared spectroscopy, electrocardiogram, electromyogram, and video monitoring [155]. However, to date, studies evaluating their efficacy are scanty, frequently conducted on small population of patients and by the same team developing the devices.

Although evidence regarding prone position as a risk factor for SUDEP is discordant, different simple preventive measures have been suggested, such as positioning or the use of antisuffocation pillow. Moreover, using early intervention, such as stimulating and turning the patient to the lateral position and suction with or without supplemental oxygen administration could help to reduce the duration of peri-ictal hypoxemia and seizure [156].

Finally, Bateman et al. found that SSRIs are associated with reduced severity of ictal hypoxemia in patients with medically refractory partial seizures [157]; however, further studies are needed to determine if SSRIs can reduce SUDEP risk.

In summary, epilepsy patients often display ANS dysfunction during interictal states that can be related to genetic, medication, and other factors. Seizures may induce acute cardiac and respiratory dysfunction. Indeed, during seizures a sinus tachycardia frequently occurs but also asystole and malignant tachyarrhythmias have been observed. Seizures can also trigger an acute respiratory dysfunction, such as central ictal and obstructive apnea related to laryngospasm. Thus, recent data suggest that the underlying autonomic dysfunction in epilepsy patients might predispose them to a sudden fatal cardio-respiratory dysfunction during a seizure, resulting in SUDEP.

References

1. Myers KA, Sivathamboo S, Perucca P. Heart rate variability measurement in epilepsy: how can we move from research to clinical practice? Epilepsia. 2018;59(12):2169–78.
2. Barot N, Nei M. Autonomic aspects of sudden unexpected death in epilepsy (SUDEP). Clin Auton Res. 2019;29(2):151–60.
3. Lugaresi E, Cirignotta F. Hypnogenic paroxysmal dystonia: epileptic seizure or a new syndrome? Sleep. 1981;4(2):129–38.
4. Lugaresi E, Cirignotta F, Montagna P. Nocturnal paroxysmal dystonia. J Neurol Neurosurg Psychiatry. 1986;49(4):375–80.
5. Tharp BR. Orbital frontial seizures. An unique electroencephalographic and clinical syndrome. Epilepsia. 1972;13(5):627–42.
6. Williamson PD, Spencer DD, Spencer SS, Novelly RA, Mattson RH. Complex partial seizures of frontal lobe origin. Ann Neurol. 1985;18(4):497–504.
7. Waterman K, Purves SJ, Kosaka B, Strauss E, Wada JA. An epileptic syndrome caused by mesial frontal lobe seizure foci. Neurology. 1987;37(4):577–82.
8. Tinuper P, Bisulli F, Cross JH, Hesdorffer D, Kahane P, Nobili L, et al. Definition and diagnostic criteria of sleep-related hypermotor epilepsy. Neurology. 2016;86(19):1834–42.
9. Scheffer IE, Bhatia KP, Lopes-Cendes I, Fish DR, Marsden CD, Andermann F, et al. Autosomal dominant frontal epilepsy misdiagnosed as sleep disorder. Lancet Lond Engl. 1994;343(8896):515–7.
10. Provini F, Plazzi G, Tinuper P, Vandi S, Lugaresi E, Montagna P. Nocturnal frontal lobe epilepsy: a clinical and polygraphic overview of 100 consecutive cases. Brain. 1999;122(6):1017–31.
11. Nobili L, Francione S, Mai R, Cardinale F, Castana L, Tassi L, et al. Surgical treatment of drug-resistant nocturnal frontal lobe epilepsy. Brain J Neurol. 2007;130(Pt 2):561–73.
12. Vignatelli L, Bisulli F, Giovannini G, Licchetta L, Naldi I, Mostacci B, et al. Prevalence of nocturnal frontal lobe epilepsy in the adult population of Bologna and Modena, Emilia-Romagna region, Italy. Sleep. 2015;38(3):479–85.
13. Mostacci B, Bisulli F, Vignatelli L, Licchetta L, Di Vito L, Rinaldi C, et al. Incidence of sudden unexpected death in nocturnal frontal lobe epilepsy: a cohort study. Sleep Med. 2015;16(2):232–6.
14. Aridon P, Marini C, Di Resta C, Brilli E, De Fusco M, Politi F, et al. Increased sensitivity of the neuronal nicotinic receptor alpha 2 subunit causes familial epilepsy with nocturnal wandering and ictal fear. Am J Hum Genet. 2006;79(2):342–50.
15. De Fusco M, Becchetti A, Patrignani A, Annesi G, Gambardella A, Quattrone A, et al. The nicotinic receptor beta 2 subunit is mutant in nocturnal frontal lobe epilepsy. Nat Genet. 2000;26(3):275–6.
16. McLellan A, Phillips HA, Rittey C, Kirkpatrick M, Mulley JC, Goudie D, et al. Phenotypic comparison of two Scottish families with mutations in different genes causing autosomal dominant nocturnal frontal lobe epilepsy. Epilepsia. 2003;44(4):613–7.
17. Heron SE, Smith KR, Bahlo M, Nobili L, Kahana E, Licchetta L, et al. Missense mutations in the sodium-gated potassium channel gene KCNT1 cause severe autosomal dominant nocturnal frontal lobe epilepsy. Nat Genet. 2012;44(11):1188–90.
18. Barcia G, Fleming MR, Deligniere A, Gazula V-R, Brown MR, Langouet M, et al. De novo gain-of-function KCNT1 channel mutations cause malignant migrating partial seizures of infancy. Nat Genet. 2012;44(11):1255–9.
19. Cataldi M, Nobili L, Zara F, Combi R, Prato G, Giacomini T, et al. Migrating focal seizures in autosomal dominant sleep-related hypermotor epilepsy with KCNT1 mutation. Seizure. 2019;67:57–60.
20. Ricos MG, Hodgson BL, Pippucci T, Saidin A, Ong YS, Heron SE, et al. Mutations in the mammalian target of rapamycin pathway regulators NPRL2 and NPRL3 cause focal epilepsy. Ann Neurol. 2016;79(1):120–31.
21. Korenke G-C, Eggert M, Thiele H, Nürnberg P, Sander T, Steinlein OK. Nocturnal frontal lobe epilepsy caused by a mutation in the GATOR1 complex gene *NPRL3*. Epilepsia. 2016;57(3):e60–3.
22. Ishida S, Picard F, Rudolf G, Noé E, Achaz G, Thomas P, et al. Mutations of DEPDC5 cause autosomal dominant focal epilepsies. Nat Genet. 2013;45(5):552–5.
23. Dibbens LM, de Vries B, Donatello S, Heron SE, Hodgson BL, Chintawar S, et al. Mutations in DEPDC5 cause familial focal epilepsy with variable foci. Nat Genet. 2013;45(5):546–51.
24. Baulac S, Ishida S, Marsan E, Miquel C, Biraben A, Nguyen DK, et al. Familial focal epilepsy with focal cortical dysplasia due to DEPDC5 mutations. Ann Neurol. 2015;77(4):675–83.
25. Carvill GL, Crompton DE, Regan BM, McMahon JM, Saykally J, Zemel M, et al. Epileptic spasms are a feature of DEPDC5 mTORopathy. Neurol Genet. 2015;1(2):e17.
26. Chen Z-H, Wang C, Zhuo M-Q, Zhai Q-X, Chen Q, Guo Y-X, et al. Exome sequencing identified a novel missense mutation c.464G>A (p.G155D) in Ca2+−binding protein 4 (CABP4) in a Chinese pedigree with autosomal dominant nocturnal frontal lobe epilepsy. Oncotarget. 2017;8(45):78940–7.
27. Peres J, Antunes F, Zonjy B, Mitchell AL, Lhatoo SD. Sleep-related hypermotor epilepsy and peri-ictal hypotension in a patient with syntaxin-1B mutation. Epileptic Disord. 2018;20(5):413–7.
28. Proserpio P, Cossu M, Francione S, Gozzo F, Lo Russo G, Mai R, et al. Epileptic motor behaviors during sleep: Anatomo-electro-clinical features. Sleep Med. 2011;12:S33–8.
29. Nobili L, Cardinale F, Magliola U, Cicolin A, Didato G, Bramerio M, et al. Taylor's focal cortical dysplasia increases the risk of sleep-related epilepsy. Epilepsia. 2009;50(12):2599–604.
30. Licchetta L, Bisulli F, Vignatelli L, Zenesini C, Di Vito L, Mostacci B, et al. Sleep-related hypermotor epilepsy: long-term outcome in a large cohort. Neurology. 2017;88(1):70–7.
31. Gibbs SA, Proserpio P, Francione S, Mai R, Cardinale F, Sartori I, et al. Clinical features of sleep-related hypermotor epilepsy in relation to the seizure-onset zone: a review of 135 surgically treated cases. Epilepsia. 2019;60(4):707–17.
32. Oldani A, Zucconi M, Ferini-Strambi L, Bizzozero D, Smirne S. Autosomal dominant nocturnal frontal lobe epilepsy: electro-clinical picture. Epilepsia. 1996;37(10):964–76.
33. Nobili L, Francione S, Mai R, Tassi L, Cardinale F, Castana L, et al. Nocturnal frontal lobe epilepsy: intracerebral recordings of paroxysmal motor attacks with increasing complexity. Sleep. 2003;26(7):883–6.
34. Nobili L, Sartori I, Terzaghi M, Tassi L, Mai R, Francione S, et al. Intracerebral recordings of minor motor events, paroxysmal arousals and major seizures in nocturnal frontal lobe epilepsy. Neurol Sci Off J Ital Neurol Soc Ital Soc Clin Neurophysiol. 2005;26(Suppl 3):S215–9.
35. Terzaghi M, Sartori I, Mai R, Tassi L, Francione S, Cardinale F, et al. Sleep-related minor motor events in nocturnal frontal lobe epilepsy. Epilepsia. 2007;48(2):335–41.
36. Nobili L, Sartori I, Terzaghi M, Stefano F, Mai R, Tassi L, et al. Relationship of epileptic discharges to arousal instability and periodic leg movements in a case of nocturnal frontal lobe epilepsy: a stereo-EEG study. Sleep. 2006;29(5):701–4.
37. Gibbs SA, Proserpio P, Terzaghi M, Pigorini A, Sarasso S, Lo Russo G, et al. Sleep-related epileptic behaviors and non-REM-related parasomnias: insights from stereo-EEG. Sleep Med Rev. 2016;25:4–20.
38. Proserpio P, Cossu M, Francione S, Tassi L, Mai R, Didato G, et al. Insular-opercular seizures manifesting with sleep-related paroxysmal motor behaviors: a stereo-EEG study: nocturnal insular-opercular seizures. Epilepsia. 2011;52(10):1781–91.
39. Mai R, Sartori I, Francione S, Tassi L, Castana L, Cardinale F, et al. Sleep-related hyperkinetic seizures: always a frontal onset? Neurol Sci. 2005;26(S3):s220–4.

40. Ryvlin P, Minotti L, Demarquay G, Hirsch E, Arzimanoglou A, Hoffman D, et al. Nocturnal hypermotor seizures, suggesting frontal lobe epilepsy, can originate in the insula. Epilepsia. 2006;47(4):755–65.
41. Rheims S, Ryvlin P, Scherer C, Minotti L, Hoffmann D, Guenot M, et al. Analysis of clinical patterns and underlying epileptogenic zones of hypermotor seizures. Epilepsia. 2008;49(12):2030–40.
42. Gibbs SA, Proserpio P, Francione S, Mai R, Cossu M, Tassi L, et al. Seizure duration and latency of hypermotor manifestations distinguish frontal from extrafrontal onset in sleep-related hypermotor epilepsy. Epilepsia. 2018;59(9):e130–4.
43. Nobili L, Francione S, Mai R, Cardinale F, Castana L, Tassi L, et al. Surgical treatment of drug-resistant nocturnal frontal lobe epilepsy. Brain. 2007;130(2):561–73.
44. Menghi V, Bisulli F, Tinuper P, Nobili L. Sleep-related hypermotor epilepsy: prevalence, impact and management strategies. Nat Sci Sleep. 2018;10:317–26.
45. Losurdo A, Proserpio P, Cardinale F, Gozzo F, Tassi L, Mai R, et al. Drug-resistant focal sleep related epilepsy: results and predictors of surgical outcome. Epilepsy Res. 2014;108(5):953–62.
46. Harnod T, Yang CCH, Hsin Y-L, Wang P-J, Shieh K-R, Kuo TBJ. Heart rate variability in patients with frontal lobe epilepsy. Seizure. 2009;18(1):21–5.
47. Tobaldini E, Nobili L, Strada S, Casali KR, Braghiroli A, Montano N. Heart rate variability in normal and pathological sleep. Front Physiol. 2013;4:294.
48. Halász P, Terzano M, Parrino L, Bódizs R. The nature of arousal in sleep. J Sleep Res. 2004;13(1):1–23.
49. Halász P, Kelemen A, Szűcs A. Physiopathogenetic interrelationship between nocturnal frontal lobe epilepsy and nrem arousal parasomnias. Epilepsy Res Treat. 2012;2012:1–8.
50. Calandra-Buonaura G, Toschi N, Provini F, Corazza I, Bisulli F, Barletta G, et al. Physiologic autonomic arousal heralds motor manifestations of seizures in nocturnal frontal lobe epilepsy: implications for pathophysiology. Sleep Med. 2012;13(3):252–62.
51. Dorantes G, Méndez M, Alba A, Gonzaáez JS, Parrino L, Milioli G. Heart rate variability in cyclic alternating pattern during sleep in healthy and nocturnal front lobe epilepsy patients. Conf Proc IEEE Eng Med Biol Soc. 2015;2015:5944–7.
52. Pal DK, Ferrie C, Addis L, Akiyama T, Capovilla G, Caraballo R, et al. Idiopathic focal epilepsies: the "lost tribe". Epileptic Disord Int Epilepsy J Videotape. 2016;18(3):252–88.
53. Baglietto MG, Battaglia FM, Nobili L, Tortorelli S, De Negri E, Calevo MG, et al. Neuropsychological disorders related to interictal epileptic discharges during sleep in benign epilepsy of childhood with centrotemporal or Rolandic spikes. Dev Med Child Neurol. 2001;43(6):407–12.
54. Wickens S, Bowden SC, D'Souza W. Cognitive functioning in children with self-limited epilepsy with centrotemporal spikes: a systematic review and meta-analysis. Epilepsia. 2017;58(10):1673–85.
55. Neumann H, Helmke F, Thiels C, Polster T, Selzer LM, Daseking M, et al. [Cognitive development in children with benign rolandic epilepsy of childhood with centrotemporal spikes – results of a current systematic database search]. Fortschr Neurol Psychiatr. 2016;84(10):617–632. (*Article in German*).
56. Chan S, Pressler R, Boyd SG, Baldeweg T, Cross JH. Does sleep benefit memory consolidation in children with focal epilepsy? Epilepsia. 2017;58(3):456–66.
57. Lemke JR, Lal D, Reinthaler EM, Steiner I, Nothnagel M, Alber M, et al. Mutations in GRIN2A cause idiopathic focal epilepsy with rolandic spikes. Nat Genet. 2013;45(9):1067–72.
58. Dimassi S, Labalme A, Lesca G, Rudolf G, Bruneau N, Hirsch E, et al. A subset of genomic alterations detected in rolandic epilepsies contains candidate or known epilepsy genes including GRIN2A and PRRT2. Epilepsia. 2014;55(2):370–8.
59. Seri S, Di Lorenzo G, Pisano T, Pinci M, Brazzo D, Betteridge H, et al. Interictal autonomic abnormalities in idiopathic Rolandic epilepsy. Epilepsy Behav. 2012;24(2):241–5.
60. Panayiotopoulos CP. Benign childhood epilepsy with occipital paroxysms: a 15-year prospective study. Ann Neurol. 1989;26(1):51–6.
61. Koutroumanidis M. Panayiotopoulos syndrome: an important electroclinical example of benign childhood system epilepsy. Epilepsia. 2007;48(6):1044–53.
62. Caraballo R, Cersósimo R, Fejerman N. Panayiotopoulos syndrome: a prospective study of 192 patients. Epilepsia. 2007;48(6):1054–61.
63. Schmitt B. Sleep and epilepsy syndromes. Neuropediatrics. 2015;46(3):171–80.
64. Beelke M, Nobili L, Baglietto MG, De Carli F, Robert A, De Negri E, et al. Relationship of sigma activity to sleep interictal epileptic discharges: a study in children affected by benign epilepsy with occipital paroxysms. Epilepsy Res. 2000;40(2–3):179–86.
65. Specchio N, Trivisano M, Claps D, Battaglia D, Fusco L, Vigevano F. Documentation of autonomic seizures and autonomic status epilepticus with ictal EEG in Panayiotopoulos syndrome. Epilepsy Behav. 2010;19(3):383–93.
66. Camfield CS, Striano P, Camfield PR. Epidemiology of juvenile myoclonic epilepsy. Epilepsy Behav. 2013;28(Suppl 1):S15–7.
67. Kasteleijn-Nolst Trenité DGA, Schmitz B, Janz D, Delgado-Escueta AV, Thomas P, Hirsch E, et al. Consensus on diagnosis and management of JME: from founder's observations to current trends. Epilepsy Behav. 2013;28(Suppl 1):S87–90.
68. Genton P, Thomas P, Kasteleijn-Nolst Trenité DGA, Medina MT, Salas-Puig J. Clinical aspects of juvenile myoclonic epilepsy. Epilepsy Behav. 2013;28(Suppl 1):S8–14.
69. Mayer TA, Schroeder F, May TW, Wolf PT. Perioral reflex myoclonias: a controlled study in patients with JME and focal epilepsies. Epilepsia. 2006;47(6):1059–67.
70. Serafini A, Rubboli G, Gigli GL, Koutroumanidis M, Gelisse P. Neurophysiology of juvenile myoclonic epilepsy. Epilepsy Behav. 2013;28(Suppl 1):S30–9.
71. Krishnan P, Sinha S, Taly AB, Ramachandraiah CT, Rao S, Satishchandra P. Sleep disturbances in juvenile myoclonic epilepsy: a sleep questionnaire-based study. Epilepsy Behav. 2012;23(3):305–9.
72. Nayak C, Sinha S, Nagappa M, Thennarasu K, Taly AB. Lack of heart rate variability during apnea in patients with juvenile myoclonic epilepsy (JME). Sleep Breath Schlaf Atm. 2015;19(4):1175–83.
73. Glauser TA, Loddenkemper T. Management of childhood epilepsy. Contin Minneap Minn. 2013;19(3 Epilepsy):656–81.
74. Pavone P, Striano P, Falsaperla R, Pavone L, Ruggieri M. Infantile spasms syndrome, west syndrome and related phenotypes: what we know in 2013. Brain Dev. 2014;36(9):739–51.
75. Guerrini R, Pellacani S. Benign childhood focal epilepsies. Epilepsia. 2012;53(Suppl 4):9–18.
76. Watanabe K, Miura K, Natsume J, Hayakawa F, Furune S, Okumura A. Epilepsies of neonatal onset: seizure type and evolution. Dev Med Child Neurol. 1999;41(5):318–22.
77. Rating D, Seidel U, Grimm B, Hanefeld F. The prognostic value of EEG patterns in epilepsies with infantile spasms. Brain Dev. 1987;9(4):361–4.
78. Kramer U, Sue WC, Mikati MA. Hypsarrhythmia: frequency of variant patterns and correlation with etiology and outcome. Neurology. 1997;48(1):197–203.
79. Fattinger S, Schmitt B, Bölsterli Heinzle BK, Critelli H, Jenni OG, Huber R. Impaired slow wave sleep downscaling in patients with

infantile spasms. Eur J Paediatr Neurol EJPN Off J Eur Paediatr Neurol Soc. 2015;19(2):134–42.
80. Huber R, Hill SL, Holladay C, Biesiadecki M, Tononi G, Cirelli C. Sleep homeostasis in Drosophila melanogaster. Sleep. 2004;27(4):628–39.
81. Kurth S, Jenni OG, Riedner BA, Tononi G, Carskadon MA, Huber R. Characteristics of sleep slow waves in children and adolescents. Sleep. 2010;33(4):475–80.
82. Wilhelm I, Diekelmann S, Molzow I, Ayoub A, Mölle M, Born J. Sleep selectively enhances memory expected to be of future relevance. J Neurosci Off J Soc Neurosci. 2011;31(5):1563–9.
83. Hancock EC, Osborne JP, Edwards SW. Treatment of infantile spasms. Cochrane Database Syst Rev. 2013;6:CD001770.
84. O'Callaghan FJK, Edwards SW, Alber FD, Cortina Borja M, Hancock E, Johnson AL, et al. Vigabatrin with hormonal treatment versus hormonal treatment alone (ICISS) for infantile spasms: 18-month outcomes of an open-label, randomised controlled trial. Lancet Child Adolesc Health. 2018;2(10):715–25.
85. Go CY, Mackay MT, Weiss SK, Stephens D, Adams-Webber T, Ashwal S, et al. Evidence-based guideline update: medical treatment of infantile spasms. Report of the Guideline Development Subcommittee of the American Academy of Neurology and the Practice Committee of the Child Neurology Society. Neurology. 2012;78(24):1974–80.
86. Møller MM, Høgenhaven H, Uldall P, Ballegaard M. Heart rate variability in infants with west syndrome. Seizure. 2015;27:10–5.
87. Gencpinar P, Kocabas A, Duman Ö, Dündar NO, Haspolat S, Kardelen F. Cardiac autonomic dysfunction in patients with infantile spasm and the effect of adrenocorticotropic hormone treatment. J Child Neurol. 2016;31(2):134–7.
88. Jansen K, Vandeput S, Van Huffel S, Lagae L. Cardiac autonomic dysfunction in west syndrome. Epilepsy Res. 2012;102(3):167–72.
89. Hattori A, Hayano J, Fujimoto S, Ando N, Mizuno K, Kamei M, et al. Cardiac vagal activation by adrenocorticotropic hormone treatment in infants with west syndrome. Tohoku J Exp Med. 2007;211(2):133–9.
90. van Rijckevorsel K. Treatment of Lennox-Gastaut syndrome: overview and recent findings. Neuropsychiatr Dis Treat. 2008;4(6):1001–19.
91. Arzimanoglou A, French J, Blume WT, Cross JH, Ernst J-P, Feucht M, et al. Lennox-Gastaut syndrome: a consensus approach on diagnosis, assessment, management, and trial methodology. Lancet Neurol. 2009;8(1):82–93.
92. Crumrine PK. Lennox-Gastaut syndrome. J Child Neurol. 2002;17(Suppl 1):S70–5.
93. Borrelli S, El Tahry R. Therapeutic approach to Lennox-Gastaut syndrome: a systematic review. Acta Neurol Belg. 2019;119(3):315–24.
94. Koenig SA, Longin E, Bell N, Reinhard J, Gerstner T. Vagus nerve stimulation improves severely impaired heart rate variability in a patient with Lennox-Gastaut-syndrome. Seizure. 2008;17(5):469–72.
95. Tassinari CA, Cantalupo G, Rios-Pohl L, Giustina ED, Rubboli G. Encephalopathy with status epilepticus during slow sleep: "the Penelope syndrome". Epilepsia. 2009;50(Suppl 7):4–8.
96. Aeby A, Poznanski N, Verheulpen D, Wetzburger C, Van Bogaert P. Levetiracetam efficacy in epileptic syndromes with continuous spikes and waves during slow sleep: experience in 12 cases. Epilepsia. 2005;46(12):1937–42.
97. Galanopoulou AS, Bojko A, Lado F, Moshé SL. The spectrum of neuropsychiatric abnormalities associated with electrical status epilepticus in sleep. Brain Dev. 2000;22(5):279–95.
98. Halász P, Bódizs R, Ujma PP, Fabó D, Szűcs A. Strong relationship between NREM sleep, epilepsy and plastic functions – a conceptual review on the neurophysiology background. Epilepsy Res. 2019;150:95–105.
99. Guzzetta F, Battaglia D, Veredice C, Donvito V, Pane M, Lettori D, et al. Early thalamic injury associated with epilepsy and continuous spike-wave during slow sleep. Epilepsia. 2005;46(6):889–900.
100. De Negri M. Electrical status epilepticus during sleep (ESES). Different clinical syndromes: towards a unifying view? Brain Dev. 1997;19(7):447–51.
101. Lesca G, Rudolf G, Bruneau N, Lozovaya N, Labalme A, Boutry-Kryza N, et al. GRIN2A mutations in acquired epileptic aphasia and related childhood focal epilepsies and encephalopathies with speech and language dysfunction. Nat Genet. 2013;45(9):1061–6.
102. Veggiotti P, Pera MC, Teutonico F, Brazzo D, Balottin U, Tassinari CA. Therapy of encephalopathy with status epilepticus during sleep (ESES/CSWS syndrome): an update. Epileptic Disord Int Epilepsy J Videotape. 2012;14(1):1–11.
103. Cockerell OC, Johnson AL, Sander JW, Hart YM, Goodridge DM, Shorvon SD. Mortality from epilepsy: results from a prospective population-based study. Lancet Lond Engl. 1994;344(8927):918–21.
104. Nashef L, So EL, Ryvlin P, Tomson T. Unifying the definitions of sudden unexpected death in epilepsy: unifying the definitions of SUDEP. Epilepsia. 2012;53(2):227–33.
105. Annegers JF. United States perspective on definitions and classifications. Epilepsia. 1997;38(11 Suppl):S9–12.
106. Nashef L. Sudden unexpected death in epilepsy: terminology and definitions. Epilepsia. 1997;38(11 Suppl):S6–8.
107. Thurman DJ, Logroscino G, Beghi E, Hauser WA, Hesdorffer DC, Newton CR, et al. The burden of premature mortality of epilepsy in high-income countries: a systematic review from the mortality task force of the international league against epilepsy. Epilepsia. 2017;58(1):17–26.
108. Harden C, Tomson T, Gloss D, Buchhalter J, Cross JH, Donner E, et al. Practice guideline summary: sudden unexpected death in epilepsy incidence rates and risk factors: report of the Guideline Development, Dissemination, and Implementation Subcommittee of the American Academy of neurology and the American Epilepsy Society. Neurology. 2017;88(17):1674–80.
109. Keller AE, Whitney R, Li S-A, Pollanen MS, Donner EJ. Incidence of sudden unexpected death in epilepsy in children is similar to adults. Neurology. 2018;91(2):e107–11.
110. Sveinsson O, Andersson T, Carlsson S, Tomson T. The incidence of SUDEP: a nationwide population-based cohort study. Neurology. 2017;89(2):170–7.
111. Doumlele K, Friedman D, Buchhalter J, Donner EJ, Louik J, Devinsky O. Sudden unexpected death in epilepsy among patients with benign childhood epilepsy with centrotemporal spikes. JAMA Neurol. 2017;74(6):645–9.
112. Sillanpää M, Riikonen R, Saarinen MM, Schmidt D. Long-term mortality of patients with west syndrome. Epilepsia Open. 2016;1(1–2):61–6.
113. DeGiorgio CM, Miller P, Meymandi S, Chin A, Epps J, Gordon S, et al. RMSSD, a measure of vagus-mediated heart rate variability, is associated with risk factors for SUDEP: the SUDEP-7 Inventory. Epilepsy Behav. 2010;19(1):78–81.
114. Walczak TS, Leppik IE, D'Amelio M, Rarick J, So E, Ahman P, et al. Incidence and risk factors in sudden unexpected death in epilepsy: a prospective cohort study. Neurology. 2001;56(4):519–25.
115. Novak JL, Miller PR, Markovic D, Meymandi SK, DeGiorgio CM. Risk assessment for sudden death in epilepsy: the SUDEP-7 Inventory. Front Neurol. 2015;6:252.
116. Shmuely S, Sisodiya SM, Gunning WB, Sander JW, Thijs RD. Mortality in Dravet syndrome: a review. Epilepsy Behav. 2016;64(Pt A):69–74.
117. Johannesen KM, Gardella E, Scheffer I, Howell K, Smith DM, Helbig I, et al. Early mortality in SCN8A-related epilepsies. Epilepsy Res. 2018;143:79–81.

118. Coll M, Oliva A, Grassi S, Brugada R, Campuzano O. Update on the genetic basis of sudden unexpected death in epilepsy. Int J Mol Sci. 2019;20(8):1979.
119. Nobili L, Proserpio P, Rubboli G, Montano N, Didato G, Tassinari CA. Sudden unexpected death in epilepsy (SUDEP) and sleep. Sleep Med Rev. 2011;15(4):237–46.
120. Purnell BS, Thijs RD, Buchanan GF. Dead in the night: sleep-wake and time-of-day influences on sudden unexpected death in epilepsy. Front Neurol. 2018;9:1079.
121. Lamberts RJ, Thijs RD, Laffan A, Langan Y, Sander JW. Sudden unexpected death in epilepsy: people with nocturnal seizures may be at highest risk. Epilepsia. 2012;53(2):253–7.
122. Ali A, Wu S, Issa NP, Rose S, Towle VL, Warnke P, et al. Association of sleep with sudden unexpected death in epilepsy. Epilepsy Behav. 2017;76:1–6.
123. Persson H, Kumlien E, Ericson M, Tomson T. Preoperative heart rate variability in relation to surgery outcome in refractory epilepsy. Neurology. 2005;65(7):1021–5.
124. Natelson BH, Suarez RV, Terrence CF, Turizo R. Patients with epilepsy who die suddenly have cardiac disease. Arch Neurol. 1998;55(6):857–60.
125. Tomson T, Kennebäck G. Arrhythmia, heart rate variability, and antiepileptic drugs. Epilepsia. 1997;38(11 Suppl):S48–51.
126. Lossius MI, Erikssen JE, Mowinckel P, Gulbrandsen P, Gjerstad L. Changes in autonomic cardiac control in patients with epilepsy after discontinuation of antiepileptic drugs: a randomized controlled withdrawal study. Eur J Neurol. 2007;14(9):1022–8.
127. Surges R, Henneberger C, Adjei P, Scott CA, Sander JW, Walker MC. Do alterations in inter-ictal heart rate variability predict sudden unexpected death in epilepsy? Epilepsy Res. 2009;87(2–3):277–80.
128. Ryvlin P, Nashef L, Lhatoo SD, Bateman LM, Bird J, Bleasel A, et al. Incidence and mechanisms of cardiorespiratory arrests in epilepsy monitoring units (MORTEMUS): a retrospective study. Lancet Neurol. 2013;12(10):966–77.
129. Espinosa PS, Lee JW, Tedrow UB, Bromfield EB, Dworetzky BA. Sudden unexpected near death in epilepsy: malignant arrhythmia from a partial seizure. Neurology. 2009;72(19):1702–3.
130. Rugg-Gunn FJ, Simister RJ, Squirrell M, Holdright DR, Duncan JS. Cardiac arrhythmias in focal epilepsy: a prospective long-term study. Lancet Lond Engl. 2004;364(9452):2212–9.
131. Nei M, Ho RT, Abou-Khalil BW, Drislane FW, Liporace J, Romeo A, et al. EEG and ECG in sudden unexplained death in epilepsy. Epilepsia. 2004;45(4):338–45.
132. Kaada BR, Jasper H. Respiratory responses to stimulation of temporal pole, insula, and hippocampal and limbic gyri in man. AMA Arch Neurol Psychiatry. 1952;68(5):609–19.
133. Seyal M, Bateman LM. Ictal apnea linked to contralateral spread of temporal lobe seizures: intracranial EEG recordings in refractory temporal lobe epilepsy. Epilepsia. 2009;50(12):2557–62.
134. Dlouhy BJ, Gehlbach BK, Kreple CJ, Kawasaki H, Oya H, Buzza C, et al. Breathing inhibited when seizures spread to the amygdala and upon amygdala stimulation. J Neurosci. 2015;35(28):10281–9.
135. Seyal M. Frontal hemodynamic changes precede EEG onset of temporal lobe seizures. Clin Neurophysiol Off J Int Fed Clin Neurophysiol. 2014;125(3):442–8.
136. Kloster R, Engelskjøn T. Sudden unexpected death in epilepsy (SUDEP): a clinical perspective and a search for risk factors. J Neurol Neurosurg Psychiatry. 1999;67(4):439–44.
137. Reay DT, Howard JD, Fligner CL, Ward RJ. Effects of positional restraint on oxygen saturation and heart rate following exercise. Am J Forensic Med Pathol. 1988;9(1):16–8.
138. Ursin R. Serotonin and sleep. Sleep Med Rev. 2002;6(1):55–69.
139. Richter DW, Manzke T, Wilken B, Ponimaskin E. Serotonin receptors: guardians of stable breathing. Trends Mol Med. 2003;9(12):542–8.
140. Bagdy G, Kecskemeti V, Riba P, Jakus R. Serotonin and epilepsy. J Neurochem. 2007;100(4):857–73.
141. Uteshev VV, Tupal S, Mhaskar Y, Faingold CL. Abnormal serotonin receptor expression in DBA/2 mice associated with susceptibility to sudden death due to respiratory arrest. Epilepsy Res. 2010;88(2–3):183–8.
142. Nakase K, Kollmar R, Lazar J, Arjomandi H, Sundaram K, Silverman J, et al. Laryngospasm, central and obstructive apnea during seizures: defining pathophysiology for sudden death in a rat model. Epilepsy Res. 2016;128:126–39.
143. McLean BN, Wimalaratna S. Sudden death in epilepsy recorded in ambulatory EEG. J Neurol Neurosurg Psychiatry. 2007;78(12):1395–7.
144. Dütsch M, Devinsky O, Doyle W, Marthol H, Hilz MJ. Cerebral autoregulation improves in epilepsy patients after temporal lobe surgery. J Neurol. 2004;251(10):1190–7.
145. Corfield DR, Meadows GE. Control of cerebral blood flow during sleep and the effects of hypoxia. Adv Exp Med Biol. 2006;588:65–73.
146. McCarter AR, Timm PC, Shepard PW, Sandness DJ, Luu T, McCarter SJ, et al. Obstructive sleep apnea in refractory epilepsy: a pilot study investigating frequency, clinical features, and association with risk of sudden unexpected death in epilepsy. Epilepsia. 2018;59(10):1973–81.
147. Gami AS, Olson EJ, Shen WK, Wright RS, Ballman KV, Hodge DO, et al. Obstructive sleep apnea and the risk of sudden cardiac death: a longitudinal study of 10,701 adults. J Am Coll Cardiol. 2013;62(7):610–6.
148. Lamberts RJ, Blom MT, Novy J, Belluzzo M, Seldenrijk A, Penninx BW, et al. Increased prevalence of ECG markers for sudden cardiac arrest in refractory epilepsy. J Neurol Neurosurg Psychiatry. 2015;86(3):309–13.
149. Roche F, Xuong ANT, Court-Fortune I, Costes F, Pichot V, Duverney D, et al. Relationship among the severity of sleep apnea syndrome, cardiac arrhythmias, and autonomic imbalance. Pacing Clin Electrophysiol PACE. 2003;26(3):669–77.
150. Yuan H, Pinto SJ, Huang J, McDonough JM, Ward MB, Lee YN, et al. Ventilatory responses to hypercapnia during wakefulness and sleep in obese adolescents with and without obstructive sleep apnea syndrome. Sleep. 2012;35(9):1257–67.
151. Malow BA. Sleep deprivation and epilepsy. Epilepsy Curr. 2004;4(5):193–5.
152. RamachandranNair R, Jack SM. SUDEP: what do adult patients want to know? Epilepsy Behav. 2016;64(Pt A):195–9.
153. Strzelczyk A, Zschebek G, Bauer S, Baumgartner C, Grond M, Hermsen A, et al. Predictors of and attitudes toward counseling about SUDEP and other epilepsy risk factors among Austrian, German, and Swiss neurologists and neuropediatricians. Epilepsia. 2016;57(4):612–20.
154. Ryvlin P, Cucherat M, Rheims S. Risk of sudden unexpected death in epilepsy in patients given adjunctive antiepileptic treatment for refractory seizures: a meta-analysis of placebo-controlled randomised trials. Lancet Neurol. 2011;10(11):961–8.
155. Zhao X, Lhatoo SD. Seizure detection: do current devices work? And when can they be useful? Curr Neurol Neurosci Rep. 2018;18(7):40.
156. Seyal M, Bateman LM, Li C-S. Impact of periictal interventions on respiratory dysfunction, postictal EEG suppression, and postictal immobility. Epilepsia. 2013;54(2):377–82.
157. Bateman LM, Li C-S, Lin T-C, Seyal M. Serotonin reuptake inhibitors are associated with reduced severity of ictal hypoxemia in medically refractory partial epilepsy. Epilepsia. 2010;51(10):2211–4.

The Postural Tachycardia Syndrome (PoTS)

20

Christopher J. Mathias, Andrew P. Owens, and Valeria Iodice

Introduction

The postural tachycardia syndrome (PoTS) has been increasingly recognised since the start of the new millennium. The term 'PoTS' was first used in 1982 [1], and subsequently in 1993 [2], when Schondorf and Low described it as the 'Postural Orthostatic Tachycardia Syndrome'. The acronym PoTS is ideal, but with exclusion of 'orthostatic' as this is superfluous. PoTS predominantly affects the young, between 13 and 40 years, with a higher prevalence in females. Although the prevalence is not accurately known, it previously has been estimated at 170 cases per 1000,000 in the general population [3].

PoTS is characterised by an abnormally elevated rise in heart rate of >30 beats per minute (bpm) or greater in adults, ≥40 bpm in adolescent or younger adults (12–19 years) within 10 minutes of head-up tilt or standing, or when the heart rate (HR) is over 120 bpm while upright (Fig. 20.1). There should be no fall in blood pressure (BP) or orthostatic hypotension, as may occur in high spinal cord injuries where HR rises due to a vagal response to falling BP (Fig. 20.2).

Descriptions suggestive of PoTS were made during the American Civil War ('irritable heart syndrome' [4]) and after the First World War ('soldier's heart', Sir Thomas Lewis, 1918 [5]). Both Da Costa and Lewis wished to separate these conditions from organic/valvular cardiac disease. PoTS probably was described previously as vasoregulatory asthenia, neurocirculatory asthenia, hyperadrenergic orthostatic hypotension, and sympathotonic orthostatic hypotension. It is important that in addition to the key defining criteria (postural tachycardia and absence of orthostatic hypotension), there is no evidence of autonomic failure or other causes that can raise HR abnormally [6]. Some have considered PoTS under hyperadrenergic or neuropathic phenotypes [7]. Dysfunction of the noradrenaline transporter gene promoter region [8], deconditioning [9], hypovolemia, and/or poor orthostatic cerebral autoregulation [10] also have been reported.

Common features in PoTS include fatigue, which often is present when patients wake up in the morning feeling unrefreshed. This is not necessarily related to, but often is associated with, sleep disturbances that include either getting to sleep or being interrupted, for reasons that could include nocturnal palpitations. Fatigue may occur even in those who sleep normally, or for prolonged periods of time. In a recent study of almost 5000 participants, lightheadedness, tachycardia, headache, and difficulty in concentration were key symptoms [11]. As this was a community-based study, it is uncertain how many were objectively diagnosed on autonomic testing and thus with a definitive diagnosis of PoTS. Associated morbidities included headache in 40%, irritable bowel syndrome in 30%, chronic fatigue in 21%, and features of the joint hypermobile form of Ehlers-Danlos syndrome (E-DS III) in 25%. The incidence of the last, E-DS III was lower and differs from our experience in London for reasons yet to be explained, the last lower and differing from our experience for reasons yet to be explained.

C. J. Mathias (✉)
Queen Square Institute of Neurology, University College London, London, UK

Autonomic & Neurovascular Medicine, Lindo Wing, St Mary's Hospital, Imperial College Healthcare Trust, London, UK

Autonomic & Neurovascular Medicine Centre, Hospital of St John & St Elizabeth, London, UK

A. P. Owens
Department of Old Age Psychiatry, Institute of Psychiatry, Psychology & Neuroscience, Kings College, London, UK

V. Iodice
Queen Square Institute of Neurology, University College London, London, UK

Autonomic & Neurovascular Medicine Centre, Hospital of St John & St Elizabeth, London, UK

Autonomic Unit, National Hospital for Neurology & Neurosurgery, Queen Square, London, UK

S. Chokroverty, P. Cortelli (eds.), *Autonomic Nervous System and Sleep*, https://doi.org/10.1007/978-3-030-62263-3_20

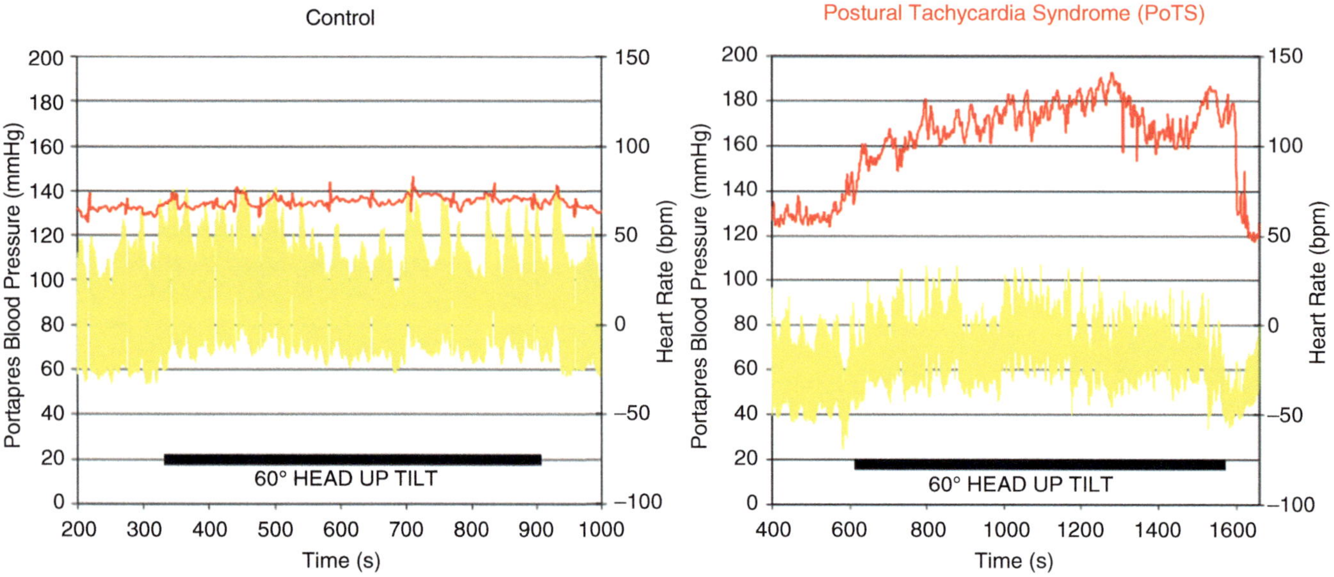

Fig. 20.1 Blood pressure (BP) and heart rate (HR) measured continuously and non-invasively in a normal subject (control) and in a subject with PoTS before, during, and after head-up tilt. PoTS is characterised by a rise in HR of >30 beats per minute (bpm) or greater within 10 minutes of head-up tilt or standing, or when HR is over 120 bpm while upright

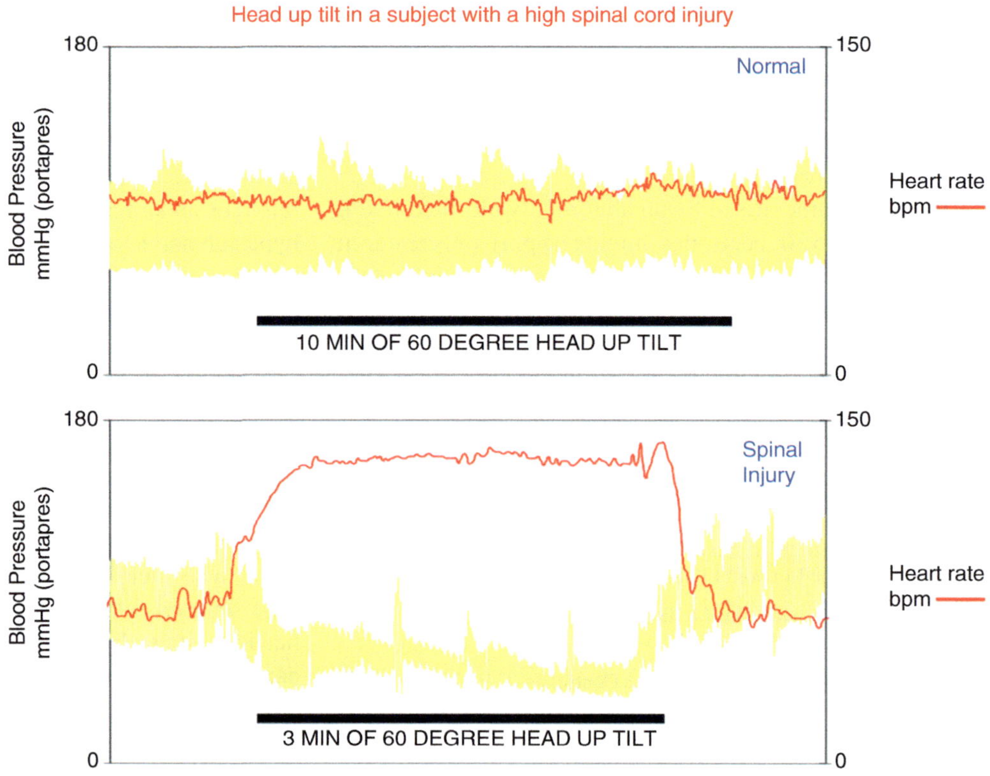

Fig. 20.2 Blood pressure (BP) and heart rate (HR) measured continuously in a normal subject (*upper panel*) and in a high spinal cord lesion (*lower panel*), before, during, and after head-up tilt. Unlike the normal subject, there is a fall in BP (orthostatic hypotension) in the tetraplegic when upright because the sympathetic efferent outflow in the spinal cord is disrupted. However, the brainstem is not affected and there is a marked rise in HR because of withdrawal of vagal nerve activity in response to the fall in BP. This differs from the HR rise in PoTS when upright, which occurs without a BP fall

Clinical Features

The history usually is of orthostatic intolerance, with presyncope and often syncope, usually after postural change from lying down to upright. Palpitations and dizziness, with postural change, are common and many patients report an onset for reasons that temporally, and in retrospect, may be difficult to pinpoint (Box 20.1). Life events that often coincide with the onset of PoTS include infection, trauma, stress or surgery. Patients often are young (below 40) and more likely to be female, although this is not exclusive, as the condition is increasingly recognised in specialist autonomic units and has improved in primary and secondary clinical practice. In addition to symptoms worsening after head-up postural change, exacerbating factors include certain foods (such as carbohydrates and even small amounts of alcohol), physical exertion and hot weather, each of which can cause vasodilatation in different vascular beds (Box 20.2). Some are aware of

Box 20.1 Symptoms of PoTS. These Symptoms Usually Occur in the Upright Position and Are Often Relieved by Lying Flat

Dizziness/light-headedness
Palpitations
Visual disturbances
Clamminess
Loss of consciousness
Nausea
Headache
Pain (stomach or chest)
Shortness of breath
Nonspecific symptoms, including fatigue, attentional deficits, brain fog

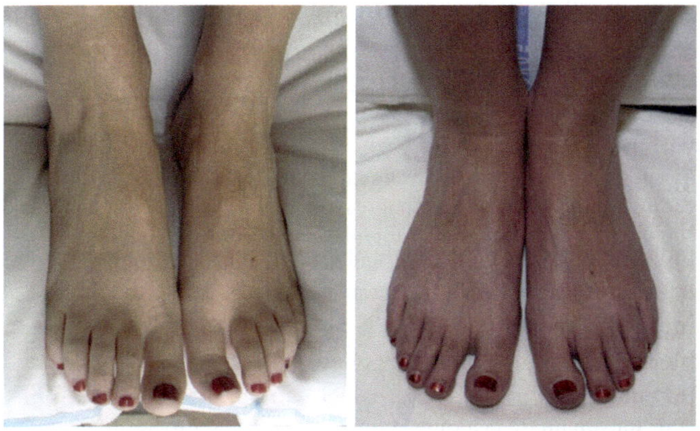

Fig. 20.3 The feet and distal lower limbs in a subject with PoTS while supine (*left panel*). There is violaceous discoloration when upright (*right panel*), which is the result of peripheral vascular pooling. This can be reversed while lying flat, emphasizing the postural component

Box 20.2 Factors that Induce or Worsen PoTS

Time of day (usually worse in the morning, especially on wakening)
Speed of positional change
Prolonged, especially stationary standing
Raised temperature (hot weather, hot bath/shower)
Dehydration
Food ingestion (in some refined carbohydrates or large meals)
Alcohol
Physical exertion
Menstrual period
Deconditioning or prolonged recumbency
Drugs that cause vasodilatation

colour changes (red/purple discoloration or mottling) in the lower limbs and especially feet, when upright (Fig. 20.3), which resolve when lying flat. Other than postural tachycardia, there usually are no abnormal cardiac findings, other than on auscultation, to suggest mitral valve prolapse.

A detailed clinical examination of various systems is essential, as they may be involved, in addition to cardiovascular autonomic features. In each of our centres, PoTS is most frequently (by coincidence or otherwise) associated with the joint hypermobile form of Ehlers-Danlos syndrome III (E-DS III), now classified as the hypermobile form of Ehlers-Danlos syndrome (hE-DS) [6]. Clinical features of hE-DS include joint hypermobility (doubled jointedness, dislocations, translocations/subluxations, clicking joints), a positive Gorlin sign (the ability to touch the nose with the tip of the tongue), lax skin and subcutaneous tissue, and paper thin (papyraceous) scars.

Patients often report cognitive difficulties, and adolescent and young adult PoTS patients can find full-time education challenging. Cognitive symptoms empirically are supported by a growing body of literature on the cognitive-affective profile of PoTS. An example is their short-term memory, with attentional and recall abilities poorer than age-matched controls and their higher score on attention deficit hyperactivity disorder indices [12, 13]. Inattention decreases over illness duration, possibly due to adaptive or treatment responses. Hyperactive traits often are not reported in childhood prior to PoTS onset, suggestive of a contributing role of PoTS to these neuropsychological symptoms. Poor quality sleep, daytime sleepiness and fatigue are also common in PoTS [14]. In PoTS with comorbid chronic fatigue syndrome, working memory, accuracy and information processing are impaired when upright, yet the cause of common 'brain fog' reported by many remains elusive, despite investigations into cerebral blood velocity, sleep quality and neurotransmitter function [15, 16].

The cause of the sleep symptoms reported in PoTS and how they relate to autonomic and neuropsychological symptoms remains unclear. Children and adolescents who sleep less than 8 hours daily are six times more likely to contract PoTS [17], and around half (55%) of adult with PoTS have a non-dipping nocturnal BP profile [18] and prolonged REM stage latency [19–21]. However, the prevalence of anecdotal fatigue and poor sleep quality reported is not reflected in polysomnography (PSG) studies, which generally are unremarkable [19, 22]. It is possible that the multisystemic nature of PoTS contributes to the sleep symptoms and fatigue reported. In a study of PoTS, a third had mild obstructive sleep apnoea (OSA) and also had E-DS III [21], which may predispose them to OSA due to upper airway collapse [23].

Diagnosis

Autonomic Investigations

As there is an overlap with other conditions, including anxiety, it is important that key investigations are performed in a dedicated autonomic laboratory [24] to be certain of the diagnosis and to determine the common underlying pathophysiology (Table 20.1). This ideally should be with continuous noninvasive techniques to record BP and HR while lying and standing, and with different homeostatic challenges. In syncope and pre-syncope BP and HR, responses to head-up tilt will also determine if the cause is autonomic in nature, thus confirming the mechanisms causing autonomic-mediated presyncope or syncope (AMS). These include the mixed form with a fall in both BP and HR (Fig. 20.4a), in the predominantly vasodepressor form with a fall in BP (Fig. 20.4b) and in some the cardio-inhibitory form (Fig. 20.4c.) The last form of AMS is of particular relevance as, although rare, it can necessitate intervention with a cardiac pacemaker. Autonomic testing also should include the response to stimuli in activities of daily living that may worsen PoTS through vasodilatation in splanchnic and muscle vascular beds, such as food and exercise. Some patients are susceptible to raised body temperature, for which facilities not widely available are needed to perform a thermoregulatory sweat test. Laboratory testing should include measurement of plasma catecholamines (plasma noradrenaline and adrenaline) to determine if the patient has the hyperadrenergic PoTS phenotype, although the experience in our departments indicates that this is not common. Moreover, elevated plasma catecholamines taken in the lab may be due to blood-injection-injury phobia (common in AMS) or 'whitecoat syndrome', and 24-hour urinary measurements of catecholamines and their metabolites should follow to confirm or exclude excessive secretion.

In addition to laboratory studies, remote measurements should include 24-hour BP/HR autonomic profiles using the Mathias et al. autonomic protocol [24], time-stamping symptoms recorded during different activities of daily living to changes in BP and HR, which have additional value other than for diagnosis (Fig. 20.5). The autonomic profiles also

Table 20.1 Autonomic investigations for PoTS. These measure the cardiovascular autonomic responses to postural change (head up tilt and standing) and determine the responsiveness of the autonomic nervous system to stimuli in daily life. They help exclude other autonomic conditions, such as those causing autonomic failure

Initial tests
Head-up tilt (at an angle of 60° for 10 min)
Standing
Pressor stimuli (to determine sympathetic vasoconstrictor function): with isometric exercise, cutaneous cold, Valsalva manoeuvre and mental arithmetic
Heart rate responses (to determine cardiac parasympathetic responsiveness): during deep breathing, the Valsalva manoeuvre, hyperventilation, standing and head up tilt
Plasma noradrenaline and adrenaline levels: supine and upright (during head up tilt or standing)
24-hour ambulatory blood pressure and heart rate monitoring
Additional tests
Prolonged head-up tilt (60° for up to 45 min)
Liquid meal challenge to determine pre-prandial and post-prandial cardiovascular autonomic responses to the transition from supine to head up tilt or standing
Graded supine exercise, to determine the cardiovascular autonomic responses while exercising while flat and to compare the responses before and after exercise and while standing

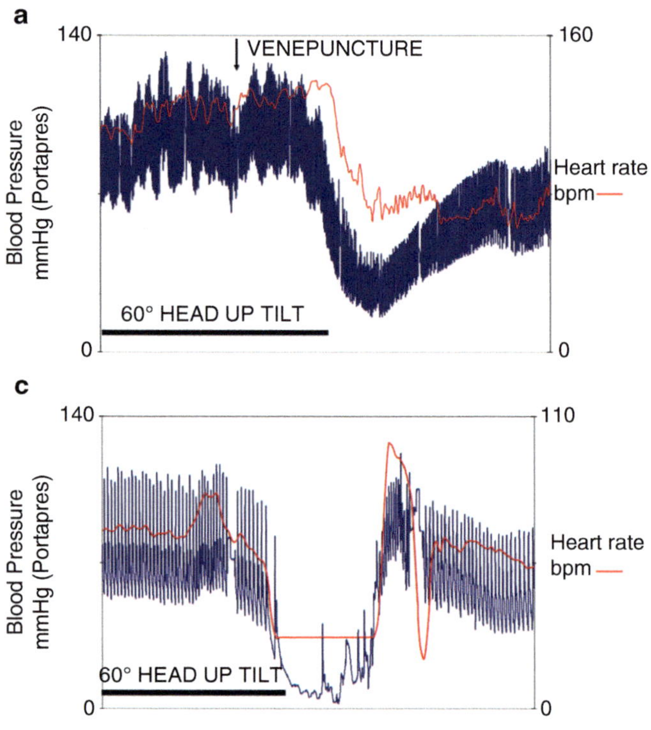

Fig. 20.4 Blood pressure (BP) and heart rate (HR) measured continuously in three different forms of autonomic-mediated syncope (AMS) induced by head-up tilt. In the mixed (cardio-inhibitory and vasodepressor) form (**a**) that is synonymous with vaso-vagal syncope, the most common form of AMS, there is a fall in both BP and HR. In the predominantly vasodepressor form (**b**), there is a fall mainly in BP. In the cardio-inhibitory form (**c**), there is a sudden fall in HR that causes the BP to fall rapidly

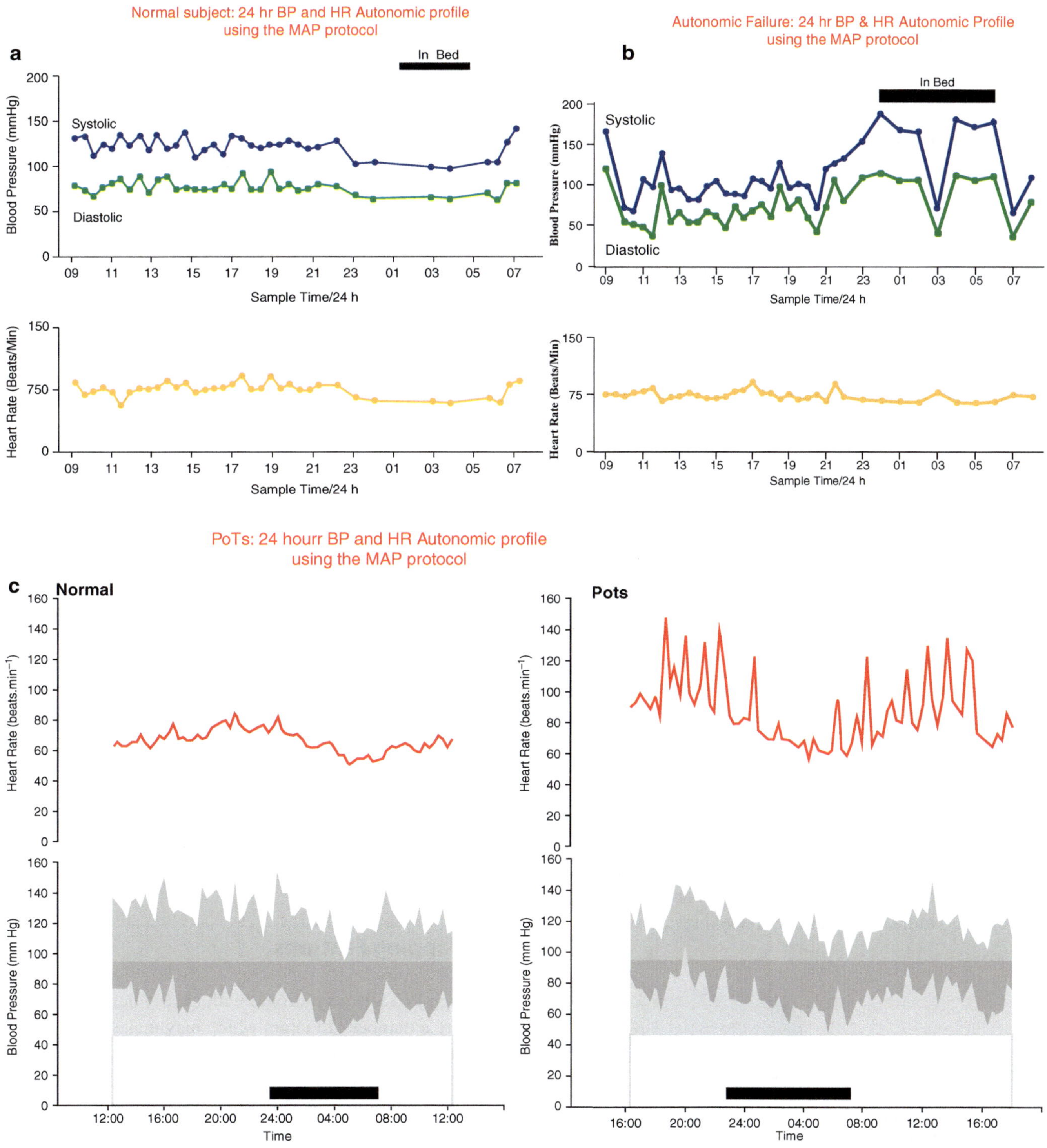

Fig. 20.5 Ambulatory blood pressure/heart rate (BP/HR) autonomic profiles using the Mathias et al. autonomic protocol (MAP) recorded during different activities and essential stimuli (postural change, food exertion and modest exertion) during a 24-hour period. There are modest changes in BP and HR responses in a normal subject (**a**), with the expected circadian fall in BP and HR at night when asleep. In a patient with autonomic failure and orthostatic hypotension (**b**), there can be marked falls in BP when upright, with hypertension while supine at night. There is a substantial fall in BP at night when the patient arose to micturate. In PoTS (**c**), there is a marked tachycardia in the day when upright, without a fall in BP

help determine the effect of non-pharmacological and pharmacological interventions by linking subjective measures and events with objective recordings.

Differential Diagnosis

A number of factors may mimic PoTS, hence there is a need for detailed autonomic investigations to confirm or exclude the diagnosis [25]. In addition to those outlined above, more investigations may be needed in some, such as to definitively exclude a phaeochromocytoma, adrenocortical deficiency/Addison's disease and other endocrine conditions such as inappropriate ADH secretion.

In the national referral centres we run in the UK, approximately 70% of confirmed PoTS patients meet the diagnostic criteria for E-DS III/hE-DS [6] (Fig. 20.6). There is an association between hE-DS and anxiety disorders (60%–68% prevalence), and in particular panic disorder [26]. Like PoTS, comorbid hE-DS and anxiety are significantly more common in young females [27]. This can make initial differential diagnosis of PoTS from an anxiety disorder challenging, particularly as comorbid psychological symptoms often are reported in PoTS [13]. However, recent evidence suggests that these psychological factors are the result rather than cause of autonomic dysfunction in PoTS [28–31]. This necessitates appropriate autonomic testing which should differentiate PoTS-related orthostatic tachycardia from psychogenic sympathetic overexcitation. Investigations of functional disability in PoTS have found day-to-day limitations closely related to catastrophising thoughts, which also mediate anxiety and somatic hypervigilance [32], the most prevalent form of anxiety in PoTS [13, 29, 31]. Therefore, although PoTS and panic disorder may share psychological (impaired concentration, health anxiety, tremulousness) and physiological (palpitations, tachycardia, chest pain, dyspnoea) features and can co-exist [33], a differentiating factor is that PoTS can be provoked by physiological challenges. These include food ingestion and exertion that cause vasodilatation when upright [6, 31] that should be exploited during diagnostic investigations.

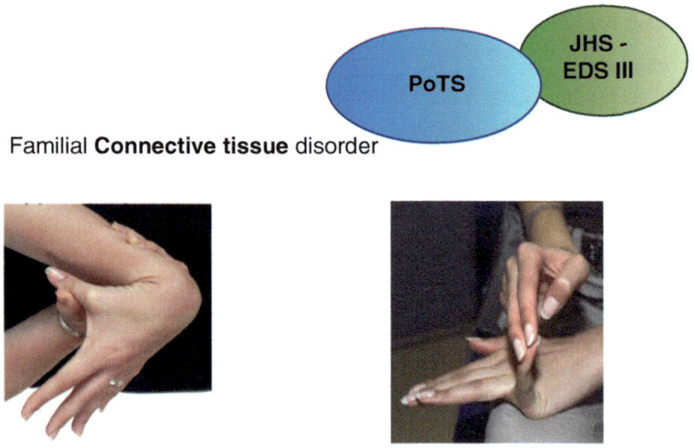

Fig. 20.6 Features of enhanced joint flexibility and hypermobility in Ehlers-Danlos syndrome (E-DS) III, now classified as the joint hypermobile form of E-DS (hE-DS)

Non-autonomic Investigations

This will depend upon the organ and system that need evaluation. They may include echocardiography or continuous 24-hour or longer periods of HR/ECG recordings, structural neuroimaging especially of the cranio-cervical junction to exclude a Chiari malformation such as that can occur in some with hE-DS, and neurophysiological studies to exclude a small fibre neuropathy. Specific testing of urinary bladder, gastrointestinal and pelvic function and anatomy also may be needed.

Pathophysiology

A number of possibilities, many of which are based on associations, as in Fig. 20.7, have been postulated. They include neural and vascular mechanisms, among others. The association with hE-DS, and in some the prominence of peripheral vascular pooling while upright (as seen in Fig. 20.3), may be a contributory factor in many. Diminished connective tissue between structures including blood vessels may be the underlying mechanism. This also may explain the worsening of features after food, exertion and heat that involve vascular regions such as the splanchnic, muscle and cutaneous beds. A number of other factors can worsen clinical features, including physical deconditioning. In some, a conditioned response causing anxiety should be considered [30].

Overlapping Features

Although PoTS is a syndrome with clearly defined features, there are a number of factors which may make the key clinical features (postural tachycardia, presyncope/syncope and fatigue) much worse. In some it can involve many systems, often with multiple comorbidities. This is especially so when associated with hE-DS, where urinary bladder features, GI dysfunction, and sudomotor abnormalities along with PoTS and fatigue occur. This now is considered under the term hypermobility spectrum disorder (HSD). Depending upon the features which are most troublesome, presentation may be to specialists in differing areas. Referral initially to an autonomic specialist is uncommon, as many in primary or even secondary care are often not aware or familiar with the complexities of this condition, and there are relatively few in the autonomic super-specialty. Patients may present to a

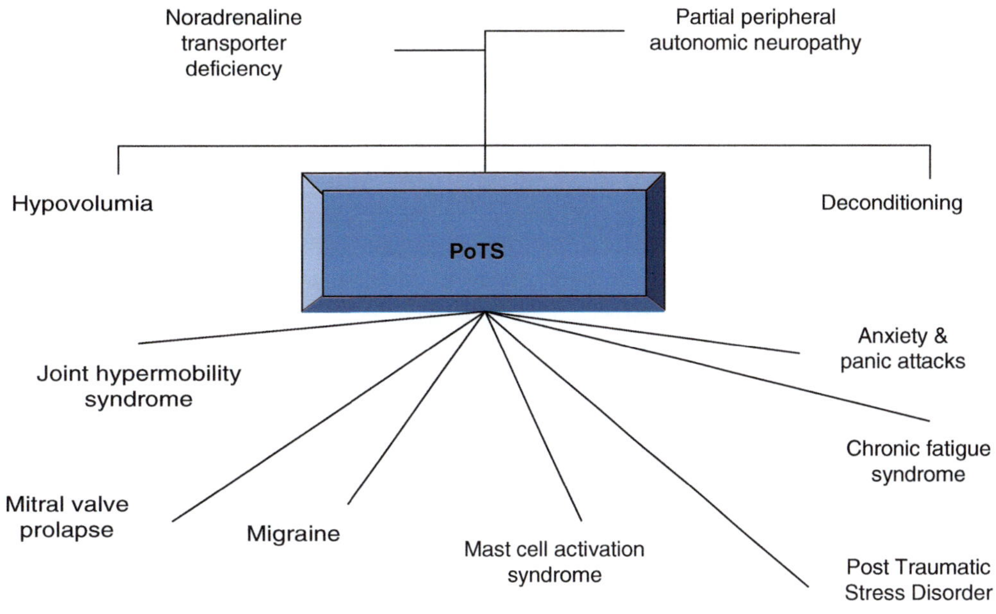

Fig. 20.7 Associations and possible causes postulated regarding the pathophysiology of PoTS. The most common association in our autonomic centres is the joint hypermobility syndrome, often with Ehlers-Danlos syndrome

variety of specialists – cardiologists because of tachycardia, neurologists because of the overlap with epilepsy, rheumatologists because of joint hypermobility and fibromyalgia, urologists because of recurrent UTIs, gastroenterologists because of a variety of GI disturbances and psychiatrists because of anxiety, among others. Overspecialisation in clinical medicine may have contributed to this issue. If autonomic testing is not carried out, patients can be diagnosed with a functional neurological disorder or with anxiety. This can result in a traumatic journey for such subjects, as the spectrum of physiological and psychological symptoms they experience is believed to be psychogenic until appropriate autonomic referral and testing is undertaken, and appropriate treatment for the physical aspects of the condition initiated.

Treatment

This should combine management of autonomic and also non-autonomic features. The latter, depending upon the specific features, often needs to be holistic and should include management of overlapping disorders. Autonomic measures are listed under non-pharmacological and pharmacological, with the first essential even if medication is to be used (Table 20.2). The choice of the initial drug, or drugs if used in combination ideally with differing mechanisms, will depend on the severity of the condition, the underlying pathophysiological basis and the initial response; hence, there is a need for prior investigation (Table 20.3). It is important that an associated disorder or condition is treated satisfactorily, as this may worsen PoTS features. An example is infection, which affects the urinary tract.

Table 20.2 Outline of key non-pharmacological measures

To be avoided
Sudden head-up postural change (especially on waking)
Prolonged recumbency
High environmental temperatures (including hot baths)
Large meals (especially of refined carbohydrate)
Alcohol
Undue exertion
Medication with vasodepressor properties
To be introduced
High salt intake
Water repletion (especially in the morning on wakening)
Small, frequent meals
Judicious regular exercise (including swimming)
Raising the head end of the bed at night
Physical manoeuvres to activate autonomic activity (such as sustained hand grip)
To be considered
Compression stockings and hosiery
Abdominal binders

Conclusion

PoTS is a condition characterised by orthostatic intolerance and tachycardia when upright. Underlying or associated disorders additionally need to be considered and addressed if contributory. The majority of patients with PoTS have no additional neurological features, but in some, such as those with a small fibre neuropathy or a Chiari malformation (albeit rare), this will need consideration. A number of patients with PoTS, especially with associated hE-DS, in addition to PoTS have other features of HSD, which include fatigue, urinary bladder, and GI dysfunction and in some,

Table 20.3 Pharmacological treatments for PoTS

Therapeutic strategy	Drug class or mechanism of action	Agent
Reducing salt loss and/ or aid plasma volume expansion	Mineralocorticoid	Fludrocortisone
Vasoconstriction	Sympathetic action on resistance vessels	Midodrine
Ganglionic nicotinic receptor stimulation	Anticholinesterase inhibitors	Pyridostigmine
Preventing vasodilation and tachycardia	β_2-Adrenoreceptor blockers, ideally cardioselective	Bisoprolol
Preventing postprandial tachycardia	Peptide release inhibitors Somatostatin analogues	Octreotide (short-acting)
Reducing tachycardia	Selective sinus node blockade	Ivabradine
Reducing raised blood pressure (if present)	Central sympatholytic	Clonidine

sudomotor abnormalities, each of which may need addressing. Many have had PoTS undiagnosed for years, often with psychological implications as a result, which will need further consideration. Thus, a holistic view to management is necessary in the majority with PoTS.

References

1. Rosen SG, Cryer PE. Postural tachycardia syndrome. Reversal of sympathetic hyperresponsiveness and clinical improvement during sodium loading. Am J Med. 1982;72(5):847–50.
2. Schondorf R, Low PA. Idiopathic postural orthostatic tachycardia syndrome: an attenuated form of acute pandysautonomia? Neurology. 1993;43(1):132–7.
3. Schondorf R, Benoit J, Wein T, Phaneuf D. Orthostatic intolerance in the chronic fatigue syndrome. J Auton Nerv Syst. 1999;75(2–3):192–201.
4. Da Costa JM. On irritable heart. A clinical study of a form of functional cardiac disorder and its consequences. Am J Med. 1951;11(5):559–67.
5. Lewis T. The soldier's heart and the effort syndrome. London: Shaw & Sons; 1918.
6. Mathias CJ, Low DA, Iodice V, Owens AP, Kirbis M, Grahame R. Postural tachycardia syndrome--current experience and concepts. Nat Rev Neurol. 2011;8(1):22–34.
7. Benarroch EE. Postural tachycardia syndrome: a heterogeneous and multifactorial disorder. Mayo Clin Proc. 2012;87(12):1214–25.
8. Esler M, Alvarenga M, Pier C, Richards J, El-Osta A, Barton D, et al. The neuronal noradrenaline transporter, anxiety and cardiovascular disease. J Psychopharmacol. 2006;20(4 Suppl):60–6.
9. Parsaik A, Allison TG, Singer W, Sletten DM, Joyner MJ, Benarroch EE, et al. Deconditioning in patients with orthostatic intolerance. Neurology. 2012;79(14):1435–9.
10. Ocon AJ, Medow MS, Taneja I, Clarke D, Stewart JM. Decreased upright cerebral blood flow and cerebral autoregulation in normocapnic postural tachycardia syndrome. Am J Physiol Heart Circ Physiol. 2009;297(2):H664–73.
11. Shaw BH, Stiles LE, Bourne K, Green EA, Shibao CA, Okamoto LE, et al. The face of postural tachycardia syndrome - insights from a large cross-sectional online community-based survey. J Intern Med. 2019;286(4):438–48.
12. Anderson JW, Lambert EA, Sari CI, Dawood T, Esler MD, Vaddadi G, Lambert GW. Cognitive function, health-related quality of life, and symptoms of depression and anxiety sensitivity are impaired in patients with the postural orthostatic tachycardia syndrome (POTS). Front Physiol. 2014;5:230. https://doi.org/10.3389/fphys.2014.00230.
13. Raj V, Haman KL, Raj SR, Byrne D, Blakely RD, Biaggioni I, et al. Psychiatric profile and attention deficits in postural tachycardia syndrome. J Neurol Neurosurg Psychiatry. 2009;80(3):339–44.
14. Bagai K, Song Y, Ling JF, Malow B, Black BK, Biaggioni I, et al. Sleep disturbances and diminished quality of life in postural tachycardia syndrome. J Clin Sleep Med. 2011;7(2):204–10.
15. Ocon AJ. Caught in the thickness of brain fog: exploring the cognitive symptoms of Chronic Fatigue Syndrome. Front Physiol. 2013;4:63. https://doi.org/10.3389/fphys.2013.00063.
16. Ross AJ, Medow MS, Rowe PC, Stewart JM. What is brain fog? An evaluation of the symptom in postural tachycardia syndrome. Clin Auton Res. 2013;23(6):305–11.
17. Lin J, Han Z, Li X, Ochs T, Zhao J, Zhang X, et al. Risk factors for postural tachycardia syndrome in children and adolescents. PLoS One. 2014;9(12):e113625.
18. Figueroa JJ, Bott-Kitslaar DM, Mercado JA, Basford JR, Sandroni P, Shen WK, et al. Decreased orthostatic adrenergic reactivity in non-dipping postural tachycardia syndrome. Auton Neurosci. 2014;185:107–11.
19. Mallien J, Isenmann S, Mrazek A, Haensch CA. Sleep disturbances and autonomic dysfunction in patients with postural orthostatic tachycardia syndrome. Front Neurol. 2014;5:118. https://doi.org/10.3389/fneur.2014.00118.
20. Pengo MF, Higgins S, Drakatos P, Martin K, Gall N, Rossi GP, Leschziner G. Characterisation of sleep disturbances in postural orthostatic tachycardia syndrome: a polysomnography-based study. Sleep Med. 2015;16(12):1457–61.
21. Miglis MG, Muppidi S, Feakins C, Fong L, Prieto T, Jaradeh S. Sleep disorders in patients with postural tachycardia syndrome. Clin Auton Res. 2016;26(1):67–73.
22. Bagai K, Peltier AC, Malow BA, Diedrich A, Shibao CA, Black BK, et al. Objective sleep assessments in patients with postural tachycardia syndrome using overnight polysomnograms. J Clin Sleep Med. 2016;12(5):727–33.
23. Guilleminault C, Primeau M, Chiu HY, Yuen KM, Leger D, Metlaine A. Sleep-disordered breathing in Ehlers-Danlos syndrome: a genetic model of OSA. Chest. 2013;144(5):1503–11.
24. Mathias CJ, Iodice V, Low DA, Bannister R. Investigation of autonomic disorders. In: Mathias CJ, Bannister R, editors. Autonomic failure: a textbook of clinical disorders of the autonomic nervous system. 5th ed. Oxford: Oxford University Press; 2013. p. 259–89.
25. Mathias CJ, Iodice I, Low DA, Galizia G. Orthostatic hypotension and orthostatic intolerance. In: Jameson JL, De Groot LJ, editors. Endocrinology adult and pediatric. 7th ed. Philadelphia: Elsevier Saunders; 2015. p. 1965–84.
26. Bulbena A, Pailhez G, Gago J. "Connective tissue" between panic disorder and dysautonomia. Am J Med. 2004;116(11):783; author reply 783–4.
27. Martín-Santos R, Bulbena A, Porta M, Gago J, Molina L, Duró JC. Association between joint hypermobility syndrome and panic disorder. Am J Psychiatry. 1998;155(11):1578–83.
28. Khurana RK. Experimental induction of panic-like symptoms in patients with postural tachycardia syndrome. Clin Auton Res. 2006;16(6):371–7.
29. Owens AP, Low DA, Iodice V, Critchley HD, Mathias CJ. The genesis and presentation of anxiety in disorders of autonomic overexcitation. Auton Neurosci. 2017;203:81–7.

30. Owens AP, Low DA, Critchley HD, Mathias CJ. Emotional orienting during interoceptive threat in orthostatic intolerance: Dysautonomic contributions to psychological symptomatology in the postural tachycardia syndrome and vasovagal syncope. Auton Neurosci. 2018;212:42–7.
31. Masuki S, Eisenach JH, Johnson CP, Dietz NM, Benrud-Larson LM, Schrage WG, et al. Excessive heart rate response to orthostatic stress in postural tachycardia syndrome is not caused by anxiety. J Appl Physiol (1985). 2007;102(3):896–903.
32. Benrud-Larson LM, Sandroni P, Haythornthwaite JA, Rummans TA, Low PA. Correlates of functional disability in patients with postural tachycardia syndrome: preliminary cross-sectional findings. Health Psychol. 2003;22(6):643–8.
33. Esler M, Alvarenga M, Lambert G, Kaye D, Hastings J, Jennings G, et al. Cardiac sympathetic nerve biology and brain monoamine turnover in panic disorder. Ann N Y Acad Sci. 2004;1018:505–14.

Congenital Central Hypoventilation Syndrome

21

Kevin S. Gipson and Christian Guilleminault

Introduction and History

Breathing is a rather unique function of the body. It is driven automatically by the respiratory centers of the central nervous system in response to physiologic and environmental perturbations but can come under volitional control when we choose to attend to it. Indeed, the conscious control of breathing is a critical aspect of speech, musicianship, exercise, and other important activities of daily life.

Congenital central hypoventilation syndrome (CCHS) is a disorder of abnormal ventilatory patterning and diffuse autonomic dysfunction associated with mutations of the gene *PHOX2B*.

Affected patients classically exhibit marked severe hypoventilation in sleep, with shallow and monotonous breathing patterns despite often markedly elevated arterial carbon dioxide ($PaCO_2$). Clinically, CCHS manifests across a spectrum of severity, but the commonest presentation is that of a newborn infant with marked hypoventilation and carbon dioxide retention in sleep, requiring long-term mechanical ventilation. These patients also commonly exhibit diffuse autonomic dysfunction, which can complicate their clinical courses and disrupt the quality of life (QOL) significantly.

CCHS was first reported in the modern medical literature by pioneering pediatric pulmonologist Robert Mellins and colleagues in 1970 [1]. At the time of this initial report, and until recently, CCHS was called by the evocative, if ill-fitting, name *Ondine's curse;* a term which had previously been used to describe patients with a loss of automatic breathing following brainstem injury. This name was used to convey, and perhaps dramatize, the loss of ventilatory automaticity seen in the classical presentations of CCHS. Of interest, though it is often presumed that the water nymph Ondine herself was the one to suffer the curse of loss of automatic respiration, or is perhaps the giver of the curse, this is a literary misconception. In the classical telling of the story, it is in fact Ondine's unfortunate lover, Hans, who is cursed by the king of the sea to this fate. In one particularly poignant passage in a 1938 interpretation of the story by Jean Giradoux, Hans describes the loss of all automatic function: "I don't see unless I tell my eyes to see… A moment of inattention and I forget to hear, to breathe…" [2, 3].

CCHS is a spectrum disorder, with severity of clinical presentation informed by the underlying *PHOX2B* mutation; however, in virtually no cases do affected patients "forget to breathe." Rather, CCHS is classically characterized as hypoventilation during sleep which is unresponsive to progressive hypercapnia. The most dramatic presentations of CCHS involve neonates who progress to respiratory insufficiency and failure shortly after birth, requiring mechanical ventilation; however, in some cases the signs of CCHS do not manifest until later in childhood or even adolescence and adulthood. With modern methods of early diagnosis and management, these patients can live long, happy, and productive lives.

Epidemiology and Genetics

CCHS is a rare disease, though there are now more than 1000 known cases associated with confirmed *PHOX2B* mutation. It is difficult to characterize the true incidence and prevalence of CCHS given limited and relatively homogenous population studies. However, current best data and expert opinion suggest an estimated incidence of approximately 1 in 148,000–200,000 births, without clear gender bias [4, 5]. Inheritance follows a predominantly autosomal dominant mode, with variable penetrance [6].

Dr. Christian Guilleminault died on 9 July 2019.

K. S. Gipson (✉)
Division of Pediatric Pulmonology and Sleep Medicine, Department of Pediatrics, Massachusetts General Hospital, Harvard Medical School, Boston, MA, USA
e-mail: kgipson@mgh.harvard.edu

C. Guilleminault (Deceased)
Stanford Sleep Medicine Center, Psychiatry and Behavioral Sciences, Stanford University, Stanford, CA, USA

S. Chokroverty, P. Cortelli (eds.), *Autonomic Nervous System and Sleep*, https://doi.org/10.1007/978-3-030-62263-3_21

Mutations of *PHOX2B* are the only known cause of CCHS, and the identification of a *PHOX2B* mutation is now considered requisite to the diagnosis of this disorder. Mutation of *PHOX2B* was first implicated in the pathogenesis of CCHS by Jeanne Amiel and her colleagues in 2003 [7]. Later, it was learned that CCHS may be caused by both polyalanine repeat mutations (PARM) of a 20-alanine repeat in exon 3 of chromosome 4p13, or by non-polyalanine repeats mutations (NPARM) which yield frameshift, missense, and nonsense mutations. PARMs reflect the majority of these mutations and are found in approximately 90% of affected patients, while NPARMs are implicated in the remaining 10% of cases [8]. As an example, a patient with two normal copies of *PHOX2B* is notated as a 20/20 genotype, and a patient with a PARM mutation of one copy of *PHOX2B* which resulted in an expansion to 26 alanines is notated as 20/26.

Genotype–Phenotype Relationship

CCHS presents with a spectrum of severity in both ventilatory and autonomic disease, and this clinical heterogeneity is determined by current understanding of the underlying *PHOX2B* mutations involved. In cases of CCHS due to PARMs, the length of the polyalanine repeat segment is correlated with the severity of the ventilatory needs and dysautonomia. For example, patients with the relatively constrained 20/25 mutation may only require ventilation at night, whereas patients with the longer 20/27 to 20/33 polyalanine repeats universally require round-the-clock invasive ventilation [8]. Patients with an NPARM mutation generally have more severe clinical presentations, with a high incidence of non-pulmonary autonomic comorbidity, and increased risk of rarer complications of *PHOX2B* mutation including Hirschsprung disease and neural crest tumors.

Clinical Manifestations and Natural History

Hypoventilation and Central Apnea in CCHS

CCHS classically presents in the newborn period, with monotonous breathing and insufficient tidal volumes leading to severe alveolar hypoventilation during sleep and, in particularly severe cases, impacted ventilation during wakefulness. Affected newborns may exhibit shallow breathing of a monotonous pattern, hypoxemia, and even cyanosis, often prompting transfer to a neonatal intensive care unit, intubation, and mechanical ventilation. Initial laboratory evaluation may reveal hypercapnia. A hallmark of CCHS is a relatively insensate response to hypercapnia and hypoxemia, and notably these neonates will frequently not exhibit any overt respiratory distress (i.e., no retractions or increased work of breathing) despite often marked hypoxemia and hypercarbia. In the most severe cases, patients may require 24/7 ventilatory support.

Many patients with CCHS can have normal and effective ventilation during wakefulness, including a relatively preserved response to exercise. A notable exception may be swimming, where the absence of normal perceptions of dyspnea may result in patients holding their breath for extended periods of time [6].

Although hypoventilation is present during all phases of sleep in CCHS patients, the relative magnitude of the ventilatory defect is state-dependent and hypoventilation is most pronounced during non-rapid eye movement (NREM) sleep [8]. Transition to sleep is a period of particular vulnerability for patients, and some vigilance is needed by parents to ensure appropriate transitions to ventilator support during sleep.

Dysautonomia in CCHS

Patients with *PHOX2B* mutation may exhibit dysautonomia of varying severity across several organ systems (Table 21.1). This dysautonomia includes both parasympathetic and sympathetic dysregulation. Notably, the cardiovascular system is frequently involved, with patients exhibiting arrhythmias (including periodic asystole in some cases) and dysregulation of blood pressure and cerebral perfusion. In cases of PARM mutation, there is a known correlation between higher-order polyalanine repeats and increased R–R interval. Children with genotypes of 20/26 and beyond may exhibit sinus pauses of 3 seconds or longer and may benefit from

Table 21.1 Features of dysautonomia associated with *PHOX2B* mutation

Respiratory	Alveolar hypoventilation Central apnea Severe breath-holding spells Absence of dyspnea or breathlessness
Cardiovascular	Decreased heart rate variability Bradyarrhythmia Sinus pauses and transient asystole Abnormal circadian modulation of blood pressure Syncope with straining effort Sudden cardiac death
Gastrointestinal	Lower esophageal dysmotility Gut dysmotility Hirschsprung disease
Ophthalmologic	Abnormal pupillary reflex and accommodation Visual acuity problems
Endocrine	Hypoglycemia
Exocrine	Sudomotor dysfunction of the sweat glands Poor heat tolerance

cardiac pacemaker implantation, and all CCHS patients will need annual cardiac screening for dysrhythmias. There are, sadly, reports of sudden cardiac death in children with CCHS. While not a pure manifestation of cardiovascular dysautonomia, children with CCHS are at particular risk for pulmonary hypertension and even cor pulmonale as a consequence of intermittent hypoxemia (although pulmonary vascular tone alteration may be multifactorial in etiology).

Aside from the relatively common cardiorespiratory sequel of CCHS, patients with CCHS are susceptible to a broad array of often subtle autonomic dysregulation. In the case of PARM mutations, the severity and the number of autonomic symptoms experienced are positively associated with the number of alanine residues [9]. Hirschsprung disease, a disorder of peristalsis in the gut, is commonly observed in cases of CCHS. Hirschsprung disease is seen in 20% of CCHS cases, but is more common in those patients with NPARM mutations, with a prevalence of 87–100% in cases of NPARM CCHS. In the literature, the co-occurrence of CCHS and Hirschsprung disease is often referred to as Haddad syndrome. Other manifestations of gastrointestinal (GI) dysmotility may be seen in CCHS, including esophageal and gut issues. Patients with CCHS have been shown to have ophthalmologic findings such as dysfunction of pupillary accommodation [10]. Affected patients may also exhibit abnormal sweating and temperature regulation.

Neurocristopathy in CCHS

PHOX2B is implicated in normal neural crest cell migration, and one critical consideration for young patients with CCHS is the development of neural crest tumors (NCT), most commonly congenital neuroblastoma, ganglioneuroblastoma, and benign ganglioneuroma. Patients with NPARM are particularly at risk with a 50% lifetime incidence of NCT [8]. These NCTs may manifest in subtle ways, including failure to thrive, abdominal pain, and fatigue, among others, and so vigilance is warranted.

Late-Onset Congenital Central Hypoventilation Syndrome

Cases of CCHS, which emerge after the newborn period are considered "late" onset. Commonly, these patients are identified after disproportionate ventilatory impairment with incidental respiratory illnesses of childhood or with anesthesia. Late-onset congenital central hypoventilation syndrome (LO-CCHS) is generally seen in the more constrained 20/24 and 20/25 PARM genotypes, though NPARM LO-CCHS has been reported.

Other Genetic Hypoventilation Syndromes Associated with Autonomic Dysfunction

Rapid-onset obesity with hypothalamic dysfunction, hypoventilation, and autonomic dysregulation (ROHHAD) bears mention in the discussion of central hypoventilation and dysautonomia. The genetic etiology of this disorder is not yet fully characterized; however, it does not involve *PHOX2B*. These patients experience a dramatic weight gain accompanied by the onset of mixed central and obstructive nocturnal hypoventilation, usually between the ages of 1.5- and 7-years old. These patients frequently have cardiac dysautonomia, and cardiac arrest is strikingly prevalent in this population. These children benefit from either nasal intermittent positive pressure ventilation (NIPPV) or tracheostomy with mechanical ventilation.

Certain forms of congenital hypoventilation with attendant dysautonomia may be seen in patients with Rhett syndrome, related to *MECP2* gene mutation, and in Prader–Willi syndrome.

Sudden Infant Death Syndrome

Sudden infant death syndrome (SIDS), a major cause of infant mortality, is thought to be related in part to dysregulation or dysmaturity of autonomic control. While SIDS is more common in the families of patients with CCHS, large case studies have not identified *PHOX2B* mutations as causative in the vast majority of SIDS.

Hypothesized Pathophysiology of *PHOX2B* Mutation

PHOX2B is a paired-like homeobox gene that codes for a homeodomain transcription factor involved in the embryonic differentiation of central and peripheral autonomic neurons in a broad array of systems, including respiratory nuclei involved in normal ventilatory patterning and chemosensory integration [6]. As a consequence, the deleterious mutation of this gene could be expected to manifest in diffuse autonomic dysfunction and respiratory dysregulation. Polyalanine (PA) tracts are found throughout the human proteome and are most commonly found in transcription factors where they are thought to impart the flexibility needed for conformational changes associated with the function of these proteins. There is evidence that PARMs disrupt the transcriptional regulation of several proteins involved in ANS development. PARMs may yield aberrant proteins, which exert either a dominant-negative or toxic gain-of-function effects [11]. Further, polyalanine repeats function as nuclear export signals, and PHOX2B aggregation and mislocalization have been reported in the context of PARMs, and could contribute to a cytotoxic effect to these mutations [12]. PARMs are associated with at least nine heritable human diseases (one notable human disease which shares this pathogenesis is oculopharyngeal muscular dystrophy), and in most cases, disease is related to the resultant dysfunction in transcription factors. The putative mechanism of PARM in CCHS is an unequal crossover between mispaired normal alleles [13]. NPARMs have experimentally demonstrated compromised transcriptional activity. NPARMs may result in dominant-negative, loss-of-function, and gain-of-function effects depending on the resultant reading frame [14].

PHOX2B is notably expressed in the retrotrapezoid nucleus (RTN) of the brainstem, a site involved in the central chemoreception of carbon dioxide (CO_2) via a pH-sensitive G-protein-coupled receptor and a hypothesized driver of the breathing pattern generators [6, 15]. Broadly, ventilation is driven by central chemoreceptor detection of $CO_2/H+$ and peripheral chemosensory response to hypoxemia, and in the normal state elevations of CO_2 drive an increase in minute ventilation. One leading theory for the pathogenesis of the ventilatory defect in CCHS is a disruption of central chemosensory integration at the RTN [6]. Presently, immunohistochemical studies locate the RTN between the seventh cranial nerve and the superior olivary nuclear complex, but this is not definitive [6]. A broad array of research into this nucleus, including *in vivo* lesion/stimulation experiments, suggests strongly that hypercapnia activates RTN cells, controlling the rate and depth of breathing [6]. RTN neurons both intrinsically sense pH changes and serve an integratory role, synthesizing inputs from peripheral chemoreceptors and central generators of respiratory drive [16]. Additionally, recent transgenic mouse work suggests that the hallmark loss of the adaptive ventilatory response to hypercapnia may be related to loss of PHOX2B-expressing neurons in the nucleus tractus solitarius, a center of integration of myriad autonomic and chemoreceptor inputs in humans including the carotid and aortic bodies, and other baroreceptor and chemoreceptor signals [17].

It is noteworthy that adult patients with CCHS exhibit respiratory-related motor cortical activity while awake, a finding not seen in normal controls, and this could imply a synergistic waking cortical mechanism that compensates for the insufficient medullary generation of automatic ventilatory drive in CCHS [18, 19]. Movement of the limbs has been shown to improve ventilatory drive during wakefulness and sleep [20].

Imaging studies have shed some light on the potential pathogenesis of ventilatory and autonomic dysfunction in CCHS. Specifically, structural injury has been observed across several centers of autonomic and ventilatory integration and regulation, including the thalamus, hypothalamus, midbrain, medulla, locus coeruleus (LC) in the pons, the nucleus of the solitary tract in the medulla, and others [21]. Additionally, there is evidence of progressive neural tissue/axonal damage over time, presumably due to intermittent hypoxemia related to the ventilatory defect and perhaps hypoperfusion and other physiologic changes secondary to dysautonomia. Of note, evidence of damage to the insula, cerebellum, and cingulate suggests a mechanism for the attenuation of breathlessness or dyspnea which may be seen in CCHS patients. However, these studies are limited by small sample size, heterogeneity of clinical severity, and practical limitations of achieving quality MRI in very young children without sedation [21]. Postmortem histopathological study of two neonatal patients with confirmed *PHOX2B* mutation, one PARM and one NPARM, suggested an abnormality of the locus coeruleus (LC), and this observation was strengthened by subsequent work by Thiago Moriera and colleagues in a humanized NPARM mouse model. This is intriguing, given the importance of the LC in autonomic control [6].

Disordered Sleep and General Dysautonomia

One novel consideration is the possible bidirectional interplay of sleep disorder in CCHS with autonomic dysfunction. There is increasing appreciation of the deeply integral role of the autonomic nervous system (ANS) in the initiation and maintenance of sleep, and in the physiologic response to the disruption of sleep [22]. While suboptimal ventilation is perhaps likely to result in fewer respiratory arousals in the context of CCHS, chronic hypercapnia and hypoxemia could theoretically disrupt sleep architecture. The use of nocturnal ventilators has the potential to cause sleep disturbance (e.g., ventilator leak alarms and other monitors, non-invasive interfaces which may disrupt sleep secondary to comfort issues). It is plausible that the autonomic dysfunction observed in CCHS, while principally related to direct effects of *PHOX2B* mutation, may also be potentiated by autonomic dysfunction induced by suboptimally managed sleep-disordered breathing. One study of neurocognitively normal adults with CCHS on optimized home nocturnal ventilation (both invasive and non-invasive) demonstrated normal sleep efficiency and architecture when compared to matched healthy adult controls; however, this study did not monitor autonomic parameters during sleep [19].

Diagnosis

The 2010 American Thoracic Society (ATS) guidelines remain perhaps the best articulation to date of the standard of care in the diagnosis of CCHS and in longitudinal management, and surveillance. Since the gene was identified in 2003, genetic testing for *PHOX2B* is the gold-standard diagnostic test in cases of suspected CCHS. Screening is accomplished via targeted analysis for pathogenic variants and identifies approximately 95% of individuals with CCHS. Yet, in the case of high clinical suspicion despite a negative screening assay, definitive diagnosis with sequence analysis is warranted to detect variants that may be missed with targeted analysis. Presently, commercial labs offer *PHOX2B* mutation testing via full gene sequence PCR-based analysis; however, care must be used in selecting these tests as not all report the polyalanine repeat details, which are important in planning surveillance studies for neural crest tumors and other issues. These labs cite a "turn-around" time for results of as long as 4 weeks, and so other diagnostic pathways may be pursued while awaiting confirmatory results.

Polysomnography

When CCHS is suspected, clinical diagnosis is made on the basis of hypoventilation and a blunted ventilatory response to hypercapnia and hypoxemia. Current expert opinion advises attended polysomnography (PSG) at the time of initial genetic diagnosis, followed by re-evaluation every 6 months until age 6 or 7 years, at which time annual PSG with as-needed ventilator titration is reasonable if the patient is otherwise stable [8]. While the diagnosis of CCHS is not made purely via the PSG, such comprehensive physiological testing is central in understanding the specific ventilatory needs of a patient within a broad spectrum of clinical severity. Ventilatory challenge during PSG may be achieved by withdrawing mechanical ventilation during NREM sleep and monitoring for end-tidal CO_2 elevations above 55 Torr for greater than 5 minutes, or above 60 Torr [23]. In one study by Huang et al., a small cohort of children with CCHS did exhibit some arousal related to hypercapnia and hypoxemia during periods off of home mechanical ventilation, and a mean duration of central apneas of 25 ± 19 seconds was observed [24]. In this study, sleep was attended by a marked drop in minute ventilation, both in respiratory rate and tidal volume, and these changes were more pronounced in non-REM (NREM) sleep. Similarly, central apnea events were more common in NREM sleep than REM. This is counter to the usual stability of ventilatory patterns in NREM sleep in the normal subject, as normally chemical control of ventilation is at its highest level in NREM sleep.

ATS guidelines recommend an assessment of a patient's response to a ventilatory challenge. A hypercapnic challenge using carbogen, a relatively available gaseous mixture of 5% CO_2 and 95% O_2, is a relatively simple assay for the presence of a normal ventilatory response to increased alveolar carbon dioxide in the eucapnic patient. In this test, the clinician monitors for a normal increase of minute ventilation in response to elevated CO_2. This bedside test is not sufficient for the diagnosis or exclusion of CCHS and should be used only as an adjunctive test.

Other Diagnostic Considerations

When there is a concern for gastrointestinal dysmotility, or when the mutation type confers particular risk for GI involvement, patients should undergo a barium enema or manometry, and rectal biopsy to assess for aganglionic colon in Hirschsprung disease should be considered in patients with NPARM mutations. Surveillance for NCTs, including serial chest and abdominal imaging, is warranted particularly in those children with either NPARM or a PARM 20/29 to 20/33 genotype [8].

Differential Diagnosis

Concurrent with genetic diagnosis, screening for other more common causes of ventilatory defects or comorbid disease should be pursued. For the critically ill neonate presenting with apnea or respiratory insufficiency, sepsis, pulmonary infections, congenital heart disease, and neurologic problems including neuromuscular disease must be quickly excluded from the differential diagnosis. ATS guidelines suggest consideration of chest imaging, comprehensive neurological and metabolic evaluation with a possible muscle biopsy, and echocardiogram during the initial diagnostic process. MRI of the brain and brainstem is warranted to rule out malformations or lesions of the centers of respiration.

Once a diagnosis of clinical CCHS and *PHOX2B* mutation is secured, the ATS expert panel suggests twice annual, then annual inpatient evaluations including characterization of ventilatory sufficiency during both wake and sleep, and a comprehensive cardiac and autonomic screen.

Current Management Strategies

The ATS expert panel on CCHS strongly suggests that affected patients be managed by multi-disciplinary centers with the experience and resources to properly evaluate and care for patients with this exceedingly rare disorder. While the need for close ventilatory management is broadly understood in the pediatric pulmonary community, the autonomic sequel of CCHS is not as fully appreciated and adequate autonomic surveillance and management is not within the purview of most of these clinicians. In practice, a hybrid approach with annual follow-up at a multi-disciplinary center and closer follow-up locally with appropriate subspecialists is appropriate [8].

Ventilatory Management

Ventilatory support is tailored to a given patient's clinical severity and is guided by annual inpatient observation and formal PSG. Many patients only require ventilation during sleep, including naps, and this may be achieved non-invasively in select older patients. Patients with extended polyalanine repeat PARM mutations or with NPARM mutations will often require 24/7 mechanical ventilation. When the genetic diagnosis is made early, tracheostomy before 1 month of age is advised to facilitate early and safe ventilatory support [8].

Pressure ventilation, a type of ventilator mode which prioritizes the delivery of a desired peak inspiratory pressure with each breath, with a back-up rate, is the recommended ventilator strategy for most CCHS patients. However, the effectiveness of any empiric ventilatory strategy must be assessed and settings iterated upon during clinical follow-ups and particularly during the annual inpatient re-evaluations. The ventilatory disorder in CCHS does not resolve spontaneously, nor is it thought to improve to any meaningful degree with age. As a consequence, ventilator settings are geared toward fully supporting a patient's ventilatory needs and weaning from the ventilator is not a usual therapeutic goal.

The ATS expert panel strongly advocates for tracheostomy with mechanical ventilation in infants and young children with CCHS, citing the importance of a secure airway and noting that non-invasive mask ventilation has the potential for displacement. However, while tracheostomy provides a relatively secure definitive airway for the infant and young child with CCHS, a tracheostomy can be complicated by airway infection and can potentially disrupt normal early childhood development (for example, speech and swallowing impairments). As such, it is reasonable to consider the transition to non-invasive ventilation via a nasal mask or pillow interface in older children (of around 7 years of age) who do not require daytime ventilation, particularly when social and family context is stable and supportive [25]. Use of mask ventilation itself has trade-offs: the interface can be uncomfortable and prone to leak or displacement. Additionally, long-term use of nasal masks in children has been associated with the development of iatrogenic mid-facial hypoplasia [26]. Treatment with supplemental oxygen alone is not sufficient, as it has little to no efficacy in alleviating hypercapnia and so will not prevent the development of pulmonary hypertension. Patients should be monitored with continuous nocturnal pulse oximetry and end-tidal CO_2. Commercially available apnea/bradycardia monitors, which work through transthoracic impedance monitoring, are not suitable for use in CCHS, as they are insufficiently sensitive to detect the hypoventilation observed in most patients.

There are several practical considerations important to successful and safe home ventilation, including the family's access to spare tracheostomy tubes, emergency back-up power (including batteries, generator, and priority status with their power company), and, when possible, a second ventilator to avoid emergency admission for ventilator malfunction. Prior to transition to college or other independent-living situations, patients must be capable of responding to high-leak alarms and other typical device management issues.

Other Ventilatory Options

Diaphragmatic pacing is a potentially effective tool in the management of CCHS and works by stimulating the patient's diaphragm via electrical pulses at the phrenic nerve bilaterally. Phrenic nerve pacing is effective in permitting children a greater freedom of movement during daytime activities, and has been successfully used in this population for children as young as 9 months of age [27]. In select cases, diaphragmatic pacing may permit discontinuation of nightly ventilatory use; however, careful screening to rule out upper airway obstruction and ongoing continuous pulse oximetry and CO_2 monitoring is critical. Generally, concurrent use of phrenic nerve pacing and cardiac pacing is possible in patients with both ventilatory defects and cardiac dysrhythmia, though the involvement of a cardiac electrophysiologist is recommended [28, 29]. Negative pressure ventilation, usually via a Cuirass-style device, is another viable option in the select patient with no comorbid upper airway obstruction. However, comfort and portability issues may complicate the use of these types of devices. Patients with CCHS do not respond to respiratory stimulant pharmacotherapy.

Management of Autonomic Nervous System Dysfunction

Autonomic nervous system dysfunction (ANSD) in CCHS outside of the hallmark ventilatory defect is common but broadly under-appreciated. ANSD can have marked quality of life and health impacts in this population and must be monitored closely during annual screening and with intercurrent illnesses. Comprehensive annual autonomic evaluation is therefore an important goal of longitudinal management. Optimally, this could include measures of autonomic function including tilt-table testing, controlled deep breathing, forced expiratory effort, and measurement of sudomotor function. Critically, children should receive annual cardiovascular screening including EKG and echocardiogram. Children with significant dysrhythmia should be considered for cardiac pacemakers, as the risk of sudden cardiac death is real in this population. Given the common pupillary dysfunction seen in CCHS, annual ophthalmologic follow-up including pupillometry is appropriate to ensure that any visual defects may be corrected.

Endocrine dysfunction including hypoglycemia has been observed in CCHS, and may be related to some combination of dysfunction of the carotid bodies (which participate in glucose-sensing through specialized cells), pancreatic islet dysfunction related to PHOX2B-dependent neural crest cells and potentially insulin hypersecretion, and may respond to diazoxide in one case report [30]. Temperature regulation is often abnormal in these patients, further complicating the response to febrile illness.

Other Management Considerations

Children with CCHS may exhibit learning disabilities. Measures of neurocognitive function may be reduced in children as young as preschool-age, and older children may have problems with working memory function and other cognitive issues [31, 32]. It is not clear if these learning issues are exclusively related to long-term intermittent hypoxemia, or perhaps also related to ventilatory loading or some other less overt intrinsic effect of *PHOX2B* mutation [33]. Annual neurocognitive testing is recommended to identify these often subtle issues in order to facilitate early intervention [34]. In addition to minimizing hypercapnia and hypoxemia, early intervention with developmental and educational surveillance and support is critical to ensuring optimal neurocognitive outcomes in these patients. As patients transition to adulthood, needs, and abilities, such as the ability to independently wake and respond to ventilator alarms, should be assessed.

Regarding exercise, CCHS patients should generally avoid vigorous or competitive swimming, even in the absence of tracheostomy, as these patients are relatively insensate to hypoxemia and so are at increased risk of drowning. More broadly, some patients will exhibit maladaptive temperature regulation, and so should take caution against overheating when playing.

Patients with CCHS may experience difficulties extubating after anesthetized procedures, and occasionally postoperative respiratory complications are a heralding sign in undiagnosed LO-CCHS [35]. When a patient is known to have CCHS, perioperative management planning and anticipation of these issues is crucial to ensuring good outcomes following invasive procedures including phrenic nerve stimulator placement. While not applicable to every anesthesia event, anesthesiologists and surgeons should consider the feasibility of regional anesthesia, the use of short-acting anesthetic agents, and avoidance of neuromuscular blocking agents during intubation [36].

In concert with direct patient care and support initiatives, the families of affected infants and children need and deserve support. It is important to be mindful of the significant stressor that chronic ventilatory disease and its attendant management may have on families. Studies of CCHS families have found worsened sleep quality and daytime function, and increased metrics of depression in the parents of affected children [37]. At minimum, these families should be directed early on to the CCHS Network family support group to connect with other families affected by this rare disease. The parents should undergo genetic counseling and subsequent testing, which may then inform family planning and drive further testing in siblings. Any identified asymptomatic carriers of the *PHOX2B* gene mutation may benefit from periodic evaluation for nocturnal hypoventilation and cardiac dysrhythmias.

Management Considerations in a Thriving CCHS Cohort

As early detection and management of CCHS have improved, children are experiencing improved health and neurocognitive outcomes, and the expected lifespan is now well into adulthood for most patients. Adult CCHS patients are themselves now having children, and it bears noting that CCHS patients have a 50% chance of passing on the *PHOX2B* mutation to their children. Polyalanine repeat mutations are relatively stable, and so the anticipation is not seen clinically. Optimally, adult patients are supported with pre-conception genetic counseling to guide reproductive decision-making, and post-conception genetic testing of the fetus to anticipate ventilatory needs for the neonate. Pregnant women with CCHS may need optimization of ventilatory support, as mechanical loading from the fetus and distention of the uterus can impair ventilation. Adolescent and adult patients should be counseled strongly about the use of alcohol and other respiratory depressants, as unfortunately there are case reports of coma and death related to alcohol ingestion in young adults with CCHS. Similar to patients with other chronic illnesses, patients with CCHS have a relatively high prevalence of anxiety and depression; and should be screened and treated for these issues.

Annual Surveillance in CCHS

The ATS expert panel outlines a clinically ambitious but appropriate plan for annual follow-up for all children with CCHS, and *the sleep physician with autonomic expertise plays a central role in the successful longitudinal evaluation of these patients.* Specifically, the ATS recommends twice annual and then annual inpatient physiologic monitoring with continuous audio–visual surveillance and recording of respiratory inductance plethysmography, ECG, pulse waveform, end-tidal CO_2, sleep staging, and temperature. Thus, PSG with adjunctive autonomic testing is the *de facto* core of this evaluation. Annual monitoring for cardiac arrhythmia and pulmonary hypertension in critical, and facilitates early interventions including cardiac pacemaker. This includes laboratory testing to rule out polycythemia and compensated chronic hypoventilation. Patients may benefit from annual ophthalmologic evaluation given the accommodative pupillary defect. In those patients with severe PARM or with NPARM mutations, chest and abdominal imaging to surveil for neural crest tumors is warranted. Barium enema or manometry may be warranted in cases of dysmotility.

Outcomes

While there is no cure for CCHS to date, timely intervention on the primary ventilatory defect, awareness and management of potentially serious autonomic comorbidities, and expert follow-up in an experienced pediatric center can prevent the most dreaded complications of this disease and ensure optimal survival and quality of life for these patients.

Future Directions in Research and Therapeutics

The study of CCHS and *PHOX2B* mutation has yielded important insight into the molecular basis and neuroanatomy of the ANS and into the neural control of ventilation. Future research will continue to characterize these complex systems, and to disentangle the congenital impact of *PHOX2B* mutation on the ANS from any ongoing effects. These mutations may have on physiologic ANS functions. Ongoing advancements in mechanical ventilation, including more sophisticated ventilatory algorithms, more sensitive home monitoring, and cloud-based management will continue to improve patient cardiopulmonary outcomes and comfort, as will the advancement of non-invasive ventilatory technologies. As CCHS is likely a principally developmental disorder, the efficacy of gene-editing technologies including CRISPR Cas-9 may be limited in their ability to modulate the ventilatory and autonomic defects seen postnatally, though it is conceivable that prenatal genetic interventions may be feasible one day. Pharmacotherapy trials are few, but one animal study suggested that the hormone desogestrel could improve resting ventilation in CCHS patients by increasing baseline respiratory frequency [38]. At the time of this writing, clinicaltrials.gov lists one ongoing international registry of CCHS patients, which is estimated to complete in 2021. Such a registry of *PHOX2B* mutations and data on clinical outcomes will be helpful in guiding future clinical research.

Conclusions

CCHS is a rare but clinically impactful disorder of ventilation and autonomic function caused by mutation of the gene *PHOX2B,* a transcription factor that is critical in the development of the ANS. The sleep clinician with autonomic expertise plays a central role in the diagnosis and management of patients with CCHS, and early intervention and effective longitudinal management of these patients have the potential to dramatically improve health and neurocognitive/functional outcomes, and to promote longevity and good quality of life.

References

1. Mellins RB, Balfour HH Jr, Turino GM, Winters RW. Failure of automatic control of ventilation (Ondine's curse). Report of an infant born with this syndrome and review of the literature. Medicine (Baltimore). 1970;49(6):487–504.
2. Severinghaus J. Ondine's curse: failure of respiratory center automaticity while awake. Clin Res. 1962;10:122.
3. Goldblatt D. Undine's course. Semin Neurol. 1995;15(2):218–23.
4. Trang H, Dehan M, Beaufils F, Zaccaria I, Amiel J, Gaultier C, et al. The French congenital central hypoventilation syndrome registry. Chest. 2005;127(1):72–9.
5. Shimokaze T, Sasaki A, Meguro T, Hasegawa H, Hiraku Y, Yoshikawa T, et al. Genotype–phenotype relationship in Japanese patients with congenital central hypoventilation syndrome. J Hum Genet. 2015;60(9):473–7.
6. Moreira TS, Takakura AC, Czeisler C, Otero JJ. Respiratory and autonomic dysfunction in congenital central hypoventilation syndrome. J Neurophysiol. 2016;116(2):742–52.
7. Amiel J, Laudier B, Attié-Bitach T, Trang H, de Pontual L, Gener B, et al. Polyalanine expansion and frameshift mutations of the paired-like homeobox gene PHOX2B in congenital central hypoventilation syndrome. Nat Genet. 2003;33(4):459–61.
8. Weese-Mayer DE, Berry-Kravis EM, Ceccherini I, Keens TG, Loghmanee DA, Trang H. An official ATS clinical policy statement: congenital central hypoventilation syndrome: genetic basis, diagnosis, and management. Am J Respir Crit Care Med. 2010;181(6):626–44.
9. Patwari PP, Loghmanee DA, Rand CM, Koliboski CM, Berry-Kravis EM, Weese-Mayer DE. Paired-like homeobox 2B (PHOX2B) gene and autonomic nervous system dysregulation (ANSD): comprehensive genotype/phenotype correlation in cohort of 98 congenital central hypoventilation syndrome (CCHS) cases. American Thoracic Society conference. A49 sleep and control of breathing. Am J Respir Crit Care Med. 2009;179:A1745.
10. Patwari PP, Stewart TM, Rand CM, Carroll MS, Kuntz NL, Kenny AS, et al. Pupillometry in congenital central hypoventilation syndrome (CCHS): quantitative evidence of autonomic nervous system dysregulation. Pediatr Res. 2012;71(3):280–5.
11. Di Lascio S, Belperio D, Benfante R, Fornasari D. Alanine expansions associated with congenital central hypoventilation syndrome impair PHOX2B homeodomain-mediated dimerization and nuclear import. J Biol Chem. 2016;291(25):13375–93.
12. Li L, Ng NKL, Koon AC, Chan HY. Expanded polyalanine tracts function as nuclear export signals and promote protein mislocalization via eEF1A1 factor. J Biol Chem. 2017;292(14):5784–800.

13. Shoubridge C, Gecz J. Polyalanine tract disorders and neurocognitive phenotypes. In: Tandem repeat polymorphisms. New York: Springer; 2012. p. 185–203.
14. Di Lascio S, Benfante R, Di Zanni E, Cardani S, Adamo A, Fornasari D, et al. Structural and functional differences in PHOX2B frameshift mutations underlie isolated or syndromic congenital central hypoventilation syndrome. Hum Mutat. 2018;39(2):219–36.
15. Nattie E. Ondine undone. New Engl J Med. 2015;373(6):573–5.
16. Guyenet PG, Bayliss DA, Stornetta RL, Ludwig MG, Kumar NN, Shi Y, et al. Proton detection and breathing regulation by the retrotrapezoid nucleus. J Physiol. 2016;594(6):1529–51.
17. Fu C, Xue J, Wang R, Chen J, Ma L, Liu Y, et al. Chemosensitive Phox2b-expressing neurons are crucial for hypercapnic ventilatory response in the nucleus tractus solitarius. J Physiol. 2017;595(14):4973–89.
18. Tremoureux L, Raux M, Hudson AL, Ranohavimparany A, Straus C, Similowski T. Does the supplementary motor area keep patients with Ondine's curse syndrome breathing while awake? PLoS One. 2014;9(1):e84534.
19. Attali V, Straus C, Pottier M, Buzare M-A, Morélot-Panzini C, Arnulf I, et al. Normal sleep on mechanical ventilation in adult patients with congenital central alveolar hypoventilation (Ondine's curse syndrome). Orphanet J Rare Dis. 2017;12(1):18.
20. Gozal D, Simakajornboon N. Passive motion of the extremities modifies alveolar ventilation during sleep in patients with congenital central hypoventilation syndrome. Am J Respir Crit Care Med. 2000;162(5):1747–51.
21. Harper RM, Kumar R, Macey PM, Ogren JA, Richardson HL. Functional neuroanatomy and sleep-disordered breathing: implications for autonomic regulation. Anat Rec. 2012;295(9):1385–95.
22. Miglis MG. Autonomic dysfunction in primary sleep disorders. Sleep Med. 2016;19:40–9.
23. Wise MS, Nichols CD, Grigg-Damberger MM, Marcus CL, Witmans MB, Kirk VG, et al. Executive summary of respiratory indications for polysomnography in children: an evidence-based review. Sleep. 2011;34(3):389–98.
24. Huang J, Colrain IM, Panitch HB, Tapia IE, Schwartz MS, Samuel J, et al. Effect of sleep stage on breathing in children with central hypoventilation. J Appl Physiol. 2008;105(1):44–53.
25. Kam K, Bjornson C, Mitchell I. Congenital central hypoventilation syndrome; safety of early transition to non-invasive ventilation. Pediatr Pulmonol. 2014;49(4):410–3.
26. Li KK, Riley RW, Guilleminault C. An unreported risk in the use of home nasal continuous positive airway pressure and home nasal ventilation in children. Chest. 2000;117(3):916–8.
27. DiMarco AF. Diaphragm pacing. Clin Chest Med. 2018;39(2):459–71.
28. Movahed MR, Jalili M, Kiciman N. Cardiovascular abnormalities and arrhythmias in patients with Ondine's curse (congenital central hypoventilation) syndrome. Pacing Clin Electrophysiol. 2005;28(11):1226–30.
29. Kolb C, Eicken A, Zrenner B, Schmitt C. Cardiac pacing in a patient with diaphragm pacing for congenital central hypoventilation syndrome (Ondine's curse). J Cardiovasc Electrophysiol. 2006;17(7):789–91.
30. Marics G, Amiel J, Vatai B, Lódi C, Mikos B, Tóth-Heyn P. Autonomic dysfunction of glucose homoeostasis in congenital central hypoventilation syndrome. Acta Paediatr. 2013;102(4):e178–e80.
31. Charnay AJ, Antisdel-Lomaglio JE, Zelko FA, Rand CM, Le M, Gordon SC, et al. Congenital central hypoventilation syndrome: neurocognition already reduced in preschool-aged children. Chest. 2016;149(3):809–15.
32. Zelko FA, Stewart TM, Brogadir CD, Rand CM, Weese-Mayer DE. Congenital central hypoventilation syndrome: broader cognitive deficits revealed by parent controls. Pediatr Pulmonol. 2018;53(4):492–7.
33. Nierat M-C, Demiri S, Dupuis-Lozeron E, Allali G, Morélot-Panzini C, Similowski T, et al. When breathing interferes with cognition: experimental inspiratory loading alters timed up-and-go test in normal humans. PLoS One. 2016;11(3):e0151625.
34. Esteso Orduña B, Seijas Gómez R, García Esparza E, Briceño EM, Melero Llorente J, Fournier Del Castillo MC. Neuropsychological profile and social cognition in congenital central hypoventilation syndrome (CCHS): correlation with neuroimaging in a clinical case. J Clin Exp Neuropsychol. 2018;40(1):75–83.
35. Mahmoud M, Bryan Y, Gunter J, Kreeger RN, Sadhasivam S. Anesthetic implications of undiagnosed late onset central hypoventilation syndrome in a child: from elective tonsillectomy to tracheostomy. Pediatr Anesth. 2007;17(10):1001–5.
36. Niazi AU, Mocon A, Varadi RG, Chan VW, Okrainec A. Ondine's curse: anesthesia for laparoscopic implantation of a diaphragm pacing stimulation system. Can J Anesth. 2011;58(11):1034.
37. Paddeu EM, Giganti F, Piumelli R, De Masi S, Filippi L, Viggiano MP, et al. Sleeping problems in mothers and fathers of patients suffering from congenital central hypoventilation syndrome. Sleep Breath. 2015;19(3):1057–64.
38. Joubert F, Perrin-Terrin AS, Verkaeren E, Cardot P, Fiamma M-N, Frugière A, et al. Desogestrel enhances ventilation in ondine patients: animal data involving serotoninergic systems. Neuropharmacology. 2016;107:339–50.

Further Reading

Moreira TS, Takakura AC, Czeisler C, Otero JJ. Respiratory and autonomic dysfunction in congenital central hypoventilation syndrome. J Neurophysiol. 2016;116(2):742–52.

Weese-Mayer DE, Marazita ML, Rand CM, Berry-Kravis EM. Congenital central hypoventilation syndrome. In: Adam MP, Ardinger HH, Pagon RA, Wallace SE, Bean LJH, Stephens K, Amemiya A, editors. GeneReviews® [Internet]. Seattle: University of Washington, Seattle; 1993–2020. 28 Jan 2004. [Last update 30 Jan 2014].

Weese-Mayer DE, Berry-Kravis EM, Ceccherini I, Keens TG, Loghmanee DA, Trang H. An official ATS clinical policy statement: congenital central hypoventilation syndrome. Am J Respir Crit Care Med. 2010;181(6):626–44.

Autonomic Dysfunction in Parasomnias of REM Sleep

22

Jennifer Zitser and Mitchell G. Miglis

Introduction

The balance of the autonomic nervous system (ANS) during sleep is highly dependent on the stage of sleep. While non-rapid eye movement (NREM) sleep is a state of parasympathetic control and metabolic recovery, rapid eye movement (REM) sleep is a more active stage of sleep and a dynamic state of autonomic balance. Periodic surges in sympathetic activity during phasic REM can lead to variability in heart rate, blood pressure, and respiration, shifting the autonomic balance toward sympathetic dominance. The fluctuating activity of this stage of sleep was recognized early in the field of sleep research, prompting Michel Jouvet to propose the term "paradoxical sleep (PS)" in 1965, well before any human or animal studies objectively analyzed such autonomic activity during REM sleep.

The discovery of REM-sleep behavior disorder (RBD) in 1986 by Carlos Schenck and Mark Mahowald expanded the clinical realm of the REM parasomnias, and subsequent longitudinal studies by these researchers and other have documented a clear association between RBD and the neurodegenerative disorders of α[alpha]-synuclein (α[alpha]-syn) deposition, collectively termed the α[alpha]-synucleinopathies—namely Parkinson's disease (PD), multiple system atrophy (MSA), dementia with Lewy bodies (DLB), and pure autonomic failure (PAF)—conditions that are associated with a high rate of autonomic dysfunction [1]. Animal studies by Jouvet and others established the dorsal pons as the primary control center of REM sleep, an area of the brainstem closely situated to cell populations integral to autonomic control. Thus, it is not surprising that disorders of REM function are also associated with disorders of autonomic function, and vice versa. This chapter will cover the available literature to date on these associations, the relevant anatomy and physiology of REM sleep and the central autonomic network (CAN), as well as the type and severity of autonomic dysfunction in REM parasomnias.

Anatomy of REM Sleep and the Central Autonomic Network

REM sleep is one of the two states of human sleep, characterized by mixed-frequency electroencephalogram (EEG) activity, rapid eye movements, and active inhibition of motor neurons, leading to near complete skeletal muscle paralysis. Multiple neurotransmitter systems are responsible for muscle atonia during REM sleep [2, 3], including brainstem glycinergic and GABAergic premotor neurons that promote inhibition of spinal (except those responsible for eye movements) and cranial motor neurons [4]. The perilocus coeruleus alpha, located in the dorsal pons, exerts an excitatory influence on the medullary reticular formation through the lateral tegmentoreticular tract. These neuronal groups hyperpolarize spinal motor neurons through the ventrolateral reticulospinal tract, leading to muscle atonia (Fig. 22.1).

Much of the knowledge of REM sleep pathophysiology comes from lesion studies, many of which were performed by Jouvet and colleagues. All structural lesions identified to date have been localized to the dorsal midbrain, pons, or medulla [5]. Neuroimaging studies of at least 20 cases of RBD have shown that lesions within or near the mesencephalic and pontine tegmentum can produce dream-enacting behaviors with loss of REM atonia [6]. More

J. Zitser
Global Brain Health Institute, Department of Neurology & Neurological Sciences, University of California, San Francisco, San Francisco, CA, USA

Movement Disorders Unit, Department of Neurology, Tel-Aviv Sourasky Medical Center, Sackler Faculty of Medicine, Tel Aviv University, Tel Aviv, Israel

M. G. Miglis (✉)
Autonomic Division, Department of Neurology and Neurological Sciences; Sleep Medicine Division, Department of Psychiatry and Behavioral Sciences, Stanford University, Palo Alto, CA, USA
e-mail: mmiglis@stanford.edu

S. Chokroverty, P. Cortelli (eds.), *Autonomic Nervous System and Sleep*, https://doi.org/10.1007/978-3-030-62263-3_22

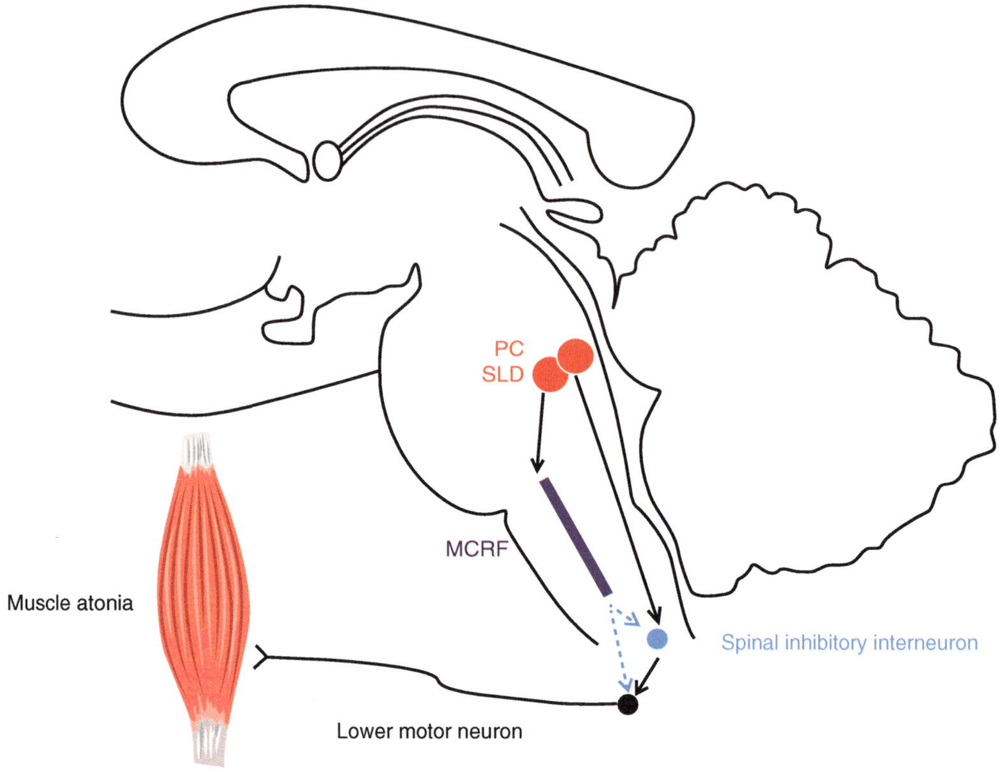

Fig. 22.1 Neuroanatomical structures involved in REM sleep (PC precoeruleus—studied in cats, SLD sublaterodorsal nucleus—studied in rats, MCRF magnocellularreticular formation)

recent neuroimaging of the voltage-gated potassium channel complex-associated RBD cases, however, have demonstrated abnormalities in the mesial temporal lobe structures and not exclusively in the brainstem [7]. These unique cases underscore the fact that while some of the networks and neurotransmitter systems involved in RBD remain unclear, most consistently relate to brainstem networks and their efferent or afferent connections.

Even though the relationship between REM parasomnias and autonomic impairment is likely anatomical, the exact pathways involved remains unclear. In addition to REM control networks, the brainstem contains much of the neural circuitry responsible for the control of nocturnal and diurnal autonomic function. The higher-order regulation system of the CAN consists of a group of interconnected areas distributed throughout the neuraxis and is involved in visceromotor, neuroendocrine, complex motor, and pain-modulating control mechanisms (Fig. 22.2) [2, 8–20]. The periaqueductal gray in the midbrain, the parabrachial nucleus of the pons and several regions in the medulla, including the dorsal motor nucleus of the vagus (DMV), the nucleus tractus solitarius (NTS), and the nucleus ambiguus, are critical components of the CAN [8]. It is significant that the CAN is state dependent, and certain pathways that are activated in the waking state are deactivated during sleep, and vice versa. The most illustrative condition of CAN and peripheral autonomic dysfunction in the REM parasomnias is RBD.

Rapid Eye Movement Sleep Behavior Disorder

RBD is a parasomnia characterized by loss of the normal skeletal muscle atonia that accompanies REM sleep. Consequently, patients may talk, gesture, punch, kick, or perform other complex motor behaviors in association with dream content [21]. RBD is common, affecting an estimated 1% of those over the age of 60 [22, 23]. In addition, over a third of patients may be unaware of their sleep behaviors, suggesting that the diagnosis may be detected secondarily when patients present with other sleep problems [24]. Much interest has arisen around the association between the α[alpha]-synucleinopathies and idiopathic RBD (iRBD), or clinically isolated RBD without signs of CNS neurodegeneration. Recent studies have documented that patients with iRBD are at substantial risk of developing a CNS α[alpha]-synucleinopathy within their lifetime, although time to phenoconversion is variable, spanning from years to decades. Most longitudinal studies of patients initially diagnosed with iRBD have demonstrated a phenoconversion rate of greater than 80%, approximately 6–10% per year from diagnosis, establishing iRBD as a clear and early marker of neurodegeneration [6, 25–28]. In a recent longitudinal, multicenter pooled cohort of 1280 patients with iRBD, the median time to phenoconversion was 8 years, with an overall phenoconversion rate of 6.25% per year. More specifically, the risk of

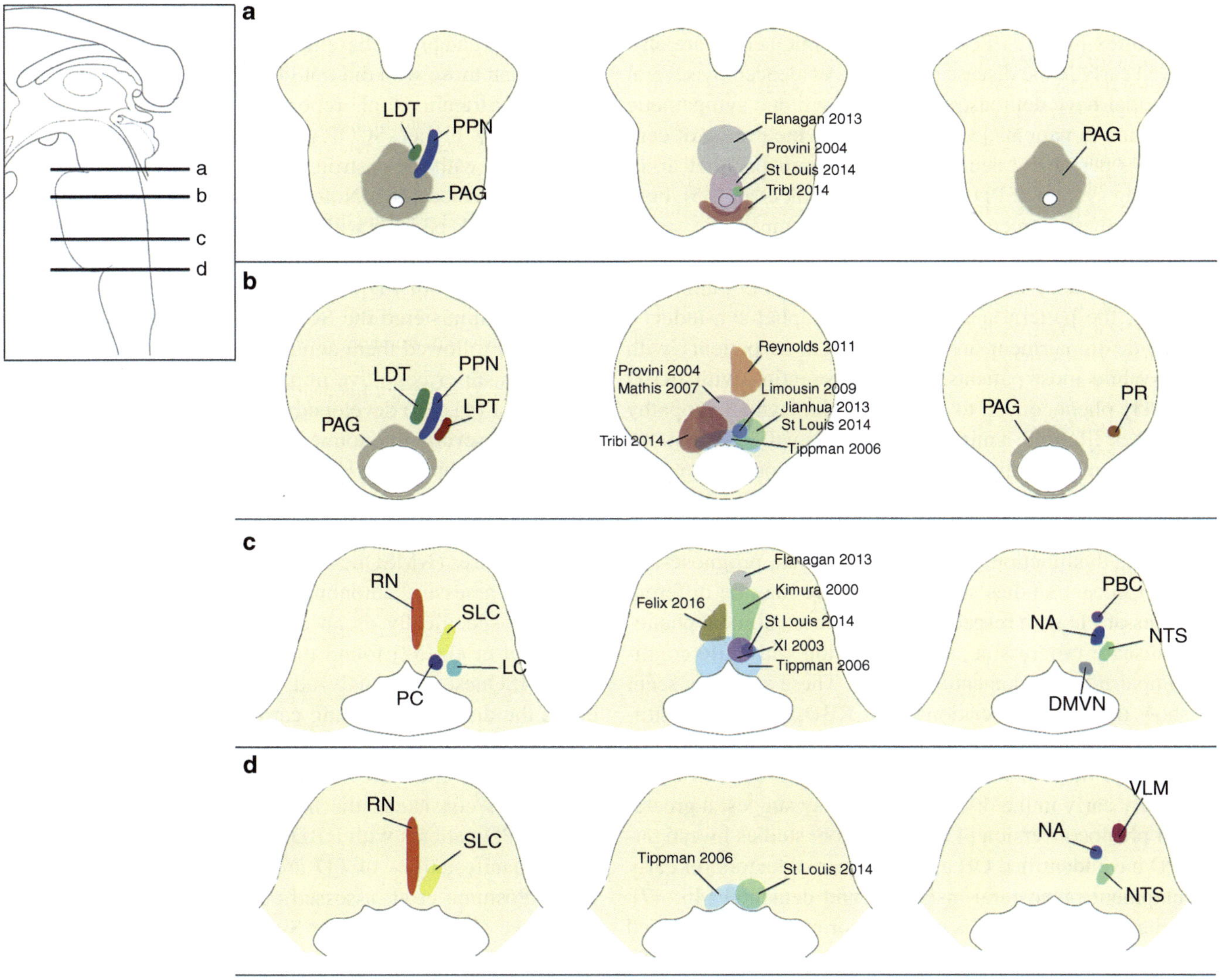

Fig. 22.2 Human brainstem templates showing the proposed nuclei involved in REM sleep control (*left column*), published cases of REM sleep behavior disorder associated with brainstem lesions and their approximate locations of the lesions based on magnetic resonance imaging data (*central column*), and the most important areas of the central autonomic network and their approximate location (*right column*). Letters represent cross-sectional views through the brain stem, with (**a**) corresponding to the ponto-mesencephalic junction, (**b**) to the upper/mid pons, (**c**) to lower/mid pons, and (**d**) just rostral to the ponto-medullary junction. Abbreviations: LDT laterodorsal tegmental nucleus, PPN pedunculopontine nucleus, PAG periaqueductal grey matter, LPT lateral pontine tegmentum, PR parabrachial region, RN raphe nucleus, PC precoeruleus, LC locus coeruleus, SLD sublaterodorsal nucleus, NA nucleus ambiguus, PBC Pre-Bötzinger complex, NTS nucleus of the tractus solitaries, DMVN dorsal motor vagal nucleus, VLM ventrolateral medulla. (Adapted from Boeve et al. [2] and Benarroch [8])

phenoconversion on Kaplan–Meier analysis was 10.6% after 2 years, 17.9% after 3 years, 31.3% after 5 years, 51.4% after 8 years, 60.2% after 10 years, and 73.5% after 12 years [28].

RBD is a common feature of all CNS α[alpha]-synucleinopathies and is often present at the time of diagnosis. It is estimated to occur in 30–50% of patients with PD, 50–80% of patients with DLB, and 80–95% of patients with MSA [5, 29]. Like RBD, autonomic impairment is extremely common in the α[alpha]-synucleinopathies. Orthostatic hypotension (OH), for example, occurs in 20–50% of patients with PD, 30–70% of patients with DLB, 80% of patients with MSA and 100% of patients with PAF [30]. The similarity between prevalence of RBD and OH in these conditions is striking.

The reason for this association is anatomical, as α [alpha]-syn-induced neurodegeneration of autonomic brainstem centers likely results in a significant portion of the disease burden seen in these patients. Neuropathological studies in patients with RBD have demonstrated α[alpha]-syn deposition in several areas of the CAN including the locus coeruleus (LC), raphe nuclei, amygdala, thalamus, and entorhinal cortex [31, 32]. Peripheral autonomic nerves are also involved early in the disease process, as evidenced by several studies that have demonstrated post-ganglionic sympathetic denervation in patients [33, 34]; however, the timing of central versus peripheral neurodegeneration remains unclear. In the staging system of PD proposed by Braak et al. [35], both parasympathetic structures (DMV) and sympathetic structures (postganglionic cardiac and sudomotor nerves) show inclusion of Lewy bodies at early stages of PD pathology. However, the pattern and severity of α[alpha]-syn-induced autonomic impairment are quite variable in patients with RBD. While most patients initially presenting with iRBD will likely phenoconvert to a CNS α[alpha]-synucleinopathy within their lifetime, a minority of patients will remain in the isolated form of the disease [36], and phenoconversion rates are variable between patients. Each of the CNS α[alpha]-synucleinopathies manifests their own unique patterns of autonomic dysfunction, and all have different prognoses. In addition, recent studies suggest that there may be different subtypes of PD with respect to disease onset, clinical phenotype, disease progression, and association with mild cognitive impairment or dementia [37–44]. These subtypes seem to show different associations with RBD, another illustration that α[alpha]-syn spread may be highly individual. For example, in those patients with PAF, the presence of RBD, especially early in the disease course, may suggest a greater risk of phenoconversion [45]. In addition, studies investigating PD have identified OH and RBD as risk factors for early development of postural instability and dementia [46, 47]. In patients with PD, OH is strongly correlated with reduced survival, falls, and an increased risk of dementia, while RBD is also associated with an increased risk of dementia and postural impairment, thus supporting the concept of the RBD-OH phenotype as a more aggressive and malignant PD subtype.

Autonomic Symptoms in Patients with RBD

Autonomic symptoms are common in RBD, reported in up to 94% of patients [33]. Furthermore, the severity of autonomic symptoms may be correlated with an accelerated rate of phenoconversion from iRBD to manifest CNS disease [27]. An early multicenter case-control study compared the presence of autonomic symptoms in 318 patients with iRBD to an equal number of sex- and age-matched controls by means of the Scale for Outcomes in PD-Autonomic (SCOPA-AUT), a self-assessment measure that addresses autonomic symptoms in patients with PD [48]. iRBD patients had substantially more symptoms of autonomic impairment when compared to controls, with the most severe symptoms in the gastrointestinal, urinary, and cardiovascular domains. In a similar study of patients with iRBD, those who converted to PD or DLB had higher baseline cardiovascular SCOPA-AUT scores than those who did not [49].

Ferini-Strambi et al. reported that iRBD patients had significantly higher SCOPA-AUT scores when compared to controls, with the gastrointestinal domain being the most severely affected [48]. Notably, constipation may be more common in PD patients with RBD than in those without RBD [50], and it is well known that constipation is an early premotor symptom of PD. In an important longitudinal study, Li et al. administered the SCOPA-AUT to 43 patients with iRBD and followed them annually until the development of parkinsonism or cognitive impairment. Eighteen patients in this cohort (41.9%) developed a synucleinopathy, and those with more severe autonomic symptoms had an accelerated rate of phenoconversion [27].

Aguirre-Mardones et al. reported that iRBD patients scored higher than controls on the Non-Motor Symptoms Questionnaire (NMSQuest), a scale that includes some questions assessing autonomic function, though it was not designed specifically as an autonomic questionnaire [51]. Schrempf et al. [52] found that when different domains of the NMSQuest were analyzed, iRBD patients scored highest in the domains assessing cardiovascular (33%), urinary (50%), gastrointestinal (17%), and sexual (22%) function.

While the literature on autonomic symptom severity in iRBD is consistent, the literature on autonomic impairment in PD patients with RBD is less so. To help determine if the manifestations of PD are related to the presence of RBD, Postuma et al. assessed autonomic impairment with subjective (Unified Multiple System Atrophy Rating Scale [UMSARS]) and objective outcome measures (1-minute active stand test) in a cohort of patients with PD [38]. Motor manifestations did not differ in patients with and without RBD; however, the presence of RBD was strongly associated with orthostatic intolerance and an orthostatic BP fall at 1 minute. There was no association between RBD and other autonomic symptoms (constipation, urinary dysfunction, or erectile dysfunction) on the UMSARS. In a later study by the same group, the authors noted that symptoms of urinary frequency were reported in iRBD patients up to 7 years before conversion to PD, with an extrapolated prodromal interval of 13 years, and erectile dysfunction was observed 7 years before disease conversion, with an extrapolated prodromal interval of 11 years [53]. In a large follow-up multicenter study, the presence of constipation increased phenoconversion risk by 1.67, and erectile dysfunction by 2.13 in those with iRBD [28].

In support of the theory that ANS functions are affected in a heterogeneous pattern in PD, and that the progression of ANS dysfunction follows an erratic rather than stepwise progression, a study of 45 PD patients found no correlation between axial motor impairment, RBD, and either autonomic symptoms (NMSQuest, SCOPA-AUT) or objective autonomic impairment (cardiovascular autonomic reflex testing) [54]. Furthermore, based on prospective investigations of RBD as a predictor of motor deterioration in PD, RBD has been associated with the progression of bradykinesia [55] but not with other motor symptoms, as measured by Hoehn and Yahr scores, conversion to postural instability gait disturbance (PIGD) subtype, worsening of tremor [55], or the development of freezing of gait or falls [56].

There are some studies that have reported greater autonomic symptom severity in PD patients with RBD, compared to those without [57]. The discrepancies reported in patients with PD + RBD (as opposed to iRBD only) may be due to several factors, including a more advanced disease state, greater cognitive impairment affecting self-reporting measures, and more confounding variables, such as a polypharmacy and medical comorbidities. Nonetheless, autonomic symptoms are common in RBD, with the most common complaints involving the gastrointestinal, genitourinary, sexual, and cardiovascular systems.

Objective Markers of Autonomic Impairment in RBD

Heart Rate Variability

It is difficult to measure autonomic fluctuations during sleep due to the uncomfortable and disruptive nature of most autonomic recording techniques. Heart rate variability (HRV) analysis of the RR interval offers an indirect, noninvasive alternative. Spectral analysis of HRV is often referenced as an estimate of sympathetic and parasympathetic tone during sleep, termed the sympathovagal balance. High-frequency (HF) RR signal (>0.15 Hz) is associated with parasympathetic tone, due to the vagal respiratory sinus arrhythmia, where heart rate increases on inspiration and decreases on expiration. Conversely, low-frequency (LF) RR signal (0.04–0.15 Hz) may be associated with sympathetic tone [58] and may be influenced by baroreceptor function. A greater LF/HF ratio is suggestive of greater sympathetic drive, while a lower LF/HF ratio is suggestive of greater parasympathetic drive. It is notable, however, that this correlation is not universally accepted and may be too simplistic a metric to capture the myriad exchanges involved in ANS balance during sleep. While HRV analysis is noninvasive and easy to perform, it is prone to artifact and is thus a nonspecific marker of cardiac autonomic impairment. Nonetheless, HRV can be easily obtained from overnight polysomnography (PSG) and has been utilized in a wealth of studies of autonomic function in various disease states including RBD.

Reduced HRV has been well-documented in RBD and has been established as one of the earliest signs of ANS impairment. Most studies in this patient population have demonstrated results consistent with sympathetic impairment [43, 59, 60], while some have demonstrated both sympathetic and parasympathetic impairment [61, 62], depending on sleep stage [62], or severity of motor dysfunction [60]. Some studies have evaluated HRV only in the waking state [43], while others assessed PSG sleep data, finding differences between REM and non-REM stages [60, 61, 63]. Reduction in the HR response to arousals or periodic limb movements has been documented in both iRBD and PD, with the HR response for the iRBD group being intermediate with respect to the control and the PD groups, with a lower LF/HF ratio in REM, suggestive of sympathetic impairment [64]. It is noteworthy that this is the opposite of what is typically seen in normal, healthy sleep and is reflective of the sympathetic impairment that these patients manifest. In addition, reduced HRV alone may be an independent risk of developing PD. In one large population-based study, a reduction in HRV was associated with a 1.5–3× risk of PD [64]. The mean interval between detection of the abnormalities and onset of PD was 18 years, suggesting that this marker has a very long lead time. This finding was not replicated in a slightly smaller study that involved a 14-year follow-up [65].

Impaired nocturnal HRV in RBD has also been associated with signs of diurnal ANS impairment. In one study, patients with iRBD had not only reduced tonic and phasic HRV during sleep, but the majority of these patients also had abnormalities in one or more tests assessing cardiovascular reflex function during wakefulness [66]. However, no significant difference was found in ANS function between iRBD patients and those with diagnosed CNS synucleinopathy. Further supporting this notion, Lanfranchi et al. evaluated 10 subjects with iRBD and compared them to 10 age-matched controls, with the hypothesis that REM-related cardiorespiratory activation is altered in subjects with iRBD [67]. The authors found that REM-related cardiac and respiratory responses were absent in subjects with iRBD, but were preserved in non-REM sleep, suggesting that iRBD preferentially affects the sympathetic control that is most active during REM.

Postuma et al. retrospectively analyzed overnight HRV in patients with iRBD and compared patients who had phenoconverted to those who had not [68]. Patients who remained as iRBD demonstrated clear evidence of cardiovascular autonomic dysfunction, as evidenced by reduction in RR-standard deviation, very low frequency (vLF) and LF spectra, again suggestive of sympathetic impairment. However, this cardiovascular autonomic dysfunction, measured at baseline, did not predict phenoconversion rates, indicating that HRV abnormalities do not predict prognosis. More recently, Barone et al. evaluated HRV in 21 patients with isolated rapid eye movement sleep without atonia (RSWA) without dream enacting behaviors and 21 patients with normal REM atonia [69]. Significant differences between groups were demonstrated in RR standard deviation, HRV power and LF spectra, suggesting that cardiovascular sympathetic impairment is present well before patients are noted to have their first RBD event.

In summary, many studies have demonstrated reduced HRV in patients with RBD, most prevalent in the sympathetic power spectra, indicative of sympathetic cardiac impairment. However, the presence of this impairment does not seem to correlate with disease severity or risk of phenoconversion from iRBD to CNS synucleinopathy, as it occurs early in the disease course for most patients and is present in both iRBD and in RBD patients with CNS disease.

Cardiac Scintigraphy

Studies utilizing metaiodobenzylguanidine (MIBG) scintigraphy in RBD offer similar findings to those of HRV studies. MIBG scintigraphy is based on evidence that norepinephrine (NE) and ^{123}I-MIBG have the same mechanisms for uptake, storage, and release [70], thus an abnormal MIBG scan suggests post-ganglionic sympathetic denervation. Results are often referenced as the heart to mediastinum (H/M) ratio, which represents the capacity of MIBG uptake in the terminal post-ganglionic sympathetic fibers, with lower ratios indicating impaired neuronal uptake [71]. Studies of cardiac MIBG scintigraphy in patients with iRBD have demonstrated abnormalities similar to those seen in PD [3, 72]. These findings have also been demonstrated in DLB with and without autonomic failure [71, 73], but less so in MSA, which tends to preferentially involve preganglionic autonomic fibers. These MIBG studies provide a direct neuroanatomical correlate of the cardiac sympathetic impairment seen in HRV studies.

Kashihara et al. performed MIBG scintigraphy in patients with iRBD and compared the findings to patients with PD and controls [74], reporting that H/M ratios were lower for iRBD patients than PD patients at Hoehn and Yahr stages 1 and 2, but equal to those at Hoehn and Yahr stages 3, 4, and 5. This suggests that the autonomic denervation responsible for reduced MIBG uptake may be more closely associated with the presence of RBD than with PD. The authors also reported that cardiac sympathetic denervation is more severe in iRBD than in early PD, suggesting that the presence of RBD might predict more widespread autonomic impairment in patients with an underlying α[alpha]-synucleinopathy.

In 2008, Oguri et al. reported on two RBD patients with differing clinical progression in whom cardiac scintigraphy was performed. One 69-year-old patient had more than a 20-year history of iRBD and demonstrated a decrease in myocardial MIBG radioactivity. The other 69-year-old patient began to manifest nocturnal behaviors at age 62, then mild parkinsonism at age 68, and demonstrated a similar decrease in myocardial MIBG radioactivity both before and after the onset of parkinsonism. These cases suggest that RBD can develop in diverse patterns of clinical progression, and that an abnormal MIBG result does not necessarily predict severity of disease [75]. Other studies have demonstrated reduced MIBG uptake in iRBD compared to early PD [74], and in PD with RBD compared to PD without RBD [76, 77], suggesting that cardiac post-ganglionic sympathetic denervation may be more closely associated with the presence of RBD than with PD. In support of this theory, Kim et al. demonstrated that PD patients with RBD were more likely to have orthostatic hypotension (OH) and reduced H/M ratios when compared to those without RBD, suggesting that cardiac sympathetic denervation could be the driving mechanism behind OH in patients with RBD [78].

While MIBG abnormalities may not predict disease severity in patients with RBD, they do seem to be much more common in the α[alpha]-synucleinopathies than in other neurodegenerative diseases. Miyamoto et al. reported on the pattern of MIBG scintigraphy abnormalities in iRBD, DLB, and MSA, and compared them to progressive supranuclear palsy (PSP), a tauopathy [79]. The results were normal in the MSA, PSP, and control groups; however, they were markedly reduced in 93.5% of the patients with iRBD, 75.0% patients with PD, and 100% patients with DLB [79]. In most cases of iRBD, a marked reduction in ^{123}I-MIBG accumulation occurred soon after the onset of the disease. Barateau et al. performed a different disease-state comparison, evaluating MIBG scintigraphy in a population of 34 patients with type-1 narcolepsy (NT1) and in 15 patients with iRBD. The authors found that reduced MIBG uptake was associated with iRBD but not with NT1, again supporting the observation that cardiac sympathetic impairment seen in RBD may be unique to the synucleinopathies [80].

In summary, like HRV, several studies have demonstrated abnormal MIBG scintigraphy in patients with RBD, indicative of sympathetic cardiac impairment. However, the presence of this impairment may not correlate with disease severity or phenoconversion rate, but it may help differentiate RBD related to an underlying α[alpha]-synucleinopathy from RBD due to other disease states, such as NT1. In addition, it may be useful in differentiating certain subtypes of synucleinopathy, such as MSA and PD.

Cardiovascular Reflex Testing and Blood Pressure Analysis

Cardiovascular reflex testing has been validated as the most quantitative and comprehensive method of assessing ANS function. Autonomic cardiovascular reflex testing can include many specialized tests, but at a minimum should include measures of HRV with paced deep breathing (cardiovagal parasympathetic), the Valsalva maneuver (sympathetic adrenergic) with Valsalva heart rate ratio (cardiovagal parasympathetic and sympathetic adrenergic), and 70° head-up tilt test (HUTT) (sympathetic adrenergic) for a minimum of 10 minutes, all performed with continuous BP and HR monitoring. Testing is performed in the autonomic laboratory under controlled conditions, and patients should refrain from large meals, alcohol, nicotine, caffeine, or any medications that might alter the test results.

The first study to investigate cardiovascular reflex testing in iRBD was by Ferrini-Strambi et al. [66]. The authors compared a cohort of 10 iRBD, one PD, one AD, and two MSA patients to controls and found that the BP response to standing was abnormal in six patients (43%). Frauscher et al. investigated autonomic function in iRBD by performing cardiovascular reflex testing in 15 iRBD patients and compared them to PD patients and controls [81]. On HUTT, BP changes were similar between iRBD patients and controls; however, OH was present in two iRBD patients, the same frequency as in the PD group. Orthostatic BP changes were more pronounced in the PD group. The Valsalva ratio was significantly lower in PD patients and iRBD patients.

In another small cohort, Lee et al. performed testing on 17 patients with iRBD. Ninety-four percent of these patients demonstrated sympathetic adrenergic and/or parasympathetic cardiovagal deficits [33]. In contrast to the earlier work by Fraucher, in which the authors found relatively little OH, 10/17 (59%) of patients in this cohort had OH. Sympathetic cholinergic dysfunction was found in 7/17 (41%) of patients with iRBD, as evidenced by abnormal QSART results [33], suggesting post-ganglionic sympathetic impairment. These results suggest widespread autonomic impairment in iRBD, with both central and peripheral autonomic involvement. Others have reported no difference in sudomotor function using the SudoScan device, which utilizes electro-chemical skin conductance (ESC) to measure the sweat gland function through reverse iontophoresis [82]. The authors of this study compared a cohort of iRBD, PD with RBD, PD without RBD, and atypical Parkinson's patients to controls, and found that ESC was reduced in PD with RBD as compared to PD without RBD and controls, while ESC in iRBD patients was no different from controls. This finding illustrates the need for further studies to investigate peripheral autonomic involvement in RBD, to better understand the spread of α[alpha]-syn in the progression of neurodegenerative disease.

In summary, while studies are limited, cardiovascular autonomic reflex testing has demonstrated clear abnormalities in both central and peripheral autonomic function in patients with iRBD and provides the most comprehensive analysis of autonomic function in the waking state.

Gastrointestinal Motility

Several studies have reported a high prevalence of gastrointestinal (GI) symptoms in iRBD cohorts, equal to that of diagnosed PD [48, 51]. One study evaluated objective measures of GI function in iRBD with GI transit time, colonic volume, and peristaltic movements and compared the results to previously published data from early stage PD patients and controls [83]. GI transit time and total colonic volume were significantly increased in iRBD patients when compared to controls, but not as severely affected as in PD patients. As the innervation of the GI tract decreases from the proximal to the distal segments, the functional consequence of neuronal death is expected to become progressively more severe. The authors of this study found a clear gradient of GI dysfunction in patients with iRBD, as measured by 3D-transit, with gradually more severe involvement from stomach to colon, thus supporting the hypothesis that intestinal neuronal innervation is affected very early in the prodromal phase of the α[alpha]-synucleinopathies.

In another study, the same authors enrolled 21 patients with iRBD and utilized functional imaging with ^{11}C-donepezil PET and computed tomography (CT) to assess cholinergic gut innervation along with MIBG cardiac scintigraphy and other imaging techniques to assess cell integrity in the locus coeruleus and striatum [84]. The authors also performed orthostatic BP measurements in their cohort. As demonstrated in prior studies, both iRBD and PD groups had reduced H/M ratios on MIBG scintigraphy, with no significant difference between groups. OH was present in 7/13 iRBD patients (54%), but there was no correlation between H/M ratios and severity of OH. Compared with controls, iRBD patients had significantly lower uptake in the small intestine, with impairment comparable to those with PD. Similar results were seen in the CNS imaging tests. Idiopathic RBD patients had significantly lower locus coeruleus: pons ratios compared to controls, but not compared to PD patients. These studies indicate that patients with iRBD demonstrate peripheral autonomic nervous system dysfunction on par with diagnosed PD, and that both central and peripheral structures are affected early in the spread of α[alpha]-synuclein-induced neurodegeneration.

Biopsy and Tissue Analysis

As the results of the studies discussed would indicate, phosphorylated α[alpha]-synuclein (pSyn) containing inclusions in neurons (Lewy bodies, LB) and nerve terminals (Lewy neurites, LN) are not confined to the CNS in RBD, but are readily found in peripheral tissues and in autonomic nerves. There is pathologic evidence that pSyn accumulation in distal autonomic axons in PD occurs early and may precede the involvement of more proximal autonomic structures [85]. This provides rationale for the use of tissue α[alpha]-syn as a biomarker in these conditions [86], to both identify patients for future clinical trials and to measure disease progression [87–89]. However, the utility of pSyn detection in tissues accessible to biopsies as a reliable biomarker in iRBD remains unclear. Most studies have focused on the detection of pSyn in PD, and only recently have investigators turned their focus to tissue biopsy in iRBD.

The GI tract was one of the first sites outside of the CNS in which α[alpha]-syn was detected, with the first descriptions of enteric nervous system involvement dating back to 1960 [90]. Several groups have subsequently demonstrated pSyn deposits in the colon of patients with PD on screening colonoscopy [91, 92]. Other studies have found pSyn in the salivary glands of iRBD patients [93], and more recently the epidermis of the skin. Skin biopsy has emerged as the most promising biopsy site to date. It is easy to perform, minimally invasive, and thus represents an ideal potential site for biomarker tissue analysis. Michell et al. first reported α[alpha]-syn in human skin biopsies in 2005. Positive samples were identified in both PD and control groups, and most samples were negative. Furthermore, the authors found no apparent correlation between the amount of α[alpha]-syn detected and diagnosis or disease severity [87]. Following up on that study, Miki et al. examined Lewy pathology in 20 patients with clinically diagnosed PD, using 6-mm punch biopsies obtained from the skin of the chest wall and leg. Abnormal accumulation of pSyn was found in the chest of 10% of patients, but not in the leg [94]. Other studies failed to localize pSyn in biopsies of the ventral forearm and distal leg in patients with PD [95, 96]. These initial studies and others used techniques optimized for CNS tissue, relied on small tissue volumes, and did not systematically study autonomic substructures, and therefore detected α[alpha]-syn in only a minority of their subjects [87, 88, 94, 97, 98].

In 2013, Donadio et al. reported novel methods of indirect immunofluorescence to detect pSyn in a group of 21 patients with chronic peripheral autonomic neuropathy, a subset of whom had acquired forms, such as diabetes, and a subset of whom had pure autonomic failure (PAF), a known α-synucleinopathy [99]. In this study the authors reported methods that would be later employed in iRBD cohorts. They performed 3-mm punch biopsies at the cervical (C7) paraspinal level and the proximal and distal leg, and immunostained with PGP 9.5 and autonomic markers, such as vasoactive intestinal peptide to localize sudomotor cholinergic fibers in sweat glands and dopamine-β-hydroxylase to localize noradrenergic vasomotor and pilomotor fibers, and co-localized with pSyn mouse antibodies. pSyn was found in the samples of all patients with pure autonomic failure (PAF) but in none of the patients with acquired autonomic neuropathy and in none of the controls. Analysis showed a higher percentage of pSyn in the proximal compared to the distal leg, and a similar percentage of pSyn in the proximal leg and cervical site. Synuclein deposits did not differ between cholinergic and adrenergic autonomic structures and did not correlate with disease duration; however, most patients in this study have similar disease duration. These findings have been confirmed by other groups in patients with PD [100, 101], and in follow-up studies, pSyn ratios were noted to higher in PD patients with autonomic failure, more advanced stages of disease, and disease of longer duration [102].

Doppler et al. performed the first study of dermal pSyn analysis in iRBD patients [103]. The authors enrolled 18 patients with PSG-confirmed iRBD and compared them to 25 patients with early PD and 20 controls. They performed biopsies at cervical (C7) and thoracic (Th10) paraspinal regions, as well as the upper and lower leg, and analyzed samples for pSyn deposits in dermal nerve fibers. Patients were considered positive if at least one biopsy site had pSyn-immunoreactive nerve fibers. In the 10 pSyn-positive iRBD patients (sensitivity 55.6%), most pSyn-positive nerve fibers were found in the cervical and thoracic sites. In the 20 pSyn-positive PD patients (sensitivity 80%), there was a trend of more pSyn-positive fibers to be found in the periphery; however, the differences of affected biopsy sites were not significant. There was no pSyn in control samples (specificity 100%).

In 2017, Antelmi et al. addressed the same question in 12 iRBD patients and compared them to 55 healthy controls [104]. Skin biopsies were taken from the cervical paraspinal region and the distal leg. pSyn deposits were detected in 9/12 (75%) patients with iRBD and in none of the controls. In iRBD, the sensitivity of the test was higher at the cervical site (67%) when compared to the leg site (58%) [104], similar to the results of Doppler et al. [103].

Observations in these skin biopsy studies support the hypothesis of peripheral nerve fiber loss as an intrinsic feature of PD, and growing evidence suggests this to be also true in iRBD [105]. As discussed in the section on Cardiac Scintigraphy, skin biopsy may also serve as a test of α[alpha]-synucleinopathy subtype. In one study, all patients with PD had pSyn depositions within at least one dermal nerve fiber innervating autonomic skin structures (sensitivity 100%), while patients with MSA did not. In fact, MSA patients exhibited a different pSyn staining pattern, with abnormal aggregates found predominantly in somatosensory skin fibers, mainly those located in the subepidermal plexus. In contrast, PD, DLB, and PAF patients demonstrated pSyn deposits in autonomic fibers and plexuses close to autonomic annexes. The patterns of staining in MSA were also different, consisting of dot-like patterns, as opposed to the more homogenous staining of PD, DLB, and PAF.

In conclusion, skin biopsy has thus far emerged as the most promising tool thus for the analysis of α[alpha]-syn. It is minimally invasive, easily reproducible, and requires minimal operator training, thus represents an exciting technique for use in future longitudinal studies of phenoconversion risk in iRBD.

Nightmare Disorder and Trauma-Associated Sleep Disorder

Nightmare disorder is characterized by nightmares occurring at least once weekly, accompanied by emotional distress and impaired daytime function [106]. The literature on autonomic impairment in nightmare disorder is limited; however, some data suggest that frequent nightmares may lead to augmentation of EMG tone during pre-REM periods [107], accompanied by reduced HF spectra, indicating lower parasympathetic tone during sleep. Several studies have also demonstrated markers of increase sympathetic tone in those with post-traumatic stress disorder (PTSD), such as elevated LF spectra and the LF/HF ratio during sleep. Others have reported elevated plasma, urinary, and cerebrospinal fluid catecholamines in PTSD patients, the levels of which correlated with the severity of the patient's symptoms [108]. The use of central alpha blockers such as prazosin for nightmare disorder speaks to the involvement of the sympathetic nervous system in the genesis or propagation of nightmares.

The observation of a shift toward a sympathetic dominant state may also be related to the complaint of dream-enacting behaviors in those with PTSD. This has led to expansion of the term PTSD into the concept of "trauma-associated sleep disorder" (TSD), defined as sleep disorders sharing characteristics of both PTSD and RBD. There are several case reports and case series of sympathetic hyperactivity, and even REM-without atonia, described in younger combat veterans, a demographic quite distinct from that of the typical α[alpha]-synucleinopathy patient [109, 110]. This implies that the pathophysiology of PTSD may involve disordered REM sleep pathways; however, the mechanism is unclear, and may be multifactorial, with fragmented sleep, substance abuse, antidepressant use, and hyperarousal all potential contributing factors in this patient population. However, there is also precedent for a neuroanatomical basis; post-mortem studies in PTSD patients have demonstrated a significant reduction in the number of locus coeruleus (LC) neurons. In addition, reduced firing rates of LC neurons may lead to disinhibition of the pedunculopontine nucleus (PPN), producing some of the symptoms of PTSD [111]; however, this reduction in noradrenergic outflow to the PPN may also result in REM without atonia. With a growing population of younger combat veterans with PTSD and nightmare disorder, the overlap with RBD deserves further investigation, and future longitudinal studies are needed in this group of patients.

Conclusions

Autonomic dysfunction is common in REM parasomnias, a fact that is not surprising given the neuroanatomical proximity of the REM and autonomic control nuclei and their reciprocal connections. This dysfunction may take the form of sympathetic adrenergic impairment in RBD, or sympathetic hyperactivity in nightmare disorder and TSD. Patients with iRBD may develop prodromal symptoms of autonomic dysfunction decades before any manifest signs of CNS disease, with the most commonly reported symptoms occurring in the urinary, gastrointestinal, sexual, and cardiovascular domains. The severity of symptoms may correlate with phenoconversion rate; however, this has not been definitely established. Patients with iRBD have clear evidence of post-ganglionic cardiac sympathetic denervation, as evidenced by HRV and cardiac scintigraphy studies, and, like autonomic symptoms, this impairment is likely present decades prior to diagnosis. The severity of these deficits has not been correlated with severity of RBD or with phenoconversion rate. While the data on cardiovascular reflex testing are limited, we believe this testing has the greatest potential to measure minor autonomic changes in individuals with iRBD. Measures of sudomotor function (QSART) may help quantify peripheral denervation and small fiber neuropathy, which may correlate with peripheral α[alpha]-synuclein deposition. Measures of HRV during wake provide a measure of cardiovagal tone, and Valsalva and HUT testing provide controlled measures of sympathetic tone and baroreceptor function. Combining such measures with quantification of dermal alpha-synuclein on skin biopsy may provide the most comprehensive assessment of autonomic function in RBD and should be considered in future longitudinal trials.

Declarations All authors report nothing to declare.
All authors have seen and approved this chapter.

References

1. Schenck CH, Bundlie SR, Ettinger MG, Mahowald MW. Chronic behavioral disorders of human REM sleep: a new category of parasomnia. Sleep. 1986;9(2):293–308.
2. Boeve BF, Silber MH, Saper CB, Ferman TJ, Dickson DW, Parisi JE, et al. Pathophysiology of REM sleep behaviour disorder and relevance to neurodegenerative disease. Brain. 2007;130(Pt 11):2770–88.
3. Luppi PH, Clement O, Sapin E, Peyron C, Gervasoni D, Leger L, et al. Brainstem mechanisms of paradoxical (REM) sleep generation. Pflugers Arch. 2012;463(1):43–52.
4. Ramaligam V, Chen MC, Saper CB, Lu J. Perspectives on the rapid eye movement sleep switch in rapid eye movement sleep behavior disorder. Sleep Med. 2013;14(8):707–13.
5. Boeve BF, Silber MH, Ferman TJ, Lin SC, Benarroch EE, Schmeichel AM, et al. Clinicopathologic correlations in 172 cases

of rapid eye movement sleep behavior disorder with or without a coexisting neurologic disorder. Sleep Med. 2013;14(8):754–62.
6. Iranzo A, Santamaria J, Tolosa E. Idiopathic rapid eye movement sleep behaviour disorder: diagnosis, management, and the need for neuroprotective interventions. Lancet Neurol. 2016;15(4):405–19.
7. Thieben MJ, Lennon VA, Boeve BF, Aksamit AJ, Keegan M, Vernino S. Potentially reversible autoimmune limbic encephalitis with neuronal potassium channel antibody. Neurology. 2004;62(7):1177–82.
8. Benarroch EE. The central autonomic network: functional organization, dysfunction, and perspective. Mayo Clin Proc. 1993;68(10):988–1001.
9. Flanagan EP, Gavrilova RH, Boeve BF, Kumar N, Jelsing EJ, Silber MH. Adult-onset autosomal dominant leukodystrophy presenting with REM sleep behavior disorder. Neurology. 2013;80(1):118–20.
10. Provini F, Vetrugno R, Pastorelli F, Lombardi C, Plazzi G, Marliani AF, et al. Status dissociatus after surgery for tegmental ponto-mesencephalic cavernoma: a state-dependent disorder of motor control during sleep. Mov Disord. 2004;19(6):719–23.
11. St Louis EK, McCarter SJ, Boeve BF, Silber MH, Kantarci K, Benarroch EE, et al. Lesional REM sleep behavior disorder localizes to the dorsomedial pons. Neurology. 2014;83(20):1871–3.
12. Tribl GG, Bor-Seng-Shu E, Trindade MC, Lucato LT, Teixeira MJ, Barbosa ER. Wilson's disease presenting as rapid eye movement sleep behavior disorder: a possible window to early treatment. Arq Neuropsiquiatr. 2014;72(9):653–8.
13. Mathis J, Hess CW, Bassetti C. Isolated mediotegmental lesion causing narcolepsy and rapid eye movement sleep behaviour disorder: a case evidencing a common pathway in narcolepsy and rapid eye movement sleep behaviour disorder. J Neurol Neurosurg Psychiatry. 2007;78(4):427–9.
14. Reynolds TQ, Roy A. Isolated cataplexy and REM sleep behavior disorder after pontine stroke. J Clin Sleep Med. 2011;7(2):211–3.
15. Limousin N, Dehais C, Gout O, Heran F, Oudiette D, Arnulf I. A brainstem inflammatory lesion causing REM sleep behavior disorder and sleepwalking (parasomnia overlap disorder). Sleep Med. 2009;10(9):1059–62.
16. Jianhua C, Xiuqin L, Quancai C, Heyang S, Yan H. Rapid eye movement sleep behavior disorder in a patient with brainstem lymphoma. Intern Med. 2013;52(5):617–21.
17. Tippmann-Peikert M, Boeve BF, Keegan BM. REM sleep behavior disorder initiated by acute brainstem multiple sclerosis. Neurology. 2006;66(8):1277–9.
18. Felix S, Thobois S, Peter-Derex L. Rapid eye movement sleep behaviour disorder symptomatic of a brain stem cavernoma. J Sleep Res. 2016;25(2):211–5.
19. Kimura K, Tachibana N, Kohyama J, Otsuka Y, Fukazawa S, Waki R. A discrete pontine ischemic lesion could cause REM sleep behavior disorder. Neurology. 2000;55(6):894–5.
20. Xi MC, Fung SJ, Yamuy J, Morales FR, Chase MH. Hypocretinergic facilitation of synaptic activity of neurons in the nucleus pontis oralis of the cat. Brain Res. 2003;976(2):253–8.
21. Schenck CH, Bundlie SR, Patterson AL, Mahowald MW. Rapid eye movement sleep behavior disorder. A treatable parasomnia affecting older adults. JAMA. 1987;257(13):1786–9.
22. Kang SH, Yoon IY, Lee SD, Han JW, Kim TH, Kim KW. REM sleep behavior disorder in the Korean elderly population: prevalence and clinical characteristics. Sleep. 2013;36(8):1147–52.
23. Haba-Rubio J, Frauscher B, Marques-Vidal P, Toriel J, Tobback N, Andries D, et al. Prevalence and determinants of rapid eye movement sleep behavior disorder in the general population. Sleep. 2018;41(2):zsx197.
24. Fernandez-Arcos A, Iranzo A, Serradell M, Gaig C, Santamaria J. The clinical phenotype of idiopathic rapid eye movement sleep behavior disorder at presentation: a study in 203 consecutive patients. Sleep. 2016;39(1):121–32.
25. Postuma RB, Trenkwalder C. Neurodegeneration in REM sleep behavior disorder: stratification keeps improving. Neurology. 2017;88(16):1486–7.
26. Schenck CH. Rapid eye movement sleep behavior disorder: current knowledge and future directions. Sleep Med. 2013;14(8):699–702.
27. Li Y, Kang W, Yang Q, Zhang L, Zhang L, Dong F, et al. Predictive markers for early conversion of iRBD to neurodegenerative synucleinopathy diseases. Neurology. 2017;88(16):1493–500.
28. Postuma RB, Iranzo A, Hu M, Hogl B, Boeve BF, Manni R, et al. Risk and predictors of dementia and parkinsonism in idiopathic REM sleep behaviour disorder: a multicentre study. Brain. 2019;142(3):744–59.
29. Iranzo A, Tolosa E, Gelpi E, Molinuevo JL, Valldeoriola F, Serradell M, et al. Neurodegenerative disease status and postmortem pathology in idiopathic rapid-eye-movement sleep behaviour disorder: an observational cohort study. Lancet Neurol. 2013;12(5):443–53.
30. Coon EA, Cutsforth-Gregory JK, Benarroch EE. Neuropathology of autonomic dysfunction in synucleinopathies. Mov Disord. 2018;33(3):349–58.
31. Murray ME, Ferman TJ, Boeve BF, Przybelski SA, Lesnick TG, Liesinger AM, et al. MRI and pathology of REM sleep behavior disorder in dementia with Lewy bodies. Neurology. 2013;81(19):1681–9.
32. Dugger BN, Murray ME, Boeve BF, Parisi JE, Benarroch EE, Ferman TJ, et al. Neuropathological analysis of brainstem cholinergic and catecholaminergic nuclei in relation to rapid eye movement (REM) sleep behaviour disorder. Neuropathol Appl Neurobiol. 2012;38(2):142–52.
33. Lee H, Cho YW, Kim HA. The severity and pattern of autonomic dysfunction in idiopathic rapid eye movement sleep behavior disorder. Mov Disord. 2015;30(13):1843–8.
34. Sakakibara R, Tateno F, Kishi M, Tsuyusaki Y, Terada H, Inaoka T. MIBG myocardial scintigraphy in pre-motor Parkinson's disease: a review. Parkinsonism Relat Disord. 2014;20(3):267–73.
35. Braak H, Del Tredici K, Rub U, de Vos RA, Jansen Steur EN, Braak E. Staging of brain pathology related to sporadic Parkinson's disease. Neurobiol Aging. 2003;24(2):197–211.
36. Miglis MG, Muppidi S, During E, Jaradeh S. A case series of REM sleep behavior disorder in pure autonomic failure. Clin Auton Res. 2017;27(1):41–4.
37. Kumru H, Santamaria J, Tolosa E, Iranzo A. Relation between subtype of Parkinson's disease and REM sleep behavior disorder. Sleep Med. 2007;8(7–8):779–83.
38. Postuma RB, Gagnon JF, Vendette M, Charland K, Montplaisir J. Manifestations of Parkinson disease differ in association with REM sleep behavior disorder. Mov Disord. 2008;23(12):1665–72.
39. Postuma RB, Gagnon JF, Vendette M, Charland K, Montplaisir J. REM sleep behaviour disorder in Parkinson's disease is associated with specific motor features. J Neurol Neurosurg Psychiatry. 2008;79(10):1117–21.
40. Selikhova M, Williams DR, Kempster PA, Holton JL, Revesz T, Lees AJ. A clinico-pathological study of subtypes in Parkinson's disease. Brain. 2009;132(Pt 11):2947–57.
41. Yoritaka A, Ohizumi H, Tanaka S, Hattori N. Parkinson's disease with and without REM sleep behaviour disorder: are there any clinical differences? Eur Neurol. 2009;61(3):164–70.
42. Jozwiak N, Postuma RB, Montplaisir J, Latreille V, Panisset M, Chouinard S, et al. REM sleep behavior disorder and cognitive impairment in parkinson's disease. Sleep. 2017;40(8):zsx101.
43. Postuma RB, Montplaisir J, Lanfranchi P, Blais H, Rompre S, Colombo R, et al. Cardiac autonomic denervation in Parkinson's

disease is linked to REM sleep behavior disorder. Mov Disord. 2011;26(8):1529–33.
44. Gagnon JF, Postuma RB, Mazza S, Doyon J, Montplaisir J. Rapid-eye-movement sleep behaviour disorder and neurodegenerative diseases. Lancet Neurol. 2006;5(5):424–32.
45. Giannini G, Calandra-Buonaura G, Asioli GM, Cecere A, Barletta G, Mignani F, et al. The natural history of idiopathic autonomic failure: the IAF-BO cohort study. Neurology. 2018;91(13):e1245–e54.
46. Postuma RB, Bertrand JA, Montplaisir J, Desjardins C, Vendette M, Rios Romenets S, et al. Rapid eye movement sleep behavior disorder and risk of dementia in Parkinson's disease: a prospective study. Mov Disord. 2012;27(6):720–6.
47. Arnaldi D, De Carli F, Fama F, Brugnolo A, Girtler N, Picco A, et al. Prediction of cognitive worsening in de novo Parkinson's disease: clinical use of biomarkers. Mov Disord. 2017;32(12):1738–47.
48. Ferini-Strambi L, Oertel W, Dauvilliers Y, Postuma RB, Marelli S, Iranzo A, et al. Autonomic symptoms in idiopathic REM behavior disorder: a multicentre case-control study. J Neurol. 2014;261(6):1112–8.
49. Postuma RB, Iranzo A, Hogl B, Arnulf I, Ferini-Strambi L, Manni R, et al. Risk factors for neurodegeneration in idiopathic rapid eye movement sleep behavior disorder: a multicenter study. Ann Neurol. 2015;77(5):830–9.
50. Nihei Y, Takahashi K, Koto A, Mihara B, Morita Y, Isozumi K, et al. REM sleep behavior disorder in Japanese patients with Parkinson's disease: a multicenter study using the REM sleep behavior disorder screening questionnaire. J Neurol. 2012;259(8):1606–12.
51. Aguirre-Mardones C, Iranzo A, Vilas D, Serradell M, Gaig C, Santamaria J, et al. Prevalence and timeline of nonmotor symptoms in idiopathic rapid eye movement sleep behavior disorder. J Neurol. 2015;262(6):1568–78.
52. Schrempf W, Katona I, Dogan I, Felbert VV, Wienecke M, Heller J, et al. Reduced intraepidermal nerve fiber density in patients with REM sleep behavior disorder. Parkinsonism Relat Disord. 2016;29:10–6.
53. Postuma RB, Gagnon JF, Pelletier A, Montplaisir J. Prodromal autonomic symptoms and signs in Parkinson's disease and dementia with Lewy bodies. Mov Disord. 2013;28(5):597–604.
54. Leclair-Visonneau L, Magy L, Volteau C, Clairembault T, Le Dily S, Preterre C, et al. Heterogeneous pattern of autonomic dysfunction in Parkinson's disease. J Neurol. 2018;265(4):933–41.
55. Bugalho P, Viana-Baptista M. REM sleep behavior disorder and motor dysfunction in Parkinson's disease--a longitudinal study. Parkinsonism Relat Disord. 2013;19(12):1084–7.
56. Lavault S, Leu-Semenescu S, Tezenas du Montcel S, Cochen de Cock V, Vidailhet M, Arnulf I. Does clinical rapid eye movement behavior disorder predict worse outcomes in Parkinson's disease? J Neurol. 2010;257(7):1154–9.
57. Zhang TM, Yu SY, Guo P, Du Y, Hu Y, Piao YS, et al. Nonmotor symptoms in patients with Parkinson disease: a cross-sectional observational study. Medicine. 2016;95(50):e5400.
58. Malliani A, Pagani M, Lombardi F, Cerutti S. Cardiovascular neural regulation explored in the frequency domain. Circulation. 1991;84(2):482–92.
59. Sorensen GL, Mehlsen J, Jennum P. Reduced sympathetic activity in idiopathic rapid-eye-movement sleep behavior disorder and Parkinson's disease. Auton Neurosci. 2013;179(1–2):138–41.
60. Sauvageot N, Vaillant M, Diederich NJ. Reduced sympathetically driven heart rate variability during sleep in Parkinson's disease: a case-control polysomnography-based study. Mov Disord. 2011;26(2):234–40.
61. Covassin N, Neikrug AB, Liu L, Maglione J, Natarajan L, Corey-Bloom J, et al. Relationships between clinical characteristics and nocturnal cardiac autonomic activity in Parkinson's disease. Auton Neurosci. 2012;171(1–2):85–8.
62. Palma JA, Urrestarazu E, Alegre M, Pastor MA, Valencia M, Artieda J, et al. Cardiac autonomic impairment during sleep is linked with disease severity in Parkinson's disease. Clin Neurophysiol. 2013;124(6):1163–8.
63. Sorensen GL, Kempfner J, Zoetmulder M, Sorensen HB, Jennum P. Attenuated heart rate response in REM sleep behavior disorder and Parkinson's disease. Mov Disord. 2012;27(7):888–94.
64. Alonso A, Huang X, Mosley TH, Heiss G, Chen H. Heart rate variability and the risk of Parkinson disease: the Atherosclerosis Risk in Communities study. Ann Neurol. 2015;77(5):877–83.
65. Jain S, Ton TG, Perera S, Zheng Y, Stein PK, Thacker E, et al. Cardiovascular physiology in premotor Parkinson's disease: a neuroepidemiologic study. Mov Disord. 2012;27(8):988–95.
66. Ferini-Strambi L, Oldani A, Zucconi M, Smirne S. Cardiac autonomic activity during wakefulness and sleep in REM sleep behavior disorder. Sleep. 1996;19(5):367–9.
67. Lanfranchi PA, Fradette L, Gagnon JF, Colombo R, Montplaisir J. Cardiac autonomic regulation during sleep in idiopathic REM sleep behavior disorder. Sleep. 2007;30(8):1019–25.
68. Postuma RB, Lanfranchi PA, Blais H, Gagnon JF, Montplaisir JY. Cardiac autonomic dysfunction in idiopathic REM sleep behavior disorder. Mov Disord. 2010;25(14):2304–10.
69. Barone DA, Ebben MR, Samie A, Mortara D, Krieger AC. Autonomic dysfunction in isolated rapid eye movement sleep without atonia. Clin Neurophysiol. 2015;126(4):731–5.
70. Yamashina S, Yamazaki J. Neuronal imaging using SPECT. Eur J Nucl Med Mol Imaging. 2007;34(Suppl 1):S62–73.
71. Taki J, Nakajima K, Hwang EH, Matsunari I, Komai K, Yoshita M, et al. Peripheral sympathetic dysfunction in patients with Parkinson's disease without autonomic failure is heart selective and disease specific. Eur J Nucl Med. 2000;27(5):566–73.
72. Miyamoto T, Miyamoto M, Inoue Y, Usui Y, Suzuki K, Hirata K. Reduced cardiac 123I-MIBG scintigraphy in idiopathic REM sleep behavior disorder. Neurology. 2006;67(12):2236–8.
73. Orimo S, Amino T, Itoh Y, Takahashi A, Kojo T, Uchihara T, et al. Cardiac sympathetic denervation precedes neuronal loss in the sympathetic ganglia in Lewy body disease. Acta Neuropathol. 2005;109(6):583–8.
74. Kashihara K, Imamura T, Shinya T. Cardiac 123I-MIBG uptake is reduced more markedly in patients with REM sleep behavior disorder than in those with early stage Parkinson's disease. Parkinsonism Relat Disord. 2010;16(4):252–5.
75. Oguri T, Tachibana N, Mitake S, Kawanishi T, Fukuyama H. Decrease in myocardial 123I-MIBG radioactivity in REM sleep behavior disorder: two patients with different clinical progression. Sleep Med. 2008;9(5):583–5.
76. Nomura T, Inoue Y, Hogl B, Uemura Y, Kitayama M, Abe T, et al. Relationship between (123)I-MIBG scintigrams and REM sleep behavior disorder in Parkinson's disease. Parkinsonism Relat Disord. 2010;16(10):683–5.
77. Miyamoto T, Miyamoto M, Iwanami M, Hirata K. Cardiac 123I-MIBG accumulation in Parkinson's disease differs in association with REM sleep behavior disorder. Parkinsonism Relat Disord. 2011;17(3):219–20.
78. Kim JS, Park HE, Oh YS, Lee SH, Park JW, Son BC, et al. Orthostatic hypotension and cardiac sympathetic denervation in Parkinson disease patients with REM sleep behavioral disorder. J Neurol Sci. 2016;362:59–63.
79. Miyamoto T, Miyamoto M, Suzuki K, Nishibayashi M, Iwanami M, Hirata K. 123I-MIBG cardiac scintigraphy provides clues to the underlying neurodegenerative disorder in idiopathic REM sleep behavior disorder. Sleep. 2008;31(5):717–23.

80. Barateau L, Jaussent I, Lopez R, Evangelista E, Chenini S, Benkiran M, et al. Cardiac sympathetic activity differentiates idiopathic and symptomatic rapid eye movement sleep behaviour disorder. Sci Rep. 2018;8(1):7304.
81. Frauscher B, Nomura T, Duerr S, Ehrmann L, Gschliesser V, Wenning GK, et al. Investigation of autonomic function in idiopathic REM sleep behavior disorder. J Neurol. 2012;259(6):1056–61.
82. Al-Qassabi A, Pelletier A, Fereshtehnejad SM, Postuma RB. Autonomic sweat responses in rem sleep behavior disorder and parkinsonism. J Parkinsons Dis. 2018;8(3):463–8.
83. Knudsen K, Fedorova TD, Hansen AK, Sommerauer M, Haase AM, Svendsen KB, et al. Objective intestinal function in patients with idiopathic REM sleep behavior disorder. Parkinsonism Relat Disord. 2019;58:28–34.
84. Knudsen K, Fedorova TD, Hansen AK, Sommerauer M, Otto M, Svendsen KB, et al. In-vivo staging of pathology in REM sleep behaviour disorder: a multimodality imaging case-control study. Lancet Neurol. 2018;17(7):618–28.
85. Orimo S, Uchihara T, Nakamura A, Mori F, Kakita A, Wakabayashi K, et al. Axonal alpha-synuclein aggregates herald centripetal degeneration of cardiac sympathetic nerve in Parkinson's disease. Brain. 2008;131(Pt 3):642–50.
86. Katz R. Biomarkers and surrogate markers: an FDA perspective. NeuroRx. 2004;1(2):189–95.
87. Michell AW, Luheshi LM, Barker RA. Skin and platelet alpha-synuclein as peripheral biomarkers of Parkinson's disease. Neurosci Lett. 2005;381(3):294–8.
88. Beach TG, Adler CH, Sue LI, Vedders L, Lue L, White Iii CL, et al. Multi-organ distribution of phosphorylated alpha-synuclein histopathology in subjects with Lewy body disorders. Acta Neuropathol. 2010;119(6):689–702.
89. Shannon KM, Keshavarzian A, Dodiya HB, Jakate S, Kordower JH. Is alpha-synuclein in the colon a biomarker for premotor Parkinson's disease? Evidence from 3 cases. Mov Disord. 2012;27(6):716–9.
90. Jager WDH, Bethlem J. The distribution of Lewy bodies in the central and autonomic nervous systems in idiopathic paralysis agitans. J Neurol Neurosurg Psychiatry. 1960;23:283–90.
91. Lebouvier T, Neunlist M, Bruley des Varannes S, Coron E, Drouard A, N'Guyen JM, et al. Colonic biopsies to assess the neuropathology of Parkinson's disease and its relationship with symptoms. PLoS One. 2010;5(9):e12728.
92. Lebouvier T, Chaumette T, Damier P, Coron E, Touchefeu Y, Vrignaud S, et al. Pathological lesions in colonic biopsies during Parkinson's disease. Gut. 2008;57(12):1741–3.
93. Beach TG, Adler CH, Dugger BN, Serrano G, Hidalgo J, Henry-Watson J, et al. Submandibular gland biopsy for the diagnosis of Parkinson disease. J Neuropathol Exp Neurol. 2013;72(2):130–6.
94. Miki Y, Tomiyama M, Ueno T, Haga R, Nishijima H, Suzuki C, et al. Clinical availability of skin biopsy in the diagnosis of Parkinson's disease. Neurosci Lett. 2010;469(3):357–9.
95. Kawada M, Tamada Y, Simizu H, Yanagishita T, Yamashita N, Ishida N, et al. Reduction in QSART and vasoactive intestinal polypeptide expression in the skin of Parkinson's disease patients and its relation to dyshidrosis. J Cutan Pathol. 2009;36(5):517–21.
96. Navarro-Otano J, Casanova-Molla J, Morales M, Valls-Sole J, Tolosa E. Cutaneous autonomic denervation in Parkinson's disease. J Neural Transm. 2015;122(8):1149–55.
97. Ikemura M, Saito Y, Sengoku R, Sakiyama Y, Hatsuta H, Kanemaru K, et al. Lewy body pathology involves cutaneous nerves. J Neuropathol Exp Neurol. 2008;67(10):945–53.
98. Beach TG, White CL, Hamilton RL, Duda JE, Iwatsubo T, Dickson DW, et al. Evaluation of alpha-synuclein immunohistochemical methods used by invited experts. Acta Neuropathol. 2008;116(3):277–88.
99. Donadio V, Incensi A, Cortelli P, Giannoccaro MP, Jaber MA, Baruzzi A, et al. Skin sympathetic fiber alpha-synuclein deposits: a potential biomarker for pure autonomic failure. Neurology. 2013;80(8):725–32.
100. Wang N, Gibbons CH. Skin biopsies in the assessment of the autonomic nervous system. Handb Clin Neurol. 2013;117:371–8.
101. Wang N, Gibbons CH, Lafo J, Freeman R. alpha-Synuclein in cutaneous autonomic nerves. Neurology. 2013;81(18):1604–10.
102. Gibbons CH, Garcia J, Wang N, Shih LC, Freeman R. The diagnostic discrimination of cutaneous alpha-synuclein deposition in Parkinson disease. Neurology. 2016;87(5):505–12.
103. Doppler K, Jentschke HM, Schulmeyer L, Vadasz D, Janzen A, Luster M, et al. Dermal phospho-alpha-synuclein deposits confirm REM sleep behaviour disorder as prodromal Parkinson's disease. Acta Neuropathol. 2017;133(4):535–45.
104. Antelmi E, Donadio V, Incensi A, Plazzi G, Liguori R. Skin nerve phosphorylated alpha-synuclein deposits in idiopathic REM sleep behavior disorder. Neurology. 2017;88(22):2128–31.
105. Doppler K, Ebert S, Uceyler N, Trenkwalder C, Ebentheuer J, Volkmann J, et al. Cutaneous neuropathy in Parkinson's disease: a window into brain pathology. Acta Neuropathol. 2014;128(1):99–109.
106. Sateia MJ. International classification of sleep disorders-third edition: highlights and modifications. Chest. 2014;146(5):1387–94.
107. Germain A, Nielsen TA. Sleep pathophysiology in posttraumatic stress disorder and idiopathic nightmare sufferers. Biol Psychiatry. 2003;54(10):1092–8.
108. Mellman TA, Kumar A, Kulick-Bell R, Kumar M, Nolan B. Nocturnal/daytime urine noradrenergic measures and sleep in combat-related PTSD. Biol Psychiatry. 1995;38(3):174–9.
109. Feemster JC, Smith KL, McCarter SJ, St Louis EK. Trauma-associated sleep disorder: a posttraumatic stress/REM sleep behavior disorder mash-up? J Clin Sleep Med. 2019;15(2):345–9.
110. Ross RJ, Ball WA, Dinges DF, Kribbs NB, Morrison AR, Silver SM, et al. Motor dysfunction during sleep in posttraumatic stress disorder. Sleep. 1994;17(8):723–32.
111. Garcia-Rill E. Disorders of the reticular activating system. Med Hypotheses. 1997;49(5):379–87.

Multiple System Atrophy

23

Roberto Vetrugno

Introduction

Multiple system atrophy (MSA) is an adult-onset, progressive, and fatal neurodegenerative disease characterized by a variable combination of parkinsonian features, cerebellar impairment, corticospinal signs, and autonomic dysfunction [1]. The latter includes orthostatic hypotension (OH) and bladder, bowel, sexual, and breathing disorders. Moreover, sleep disorders are frequent and severe in MSA, consisting of insomnia, daytime sleepiness, restless legs syndrome (RLS), REM sleep behavior disorder (RBD), and sleep disordered breathing (SDB).

MSA is a unifying term introduced by Graham and Oppenheimer in 1969 [2] to bring together a group of neurodegenerative syndromes with overlapping clinical features and brain pathology, i.e., olivopontocerebellar atrophy (OPCA) [3], striatonigral degeneration (SND) [4], and Shy-Drager syndrome (SDS, parkinsonism with autonomic failure) [5]. The clinical abnormalities are due to a complex pathophysiology that reflects neurodegeneration of cortical areas, the basal ganglia, brainstem, and cerebellum [6–10]. Widespread neuronal degeneration results in a short median survival time, ranging across studies from 6 to 10 years [11].

Although MSA is regarded as a sporadic disease, genetic factors have been implicated in the etiology of this disorder in some cases. These include copy number loss of C-terminal Src homology 2 Adapter Protein 2 (*SHC2*) [12], *SNCA gene* (synuclein alpha) single-nucleotide polymorphisms [13, 14], and mutation in the *CoQ2 gene* which encodes for 4 hydroxbenzoate polyprenyltransferase, an enzyme involved in coenzyme Q10 biosynthesis [15, 16]. Notably, a genome-wide association study in MSA identified single nucleotide polymorphisms in four genes which did not include SNCA or CoQ2 [17].

According to clinical diagnostic criteria, two major subtypes may be distinguished by their predominant motor features. The variant characterized by parkinsonian features is designed MSA-P (parkinsonian subtype), while cerebellar ataxia is the main motor presentation in MSA-C (cerebellar subtype) [7, 18]. Nevertheless, autonomic failure is observed almost universally in both motor presentations [1].

The pathologic hallmark is the accumulation of aggregated alpha-synuclein (α-syn), which qualifies MSA as a synucleinopathy together with Parkinson's disease (PD) and dementia with Lewy bodies (DLB). In Lewy body diseases (PD and DLB), α-syn aggregates in neurons such as Lewy bodies (LBs) and Lewy neurites. In contrast, MSA is characterized by the accumulation of α-syn in oligodendrocytes as glial cytoplasmic inclusions (GCIs). Moreover, it seems that pathological α-syn such as GCIs and LBs (GCI-α-syn and LB-α-syn) are conformationally and biologically distinct, with GCI-α-syn forming more compact structures and being ~1000-fold more potent than LB-α-syn in seeding α-syn aggregation, which is consistent with the highly aggressive nature of MSA [19, 20].

Epidemiology and Natural History

MSA affects 3–5 people out of every 100,000 in the general population [7]. The estimated annual incidence of MSA in the population >50 years old is approximately 3 per 100,000 [21]. The estimated prevalence of MSA is between 2 and 5 cases per 100,000 population [22, 23]. There is no specific racial predilection, and the disease has been reported in Caucasian, African, and Asian populations.

Retrospective and prospective studies report survival between 6.2 and 10 years in MSA [24–27], with average age of onset ranging from 53 to 63 years [26–28]. Few patients have been reported surviving more than 15 years [29].

The onset of MSA before 40 is referred to as young-onset MSA [30], and some specific clues (e.g., the presence of

R. Vetrugno (✉)
Department of Neurology–Neurophysiology, Casa di Cura Madre Fortunata Toniolo, Bologna, Italy

S. Chokroverty, P. Cortelli (eds.), *Autonomic Nervous System and Sleep*, https://doi.org/10.1007/978-3-030-62263-3_23

dystonia, myoclonus, or pyramidal signs) may help identify these young-onset MSA patients [31]. A great variability in clinical factors have been reported as predictive of shortened survival. In particular, older age of onset [24, 32–35], gender (male or female) [25, 32, 34], MSA-P subtype [24, 25, 36, 37], and early or initial autonomic symptoms [27, 28, 34, 35, 38] seem to be associated with worse survival, while late development of autonomic failure has been reported as a favorable prognostic factor [29, 39]. However, with regard to the natural history of the disease whether there are any differences between the MSA-P and MSA-C subtypes remains a matter of debate [11]. In this regard, Coon and co-workers investigated the role of autonomic testing as a mean of evaluating survival in a large number of patients with MSA ($n = 685$) and concluded that the results of such tests can serve as a prognostic marker [40]. All MSA patients underwent comprehensive standardized autonomic testing. The median survival was 7.51 years with no difference between MSA subtype and gender. Older age of onset and both motor and autonomic clinical features predicted shorter survival. In particular, motor symptoms of falls within 3 years, autonomic manifestations of bladder symptoms (e.g., urinary catheterization) within 3 years, and symptoms related to orthostatic intolerance developing within a year from the onset were the strongest predictors of shorter survival. The finding that early and generalized autonomic dysfunction over the disease course (though not the prevalent motor phenotype) is associated with shorter survival in MSA underscores the importance of standardized autonomic testing not only as a means of identifying this disease but also as an important prognostic indicator.

Clinical Features

Bradykinesia and rigidity, postural instability and freezing (akinetic rigid form) characterizes the motor presentation of the parkinsonian subtype of MSA. The presence of classical pill rolling rest tremor, which is common in Parkinson's disease, is unusual in MSA patient, whereas postural action tremor with superimposed jerks is seen in half of all patients. In particular, abnormal hand and finger movements in patients with MSA-P are a form of postural and action myoclonus described as mini-polymyoclonus [41]. Postural stability is massively impaired, and freezing of gait may be observed in the majority of MSA patients still ambulant [18]. Other warning signs that herald parkinsonism in MSA include falls usually within 3 years of motor onset, pyramidal signs with extensor plantar response, and rapid progression regardless of dopaminergic treatment [42].

Cerebellar ataxia dominates the motor disorder of MSA-C patients, but it is also present in nearly half of MSA-P patients, underpinning the multisystem character of this disease [18]. Cerebellar dysfunctions manifest as gait ataxia, limb ataxia, ataxic dysarthria, and cerebellar-type of abnormal eye movement disorders, i.e., gaze-evoked nystagmus, impaired smooth pursuit with saccadic intrusion, and ocular dysmetria.

"Abnormal postures" may be associated with the motor presentation of MSA in 16–42% patients and include Pisa syndrome (reversible lateral bending of the trunk), disproportionate antecollis and/or contractures of hand or feet (excluding Dupuytren disease or contracture due to other known cause) [43].

The speech pattern in patients with MSA is also characteristic. In addition to the hypophonic monotony, patients with MSA-P also have an increase in pitch and quivering, strained element to their speech. By contrast, patients with MSA-C have a more typical cerebellar scanning dysarthria [11].

Dysphagia is prominent in both MSA-P and MSA-C. The characteristics of dysphagia in MSA-P are consistent with the parkinsonian syndrome, which manifests as swallowing dysfunction in the oral phase, such as delayed bolus transport from the oral cavity to the pharynx and disturbance of bolus holding in the oral cavity. This is as a result of bradykinesia and rigidity of the tongue, which is related to parkinsonism [44, 45]. In addition to the oral phase, parkinsonism disrupts the normal sequencing of the pharyngeal phase, causing a reduction or absence of relaxation of the cricopharyngeal muscle [46–48]. On the other hand, in MSA-C, disturbed coordination of tongue movement by cerebellar dysfunction, rather than parkinsonism, results in swallowing dysfunction in the oral phase [45]. Patients with MSA-P commence diet modification earlier than those with MSA-C, despite no significant difference in the latency to onset of tube feeding. Deterioration of dysphagia may be more pronounced in the oral function (such as lip, tongue, and masticatory function) of MSA patients [49].

Dysautonomia is a core clinical criterion for MSA [50]. Autonomic dysfunction can precede the onset of motor symptoms of MSA in up to 50% of patients [51]. Urinary dysfunction and orthostatic hypotension (OH) are the most frequent dysautonomic symptoms of MSA, with an earlier onset of urinary symptoms particularly in the cerebellar phenotype [51, 52]. In MSA, severe dysautonomia and the early combination of dysautonomic and motor symptoms are poor prognostic factors, regardless of the phenotype [40, 53].

OH, the main clinical feature of cardiovascular autonomic dysfunction, is defined as sustained drop in systolic pressure of at least 20 mm Hg or a sustained diastolic drop of at least 10 mm Hg within the first 3 min after standing up [54]. This time cutoff might not be sensitive for α-synucleinopathies, in which the presentation is most commonly that of delayed OH; therefore, measuring blood pressure for at least 10 min has been recommended. Delayed OH has been documented as a risk factor for MSA, which frequently progresses to OH with a high mortality [55]. OH affects around 43% of patients with MSA from early stages of the disease, and of these, 50% also display post-prandial hypotension as well as nocturnal and supine hypertension [51, 56, 57]. This condition is more frequent and more severe in the cerebellar subtype of MSA when compared to the parkinsonian subtype [58].

Constipation is defined as a frequency of less than three bowel movements in 1 week [59]. Constipation has been reported in MSA and may precede up to 10 years the onset of motor symptoms [60].

Up to 96% of MSA patients display urinary symptoms (i.e., nocturia, altered urinary frequency, urinary incontinence, and detrusor hyperactivity), which tend to be more severe than in PD. In 60% of MSA patients, urinary symptoms start before the onset of motor symptoms (with a mean of 4 years before diagnosis), mostly with post-residual volume alterations [56, 61, 62].

Erectile dysfunction, defined as the incapacity to achieve or maintain a penile erection long enough to allow a sexual relation [63], is present in up to 97% of men diagnosed with MSA. It is the initial symptom in 48% of male patients, preceding motor symptoms for as long as a decade [51, 60, 62].

Sleep and breathing disorders in MSA are frequent and severe. Their consequences on life quality and life expectancy are very important and justify a precise and efficacious management [64–66]. MSA patients complain about insomnia, daytime sleepiness, restless legs syndrome (RLS), rapid eye movement (REM) sleep behavior disorder (RBD), and breathing disorders mainly sleep disordered breathing (SDB). Sleep recordings (i.e., videopolysomnography – VPSG) confirm these disorders and show their severity.

RLS is an urge to move mostly the legs, usually associated with paresthesia that occurs or worsens at rest and during the evening or the night and is relieved by activity. RLS prevalence in MSA varies from 4.7% to 28% [67–70]. This prevalence may be overestimated since many symptoms of MSA may mimic those of RLS, including wearing off, dystonic and overnight motor symptoms, or akathisia. A diagnosis of RLS in MSA may therefore be quite challenging even when applying well-established diagnostic criteria [71]. On the other hand, RLS in MSA could be sometimes underestimated since almost a third of the patients explored undergoing a VPSG study presents RLS features with obvious restlessness at night, but without ever reporting it before in most of the cases [72]. Moreover, even if the prevalence of RLS seems to be increased in MSA compared to that in the general population, its pathophysiology remains unclear.

Periodic limb movements during sleep (PLMS) are stereotypic, repetitive, non-epileptiform movements of the legs, usually consisting of dorsiflexion of the ankle. They are usually reported by the co-sleeper and confirmed on the sleep recordings. They often increase sleep fragmentation. In MSA, PLM indexes (asleep, asleep with awakenings, and while awake) vary a lot across the studies [73–75]. The high indexes observed in some studies could be the result of the degeneration of the spinocerebellar pathways involved in PLM generation, probably more affected in MSA than in PD patients. Moreover, a decrease in the cortical and autonomic arousal responses to PLMS has been reported in MSA patients [76].

The most frequent abnormal movement disorder during sleep observed in MSA is RBD. RBD is a parasomnia characterized by the abnormal persistence of muscular tone during REM sleep allowing prominent motor activity accompanying dreaming, e.g., laughing, talking, shouting, kicking, fighting [77]. The dream-enacting behaviors can be violent leading to self or co-sleeper injuries [78] (Fig. 23.1). RBD can be idiopathic, but follow-up studies have shown that most patients tend to develop a neurodegenerative disorder, synucleinopathies most of the time (PD, DLB, or MSA) [79]. A recent meta-analysis has explored the prevalence of RBD in MSA and has shown very high summary prevalence of clinically suspected RBD with 73% in a total sample of 324 patients and a summary prevalence of VPSG-confirmed RBD even higher of 88% in a total sample of 217 patients [80]. This prevalence is much higher than that in PD where prevalence of RBD is usually reported in about 50% of the patients. The natural course of RBD in patients with MSA has been compared to patients with PD [81]. RBD symptoms in patients with MSA displayed a limited appearance in the period shortly before the onset of other neurological symptoms, but mostly disappeared within a few years after the onset of neurological symptoms. The number of MSA patients with RBD symptoms did not increase with the course of the disease. In PD, on the contrary, RBD symptoms seemed to increase with the course of the disease. As brain lesions in MSA spread more rapidly and widely than those in PD [82], RBD symptoms in MSA patients could disappear due to progressive neurodegeneration of the brainstem structures responsible for RBD. This could be linked to the occurrence of status dissociatus evolving from RBD over the course of the disease as previously reported [83].

Stridor is a harsh, high-pitched inspiratory sound due to a laryngeal narrowing, which may appear first during sleep in MSA patients and as the initial manifestation of the disease (Fig. 23.2). Specifically, stridor could be also expiratory when it is caused by an obstruction in the intrathoracic region, whereas inspiratory stridor is due to an extrathoracic obstruction in the upper airway. The reported prevalence of stridor in MSA varies from 15% to 40% of patients, depending on the methods of assessment [84]. Stridor is a red flag for the diagnosis of MSA with a high diagnostic positive predicted value [7, 85, 86] because it is rarely observed in other parkinsonian syndromes such as PD or progressive supranuclear palsy. Laryngoscopy is

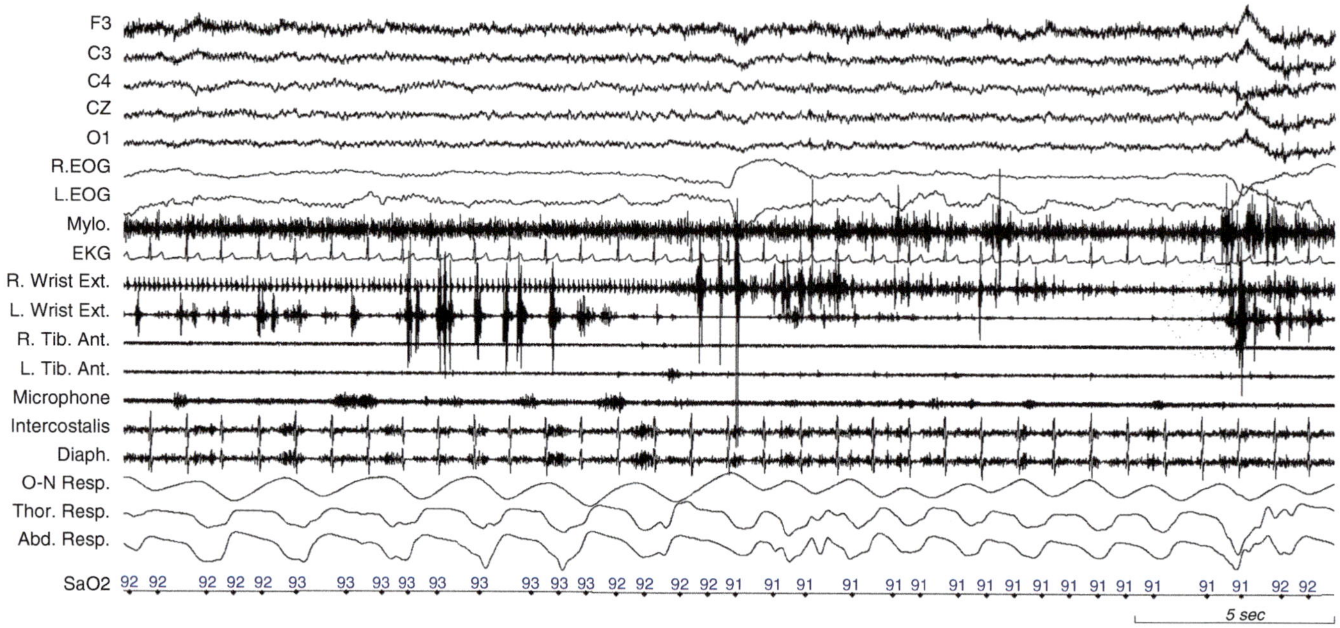

Fig. 23.1 Abnormal behavior with vigorous, mainly upper limb (*Wrist Ext.*), movements and vocalization (*Microphone*) emerging during REM sleep consistent with REM sleep behavior disorders in a multiple system atrophy patient with predominant parkinsonism (MSA-P). (EOG electro-oculogram, Mylo. mylohyoideus muscle, EKG electrocardiogram, Wrist Ext. wrist extensor muscle, Tib. Ant tibialis anterior muscle, Intercostalis intercostalis muscle, Diaph. diaphragmatic muscle, O-N Resp. oro-nasal respiratory trace, Thor. Resp. thoracic respiratory trace, Abd. Resp. abdominal respiratory trace, SaO_2 oxyhaemoglobin saturation)

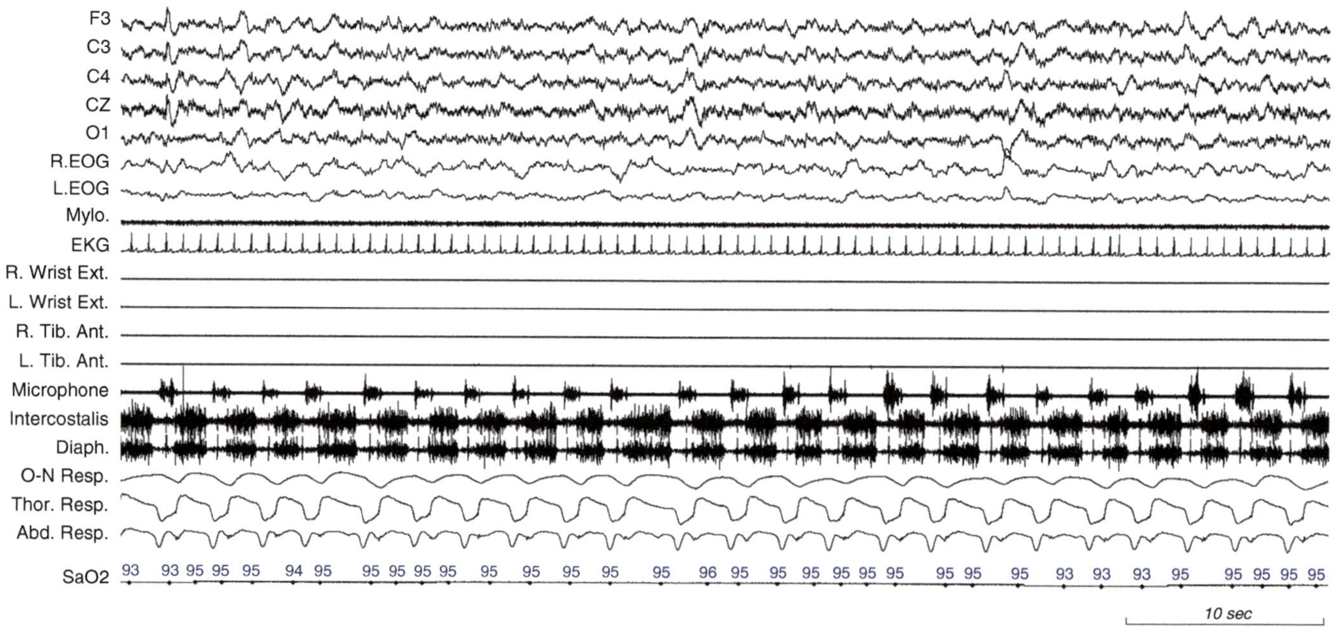

Fig. 23.2 NREM sleep recording (excerpts) in a multiple system atrophy patient with predominant cerebellar ataxia (MSA-C) and inspiratory stridor (*Microphone*). The activity of the microphone is in phase with the downward (inspiratory) deflection of the respiratory tracks. Dystonic subcontinuous muscle recruitment patterns are also seen in intercostalis and diaphragm muscles spanning almost continuously across the entire respiratory cycle (the inspiratory and especially expiratory phases). Note the absence of significant oxyhemoglobin saturation (SaO_2) changes. (EOG electro-oculogram, Mylo. mylohyoideus muscle, EKG electrocardiogram, Wrist Ext. wrist extensor muscle, Tib. Ant tibialis anterior muscle, Intercostalis intercostalis muscle*, Diaph. diaphragmatic muscle†, O-N Resp. oro-nasal respiratory trace, Thor. Resp. thoracic respiratory trace, Abd. Resp. abdominal respiratory trace)

*Intercostalis electrodes are placed at least 2 cm apart on the second anterior intercostal space lateral to the sternum

†Diaphragmatic electrodes are placed at the seventh intercostal space on the anterior axillary line on the right to reduce cardiac artifact

very useful in the diagnosis of stridor showing the reduction of the glottis aperture in the larynx, paradoxical cord movements, and floppy epiglottis [87]. Serial examination may be needed because of the fluctuation of the symptom. The partial or complete reduction of the vocal cord abduction has been attributed to denervation of laryngeal muscles [85] or to adduction dystonia of vocal cords [88]. Stridor is a life-threatening condition as it may lead to acute respiratory failure and sudden death. Tracheostomy or continuous positive airway pressure (CPAP) are the two main options to treat stridor [89–91]. Both treatments are effective but CPAP as a noninvasive therapy is usually considered first. In cases where CPAP is not well tolerated, if stridor is present during the daytime and if immobile vocal cords on laryngoscopy appear, tracheostomy should be preferred. It has been reported that tracheostomy may increase central sleep apneas in some cases [92]. However, in a recent study based on a large number of MSA patients with stridor (n = 136), Giannini et al. have shown that treatment is associated with longer survival and that tracheostomy tends to increase life expectancy in patients more than CPAP [66]. Botulinum toxin, unilateral cordectomy, and laser arytenoidectomy have also been proposed [89]. Giannini et al. again in their large study have demonstrated that it was not the presence of stridor but its presence in early stage of the disease that was an independent risk factor for shorter survival [66]. Early stridor may be indeed the harbinger for severe early change in autonomic centers controlling respiration and other vital functions, accounting for the reduction in life expectancy in MSA [88, 93, 94].

Central breathing disorders in MSA include central apnea, Cheyne-Stokes breathing during sleep, sometimes wakefulness, and sleep-related dysrhythmic breathing patterns [95]. These disorders are usually observed in later stages of MSA but may be a presenting feature [96]. Moreover, obstructive disorders can become central in the evolution of the disease [97]. Central sleep apnea may be a manifestation of impaired ventilatory chemosensitivity but, despite its potential pathophysiological significance, ventilatory chemosensitivity has rarely been studied systematically in MSA. Diminished ventilatory response to hypercapnia has been reported in one MSA case [98], whereas impaired ventilatory responses to hypoxia, but not to hypercapnia, have been documented in cerebellar predominant MSA cases [99]. Patients with MSA may also exhibit dysrhythmic breathing [100, 101], including Cheyne-Stokes respiration [98], cluster breathing [102], periodic inspiratory gasps [83, 103], and arrhythmic respiration with central alveolar hypoventilation [104]. Central breathing disorders in MSA result from the neurodegeneration of the brain stem causing dysfunction of the centers for regulation of respiration [93]. In patients with central breathing disorders, CPAP therapy may not be beneficial and the use of adaptive servo-ventilation is also recommended.

In MSA, obstructive sleep apnea (OSA) occurs more frequently than central sleep apnea, ranging from 15% to 37% of the cases [74, 105]. OSA results from narrowing of the upper airway at the level of the vocal cords, laryngeal inlet, base of the tongue, and soft palate [106]. Hypokinesia, rigidity, dystonia, and paralysis of the upper airway muscles may also predispose to OSA in MSA [107]. CPAP may be an effective treatment for eliminating obstructive sleep apnea in MSA patients [65, 90, 108], mainly in patients at early stages of the disease. Adaptation to CPAP may be difficult in advanced cases [108]. Moreover, floppy epiglottis can be a contraindication of CPAP in patients with MSA. A floppy epiglottis may indeed cause laryngeal obstruction when the epiglottis is sucked into the laryngeal inlet during inspiration, and CPAP may exacerbate upper airway obstruction by further promoting the downward displacement of the epiglottis into the laryngeal inlet [109]. Moreover, MSA patients could experience sudden death despite CPAP use [110].

Clinical Assessment of MSA

Clinical tests designed to measure the end-organ responses to the autonomic nervous systems can be used to quantitatively analyze autonomic dysfunction, playing an important role in the clinical assessment of MSA. Tests of cardiovagal function include heart rate variability with deep breathing, postural changes (such as the head-up tilt test), or the Valsalva maneuver, in which the patient forcefully exhales into a sphygmomanometer with an open glottis at a pressure of 40 mmHg for 15 s. Sympathetic adrenergic function can be assessed by measuring blood pressure response to postural change, Valsalva maneuver or isometric exercise, as well as by the cold pressor test, in which the subject is instructed to immerse his or her hand in ice water for 1 min [111]. The decrease of heart rate and blood pressure variability can be accurately demonstrated through power spectrum techniques, which provide a quantitative assessment of such variability [112]. Ambulatory blood pressure monitoring can also provide sensitive markers of autonomous nervous system failure, such as post-prandial hypotension and nocturnal/supine hypertension [113, 114]. Clinical assessments of sudomotor function include thermoregulatory sweat testing, quantitative sudomotor axon reflex testing, silicone impression, sympathetic skin response, acetylcholine sweat-spot test, and quantitative direct and indirect axon reflex testing, as well as electromyographic skin potentials [115–117]. Cutaneous autonomic pilomotor testing, in which iontophoresis of phenylephrine induces a local neurogenic pilomotor erection ("goose bumps") as a measure of functional integrity of autonomic skin nerve fibers, is an approach to capture the progression of autonomic nerve dysfunction and α-synuclein deposition [118]. Differential diagnosis of the parkinsonian subtype of MSA and PD or other parkinsonian syndromes is mostly based on the evaluation of autonomic dysfunction [51, 119]. Clinical autonomic cardiovascular tests can distinguish MSA and PD with a sensitivity of 91% and a specificity of 92%. 123-I-myocardial metaiodobenzylguanidine ($^{123\text{-}I}$MIBG) scintigraphy can distinguish these entities with a sensitivity of 90% and specificity of 82% [51, 120]. Cardiovagal baroreflex is also sensitive for the differentiation between MSA and PD, being disproportionally affected in MSA [121]. Added sweating and thermoregulation tests have also been found to improve differential diagnostic reliability [122, 123].

Current consensus guidelines include neuroimaging criteria for the diagnosis of possible MSA [7] (Table 23.1). These include the presence of atrophy of the putamen, middle cerebellar peduncle, pons, or cerebellum on brain magnetic resonance imaging (MRI), and putamen, brainstem, or cerebellum hypometabolism on brain fluorodeoxyglucose (FDG) positron emission tomography (PET), as well as dopaminergic denervation on PET or single photon emission computed tomography (SPECT) [124].

As sleep disorders in MSA are frequent and severe, sleep recordings should be recommended to all patients with MSA, sometimes without delay when stridor is suspected. Explorations should be repeated in time since sleep disorders can vary with the evolution of the disease.

The latest consensus diagnostic criteria for MSA consider dementia as a non-supporting feature of the disease [7]. There is increasing evidence, however, showing that cognitive impairment may be an integral part of the disease [125–127]. Cognitive disturbances in MSA occur across a wide spectrum ranging from mild single domain deficits to impairments in multiple domains and even to frank dementia in rare cases. Frontal-executive dysfunction is the most common presentation, while memory and visuospatial abilities may also be impaired [126, 128]. Thus, all patients with MSA should be screened for cognitive impairment with a standardized test, even if operational guidelines for the diagnosis and treatment of cognitive impairment in MSA are lacking.

Table 23.1 Current consensus criteria for the diagnosis of multiple system atrophy (MSA)

Criteria for definite MSA include neuropathological findings during postmortem examination of:
(a) Widespread and abundant cerebral α-synuclein-positive glial cytoplasmic inclusions
(b) Neurodegenerative changes in striatonigral or olivopontocerebellar region
Criteria for probable MSA include a sporadic progressive adult (>30 years old) onset disease characterized by the following:
(a) Autonomic failure involving urinary incontinence (inability to control the release of urine from the bladder with erectile dysfunction in males) or an orthostatic decrease of blood pressure within 3 min of standing by at least 30 mm Hg systolic or 15 mm Hg diastolic, *and*
(b) Poor levodopa-responsive parkinsonism (bradykinesia with rigidity, tremor, or postural instability), *or*
(c) A cerebellar syndrome (gait ataxia with cerebellar dysarthria, limb ataxia, or cerebellar oculomotor dysfunction)
Criteria for possible MSA include a sporadic progressive adult (>30 years old) onset disease characterized by the following:
(a) Parkinsonism (bradykinesia with rigidity tremor or postural instability), *or*
(b) Cerebellar syndrome (gait ataxia with cerebellar dysarthria limb ataxia or cerebellar oculomotor dysfunction), *and*
(c) At least one feature suggesting autonomic dysfunction (otherwise unexplained urinary urgency frequency or incomplete bladder emptying, erectile dysfunction in males, or significant orthostatic blood pressure decline that does not meet the level required in probable MSA), *and*
(d) At least one of the following features:
Babinski sign with hyperreflexia
Stridor
Rapidly progressive parkinsonism
Poor response to levodopa
Postural instability within 3 years of motor onset
Gait ataxia, cerebellar dysarthria, limb ataxia, or cerebellar oculomotor dysfunction
Dysphagia within 5 years of motor onset
Atrophy on MRI of putamen middle cerebellar peduncle, pons, or cerebellum
Hypometabolism on FDG-PET in putamen, brainstem, or cerebellum
Presynaptic nigrostriatal dopaminergic denervation on SPECT or PET

MRI magnetic resonance imaging, *FDG-PET* fluorodeoxyglucose-positron emission tomography, *SPECT* single photon emission computed tomography

Diagnosis

Due to overlapping clinical presentations, the distinction between early-stage MSA, PD, and atypical parkinsonian disorders (including pure autonomic failure or adult-onset cerebellar ataxia) may be difficult [129–133]. Revised consensus guidelines define three degrees of certainty of the clinical diagnosis of MSA: definite, probable, and possible [7] (Table 23.1).

Definite MSA requires postmortem evidence of widespread α-syn positive inclusions with concomitant SND or OPCA [6].

Probable MSA is defined as a sporadic, progressive disorder in adults, clinically characterized by severe autonomic failure, urinary dysfunction, and poor levodopa-responsive parkinsonism or cerebellar ataxia.

Possible MSA can be diagnosed, when a sporadic, progressive adult-onset disorder with parkinsonism or cerebellar ataxia is accompanied by at least one of the additional features suggesting autonomic or urogenital dysfunction plus one other clinical or neuroimaging abnormality.

Recognition of patients with early or possible MSA may be supported by including one or more "red flags" (warning signs); two or more out of six red flags had a specificity of 98.3% and a sensitivity of 84.2% [18, 31, 43].

No reliable diagnostic and prognostic fluid biomarkers are currently available, although many studies suggest that a combination of CSF biomarkers, such as DJ-1, phospho-tau, light chain neurofilament protein, and $A\beta_{42}$ may be helpful in the differential diagnosis between MSA and other parkinsonian disorders [134, 135].

As cardiac sympathetic postganglionic denervation distinguishes PD from MSA patients showing intact innervation, $^{123\text{-}I}$MIBG scan can help differentiate the two disorders [136]. Despite some overlap with PD (reduced $^{123\text{-}I}$MIBG uptake), the presence of normal or only mildly reduced tracer uptake supports the diagnosis of MSA-P [137]. In patients with isolated autonomic failure, $^{123\text{-}I}$MIBG myocardial scintigraphy may be a valuable predictor of conversion to MSA [138].

Odor identification tests showing severe loss of smell may exclude MSA [139], separating PD from MSA with a sensitivity of 76.7% and a specificity of 95.7% [140].

MRI abnormalities including the "hot-cross bun" sign, a cruciform hyperintensity in the pons [141], and the "putaminal rim sign" (that marks hyperintensity bordering the dorsolateral margin of the putamen in T2-weighted MRI reflecting degeneration and iron Fe^{3+} deposition) may differentiate MSA-P from PD [142–144]. They are, however, non-specific signs and, therefore, not included in the recent consensus criteria [7], while putaminal atrophy shows 92.3% specificity but low sensitivity (44.4%) for distinguishing MSA-P from PD [145]. The combination of "swallow-tail" sign and putaminal hypointensity can increase the accuracy of discrimination between MSA and idiopathic PD [146].

Ancillary investigations for MSA have been summarized recently [1]. Skin biopsy is a promising diagnostic tool for the in vivo diagnosis of synucleinopathies, and in MSA, a peculiar pattern of skin misfolded α-syn aggregates has been reported [147–150].

Current Therapies

Although symptomatic therapies are available for parkinsonism and autonomic failures, their response is often poor if not absent, and no effective disease-modifying therapies are currently available. However, due to remarkable progress in our understanding of the etiopathogenesis of MSA, novel therapeutic targets have emerged from preclinical studies and interventional trials [1, 151]. Levodopa responsiveness has been reported initially in 83% of MSA-P patients, but the effect is usually transient and only 31% showed a response for a period of 3.5 years. According to international diagnostic criteria, a "poor" levodopa response is indeed the hallmark of probable MSA with predominant parkinsonism (MSA-P), while a "good" and sustained response is diagnostic for PD. At this regard, estimation of pharmacodynamic variables after a subacute low levodopa dose test may be also a simple and practical clinical tool to aid the differential diagnosis between MSA-P and PD [152].

In some patients, motor fluctuations with wearing-off phenomena or off-bound dystonia have been observed. Deep brain stimulation could not be recommended for MSA [153], while active immunization against α-syn and combination with anti-inflammatory treatment may be promising therapeutic strategies [154]. Clarifying the pathogenic mechanisms of MSA will improve the therapeutic approach to disease.

References

1. Fanciulli A, Wenning GK. Multiple-system atrophy. N Engl J Med. 2015;372(3):249–63.
2. Graham JG, Oppenheimer DR. Orthostatic hypotension and nicotine sensitivity in a case of multiple system atrophy. J Neurol Neurosurg Psychiatry. 1969;32(1):28–34.
3. Dejerine TA. L'atrophie olivo-ponto-cérébelleuse. Nouvelle Iconographie de la Salpêtrière: Clinique des Maladies du Système Nerveux. 1900;13:330–70.
4. Adams R, Van Bogaert L, van der Eecken H. [Nigro-striate and cerebello-nigro-striate degeneration. (Clinical uniqueness and pathological variability of presenile degeneration of extrapyramidal rigidity type)]. Psychiatr Neurol (Basel). 1961;142:219–59. [*Article in French*].
5. Shy GM, Drager GA. A neurological syndrome associated with orthostatic hypotension: a clinical-pathologic study. Arch Neurol. 1960;2:511–27.
6. Trojanowski JQ, Revesz T. Proposed neuropathological criteria for the post mortem diagnosis of multiple system atrophy; Neuropathology Working Group on MSA. Neuropathol Appl Neurobiol. 2007;33:615–20.
7. Gilman S, Wenning GK, Low PA, Brooks DJ, Mathias CJ, Trojanowski JQ, et al. Second consensus statement on the diagnosis of multiple system atrophy. Neurology. 2008;71(9):670–6.
8. Bologna M, Marsili L, Khan N, Parvez AK, Paparella G, Modugno N, et al. Blinking in patients with clinically probable multiple system atrophy. Mov Disord. 2014;29(3):415–20.
9. Suppa A, Marsili L, Di Stasio F, Latorre A, Parvez AK, Colosimo C, et al. Primary motor cortex long-term plasticity in multiple system atrophy. Mov Disord. 2014;29(1):97–104.
10. Cykowski MD, Coon EA, Powell SZ, Jenkins SM, Benarroch EE, Low P, et al. Expanding the spectrum of neuronal pathology in multiple system atrophy. Brain. 2015;138(Pt 8):2293–309.
11. Wenning GK, Colosimo C, Geser F, Poewe W. Multiple system atrophy. Lancet Neurol. 2004;3(3):93–103. Review. Erratum in Lancet Neurol. 2004;3(3):137.
12. Ferguson MC, Garland EM, Hedges L, Womack-Nunley B, Hamid R, Phillips JA 3rd, et al. SHC2 gene copy number in multiple system atrophy (MSA). Clin Auton Res. 2014;24(1):25–30.

13. Scholz SW, Houlden H, Schulte C, Sharma M, Li A, Berg D, et al. SNCA variants are associated with increased risk for multiple system atrophy. Ann Neurol. 2009;65(5):610–4.
14. Al-Chalabi A, Dürr A, Wood NW, Parkinson MH, Camuzat A, Hulot JS, et al.; NNIPPS Genetic Study Group. Genetic variants of the alpha-synuclein sene SNCA are associated with multiple system atrophy. PLoS One. 2009;4(9):e7114.
15. Multiple-System Atrophy Research Collaboration. Mutations in COQ2 in familial and sporadic multiple-system atrophy. N Engl J Med. 2013;369(3):233–44.
16. Stefanova N, Reindl M, Neumann M, Haass C, Poewe W, Kahle PJ, Wenning GK. Oxidative stress in transgenic mice with oligodendroglial alpha-synuclein overexpression replicates the neuropathology of multiple system atrophy. Am J Pathol. 2005;166(3):869–76.
17. Sailer A, Scholz SW, Nalls MA, Schulte C, Federoff M, Price TR, et al.; European Multiple System Atrophy Study Group and the UK Multiple System Atrophy Study Group. A genome-wide association study in multiple system atrophy. Neurology. 2016;87(15):1591–8.
18. Kollensperger M, Geser F, Ndaysaba JP, Boesch S, Seppi K, Ostergaard K, et al.; EMSA-SG. Presentation, diagnosis, and management of multiple system atrophy in Europe: final analysis of the European multiple system atrophy registry. Mov Disord. 2010;15;25(15):2604–12.
19. Peng C, Gathagan RJ, Covell DJ, Medellin C, Stieber A, Robinson JL, et al. Cellular milieu imparts distinct pathological α-synuclein strains in α-synucleinopathies. Nature. 2018;557(7706):558–63.
20. Breen DP, Fasano A. α-Synuclein strains in multiple system atrophy: a product of their environment? Mov Disord. 2018;33(8):1270.
21. Bower JH, Maraganore DM, McDonnell SK, Rocca WA. Incidence of progressive supranuclear palsy and multiple system atrophy in Olmsted County, Minnesota, 1976-1990. Neurology. 1997;49(5):1284–8.
22. Schrag A, Ben-Shlomo Y, Quinn NP. Prevalence of progressive supranuclear palsy and multiple system atrophy: a cross-sectional study. Lancet. 1999;354(9192):1771–5.
23. Tison F, Yekhlef F, Chrysostome V, Sourgen C. Prevalence of multiple system atrophy. Lancet. 2000;355(9202):495–6.
24. Ben-Shlomo Y, Wenning GK, Tison F, Quinn NP. Survival of patients with pathologically proven multiple system atrophy: a meta-analysis. Neurology. 1997;48(2):384–93.
25. Kim HJ, Jeon BS, Lee JY, Yun JY. Survival of Korean patients with multiple system atrophy. Mov Disord. 2011;26(5):909–12.
26. Wenning GK, Geser F, Krismer F, Seppi K, Duerr S, Boesch S, et al.; European Multiple System Atrophy Study Group. The natural history of multiple system atrophy: a prospective European cohort study. Lancet Neurol. 2013;12(3):264–74.
27. Low PA, Reich SG, Jankovic J, Shults CW, Stern MB, Novak P, et al. Natural history of multiple system atrophy in North America: a prospective cohort study. Lancet Neurol. 2015;14(7):710–9.
28. Watanabe H, Saito Y, Terao S, Ando T, Kachi T, Mukai E, et al. Progression and prognosis in multiple system atrophy: an analysis of 230 Japanese patients. Brain. 2002;125(Pt 5):1070–83.
29. Petrovic IN, Ling H, Asi Y, Ahmed Z, Kukkle PL, Hazrati LN, et al. Multiple system atrophy-parkinsonism with slow progression and prolonged survival: a diagnostic catch. Mov Disord. 2012;27(9):1186–90.
30. Kim HJ, Jeon BS, Lee JY, Yun JY, Kim YE, Paek SH. Young-onset multiple system atrophy. J Neurol Sci. 2012;319(1–2):168–70.
31. Batla A, De Pablo-Fernandez E, Erro R, Reich M, Calandra-Buonaura G, Barbosa P, et al. Young-onset multiple system atrophy: clinical and pathological features. Mov Disord. 2018;33(7):1099–107.
32. Wenning GK, Ben Shlomo Y, Magalhaes M, Daniel SE, Quinn NP. Clinical features and natural history of multiple system atrophy. An analysis of 100 cases. Brain. 1994;117(Pt 4):835–45.
33. Klockgether T, Lüdtke R, Kramer B, Abele M, Bürk K, Schöls L, et al. The natural history of degenerative ataxia: a retrospective study in 466 patients. Brain. 1998;121(Pt 4):589–600.
34. O'Sullivan SS, Massey LA, Williams DR, Silveira-Moriyama L, Kempster PA, Holton JL, et al. Clinical outcomes of progressive supranuclear palsy and multiple system atrophy. Brain. 2008;131(Pt 5):1362–72.
35. Figueroa JJ, Singer W, Parsaik A, Benarroch EE, Ahlskog JE, Fealey RD, et al. Multiple system atrophy: prognostic indicators of survival. Mov Disord. 2014;29(9):1151–7.
36. Saito Y, Matsuoka Y, Takahashi A, Ohno Y. Survival of patients with multiple system atrophy. Intern Med. 1994;33(6):321–5.
37. Schulz JB, Klockgether T, Petersen D, Jauch M, Müller-Schauenburg W, Spieker S, et al. Multiple system atrophy: natural history, MRI morphology, and dopamine receptor imaging with 123IBZM-SPECT. J Neurol Neurosurg Psychiatry. 1994;57(9):1047–56.
38. Tada M, Onodera O, Tada M, Ozawa T, Piao YS, Kakita A, et al. Early development of autonomic dysfunction may predict poor prognosis in patients with multiple system atrophy. Arch Neurol. 2007;64(2):256–60.
39. Calandra-Buonaura G, Guaraldi P, Sambati L, Lopane G, Cecere A, Barletta G, et al. Multiple system atrophy with prolonged survival: is late onset of dysautonomia the clue? Neurol Sci. 2013;34(10):1875–8.
40. Coon EA, Sletten DM, Suarez MD, Mandrekar JN, Ahlskog JE, Bower JH, et al. Clinical features and autonomic testing predict survival in multiple system atrophy. Brain. 2015;138(Pt 12):3623–31.
41. Salazar G, Valls-Solé J, Martí MJ, Chang H, Tolosa ES. Postural and action myoclonus in patients with parkinsonian type multiple system atrophy. Mov Disord. 2000;15(1):77–83.
42. Quinn NP. How to diagnose multiple system atrophy. Mov Disord. 2005;20(Suppl 12):S5–S10.
43. Köllensperger M, Geser F, Seppi K, Stampfer-Kountchev M, Sawires M, Scherfler C; European MSA Study Group. Red flags in multiple system atrophy. Mov Disord. 2008;23(8):1093–9.
44. Higo R, Tayama N, Watanabe T, Nitou T, Ugawa Y. Videofluoroscopic and manometric evaluation of swallowing function in patients with multiple system atrophy. Ann Otol Rhinol Laryngol. 2003;112(7):630–6.
45. Higo R, Nito T, Tayama N. Swallowing function in patients with multiple-system atrophy with a clinical predominance of cerebellar symptoms (MSA-C). Eur Arch Otorhinolaryngol. 2005;262(8):646–50.
46. Alfonsi E, Versino M, Merlo IM, Pacchetti C, Martignoni E, Bertino G, et al. Electrophysiologic patterns of oral-pharyngeal swallowing in parkinsonian syndromes. Neurology. 2007;68(8):583–9.
47. Pfeiffer RF. Gastrointestinal dysfunction in Parkinson's disease. Lancet Neurol. 2003;2(2):107–16. Review.
48. Hunter PC, Crameri J, Austin S, Woodward MC, Hughes AJ. Response of parkinsonian swallowing dysfunction to dopaminergic stimulation. J Neurol Neurosurg Psychiatry. 1997;63(5):579–83.
49. Do HJ, Seo HG, Lee HH, Oh BM, Kim Y, Kim A, et al. Progression of oropharyngeal dysphagia in patients with multiple system atrophy. Dysphagia. 2019; https://doi.org/10.1007/s00455-019-09990-z. [Epub ahead of print].
50. Laurens B, Vergnet S, Lopez MC, Foubert-Samier A, Tison F, Fernagut PO, Meissner WG. Multiple system atrophy - state of the art. Curr Neurol Neurosci Rep. 2017;17(5):41.

51. Bhatia KP, Stamelou M. Nonmotor features in atypical Parkinsonism. Int Rev Neurobiol. 2017;134:1285–301.
52. Zheng J, Yang X, Chen Y, Zhao Q, Tian S, Huang H, et al. Onset of bladder and motor symptoms in multiple system atrophy: differences according to phenotype. Clin Auton Res. 2017;27(2):103–6.
53. Glasmacher SA, Leigh PN, Saha RA. Predictors of survival in progressive supranuclear palsy and multiple system atrophy: a systematic review and meta-analysis. J Neurol Neurosurg Psychiatry. 2017;88(5):402–11.
54. Scorza FA, Fiorini AC, Scorza CA, Finsterer J. Cardiac abnormalities in Parkinson's disease and parkinsonism. J Clin Neurosci. 2018;53:1–5.
55. Gibbons CH, Freeman R. Clinical implications of delayed orthostatic hypotension. Neurology. 2015;85(16):1362–7.
56. Sakakibara R, Hattori T, Uchiyama T, Kita K, Asahina M, Suzuki A, Yamanishi T. Urinary dysfunction and orthostatic hypotension in multiple system atrophy: which is the more common and earlier manifestation? J Neurol Neurosurg Psychiatry. 2000;68(1):65–9.
57. Fanciulli A, Göbel G, Ndayisaba JP, Granata R, Duerr S, Strano S, et al. Supine hypertension in Parkinson's disease and multiple system atrophy. Clin Auton Res. 2016;26(2):97–105.
58. Wenning GK, Granata R, Krismer F, Dürr S, Seppi K, Poewe W, et al. Orthostatic hypotension is differentially associated with the cerebellar versus the parkinsonian variant of multiple system atrophy: a comparative study. Cerebellum. 2012;11(1):223–6.
59. Andy UU, Vaughan CP, Burgio KL, Alli FM, Goode PS, Markland AD. Shared risk factors for constipation, fecal incontinence, and combined symptoms in older U.S. adults. J Am Geriatr Soc. 2016;64(11):e183–8.
60. Savica R, Bradley BF, Mielke MM. When do α-ynucleinopathies start? An epidemiological timeline: a review. JAMA Neurol. 2018;75(4):503–9.
61. Sakakibara R, Tateno F, Yamamoto T, Uchiyama T, Yamanishi T. Urological dysfunction in synucleinopathies: epidemiology, pathophysiology and management. Clin Auton Res. 2018;28(1):83–101.
62. McKay JH, Cheshire WP. First symptoms in multiple system atrophy. Clin Auton Res. 2018;28(2):215–21.
63. Shamloul R, Ghanem H. Erectile dysfunction. Lancet. 2013;381(9861):153–65.
64. Schrag A, Geser F, Stampfer-Kountchev M, Seppi K, Sawires M, Köllensperger M, et al.; European MSA-Study Group. Health-related quality of life in multiple system atrophy. Mov Disord. 2006;21(6):809–15.
65. Iranzo A, Santamaria J, Tolosa E, Vilaseca I, Valldeoriola F, Martí MJ, Muñoz E. Long-term effect of CPAP in the treatment of nocturnal stridor in multiple system atrophy. Neurology. 2004;63(5):930–2.
66. Giannini G, Calandra-Buonaura G, Mastrolilli F, Righini M, Bacchi-Reggiani ML, Cecere A, et al. Early stridor onset and stridor treatment predict survival in 136 patients with MSA. Neurology. 2016;87(13):1375–83.
67. Moreno-López C, Santamaría J, Salamero M, Del Sorbo F, Albanese A, Pellecchia MT, et al. Excessive daytime sleepiness in multiple system atrophy (SLEEMSA study). Arch Neurol. 2011;68(2):223–30.
68. Bhalsing K, Suresh K, Muthane UB, Pal PK. Prevalence and profile of restless legs syndrome in Parkinson's disease and other neurodegenerative disorders: a case-control study. Parkinsonism Relat Disord. 2013;19(4):426–30.
69. Ghorayeb I, Dupouy S, Tison F, Meissner WG. Restless legs syndrome in multiple system atrophy. J Neural Transm. 2014;121(12):1523–7.
70. Gama RL, Távora DG, Bomfim RC, Silva CE, de Bruin VM, de Bruin PF. Sleep disturbances and brain MRI morphometry in Parkinson's disease, multiple system atrophy and progressive supranuclear palsy - a comparative study. Parkinsonism Relat Disord. 2010;16(4):275–9.
71. Chokroverty S. Differential diagnoses of restless legs syndrome/Willis-Ekbom disease: mimics and comorbidities. Sleep Med Clin. 2015;10(3):249–62.
72. Muntean M-L, Sixel-Döring F, Trenkwalder C. No difference in sleep and RBD between different types of patients with multiple system atrophy: a pilot video-polysomnographical study. Sleep Disord. 2013;2013:258390.
73. Wetter TC, Collado-Seidel V, Pollmächer T, Yassouridis A, Trenkwalder C. Sleep and periodic leg movement patterns in drug-free patients with Parkinson's disease and multiple system atrophy. Sleep. 2000;23(3):361–7.
74. Vetrugno R, Provini F, Cortelli P, Plazzi G, Lotti EM, Pierangeli G, et al. Sleep disorders in multiple system atrophy: a correlative video-polysomnographic study. Sleep Med. 2004;5(1):21–30.
75. Cochen De Cock V, Debs R, Oudiette D, Leu-Semenescu S, Radji F, Tiberge M, et al. The improvement of movement and speech during rapid eye movement sleep behaviour disorder in multiple system atrophy. Brain. 2011;134(Pt 3):856–62.
76. Vetrugno R, D'Angelo R, Cortelli P, Plazzi G, Vignatelli L, Montagna P. Impaired cortical and autonomic arousal during sleep in multiple system atrophy. Clin Neurophysiol. 2007;118(11):2512–8.
77. Schenck CH, Mahowald MW. REM sleep behavior disorder: clinical, developmental, and neuroscience perspectives 16 years after its formal identification in SLEEP. Sleep. 2002;25(2):120–38.
78. Comella CL, Nardine TM, Diederich NJ, Stebbins GT. Sleep-related violence, injury, and REM sleep behavior disorder in Parkinson's disease. Neurology. 1998;51(2):526–9.
79. Iranzo A, Santamaria J, Tolosa E. Idiopathic rapid eye movement sleep behaviour disorder: diagnosis, management, and the need for neuroprotective interventions. Lancet Neurol. 2016;15(4):405–19.
80. Palma JA, Fernandez-Cordon C, Coon EA, Low PA, Miglis MG, Jaradeh S, et al. Prevalence of REM sleep behavior disorder in multiple system atrophy: a multicenter study and meta-analysis. Clin Auton Res. 2015;25(1):69–75.
81. Nomura T, Inoue Y, Högl B, Uemura Y, Yasui K, Sasai T, et al. Comparison of the clinical features of rapid eye movement sleep behavior disorder in patients with Parkinson's disease and multiple system atrophy. Psychiatry Clin Neurosci. 2011;65(3):264–71.
82. Benarroch EE. Brainstem in multiple system atrophy: clinicopathological correlations. Cell Mol Neurobiol. 2003;23(4–5):519–26.
83. Vetrugno R, Alessandria M, D'Angelo R, Plazzi G, Provini F, Cortelli P, et al. Status dissociatus evolving from REM sleep behaviour disorder in multiple system atrophy. Sleep Med. 2009;10(2):247–52.
84. Ghorayeb I, Yekhlef F, Chrysostome V, Balestre E, Bioulac B, Tison F. Sleep disorders and their determinants in multiple system atrophy. J Neurol Neurosurg Psychiatry. 2002;72(6):798–800.
85. Ozawa T, Sekiya K, Aizawa N, Terajima K, Nishizawa M. Laryngeal stridor in multiple system atrophy: clinicopathological features and causal hypotheses. J Neurol Sci. 2016;361:243–9.
86. Osaki Y, Ben-Shlomo Y, Lees AJ, Wenning GK, Quinn NP. A validation exercise on the new consensus criteria for multiple system atrophy. Mov Disord. 2009;24(15):2272–6.
87. Isozaki E, Naito A, Horiguchi S, Kawamura R, Hayashida T, Tanabe H. Early diagnosis and stage classification of vocal cord abductor paralysis in patients with multiple system atrophy. J Neurol Neurosurg Psychiatry. 1996;60(4):399–402.
88. Vetrugno R, Liguori R, Cortelli P, Plazzi G, Vicini C, Campanini A, et al. Sleep-related stridor due to dystonic vocal cord motion and neurogenic tachypnea/tachycardia in multiple system atrophy. Mov Disord. 2007;22(5):673–8.
89. Iranzo A, Santamaría J, Rye DB, Valldeoriola F, Martí MJ, Muñoz E, et al. Characteristics of idiopathic REM sleep behav-

ior disorder and that associated with MSA and PD. Neurology. 2005;65(2):247–52.
90. Iranzo A, Santamaria J, Tolosa E. Continuous positive air pressure eliminates nocturnal stridor in multiple system atrophy. Lancet. 2000;356(9238):1329–30.
91. Yamaguchi M, Arai K, Asahina M, Hattori T. Laryngeal stridor in multiple system atrophy. Eur Neurol. 2003;49(3):154–9.
92. Jin K, Okabe S, Chida K, Abe N, Kimpara T, Ohnuma A, et al. Tracheostomy can fatally exacerbate sleep-disordered breathing in multiple system atrophy. Neurology. 2007;68(19):1618–21.
93. Benarroch EE. Brainstem respiratory control: substrates of respiratory failure of multiple system atrophy. Mov Disord. 2007;22(2):155–61.
94. Tada M, Kakita A, Toyoshima Y, Onodera O, Ozawa T, Morita T, et al. Depletion of medullary serotonergic neurons in patients with multiple system atrophy who succumbed to sudden death. Brain. 2009;132(Pt 7):1810–9.
95. Iranzo A. Sleep and breathing in multiple system atrophy. Curr Treat Options Neurol. 2007;9(5):347–53.
96. Garcia-Sanchez A, Fernandez-Navarro I, Garcia-Rio F. Central apneas and REM sleep behavior disorder as an initial presentation of multiple system atrophy. J Clin Sleep Med. 2016;12(2):267–70.
97. Ohshima Y, Nakayama H, Matsuyama N, Hokari S, Sakagami T, Sato O, et al. Natural course and potential prognostic factors for sleep-disordered breathing in multiple system atrophy. Sleep Med. 2017;34:13–7.
98. Chokroverty S, Sharp JT, Barron KD. Periodic respiration in erect posture in Shy-Drager syndrome. J Neurol Neurosurg Psychiatry. 1978;41(11):980–6.
99. Tsuda T, Onodera H, Okabe S, Kikuchi Y, Itoyama Y. Impaired chemosensitivity to hypoxia is a marker of multiple system atrophy. Ann Neurol. 2002;52(3):367–71.
100. Glass GA, Josephs KA, Ahlskog JE. Respiratory insufficiency as the primary presenting symptom of multiple system atrophy. Arch Neurol. 2006;63(7):978–81.
101. McNicholas WT, Rutherford R, Grossman R, Moldofsky H, Zamel N, Phillipson EA. Abnormal respiratory pattern generation during sleep in patients with autonomic dysfunction. Am Rev Respir Dis. 1983;128(3):429–33.
102. Lockwood AH. Shy-Drager syndrome with abnormal respirations and antidiuretic hormone release. Arch Neurol. 1976;33(4):292–5.
103. Bannister R, Oppenheimer DR. Degenerative diseases of the nervous system associated with autonomic failure. Brain. 1972;95(3):457–74.
104. Castaigne P, Laplane D, Autret A, Bousser MG, Gray F, Baron JC. [Shy-Drager syndrome with disturbances of the respiratory rhythm and consciousness. A propos of an anatomo-clinical case]. Rev Neurol (Paris). 1977;133(8–9):455–466. [*Article in French*].
105. Plazzi G, Corsini R, Provini F, Pierangeli G, Martinelli P, Montagna P, Lugaresi E, Cortelli P. REM sleep behavior disorders in multiple system atrophy. Neurology. 1997;48(4):1094–7.
106. Shimohata T, Shinoda H, Nakayama H, Ozawa T, Terajima K, Yoshizawa H, Matsuzawa Y, et al. Daytime hypoxemia, sleep-disorder breathing, and laryngopharyngeal findings in multiple system atrophy. Arch Neurol. 2007;64(6):856–61.
107. Vincken WG, Gauthier SG, Dollfuss RE, Hanson RE, Darauay CM, Cosio MG. Involvement of upper-airway muscles in extrapyramidal disorders. A cause of airflow limitation. N Engl J Med. 1984;311(7):438–42.
108. Ghorayeb I, Yekhlef F, Bioulac B, Tisfon F. Continuous positive airway pressure for sleep-related breathing disorders in multiple system atrophy: long term acceptance. Sleep Med. 2005;6(4):359–62.
109. Shimohata T, Tomita M, Nakayama H, Aizawa N, Ozawa T, Nishizawa M. Floppy epiglottis as a contraindication of CPAP in patients with multiple system atrophy. Neurology. 2011;76(21):1841–2.
110. Shimohata T, Ozawa T, Nakayama H, Tomita M, Shinoda H, Nishizawa M. Frequency of nocturnal sudden death in patients with multiple system atrophy. J Neurol. 2008;255(10):1483–5.
111. Freeman R, Chapleau MW. Testing the autonomic nervous system. Handb Clin Neurol. 2013;115:115–36. Review.
112. Barbic F, Perego F, Canesi M, Gianni M, Biagiotti S, Costantino G, et al. Early abnormalities of vascular and cardiac autonomic control in Parkinson's disease without orthostatic hypotension. Hypertension. 2007;49(1):120–6.
113. Pavy-Le Traon A, Piedvache A, Perez-Lloret S, Calandra-Buonaura G, Cochen-De Cock V, Colosimo C, et al. New insights into orthostatic hypotension in multiple system atrophy: a European multicentre cohort study. J Neurol Neurosurg Psychiatry. 2016;87(5):554–61.
114. Fanciulli A, Jordan J, Biaggioni I, Calandra-Buonaura G, Cheshire WP, Cortelli P, et al. Consensus statement on the definition of neurogenic supine hypertension in cardiovascular autonomic failure by the American Autonomic Society (AAS) and the European Federation of Autonomic Societies (EFAS): endorsed by the European Academy of Neurology (EAN) and the European Society of Hypertension (ESH). Clin Auton Res. 2018;28(4):355–62.
115. Illigens BMW, Gibbons CH. Sweat testing to evaluate autonomic function. Clin Auton Res. 2009;19(2):79–87.
116. Buchmann SJ, Penzlin AI, Kubasch ML, Illigens BM, Siepmann T. Assessment of sudomotor function. Clin Auton Res. 2018;29(1):41–53.
117. Vetrugno R, Liguori R, Cortelli P, Montagna P. Sympathetic skin response: basic mechanisms and clinical applications. Clin Auton Res. 2003;13(4):256–70.
118. Siepmann T, Pintér A, Buchmann SJ, Stibal L, Arndt M, Kubasch AS, et al. Cutaneous autonomic pilomotor testing to unveil the role of neuropathy progression in early Parkinson's disease (CAPTURE PD): protocol for a multicenter study. Front Neurol. 2017;8:212. https://doi.org/10.3389/fneur.2017.00212.
119. Baschieri F, Calandra-Buonaura G, Doria A, Mastrolilli F, Palareti A, Barletta G, et al. Cardiovascular autonomic testing performed with a new integrated instrumental approach is useful in differentiating MSA-P from PD at an early stage. Parkinsonism Relat Disord. 2015;21(5):477–82.
120. Merola A, Espay AJ, Zibetti M, Romagnolo A, Rosso M. Pure autonomic failure versus prodromal dysautonomia in Parkinson' s disease: insights from the bedside. Mov Disord. 2016;4(1):141–4.
121. Roy S, Jaryal AK, Srivastava AK, Deepak KK. Cardiovagal baroreflex sensitivity in Parkinson's disease and multiple-system atrophy. J Clin Neurol. 2016;12(2):218–23.
122. Pavy-LeTraon A, Brefel-Courbon C, Dupouy J, Ory-Magne F, Rascol O, Senard JM. Combined cardiovascular and sweating autonomic testing to differentiate multiple system atrophy from Parkinson's disease. Neurophysiol Clin. 2018;48(2):103–10.
123. Augustis S, Saferis V, Jost WH. Autonomic disturbances including impaired hand thermoregulation in multiple system atrophy and Parkinson's disease. J Neural Transm. 2017;124(8):965–72.
124. Palma JA, Norcliffe-Kaufmann L, Kaufmann H. Diagnosis of multiple system atrophy. Auton Neurosci. 2018;211:15–25.
125. Stanzani-Maserati M, Gallassi R, Calandra-Buonaura G, Alessandria M, Oppi F, Poda R, et al. Cognitive and sleep features of multiple system atrophy: review and prospective study. Eur Neurol. 2014;72(5–6):349–59.
126. Stankovic I, Krismer F, Jesic A, Antonini A, Benke T, Brown RG, et al. Cognitive impairment in multiple system atrophy: a position statement by the Neuropsychology Task Force of the MDS Multiple System Atrophy (MODIMSA) study group. Mov Disord. 2014;29(7):857–67.

127. Koga S, Parks A, Uitti RJ, van Gerpen JA, Cheshire WP, Wszolek ZK, Dickson DW. Profile of cognitive impairment and underlying pathology in multiple system atrophy. Mov Disord. 2017;32(3):405–13.
128. Brown RG, Lacomblez L, Landwehrmeyer BG, Bak T, Uttner I, Dubois B, et al.; NNIPPS Study Group. Cognitive impairment in patients with multiple system atrophy and progressive supranuclear palsy. Brain. 2010;133(Pt 8):2382–93.
129. Kim HJ, Jeon BS, Jellinger KA. Diagnosis and differential diagnosis of MSA: boundary issues. J Neurol. 2015;262(8): 1801–13.
130. Kim HJ, Stamelou M, Jeon B. Multiple system atrophy-mimicking conditions: diagnostic challenges. Parkinsonism Relat Disord. 2016;22(Suppl 1):S12–5.
131. Koga S, Aoki N, Uitti RJ, van Gerpen JA, Cheshire WP, Josephs KA, et al. When DLB, PD, and PSP masquerade as MSA: an autopsy study of 134 patients. Neurology. 2015;85(5):404–12.
132. Mestre TA, Gupta A, Lang AE. MRI signs of multiple system atrophy preceding the clinical diagnosis: the case for an imaging-supported probable MSA diagnostic category. J Neurol Neurosurg Psychiatry. 2016;87(4):443–4.
133. Rizzo G, Copetti M, Arcuti S, Martino D, Fontana A, Logroscino G. Accuracy of clinical diagnosis of Parkinson disease: a systematic review and meta-analysis. Neurology. 2016;86(6):566–76.
134. Koga S, Dickson DW. Recent advances in neuropathology, biomarkers and therapeutic approach of multiple system atrophy. J Neurol Neurosurg Psychiatry. 2018;89(2):175–84.
135. Laurens B, Constantinescu R, Freeman R, Gerhard A, Jellinger K, Jeromin A, et al. Fluid biomarkers in multiple system atrophy: a review of the MSA biomarker initiative. Neurobiol Dis. 2015;80:29–41.
136. Treglia G, Stefanelli A, Cason E, Cocciolillo F, Di Giuda D, Giordano A. Diagnostic performance of iodine-123-metaiodobenzylguanidine scintigraphy in differential diagnosis between Parkinson's disease and multiple-system atrophy: a systematic review and a meta-analysis. Clin Neurol Neurosurg. 2011;113(10):823–9.
137. Nagayama H, Ueda M, Yamazaki M, Nishiyama Y, Hamamoto M, Katayama Y. Abnormal cardiac [(123)I]-meta-iodobenzylguanidine uptake in multiple system atrophy. Mov Disord. 2010;25(11):1744–7.
138. Baschieri F, Calandra-Buonaura G, Cecere A, Barletta G, Contin M, Parchi P, Cortelli P. Iodine-123-meta-iodobenzylguanidine myocardial scintigraphy in isolated autonomic failure: potential red flag for future multiple system atrophy. Front Neurol. 2017;8:225. https://doi.org/10.3389/fneur.2017.00225.
139. Krismer F, Pinter B, Mueller C, Mahlknecht P, Nocker M, Reiter E, Djamshidian-Tehrani A, et al. Sniffing the diagnosis: olfactory testing in neurodegenerative parkinsonism. Parkinsonism Relat Disord. 2017;35:36–41.
140. Abele M, Riet A, Hummel T, Klockgether T, Wullner U. Olfactory dysfunction in cerebellar ataxia and multiple system atrophy. J Neurol. 2003;250(12):1453–5.
141. Schrag A, Good CD, Miszkiel K, Morris HR, Mathias CJ, Lees AJ, Quinn NP. Differentiation of atypical parkinsonian syndromes with routine MRI. Neurology. 2000;54(3):697–702.
142. Ramli N, Nair SR, Ramli NM, Lim SY. Differentiating multiple-system atrophy from Parkinson's disease. Clin Radiol. 2015;70(5):555–64.
143. Sugiyama A, Ito S, Suichi T, Sakurai T, Mukai H, Yokota H, et al. Putaminal hypointensity on T2*-weighted MR imaging is the most practically useful sign in diagnosing multiple system atrophy: a preliminary study. J Neurol Sci. 2015;349(1–2):174–8.
144. Deguchi K, Ikeda K, Kume K, Takata T, Kokudo Y, Kamada M, et al. Significance of the hot-cross bun sign on T2*-weighted MRI for the diagnosis of multiple system atrophy. J Neurol. 2015;262(6):1433–9.
145. Feng JY, Huang B, Yang WQ, Zhang YH, Wang LM, Wang LJ, Zhong XL. The putaminal abnormalities on 3.0T magnetic resonance imaging: can they separate parkinsonism-predominant multiple system atrophy from Parkinson's disease? Acta Radiol. 2015;56(3):322–8.
146. Wang N, Yang H, Li C, Fan G, Luo X. Using 'swallow-tail' sign and putaminal hypointensity as biomarkers to distinguish multiple system atrophy from idiopathic Parkinson's disease: a susceptibility-weighted imaging study. Eur Radiol. 2017;27(8):3174–80.
147. Nakamura K, Mori F, Kon T, Tanji K, Miki Y, Tomiyama M, et al. Accumulation of phosphorylated alpha-synuclein in subpial and periventricular astrocytes in multiple system atrophy of long duration. Neuropathology. 2015;36(2):157–67.
148. Doppler K, Weis J, Karl K, Ebert S, Ebentheuer J, Trenkwalder C, et al. Distinctive distribution of phospho-alpha-synuclein in dermal nerves in multiple system atrophy. Mov Disord. 2015;30(12):1688–92.
149. Zange L, Noack C, Hahn K, Stenzel W, Lipp A. Phosphorylated alpha-synuclein in skin nerve fibres differentiates Parkinson's disease from multiple system atrophy. Brain. 2015;138(Pt 8):2310–21.
150. Donadio V, Incensi A, El-Agnaf O, Rizzo G, Vaikath N, Del Sorbo F, et al. Skin α-synuclein deposits differ in clinical variants of synucleinopathy: an in vivo study. Sci Rep. 2018;8(1):14246.
151. Krismer F, Wenning GK. Multiple system atrophy: insights into a rare and debilitating movement disorder. Nat Rev Neurol. 2017;13(4):232–43.
152. Calandra-Buonaura G, Doria A, Lopane G, Guaraldi P, Capellari S, Martinelli P, et al. Pharmacodynamics of a low subacute levodopa dose helps distinguish between multiple system atrophy with predominant Parkinsonism and Parkinson's disease. J Neurol. 2016;263(2):250–6.
153. Meissner WG, Laurencin C, Tranchant C, Witjas T, Viallet F, Guehl D, et al. Outcome of deep brain stimulation in slowly progressive multiple system atrophy: a clinico-pathological series and review of the literature. Parkinsonism Relat Disord. 2016;24:69–75.
154. Valera E, Monzio Compagnoni G, Masliah E. Review: novel treatment strategies targeting alpha-synuclein in multiple system atrophy as a model of synucleinopathy. Neuropathol Appl Neurobiol. 2016;42(1):95–106.

Pure Autonomic Failure

24

Ramesh K. Khurana

Introduction

Wagner cited the first clinical account of orthostatic hypotension by Piorry in 1826 [1]. In 1925, Bradbury and Eggleston described, in exquisite detail, three men with severe orthostatic hypotension and anhidrosis of over 3 years' duration [2]. The authors described clinical, physiological, and pharmacological observations in the patients and tried symptomatic treatment. They reported that one patient had transient shortness of breath, dizziness, and blindness upon climbing stairs. Another patient reported dizziness upon standing which improved by crouching in a chair and pressing the folded arms over the abdomen. All three suffered from recurrent syncope, more often in the morning, during or after exertion, or even after standing for several minutes. Additional complaints were loss of sweating even in a Turkish bath, weakness, exhaustion, loss of sexual power, and increased nocturnal urinary excretion. Case one had marked constipation for many years, 26 lb. weight loss in 1 year, and a period of profuse sweating preceding loss of perspiration. The authors described "slight and indefinite changes" in the nervous system. Case two showed brisker right knee jerk and case three demonstrated hyperactive knee jerks with bilateral Babinski signs. There was no progression noted during the "several" years of follow-up.

All patients demonstrated severe orthostatic hypotension. Case two had supine hypertension (165/100 mm Hg). Case one developed syncope following exercise with dilated pupils, convulsive limb movements, pallor, unconsciousness, and imperceptible radial pulse during the spell. He regained consciousness with blood pressure of 60/40 mm Hg at 10 minutes. The heart rate was slow and was essentially unchanged by the changes in blood pressure. A 40° head-up tilt in case two caused a decline in blood pressure from 156/106 to 90/78 with a pulse rate change from 56 to 52 beats/minute. Conversely, a 40° head-down tilt increased the blood pressure from 158/108 to 180/122 mm Hg with little change in heart rate, suggesting cardiovagal impairment. Markedly increased urine output was documented when supine and especially at night. Lowered basal metabolism was also observed. Subcutaneous or intramuscular administration of 2.5 mg atropine did not increase the heart rate. The rate of phenolsulfonphthalein excretion in urine was higher when supine than in erect position. Although patients did not sweat in response to hot environment, 6 mg pilocarpine administration resulted in profuse sweating, indicating an intact end organ.

Pharmacologic management of case one with thyroxine, digitalis, atropine, strychnine, pituitrin, and dried suprarenal substance was without benefit. Hypodermic epinephrine reduced orthostatic hypotension and improved the patient's capacity to ambulate. In case two, application of abdominal binder and tight bandages around the lower limbs allowed the patient to walk for several hours.

The authors concluded that failure of these patients to maintain blood pressure in the head-up and head-down positions was due to dysfunction of sympathetic vasoconstrictor endings and cardiac acceleration. In addition, these patients had cardiovagal impairment and anhidrosis with pharmacologically intact sweat glands. In brief, the authors described neurogenic orthostatic hypotension of "unknown" etiology with sympathetic adrenergic, sympathetic cholinergic, and cardiovagal dysfunction.

Over the next three decades, additional cases of orthostatic hypotension of known and unknown etiology were reported. Known causes included endocrinologic-metabolic disorders such as adrenal or pituitary insufficiency and diabetes mellitus, and diseases of the peripheral or central nervous system. Examples of neurological disorders included diabetic neuropathy, amyloidosis, tabes dorsalis, syringomyelia, acute and chronic cervical/thoracic spinal cord transection, brain tumor in the floor of the fourth ventricle, and parkinsonism

R. K. Khurana (✉)
Neurology Division, Department of Medicine, MedStar Union Memorial Hospital, Baltimore, MD, USA
e-mail: ramesh.khurana@medstar.net

S. Chokroverty, P. Cortelli (eds.), *Autonomic Nervous System and Sleep*, https://doi.org/10.1007/978-3-030-62263-3_24

[1]. Barker reviewed 13 cases of unknown etiology from the literature and added one patient of his own. The most consistent features in these patients were orthostatic hypotension (orthostatic fall of systolic blood pressure by >50 mm Hg) and anhidrosis. Autonomic function tests suggested predominantly efferent sympathetic failure [3]. Luft and Von Euler demonstrated reduced urinary excretion of norepinephrine [4]. Parasympathetic dysfunction was evident by the absence of atropine-induced tachycardia, absence of bradycardia during norepinephrine administration, failure of hypoglycemia to increase gastric acidity, and erectile failure in men. Treatment included underlying disease management (e.g., penicillin for tabes dorsalis), plasma volume expansion with normal saline infusion, and ephedrine by mouth. Hickler and co-workers introduced treatment with 9-alpha-fluorohydrocortisone [5]. In summary, two separate forms of chronic orthostatic hypotension were recognized, the secondary variety and the primary or idiopathic type.

Primary or idiopathic orthostatic hypotension of insidious onset with progression associated with somatic neurologic symptoms and signs was described by several authors. Young, for example, stated that this is a disorder of the nervous system, probably in the hypothalamic region, exerting depressing effect on the function of the sympathetic nervous system [6]. He did not link idiopathic orthostatic hypotension with somatic neurologic deficit. However, Shy and Drager, in 1960, described clinical features of two men who developed genitourinary dysfunction and orthostatic hypotension followed by somatic central nervous system (CNS) dysfunction [7] (see Chap. 23). Their second patient complained of impotence and nocturia at age 49 years followed by orthostatic dizziness in a course of a few months. Slowness of movements, fainting spells, and worsening bladder function developed within the next 18 months; staggering gait and were noted by the third year. Six years after the onset, the patient demonstrated severe orthostatic hypotension with fixed heart rate, unequal sluggishly reactive pupils, iris atrophy, weak medial recti muscles, paucity of facial expression, slow tongue movements, slurred speech, increased muscle tone, resting tremor, equivocal Babinski response, unsteady gait, falling backward with eyes closed, impaired coordination, atonic bladder, and relaxed anal sphincter. Sensation was intact. Laboratory tests revealed several abnormalities: pneumoencephalography demonstrating cortical atrophy; muscle biopsy of the vastus lateralis showing neurogenic atrophy; cold pressor test showing no response to BP and HR; phentolamine test revealing severe decrease in blood pressure; skin resistance test showing absent response below T10; and sweat test showing sweating only over the upper lip and axillae. The patient died after 6.5 years. Neuropathological examination displayed widespread neuronal cell loss and gliosis in the following regions: autonomic ganglia, intermediolateral, and Clarke's cell columns of the spinal cord; inferior olives, dorsal motor and ambiguus nuclei of the vagus nerves, hypoglossal nucleus and the lateral cuneate nucleus of the medulla; Purkinje cells of the cerebellum; tegmentum and locus caeruleus of the pons; substantia nigra, oculomotor nucleus, and Edinger-Westphal nucleus of the midbrain; nucleus intercalatus of mammillary body and posterior region of hypothalamus; and putamen and globus pallidus region of the basal ganglia. The authors concluded that this constellation of features involving autonomic and somatic nervous system plus neuropathological findings constituted "a definite disorder of the nervous system . . . which may be one of the etiological factors of orthostatic hypotension." In brief, these two authors were the first to relate the clinical and neuropathological features of this syndrome to a primary neuronal degeneration disorder, hence the designation Shy-Drager syndrome [7]. In 1966, Johnson et al. described two cases of idiopathic orthostatic hypotension with neuropathological data. They performed a quantitative study of the intermediolateral column cells demonstrating 70–90% loss of neurons, and attributed orthostatic hypotension to the degeneration of preganglionic sympathetic neurons. In addition, case one had Lewy body inclusions in substantia nigra, locus coeruleus, and dorsal vagal nucleus. Case two displayed pathological features of olivopontocerebellar degeneration [8]. Graham and Oppenheimer reviewed the clinicopathological data of eight cases, including two with autonomic failure and parkinsonism, and suggested the term multiple system atrophy (MSA) to encompass overlapping multisystem degenerations [9].

Physiological and morphological evidence incriminated central or efferent sympathetic dysfunction as a cause of orthostatic hypotension. Biochemical data provided further elucidation. Infusion of precursor of nonadrenaline, 3-hydroxytyramine-2-^{14}C, in three idiopathic orthostatic hypotension patients was followed by a marked decrease in the urinary excretion of radioactive nonadrenaline, suggesting reduced biosynthesis of nonadrenaline [10]. In Shy-Drager syndrome, intra-arterial administration of tyramine produced a normal vasoconstrictor response and norephinephrine infusion did not provide evidence of denervation supersensitivity, suggesting intact postganglionic function. In contrast, idiopathic orthostatic hypotension patients showed absence of vasoconstrictor response to tyramine and supersensitivity to norepinephrine, indicating a postganglionic defect. This finding was confirmed by absence of the catecholamine-specific fluorescence in the walls of blood vessels from the deltoid muscle biopsy [11]. Ziegler and colleagues measured catecholamine levels supine and after 5–10 minutes of standing in six patients with MSA and four patients with idiopathic orthostatic hypotension. In patients with MSA, plasma norepinephrine levels were normal when patients were supine but did not increase upon standing.

In patients with idiopathic orthostatic hypotension without central neurologic signs, plasma norepinephrine levels were low when the patient was supine and did not increase upon standing, indicating peripheral sympathetic dysfunction [12]. In brief, these studies distinguished two different forms of orthostatic hypotension, central and peripheral. The central form, designated MSA, was characterized by autonomic dysfunction, parkinsonism, and ataxia in any combination. The peripheral form characterized by isolated autonomic failure became known as pure autonomic failure (PAF). Recent clinical and neuropathological data, however, challenge the "purity" of PAF [13].

The Consensus Committee of the American Autonomic Society and the American Academy of Neurology defined PAF as an idiopathic, sporadic disorder characterized by orthostatic hypotension usually with evidence of more widespread autonomic failure. Reduced supine plasma norepinephrine levels are considered characteristic of PAF. No other neurological features are present [14].

Clinical Features

Symptoms

In PAF, autonomic dysfunction afflicts middle-aged or older individuals of either sex. The condition progresses slowly and may plateau for a few years. Orthostatic hypotension and sudomotor impairment may precede gastrointestinal, genitourinary, and ocular symptoms. Orthostatic hypotension, a manifestation of sympathetic vasoconstrictor failure, can be disabling enough to cause the patient to seek medical attention. Orthostatic hypotension may be asymptomatic; but these patients become symptomatic when exposed to stress such as physical exertion, eating, warming or symptomatic with any orthostatic stress leading to lightheadedness and frank syncope. Severity may vary in the same individual on different occasions [15–18]. Mathias and colleagues reported dizziness, syncope, visual disturbances, and coat-hanger ache as common symptoms of orthostatic hypotension caused by PAF [19]. Patients develop headache, provoked by upright posture, that affects the entire cranium, occipital region, nape, and shoulders in a coat-hanger configuration. This headache may be attributable to ischemia of neck muscles, nociceptive input from the infratentorial arteries and dura mater of the posterior fossa, epidural hypotension, or altered headache threshold due to vagal dysfunction. Coat-hanger ache may develop within 3–5 minutes of standing or after 10 minutes to 2 hours of sitting. It is reported more often during daily activities than during a head-up tilt test. Some patients may present with buckling of knees and falls [20, 21]. For quantitative assessment, Kaufmann and colleagues designed a 10-item questionnaire which included six items pertaining to symptoms of dizziness/lightheadedness, vision disturbance, weakness, fatigue, trouble concentrating, and head/neck discomfort. Four items evaluate activities of daily living (e.g., standing short or long time as well as walking short or long time) [22].

Sudomotor dysfunction usually presents with heat intolerance. Episodic unprovoked sweating of asymmetrical compensatory hyperhidrosis may precede the development of anhidrosis [23]. Gastrointestinal symptoms include dysphagia, early satiety, diarrhea, and constipation. Occasionally, PAF may present with chronic intestinal pseudo obstruction [24]. Urinary disturbances may manifest as hesitancy, urgency, retention, and overflow incontinence [25]. In men, parasympathetically mediated penile erection and sympathetically mediated ejaculation are impaired. Ocular symptoms of hypoperfusion such as white out, gray out, enhanced brightness, and tunnel vision can also occur.

Sleep disturbance due to nocturia is common in PAF patients. They wait to empty the bladder before going to bed and wake up frequently to void urine. Daytime hypersomnolence/nocturnal vocalization and vivid dreams have been reported [26–28]. A 1991 study of four PAF patients described a prolonged and highly variable sleep latency and increased stage 3 sleep [29]. Recently, occurrence of rapid eye movement sleep behavior disorder (RBD) in PAF has acquired clinical significance. Plazzi and colleagues studied 10 PAF patients with polysomnography and followed them for a period of two to seven (mean 4.8) years. Four patients developed MSA, including one in whom RBD symptoms began 20 years after the onset of autonomic failure. The authors noted that RBD provided a clear separation between PAF and MSA, whereas supine norepinephrine levels showed an overlap. The authors concluded that RBD was confined to MSA [30]. In another case series of three PAF patients, RBD was confirmed with video-polysomnography. These patients had a disease duration of 3–7 years [31]. The latest report contains a series of eight PAF patients with autonomic failure of 11.2 years duration in whom video-polysomnography was performed to evaluate symptoms of excessive daytime sleepiness. It showed sleep fragmentation, snoring, dream enactment, and RBD. Mean duration of RBD was 3.75 years. According to the authors, the timing of emergence of RBD versus autonomic symptoms may help distinguish PAF from other synucleinopathies [32]. Since the neural circuitry of RBD is localized in the brainstem (pedunculopontine nucleus, sublaterodorsal tegmental nucleus, and medullary magnocellular reticular formation), occurrence of RBD is considered a harbinger of the appearance of other central nervous system manifestations [33, 34]. Because of its importance, the patient should be asked about dream enactment behavior during sleep. It may range from simple repetitive jerking to complex and seemingly purposeful activity such as punching, kicking, or falling out of bed.

The patients may shout or yell as well. They are unaware of the episode except upon awakening; they become alert and recall the dream. The history of RBD can be best obtained from the bed partner.

Signs

A carefully taken history should precede bedside examination. Patients may appear pale and younger than stated age [2]. Loss of sweating should be assessed by gliding the back of a spoon over the skin to detect friction [35]. A distended bladder is readily palpable as a suprapubic swelling. Stomach fullness, character of bowel sounds, and anal tone may provide useful information. Reduced anal tone should raise suspicion of MSA [36].

Orthostatic hypotension is the most important and easily documentable component of the evaluation. It is defined as a fall in blood pressure of >20 mm Hg systolic and >10 mm Hg diastolic within 3 minutes of standing or during head-up tilt of at least 60° [37]. In patients with supine hypertension, a sustained reduction in systolic blood pressure of 30 mm Hg is considered a more appropriate criterion [37]. The cardinal test for orthostatic hypotension is measurement of change in blood pressure from supine to standing. Blood pressure and heart rate should be measured after 5 minutes supine rest and after 1 and 3 minutes of standing. The author prefers to extend the recording of blood pressure after 5, 7, and 10 minutes of standing to identify patients with delayed orthostatic hypotension. Measuring heart rate change from supine to standing also provides evidence of neurogenic involvement. Heart rate increase upon standing depends on withdrawal of vagal activity and sympathetic activation. Heart rate increase of <15 beats per minute during orthostatic hypotension suggests neurogenic orthostatic hypotension [14, 16, 37].

Supine hypertension, observed initially by Bradbury and Eggleston in 1925, is seen in over 50% of patients [38]. It is defined as systolic blood pressure ≥150 mm Hg and diastolic blood pressure ≥90 mm Hg while in supine position. Supine hypertension is an important manifestation from management perspective. It can be exacerbated by drugs used to treat orthostatic hypotension. Hypertension when supine at night can contract blood volume through natriuresis and worsen orthostatic hypotension in the morning. Furthermore, hypertension when supine at night can cause end-organ damage such as left ventricular hypertrophy and renal impairment [39, 40]. Although one can record blood pressure at night, the frequency and severity of supine hypertension can be better diagnosed with 24-hour ambulatory blood pressure monitoring [41].

A standard neurologic examination may reveal abnormalities of memory recall, nominal, and calculation functions [42]. Hyposmia can be a feature of PAF but to a lesser degree than found in Parkinson's disease (PD) [43]. The presence of obvious or even subtle parkinsonian, cerebellar, or pyramidal signs should exclude the diagnosis of PAF in favor of other synucleinopathies.

Pathology

The clinical phenotype of PAF is characterized by severe orthostatic hypotension in association with other features of autonomic failure and at least a five-year history without development of other neurological signs to diminish the probability of the diagnosis of MSA, PD, or dementia with Lewy bodies [44]. Less than a dozen neuropathological studies have been reported. Bradbury and Eggleston, in 1927, reported autopsy findings on their second patient. Brain and spinal cord were not examined; adrenal and thyroid glands were normal [2, 45]. Case one of Johnson et al. demonstrated severe intermediolateral column cell loss, Lewy bodies in the brain and spinal cord, preserved pigmented brainstem nuclei, and occasional degenerating fibers in the sympathetic ganglia [8]. Vanderhaeghen et al. (Case 1) described cell loss and Lewy bodies in the substantia nigra, locus coeruleus, intermediolateral column, dorsal nuclei of vagus, and sympathetic ganglia [46]. Both cases, however, survived less than 5 years after the onset of symptoms. A patient reported by Roessmann et al. had symptoms exceeding 11 years, but the patient had embolic strokes and showed blood pressure rise in response to cold pressor test and mental arithmetic test [47]. A review of the pertinent literature reveals seven cases with symptoms duration of 5–15 years (Table 24.1) [48–53]. The brain and spinal cord were examined for pathological changes with emphasis on substantia nigra, locus coeruleus, dorsal nuclei of vagus, thoracolumbar intermediolateral columns, and sympathetic ganglia. Neurons of the craniosacral outflow, previsceral or terminal ganglia, and myentertic plexus were infrequently examined. Two significant pathological changes reported were neuronal loss and Lewy bodies (see Table 24.1). Loss of neurons was consistently observed in the cells of intermediolateral column. The relationship between the degree of preganglionic neuronal loss and severity of orthostatic hypotension was described by Johnson et al. [8]. The case reported by Rajput and colleagues showed minimal neuronal loss in the intermediolateral cell column and marked cell loss in the sympathetic ganglia [51]. Matthews, in a histopathological examination of sympathetic ganglia, found a significant reduction in the packing density of ganglionic neurons [54]. Rajput and Rozdilsky concluded that the lesions of the sympathetic ganglia may play a major role in the production of orthostatic hypotension [51]. Neuronal cytoplasmic inclusions (Lewy body) containing insoluble deposits of 140 amino acid protein α-synuclein constitute the characteristic histopathological finding, making PAF a synucleinopathy.

Table 24.1 Neuropathological findings (cell loss and Lewy bodies) in seven patients with pure autonomic failure

Author/year	Duration of illness (y)	Cerebral cortex		Substantia nigra		Locus coeruleus		Intermedio-lateral column		Dorsal nucleus of vagus		Sympathetic ganglia		Other sites of pathology
		Cell loss	Lewy bodies	Cell loss	Lewy bodies	Cell loss	Lewy bodies	Cell loss	Lewy bodies	Cell loss	Lewy bodies	Cell loss	Lewy bodies	
Oppenheimer, 1980 [48]	5	–	–	–	+	+	+	+	+	+	+	–	–	
Van Ingelghem et al., 1994 [49]	7	–	–	–	–	–	–	+	+	–	–	+	+	
Terao et al., 1993 [50]	8	–	+	+	+	+	+	+	+	–	+	–	+	Lewy bodies in the Auerbach plexus
Hishikawa et al., 2000 [27]	8	–	–	–	+	+	+	+	+	+	+	–	+	
Rajput and Rozdisky, 1976 [51]	14	–	–	+	+	+	+	+	–	+	+	+	+	
Hague et al., 1997 [52]	15	–	–	–	+	–	+	+	+	–	–	–	+	Lewy bodies in sacral spinal cord, ubiquitin positive nerves in muscularis of the urinary bladder, epimyocardial fat, and adrenal capsule
Arai et al., 2000 [53]	15	–	–	+	–	–	+	+	+	+	+	–	+	Cell loss in the sacral intermediolateral column Lewy bodies in Edinger-Westphal nucleus, ciliary ganglia, and myenteric neurons

In 2017, Isonaka and colleagues reported a 50-year-old man with severe orthostatic hypotension, exertional chest pain, heat intolerance, constipation, and dream enactment behavior. Neurologic examination displayed somnolence and mild neuropathy. Neurogenic orthostatic hypotension was documented with blood pressure responses to head-up tilt and the Valsalva maneuver. Norepinephrine and its intraneuronal metabolite 3,4-dihydroxyphenylglycol levels were low in the plasma and cerebrospinal fluid. Plasma levels of norepinephrine and its metabolite further declined after 3 years. Thoracic 6-[18F]fluorodopamine positron emission tomography showed reduced radioactivity in the left ventricular apex. Tyrosine hydroxylase immunoreactivity was diminished in arrector pili muscle of the skin. Contrary to expectation in a patient with neuropathy, quantitative sudomotor axon reflex test was normal. Approximately 10 years after the onset of symptoms, postmortem study failed to show Lewy bodies, Lewy neurites, or α-synuclein deposits in the brain, brainstem, or sympathetic ganglia. Neurochemical and immunofluorescence studies of the harvested tissues demonstrated generalized sympathetic noradrenergic denervation involving myocardium and sympathetic ganglia. Putamen dopamine and 3,4-dihydroxyphenylacetic acid contents were also reduced [26]. This case differs from the previous seven cases and highlights the possibilities that biochemical changes may precede the development of structural pathology and that PAF may be a heterogeneous disorder.

Antemortem Pathology

Severe orthostatic hypotension is an early feature of PAF and three other synucleinopathies: diffuse Lewy body dementia (DLBD), PD, and MSA. Each of them has a different clinical course, response to pharmacotherapy, and prognosis. A long follow-up is required to exclude central neurodegeneration to ensure that autonomic failure is indeed isolated. In vivo pathology may help exclude autonomic failure of secondary origin and to differentiate PAF from other synucleinopathies at an early stage. Biopsies of muscle, sural nerve, gastrointestinal tract, skin, and superficial veins have been studied for demonstration of α-synuclein protein and for the morphology and biochemical physiology of autonomic innervation.

Muscle Biopsy In 1975, Kontos et al. provided an early histochemical demonstration of absence of catecholamine-specific fluorescence in the adrenergic vasomotor nerves from the deltoid muscle biopsy of four PAF patients compared with four normal subjects [11]. Bannister and colleagues studied perivascular sympathetic nerve plexus from quadriceps muscle biopsy of two PAF patients [55]. Electron microscopy revealed intact nerve endings but with reduced number of catecholamine-containing vesicles. Histochemistry showed almost complete absence of catecholamine fluorescence. Both these studies were consistent with efferent sympathetic adrenergic dysfunction.

Sural Nerve Biopsy An ultrastructural study of sural nerve biopsy in seven Japanese patients with PAF demonstrated reduction of unmyelinated nerve fiber density by 40% of control values. In addition, increased numbers of clusters of collagen pockets with missing unmyelinated axons were observed in five of seven patients. The authors postulated existence of postganglionic sympathetic efferents in sural nerves and their loss resulting in clusters of collagen pockets [56].

Gastrointestinal Tract Gastric and colonic tissues resected for suspected malignancy in PAF patients have demonstrated α-synuclein deposits. Symptoms of autonomic failure ranged from 6 months to 15 years [57, 58].

Skin Skin is an easily accessible tissue containing a large number of sympathetic adrenergic (arrector pili muscle) and sympathetic cholinergic (sweat glands) fibers. It can serve as a biomarker for the diagnosis of synucleinopathy-related PAF, differentiate it from other causes of sympathetic efferent dysfunction such as amyloidosis, and allow for a longitudinal follow-up. A study used immunofluorescent analysis of skin biopsy to compare autonomic innervation of PAF with MSA showing marked sympathetic denervation in PAF patients [59]. In 2010, Shishido and colleagues reported phosphorylated α-synuclein accumulation in the unmyelinated nerve fibers and around blood vessels in the dermis and subcutaneous tissue of a 73-year-old PAF patient. Sympathetic failure was supported by the evidence of lack of tyrosine hydroxylase immunoreactivity in nerve fascicles and blood vessel walls [60]. Subsequently, other authors demonstrated phosphorylated α-synuclein deposits in the postganglionic sympathetic adrenergic and cholinergic neurites from proximal (paravertebral C-8) and distal (thigh and leg) locations. Immunostaining for native and misfolded phosphorylated α-synuclein demonstrated that antibodies against α-synuclein phosphorylated at Ser 129 provided the highest sensitivity and specificity in detecting α-synuclein aggregates in the cutaneous nerves [61, 62]. The authors compared the innervation pattern and spatial distribution of P-syn inclusions of idiopathic PD patients with those of PAF patients. The idiopathic PD patients showed a proximal-distal gradient with highest positivity (100%) at the cervical level and only 31% staining rate at the leg. In contrast, PAF patients showed 100% positive staining at the proximal and distal sites, thus differentiating the two disorders [63].

Veins Ultrastructural and histochemical studies of blood vessels within the muscle and skin have been commonly studied. Direct studies of biopsies of accessible veins, although limited, provide a unique ability to evaluate abnormalities in metabolism, storage, and release of norepinephrine. Klein and colleagues studied the ultrastructure of saphenous vein, a major capacitance vessel with rich adrenergic innervation. They observed the presence of very few noradrenergic axons and terminals with sparse vesicles [64]. In a 2018 neurochemical study, forearm subcutaneous vein biopsies from 11 PAF patients were compared with MSA patients and control subjects. PAF patients showed abundance of the norepinephrine transporter protein (low or absent in sympathetic denervation), very low levels of tyrosine hydroxylase (rate-limiting enzyme in catecholamine synthesis), reduced vesicular monoamine transporter 2 (VMAT 2), and a significantly higher ratio of plasma 3, 4-dihyroxyphenylglycol (DHPG):norepinephrine. These findings suggest intact sympathetic nerves but reduced norepinephrine synthesis with a shift toward intraneuronal metabolism over sequestration into sympathetic nerve vesicles [65]. This study complimented the study by Isonaka and colleagues in supporting the possibility that biochemical sympathetic dysfunction precedes structural denervation.

Diagnosis

Patients usually present with inability to tolerate upright posture because of typical symptoms of dizziness, visual disturbance, presyncope, or syncope. However, others may present with subtle symptoms such as fatigue, legs buckling, and coat-hanger ache. Orthostatic hypotension can be easily diagnosed by measuring blood pressure supine and after 3–10 minutes of standing. Concomitant measurements of heart rate are important. Inadequate compensatory heart rate rise is typical of neurogenic orthostatic hypotension, whereas exaggerated heart rate increase suggests possibly reversible etiologies such as drugs, dehydration, and deconditioning. Drugs are perhaps the most common cause of orthostatic hypotension, especially diuretics, antihypertensives, tricyclic antidepressants, tizanidine, and tamsulosin. One should identify reversible causes and withdraw "suspicious" drugs. If orthostatic hypotension persists, then patients should be investigated for chronic autonomic failure.

Chronic autonomic failure implies impaired regulation not only of circulation but also of other visceral functions including sphincter control, sexual function, and sweating. Symptoms of chronic autonomic failure are similar whether they are caused by conditions such as diabetes mellitus, amyloidosis, and Addison's disease or by primary neurologic disorders. Central neurologic signs such as ataxia, rigidity, and bradycardia help distinguish other syncleinopathies from PAF. However, PAF can be the initial presentation of central neurodegenerative disorders.

Therefore, the goals of autonomic evaluation are as follows:

1. To document that orthostatic hypotension is due to efferent adrenergic failure
2. To document abnormality of other visceral functions if needed
3. To exclude other causes of autonomic dysfunction such as endocrinopathies, paraneoplastic disorders, and other autoimmune autonomic neuropathies
4. To differentiate PAF from other syncleinopathies presenting with neurogenic orthostatic hypotension to provide presumptive diagnosis, appropriate treatment, and approximate prognosis.

Orthostatic Hypotension due to Adrenergic Failure

The neurogenic origin of orthostatic hypotension was ascertained by Bradbury and Eggleston by documenting severe orthostatic hypotension without rise in pulse rate during head-up tilt, increased blood pressure without decrease in heart rate during head-down tilt, and absence of tachycardia following parenteral administration of 2.5 mg atropine [2, 66]. Since then, advances in technology and science have allowed the development of a standard battery of noninvasive, relatively precise, and quantifiable tests. The neural pathways and normal and impaired responses of these tests are shown in Table 24.2 [66–76]. Head-up tilt test and Valsalva maneuver evaluate baroreflex-mediated adrenergic functions. Blood pressure response to the cold face test utilizes a different afferent pathway without engaging baroreceptors for the assessment of adrenergic function. Mental arithmetic test does not involve the afferent pathway. Patients with efferent sympathetic dysfunction should demonstrate orthostatic hypotension with subnormal rise in heart rate in response to head-up tilt and reduced to absent blood pressure responses to Valsalva maneuver, mental arithmetic, and cold face test. Heart rate responses to Valsalva maneuver, deep breathing, and cold face test assess cardiovagal function. Valsalva ratio is baroreflex mediated and based on heart rate reciprocating blood pressure alterations. Heart rate response to deep breathing and cold face test assess cardiovagal function via different afferent pathways. These tests, in combination, allow the investigator to localize cardiovagal dysfunction to the central or efferent pathway. Thermoregulatory sweat test evaluates the integrity of central and efferent (preganglionic and post ganglionic) sympathetic pathways. The patterns of sweat loss depend on the site of the lesion along the sudomotor pathway. These noninvasive tests document efferent sympathetic, cardiovagal, and sudomotor abnormalities.

Additional Visceral Involvement

The term PAF has become synonymous with efferent adrenergic failure almost to the exclusion of cholinergic/parasympathetic dysfunction. Bradbury and Eggleston [2] documented cardiovagal and sudomotor impairments in their patients. Barker and colleagues [3] reported lack of hypoglycemia-induced increase in gastric acidity and erectile failure as components of cholinergic dysfunction. Neuropharmacological investigations by Polinsky and colleagues demonstrated impaired pancreatic polypeptide response to insulin-induced hypoglycemia and elevated fasting gastrin levels as indices of cholinergic dysfunction in PAF [77, 78]. These studies revealed significant cholinergic parasympathetic dysfunction. Unfortunately, there have been no further studies in this area.

Autonomic dysfunction in patients with Shy-Drager syndrome was also attributed almost entirely to efferent adrenergic failure. A study of two patients with Shy-Drager syndrome revealed widespread cholinergic dysfunction. Postmortem pathology was consistent with Shy-Drager syndrome or MSA. Subsequently, a prospective study of 11 MSA patients confirmed cholinergic dysfunction involving lacrimal glands, salivary glands, esophagus, urinary bladder, and sweat glands. Subcutaneous administration of bethanechol chloride demonstrated hyperresponsiveness and transient reversal of cholinergic dysfunction [79, 80]. In 2006, Ogata and colleagues reported a possible case of PAF with complaints of dry mouth, difficulty in urination, impotence, and progressive constipation. Cevimeline hydrochloride, a muscarinic agonist, improved these functions [81]. These data indicate the need for further investigations in this area.

Although orthostatic hypotension is the cardinal manifestation, chronic autonomic failure affects several additional organs requiring multidisciplinary evaluation. Therefore, autonomic evaluation should be individualized by using several diverse tests, based on clinical assessment, to complement the described battery (see Table 24.2) and to quantify the autonomic deficit in terms of severity and organ involvement [25, 43, 82–86].

Exclusion of Other Causes of Autonomic Dysfunction

There are many causes of chronic autonomic failure. Clinical evaluation can guide the selection of laboratory tests to detect potentially treatable disorders before labeling a patient with PAF. Uncommon presentations of common disorders such

Table 24.2 Tests to document efferent sympathetic, cardiovagal, and sudomotor dysfunction

Test	Pathway	Response Normal	Autonomic failure
Head -up tilt >60°	Aortic and carotid baroreceptor afferents → medulla →sympathetic and cardiovagal efferents	Varies based upon duration and angle of tilt. At 90° tilt: 3 min: SBP 13.05 ± 6.68 mm Hg, DBP 10.26 ± 3.94 mm Hg, HR 18.21 ± 3.09 bpm 10 min: SBP 5.74 ± 7.09 mm Hg, DBP 10.95 ± 3.33 mm Hg, HR 18.79 ± 2.27 bpm	Sustained drop in SBP ≥ 20 mm Hg and DBP ≥ 10 mm Hg. HR increase <15 bpm [37, 68]
Valsalva maneuver	Strain → baroreceptor afferents → medulla → sympathetic efferents	SBP recovery time 2.00 ± 1.98 s	Markedly prolonged, usually >10 s [69]
	Release → baroreceptor afferents → medulla → vagal efferents	Mean IV phase SBP overshoot: 38.1 mm Hg	Markedly reduced or absent [70]
		Valsalva ratio (cardiovagal index): 1.8 ± 0.3 SD (declines with age)	Markedly reduced or absent [71]
Mental arithmetic	Cerebrum → brainstem → sympathetic efferents	Mean arterial pressure elevated by about 15%	Reduced or absent [72]
Cold face test	Trigeminal afferents →brain stem → sympathetic and vagal efferents	Latency of SBP rise 13.8 ± 16.6 s, SBP rise 15.5 ± 15.5%	Reduced or absent [73, 74]
		Latency of bradycardia 5.6 ± 4.6 s bradycardia 16.6 ± 4.3%	Markedly reduced or absent
Heart rate response to deep breathing	Vagal afferents → medulla → vagal efferents	Declines with age; > 60 y: 11.8 ± 5.4 bpm	Reduced significantly [75]
Thermoregulatory sweat test	Increased blood temperature → hypothalamus → sympathetic efferents →postganglionic cholinergic nerve endings	Moisture from sweat alters the color of the indicator Generalized and symmetrical sweating.	Loss of sweating Pattern of anhidrosis may localize the site of pathology along the efferent sudomotor pathway [76]

DBP diastolic blood pressure, *HR* heart rate, *SBP* systolic blood pressure, *SD* standard deviation

as diabetes mellitus, amyloidosis, and Sjogren's syndrome should be kept in mind [87, 88]. Paraneoplastic disorders, especially those caused by small cell lung cancer and immune-mediated autonomic neuropathies, may mimic PAF [89, 90]. For example, Goldstein and colleagues described a patient who had pandysautonomia and weight loss of more the 30 lbs over several months. Laboratory data showed circulating antibody to the ganglionic nicotinic acetylcholine receptor and normal myocardial sympathetic innervation consistent with the diagnosis of autoimmune autonomic ganglionopathy [91]. One can speculate that case one of Bradbury and Eggleston [2], who lost 26 lbs in 1 year, may have had paraneoplastic or autoimmune disorder.

Distinguishing Postganglionic (e.g., PAF) from Preganglionic/Central Autonomic Failure (e.g., MSA)

The biochemical, pharmacologic, and pathologic studies have supported the hypothesis that PAF is a primary disorder of postganglionic sympathetic neurons in contrast to the preganglionic/central pathology of MSA. In 1959, a subnormal rise in norepinephrine upon standing and hyper-responsiveness of the blood pressure to an intravenous infusion of levarterenol were reported [5]. Other investigators described PAF patients lacking vasoconstriction in response to tyramine, an indirectly acting amine that must release norepinephrine from sympathetic nerve endings and denervation supersensitivity to intravenously administered norepinephrine. These patients also showed marked depletion of catecholamine-specific fluorescence in the wall of the blood vessels from muscle biopsies [92]. Polinsky and colleagues observed that the increased slope of pressor response to intravenous norepinephrine was due to deficient baroreflex modulation, but PAF patients did exhibit a shift to the left of their dose-response curve characteristic of denervation supersensitivity [93]. This was recently supplemented by the demonstration of cutaneous postganglionic denervation in PAF [59].

Clinician investigators developed tests to advance the concept of separating postganglionic PAF from preganglionic/central disorders represented by MSA and other synucleinopathies. Table 24.3 [94–101] provides an overview of commonly employed tests. Low plasma norepinephrine levels under standard resting conditions that fail to rise with upright posture, abnormal QSART response, and cardiac sympathetic denervation demonstrated by MIBG SPECT affirm postganglionic sympathetic dysfunction consistent with PAF. Hypotension-induced rise of vasopressin and increase of growth hormone during clonidine infusion indi-

Table 24.3 Tests differentiating central/preganglionic from postganglionic autonomic failure

Test	Pathway	Response	
		Normal	Autonomic failure
Quantitative sudomotor axon reflex test (QSART)	Axon reflex stimulated sweat output	Presence of sweating indicates intact postganglionic pathway	Prolonged latency and diminished to absent sweat output in postganglionic lesions [94, 95]
Plasma norepinephrine levels	Baroreceptors →medulla →sympathetic neuronal activity →release of norepinephrine from adrenergic nerve terminals	Recumbent levels: 250–350 pg/mL A twofold to threefold rise on standing	Low levels of supine and no rise when standing in postganglionic lesions Normal levels of supine and no rise when standing suggests preganglionic dysfunction [12]
^{123}I-MIBG myocardial scintigraphy	MIBG taken up by postganglionic presynaptic nerve endings via the norepinephrine transporter mechanism and stored in vesicles	Correlates with adrenergic innervation density	Markedly reduced or absent in PAF. Normal in MSA [96, 97]
Hypotension-induced plasma vasopressin levels	Hypotension → stretch receptors left atrium → brainstem → paraventricular nucleus of hypothalamus → posterior hypophysis →vasopressin release in systemic circulation	Increase $1.3 \pm 0.2 \rightarrow 3.2 \pm 0.3$ pmol/L	Small rise in central autonomic failure 0.5 ± 0.1 to 1.5 ± 0.3 pmol/L Marked rise in postganglionic autonomic failure 1.1 ± 0.3 to 38.0 ± 8.0 pmol/L (indicates normal central afferent baroreceptor pathway) [98, 99]
Clonidine infusion test	An α2-adrenoreceptor agonist stimulates GHRH neurons in the hypothalamus → anterior pituitary → growth hormone	Growth hormone rise peaked at 60 minutes in normal subjects	Growth hormone rise in postganglionic failure. Absent response in preganglionic involvement [100, 101]

GHRH growth hormone releasing hormone, *MSA* multiple system atrophy, *PAF* pure autonomic failure

cate sparing of central autonomic pathways in PAF patients. These tests, however, are not foolproof. Plasma norepinephrine levels when supine may be normal in PAF patients [102]. Plasma kinetics using tritiated norepinephrine reveal that norepinephrine levels may rise with head-up tilt because of reduced clearance from plasma [103]. PAF patients who demonstrate generalized anhidrosis with thermoregulatory sweat test may have normal QSART suggesting preganglionic dysfunction, whereas MSA patients who display anhidrosis with thermoregulatory sweat test may have absent QSART, indicating postganglionic involvement, presumably due to transsynaptic dysfunction [102]. The clonidine infusion test, although highly sensitive, lacks specificity to be a diagnostic test [104]. Hypotension-induced vasopressin rise may differentiate PAF from MSA [99], but its specificity has not been studied.

In summary, several tests are available to differentiate postganglionic PAF from preganglionic/central synucleinopathies, but none of them are so specific as to be a diagnostic test. Traditionally neuropathological data provide confirmation of diagnosis. Table 24.2, however, shows that neuropathologic studies rarely show isolated involvement of sympathetic ganglia and postganglionic structures.

Other tests that assess the odds of phenoconversion of PAF into other synucleinopathies are also relevant. A University of Pennsylvania Smell Identification Test may show impairment in PAF and PD patients, whereas it is normal in MSA patients. Hyposmia is also a feature of PAF, but to a lesser degree than in PD [43, 82]. Video polysomnography documents rapid eye movement sleep behavior disorder (RBD). As described in the symptoms section, RBD may occur in PAF patients less frequently and usually after the onset of orthostatic hypotension. Micturition disturbances are common. If post-micturition bladder scan shows >100 ml of urine volume, urodynamic studies should be obtained to delineate the type of urinary dysfunction [25]. Urethral sphincter electromyography is more likely to be abnormal in MSA than in PD or PAF [83]. Based on gastrointestinal symptoms, patients may need esophageal manometry, gastric emptying, colonic transit time, anorectal manometry, or anal sphincter electromyography. Electromyography showing reinnervation of the anal sphincter during the early stages of PAF may favor MSA [84, 85]. Brain magnetic resonance imaging can help in the diagnosis of MSA. Hot cross-bun sign representing the degeneration of the pons and pontocerebellar fibers with the preservation of corticospinal tracts produces a cruciform shape of T2 signal hyperintensity. A hyperintense rim to the putamen on T2-weighted imaging (putaminal rim sign), hyperintensity of the middle cerebellar peduncle, and atrophy of the cerebellum and brainstem are additional features of MSA [86].

Phenoconversion and Predictors

Recently, the Autonomic Disorders Consortium reported a prospective 4-year follow-up of 74 PAF patients. One-third of patients (34%) phenoconverted: 13 to dementia with Lewy bodies, 6 to PD, and 6 to MSA [44]. Kaufmann and colleagues had previously described a patient with isolated autonomic failure who developed PD after 20 years [105]. Therefore, the diagnosis of PAF should remain tentative until more specific biomarkers become available. In the meantime, information combined from history, physical examination, sleep data, smell identification test, autonomic data, and neuroimaging can provide a tentative diagnosis for management and approximate prognosis. In PAF, fainting or sudomotor dysfunction precedes constipation and urinary dysfunction [106]. MSA patients are likely to be of younger age at onset, display dream enactment behavior during sleep, and suffer from severe bowel or bladder dysfunction. The combination of normal myocardial MIBG uptake with genitourinary dysfunction favors the diagnosis of MSA [107]. Neurological examination is normal in PAF patients. MSA patients may show subtle motor signs with preserved olfaction. RBD (although described in PAF patients) is more likely to occur in other synucleinopathies such as MSA, DLBD, or PD. Autonomic data favoring conversion from PAF to MSA includes preganglionic sweat loss, supine norepinephrine levels >100 pg/mL, mild cardiovagal impairment, and severe bladder dysfunction [108]. Neuroimaging yields characteristic features of putaminal and brainstem involvement in MSA.

Box 24.1 Nonpharmacologic Measures to Treat Patients with Mild-moderate PAF

- Avoid getting out of bed rapidly, especially in the morning. Arise slowly and in stages (e.g., sitting with dangling of feet, standing, and walking).
- Avoid standing motionless especially in shower stalls.
- Avoid straining at stool or lifting heavy objects.
- Avoid not only strenuous exercise but also physical inactivity or prolonged supine bed rest.
- Avoid excessive heat. Stay in air-conditioned surroundings in the summer.
- Avoid large meals. Frequent small meals reduce orthostatic symptoms. Drinking coffee with meals may be helpful.
- Sleep with head elevated by 6 inches, which may improve orthostatic tolerance by reducing nocturia and supine hypertension [110].
- Use derby chair when needed. It is a cane when folded and a chair when unfolded.
- Avoid potential physical injury by learning to recognize symptoms of presyncope.
- Contact your physician immediately if you have diarrhea or vomiting.

Treatment

PAF is a slowly progressive disorder. Although orthostatic intolerance is the most disabling manifestation, other autonomic symptoms such as bowel or bladder dysfunction may also adversely affect quality of life and require active management. There is no treatment to slow or halt progression of disease. Symptomatic treatment is intended to reduce symptom burden and improve daily functioning.

Nonpharmacologic treatment may be effective in patients with mild to moderate symptoms and may significantly delay the use of medications. It also provides psychological benefit by making the patient an active partner in his/her management. Box 24.1 lists instructions which may be helpful to the patient [109]:

Additionally, patients should be made aware of the benefits of increased salt intake, rapid water drinking, abdominal compression, and physical counter maneuvers. Salt intake can be increased up to 12 capsules of 10 mmol sodium chloride/day to expand intravascular volume and can be monitored in an individual by obtaining 24-hour urine for sodium. In general, a 24-hour urinary sodium >170 mmol/day is considered adequate [111, 112]. A rapid ingestion of 480 ml of water may improve systolic blood pressure by 37 ± 7 mm Hg within about 5 minutes and benefit may persist for up to 50 minutes. Water, being hyposmolar, stimulates osmosensitive afferent neurons in the portal tract and reflexively increases norepinephrine levels. Water consumption in the morning and before meals can be helpful but it should be avoided before bedtime [113]. As described by Bradbury and Eggleston [2], abdominal compression improves orthostatic blood pressure. Compression of legs and thighs may provide added benefit [114]. Physical counter-maneuvers are an excellent addition to our physiologic management. They are effective, easy to apply, can be applied when needed, and can be unobtrusive. Leg crossing (crossing one leg in direct contact with the other while actively standing on both legs) and active muscle tensing for 30–60 seconds raise blood pressure to improve cerebral perfusion [115, 116].

Pharmacologic Interventions

Orthostatic hypotension in the absence of symptoms does not require drug therapy. When orthostatic hypotension is symptomatic, nonpharmacologic intervention should be the first-line management. Pharmacotherapy should be offered when response to nonpharmacologic treatment is insufficient. It should be aimed at improving orthostatic tolerance and not just correcting blood pressure values to "normal range." Usually small blood pressure increase of 10–15 mm

Hg may shift mean arterial pressure from just below to just above the critical level of cerebral perfusion.

Several drugs are available, but none mimics the physiologic effects of norepinephrine, which is released by the body in proportion to demand (more is released with upright posture). Uncertain bioavailability of drugs due to decreased gastrointestinal motility and impaired drug absorption, reduced orthostatic hepatic perfusion altering drug metabolism, variable degeneration of adrenergic nerve terminals affecting storage and release of neurotransmitters, and lack of baroreflex modulation pose a challenge for the physician and the patient. A small group of patients remain refractory to multiple therapeutic modalities.

A variety of drugs have been prescribed off-label on the basis of pharmacologic mechanisms to raise blood pressure. The 2006 European Federation of Neurological Societies Guidelines for orthostatic hypotension recommended fludrocortisone as a first-line drug and sympathomimetics such as midodrine and droxidopa as second-line drugs. In the USA, only two pressor agents have received approval by the US Food and Drug Administration (FDA), the sympathomimetic midodrine and the norepinephrine-producing droxidopa. These three drugs, however, lack long-term evidence-based data. For information on other drugs, the reader is referred to Table 24.4 and to recent reviews on these drugs.

Fludrocortisone Acetate Fludrocortisone acetate is a mineralocorticoid analog used for the treatment of orthostatic hypotension since 1959 [5]. This drug is not FDA approved for treatment of neurogenic orthostatic hypotension. It increases sodium reabsorption in distal renal tubules, decreases urinary sodium excretion, and expands plasma volume. Schmid and colleagues reported increased vascular responses of the human forearm to norepinephrine infusion after fludrocortisone treatment [117]. Chobanian and colleagues observed blood pressure elevation with sodium retention and plasma volume expansion during the first 10 days of treatment. After 6 months of treatment, plasma volume had decreased to control levels despite further rise in blood pressure. Plasma catecholamines were not affected [118]. The drug is available as an oral tablet of 0.1 mg. It is prescribed at doses of 0.1–0.3 mg daily. Its clinical benefit is evident within 1–2 weeks, but blood pressure response may continue to increase over a long period, requiring dose adjustments. Patients should be watched for breathlessness and peripheral edema. The drug can cause hypokalemia even in the first week of treatment. In a recent study, fludrocortisone was associated with increased risk of all-cause hospitalizations, especially among patients with congestive heart failure [119]. Additional side effects include headache, supine hypertension, hypertensive retinopathy, cardiac fibrosis, and muscle weakness. Combining head-up tilt during sleep with fludrocortisone provides further benefit [120]. Concurrent use of desmopressin may increase the risk of hyponatremia. Periodic monitoring of serum electrolytes and supine, as well as standing blood pressure, is recommended.

Table 24.4 Pharmacologic approaches to the treatment of neurogenic orthostatic hypotension

Expand intravascular volume	Promote vasoconstriction	Diminish vasodilatation
Fludrocortisone	Midodrine hydrochloride	Indomethacin
Desmopressin acetate	Droxidopa	Metoclopramide hydrochloride
Erythropoietin	Pyridostigmine bromide	
	Atomoxetine hydrochloride	
	Ephedrine	
	Pseudoephedrine hydrochloride	
	Yohimbine	
	Phenylpropanolamine hydrochloride	
	Dihydroergotamine	
	Octreotide acetate	

Midodrine Hydrochloride Midodrine is a direct alpha-1 agonist approved by the FDA in 1996. It raises blood pressure by causing arteriolar constriction and venoconstriction of the capacitance vessels. It is devoid of central nervous system side effects because it does not cross the blood–brain barrier. It is a prodrug that is hydrolyzed in the liver to its active form, desglymidodrine. The half-life of midodrine is ~30 minutes, but the half-life of its active metabolite is ~4 hours. Its peak effect is evident at 1 hour with a duration of action of 4–6 hours. The drug is available as an oral tablet, 2.5 mg, 5 mg, and 10 mg. It should be dosed three times a day. The author has prescribed it for intermittent use in patients with anticipated exacerbation of mild to moderate orthostatic hypotension. It improves not only symptoms of orthostatic intolerance but also fatigue, low energy level, and feelings of depression [121]. No differences were noted in pressor responses to 10 mg dose in patients with preganglionic versus postganglionic lesions [122]. Therefore, the starting dose can be the same in both. However, dosage should be individualized. Dosage should be reduced in patients with hepatic or renal dysfunction. The side effects are pruritus of scalp, chills, paresthesiae, and urinary retention. The frequency and severity of side effects are dose dependent. Occurrence or aggravation of supine hypertension is another important side effect. Therefore, midodrine should not be administered after the evening meal or less than 4 hours before bedtime.

Droxidopa L-threo-3,4-dihydroxyphenyl serine, a synthetic amino acid (droxidopa) is an orally active prodrug of norepinephrine approved for use in Japan since 1989. The US FDA approved it in 2014 for use in neurogenic orthostatic hypotension based on improvement in symptoms rather than just improvement in orthostatic blood pressure. Unlike norepinephrine, droxidopa crosses the blood–brain barrier. It is converted into norepinephrine both centrally and peripherally by aromatic L-amino acid decarboxylase and may exert its effects as central stimulant of sympathetic activity, as a peripheral sympathetic neurotransmitter, or as a circulating hormone [123]. It acts by increasing sympathetic muscle tone as measured by microneurography and increased forearm vascular resistance [124]. Short-term placebo-controlled clinical trials demonstrated significant reduction in orthostatic hypotension, but long-term studies showed conflicting results [125]. The drug is available as an oral capsule, 100 mg, 200 mg, and 300 mg. Treatment should be initiated at 100 mg three times daily and titrated in increments of 100 mg three times daily every 48 hours to a maximum dose of 1800 mg/day. Patients with supine plasma norepinephrine levels below 220 pg/mL seemed to show a more robust pressor response. Headache, dizziness, nausea, fatigue, and hypertension are common side effects. A 1 year of follow-up of 350 patients receiving droxidopa revealed cardiovascular side effects (24%), but these effects were not attributed to the drug [126]. The prescriber should monitor supine blood pressure before and during treatment to manage hypertension and avoid co-prescribing tricyclic antidepressants and monoamine oxidase inhibitors. The FDA has alerted prescribers by a black box warning about the increased risk of supine hypertension.

The subset of patients who do not respond to a single agent may benefit from a combination of drugs and from stricter adherence to nonpharmacologic therapy. Those who do not respond to commonly prescribed therapy deserve a trial with adjunct medications (see Table 24.4) [127–130]. In general, the data regarding the efficacy of these drugs are inconsistent and the quality of evidence is low.

Two co-morbidities, postprandial hypotension and supine hypertension, are often overlooked and usually require additional management. The impact of postprandial hypotension can be minimized by timing the meal about an hour after taking midrodrine or droxidopa, by rapidly drinking 480 mL of water 5–10 minutes before meals, and by consuming coffee with the meal. If postprandial hypotension is too severe to respond to these approaches, then a trial of the α-glucosidase inhibitor acarbose or the somatostatin analog octreotide may be warranted. The severity and frequency of supine hypertension, if suspected, should be confirmed with 24-hour ambulatory blood pressure monitoring. Mild to moderate supine hypertension may respond to adjustment of timing/dose of the prescribed vasopressor agent by having the patient consume the meal just before bedtime [131] and by sleeping in a reclining chair. In patients with severe and sustained hypertension, short-acting antihypertensive agents such as the angiotensin receptor antagonist losartan potassium, calcium channel antagonist nifedipine, or transdermal nitroglycerine may prove helpful.

Although symptomatic orthostatic hypotension is the most consistent, disabling, and often the presenting manifestation of PAF, other features such as bowel and bladder disturbances, impaired thermal regulation, sexual dysfunction, and RBD may adversely affect quality of life at various stages of the illness. Bowel disturbances may range from mild gastroparesis and constipation to occasional presentation with chronic intestinal pseudo-obstruction [24]. Mild gastroparesis may respond to intake of frequent small meals. However, metoclopramide should not be used to promote motility because of extrapyramidal side effects. Dietary alterations with increased roughage and use of bulk laxatives such as psyllium husk may improve constipation. Urinary dysfunction may initially respond to regular voiding habit. RBD may be severe enough to injure the patient or the bed partner. Awareness and frequent inquiry of these symptoms from the patient and the bed partner should aid the treating physician in seeking specialty consultations for appropriate management [132].

Conclusion

It took almost 70 years after the original description by Bradbury and Eggleston [2] to define the entity of PAF. However, the deconstruction of this entity had already started with the publication of a clinical neuropathological study by Johnson and colleagues reporting Lewy bodies in the substantia nigra [8]. Subsequent studies demonstrating RBD [32] and central dopamine deficiency [133] added to the presence of central nervous system abnormalities. Postmortem findings and antemortem biopsy data showing synuclein pathology in the peripheral and central autonomic structures linked PAF, idiopathic PD, and dementia with Lewy body disease. Editorials labeling PAF as an immaculate misconception and a restricted Lewy body synucleinopathy [13, 134] declared that PAF was an entity with a disappearing identity. The clinical picture, response to pharmacotherapy, and prognosis of PAF differ significantly from other synucleinopathies. One cannot be certain that the strains of synuclein found in PAF, idiopathic PD, dementia with Lewy body disease, and MSA are identical [135] or that α-synuclein is the culprit when PAF cases without synuclein pathology are discovered [26]. Instead of labeling PAF as an entity in search of an identity, these factors as discussed above should provide us with an impetus to revise the diagnostic criteria, identify promising predictors, and develop biomarkers to diagnose PAF before the development of structural pathology.

Acknowledgments I thank Jacqueline Taylor for typing the manuscript and Lyn Jones, MA, ELS, for editorial assistance.

References

1. Wagner HN Jr. Orthostatic hypotension. Bull Johns Hopkins Hosp. 1959;105:322–59.
2. Bradbury S, Eggleston C. Postural hypotension: a report of 3 cases. Am Heart J. 1925;1(1):74–86.
3. Barker NW. Postural hypotension: report of a case and review of the literature. Med Clin North Am. 1933;16:1301–12.
4. Luft R, Von Euler US. Two cases of postural hypotension showing a deficiency in release of nor-epinephrine and epinephrine. J Clin Invest. 1953;32:1065–9.
5. Hickler RB, Thompson GR, Fox LM, Hamlin JT III. Successful treatment of orthostatic hypotension with 9-alpha fluorohydrocortisone. N Engl J Med. 1959;261:788–91.
6. Young RH. Association of postural hypotension with sympathetic nervous system dysfunction: case report, with review of neurologic features associated with postural hypotension. Ann Intern Med. 1941;15:910–6.
7. Shy AM, Drager GA. A neurological syndrome associated with orthstatic hypotension. A clinical-pathological study. Arch Neurol. 1960;2:511–27.
8. Johnson RM, Lee CJ, Oppenheimer DR, Spalding JM. Autonomic failure with orthostatic hypotension due to intermediolateral column degeneration. Q J Med. 1966;35(138):276–95.
9. Graham JG, Oppenheimer DR. Orthostatic hypotension and nicotine sensitivity in a case of multiple system atrophy. J Neurol Neurosurg Psychiatry. 1969;32(1):28–34.
10. Goodall MC, Harlan WR Jr, Alton H. Decreased noradrenaline (norepinephrine) synthesis in neurogenic orthostatic hypotension. Circulation. 1968;38(3):592–603.
11. Kontos HA, Richardson DW, Norrell JE. Norephinephrine depletion in idiopathic orthostatic hypotension. Ann Intern Med. 1975;82(3):336–61.
12. Ziegler MG, Lake CR, Kopin IJ. The sympathetic-nervous-system defect in primary orthostatic hypotension. N Engl J Med. 1977;296(6):293–7.
13. Freeman R. Pure autonomic failure: an immaculate misconception? Neurology. 2004;63(6):953–4.
14. Consensus statement on the definition of orthostatic hypotension, pure autonomic failure, and multiple system atrophy. The Consensus Committee of the American Autonomic Society and the American Academy of Neurology. Neurology. 1996;46(5):1470.
15. Arbogast SD, Alshekhlee A, Hussain Z, McNeeley K, Chelimsky TC. Hypotension unawareness in profound orthostatic hypotension. Am J Med. 2009;122(6):574–80.
16. Khurana RK. Orthostatic hypotension. NY State J Med. 1988;88(11):570–2.
17. Chaudhuri KR, Maule S, Thomaides T, Pavitt D, Mathias CJ. Alcohol ingestion lowers supine blood pressure, causes splanchnic vasodilatation and worsens postural hypotension in primary autonomic failure. J Neurol. 1994;241(3):145–52.
18. Low PA, Opfer-Gehrking TL, McPhee BR, Fealey RD, Benarroch EE, Willner CL, et al. Prospective evaluation of clinical characteristics of orthostatic hypotension. Mayo Clin Proc. 1995;70(7):617–22.
19. Mathias CJ, Mallipeddi R, Bleasdale-Barr K. Symptoms associated with orthostatic hypotension in pure autonomic failure and multiple system atrophy. J Neurol. 1999;246(10):893–8.
20. Robertson D, Kincaid DW, Haile V, Robertson RM. The head and neck discomfort of autonomic failure: an unrecognized aetiology of headache. Clin Auton Res. 1994;4(3):99–103.
21. Khurana RK. Coat-hanger ache in orthostatic hypotension. Cephalalgia. 2012;32(10):731–7.
22. Kaufmann H, Malamut R, Norcliffe-Kaufmann L, Rosa K, Freeman R. The Orthostatic Hypotension Questionnaire (OHQ): validation of a novel symptom assessment scale. Clin Auton Res. 2012;22(2):79–90.
23. Gil-Diaz A, Conde-Martel A, Betancor-Leon P. A 69-year-old man with excessive sweating of the right hemithorax. BMJ Case Rep. 2011;2011:bcr0320113970.
24. Yamanaka Y, Sakakibara R, Asahina M, Uchiyama T, Liu Z, Yamamoto T, et al. Chronic intestinal pseudo-obstruction as the initial feature of pure autonomic failure. J Neurol Neurosurg Psychiatry. 2006;77(6):800.
25. Sakakibara R, Hattori T, Uchiyama T, Asahina M, Yamanishi T. Micturitional disturbance in pure autonomic failure. Neurology. 2000;54(2):499–501.
26. Isonaka R, Holmes C, Cook GA, Sullivan P, Sharabi Y, Goldstein DS. Pure autonomic failure without synucleinopathy. Clin Auton Res. 2017;27(2):97–101.
27. Hishikawa N, Hashizume Y, Hirayama M, Imamura K, Washimi Y, Koike Y, et al. Brainstem-type Lewy body disease presenting with progressive autonomic failure and lethargy. Clin Auton Res. 2000;10(3):139–43.
28. Kashihara K, Ohno M, Kawada S, Imamura T. Frequent nocturnal vocalization in pure autonomic failure. J Int Med Res. 2008;36(3):489–95.
29. Tulen JHM, Man in't Veld AJ, van Steemis HG, Mechelse K. Sleep patterns and blood pressure variability in patients with pure autonomic failure. Clin Auton Res. 1991;1(4):309–15.
30. Plazzi G, Cortelli P, Montagna P, De Monte A, Corsini R, Contin M, et al. REM sleep behaviour disorder differentiates pure autonomic failure from multiple system atrophy with autonomic failure. J Neurol Neurosurg Psychiatry. 1998;64(5):683–5.
31. Weyer A, Minnerop M, Abele M, Klockgether T. REM sleep behavioral disorder in pure autonomic failure (PAF). Neurology. 2006;66(4):608–9.
32. Miglis MG, Muppidi S, During E, Jaradeh S. A case series of REM sleep behavior disorder in pure autonomic failure. Clin Auton Res. 2017;27(1):41–4.
33. St Louis EK, Boeve AR, Boeve BF. REM sleep behavior disorder in Parkinson's Disease and other synucleinopathies. Mov Disord. 2017;32(5):645–58.
34. Barone DA, Henchcliffe C. Rapid eye movement sleep behavior disorder and the link to alpha-synucleinopathies. Clin Neurophysiol. 2018;129(8):1551–64.
35. Khurana RK, Russell C. The spoon test: a valid and reliable bedside test to assess sudomotor function. Clin Auton Res. 2017;27(2):91–5.
36. Mannen T, Iwata M, Toyokura Y, Nagashima K. The Onuf's nucleus and the external anal sphincter muscles in amyotrophic lateral sclerosis and Shy-Drager syndrome. Acta Neuropathol. 1982;58(4):255–60.
37. Gibbons CH, Schmidt P, Biaggioni I, Frazier-Mills C, Freeman R, Isaacson S, et al. The recommendations of a consensus panel for the screening, diagnosis, and treatment of neurogenic orthostatic hypotension and associated supine hypertension. J Neurol. 2017;264(8):1567–82.
38. Shannon J, Jordan J, Costa F, Robertson RM, Biaggioni I. The hypertension of autonomic failure and its treatment. Hypertension. 1997;30(5):1062–7.
39. Vagaonescu TD, Saadia D, Tuhrim S, Phillips RA, Kaufmann H. Hypertensive cardiovascular damage in patients with primary autonomic failure. Lancet. 2000;355(9205):725–6.
40. Garland EM, Gamboa A, Okamoto L, Raj SR, Black BK, Davis TL, et al. Renal impairment of pure autonomic failure. Hypertension. 2009;54(5):1057–61.
41. Norcliffe-Kaufmann L, Kaufmann H. Is ambulatory blood pressure monitoring useful in patients with chronic autonomic failure? Clin Auton Res. 2014;24(4):189–92.
42. Heims HC, Critchley HD, Martin NH, Jager HR, Mathias CJ, Cipolotti L. Cognitive functioning in orthostatic hypotension due to pure autonomic failure. Clin Auton Res. 2006;16(2):113–20.

43. Silveira-Moriyama L, Mathias C, Mason L, Best C, Quinn NP, Lees AJ. Hyposmia in pure autonomic failure. Neurology. 2009;72(19):1677–81.
44. Kaufmann H, Norcliffe-Kaufmann L, Palma JA, Biaggioni I, Low PA, Singer W, et al. Natural history of pure autonomic failure: a United States prospective cohort. Ann Neurol. 2017;81(2):287–97.
45. Bradbury S, Eggleston C. Postural hypotension: an autopsy upon a case. Am Heart J. 1927;3:105–6.
46. Vanderhaeghen JJ, Perier O, Sternon JE. Pathological findings in idiopathic orthostatic hypotension. Its relationship with Parkinson's disease. Arch Neurol. 1970;22(3):207–14.
47. Roessmann U, Van den Noort S, McFarland DE. Idiopathic orthostatic hypotension. Arch Neurol. 1971;24(6):503–10.
48. Oppenheimer DR. Lateral horn cells in progressive autonomic failure. J Neurol Sci. 1980;46(3):393–404.
49. van Ingelghem E, van Zandijcke M, Lammens M. Pure autonomic failure: a new case with clinical, biochemical, and necropsy data. J Neurol Neurosurg Psychiatry. 1994;57(6):745–7.
50. Terao Y, Takeda K, Sakuta M, Nemoto T, Takemura T, Kawai M. Pure progressive autonomic failure: a clinicopathological study. Eur Neurol. 1993;33(6):409–15.
51. Rajput AH, Rozdilsky B. Dysautonomia in parkinsonism: a clinicopathological study. J Neurol Neurosurg Psychiatry. 1976;39(11):1092–100.
52. Hague K, Lento P, Morgello S, Caro S, Kaufmann H. The distribution of Lewy bodies in pure autonomic failure: autopsy findings and review of the literature. Acta Neuropathol. 1997;94(2):192–6.
53. Arai K, Kato N, Kashiwado K, Hattori T. Pure autonomic failure in association with human alpha-synucleinopathy. Neurosci Lett. 2000;296(2–3):171–3.
54. Matthews MR. Assessing the peripheral ganglia in autonomic failure. In: Bannister R, editor. Autonomic failure: a textbook of clinical disorders of the autonomic nervous system. 2nd ed. Oxford UK: Oxford University Press; 1988. p. 511–43.
55. Bannister R, Crowe R, Eames R, Burnstock G. Adrenergic innervation in autonomic failure. Neurology. 1981;31(12):1501–6.
56. Kanda T, Tomimitsu H, Yokota T, Ohkoshi N, Hayashi M, Mizusawa H. Unmyelinated nerve fibers in sural nerve in pure autonomic failure. Ann Neurol. 1998;43(2):267–71.
57. Kurashiki-Osaka T, Adachi T, Nakayasu H, Nakashima K. Alpha-synuclein accumulation in a patient with Auerbach's plexus of pure autonomic failure. Intern Med. 2014;53(19):2261.
58. Masuda H, Asahina M, Oide T, Wakita H, Sekiguchi Y, Araki N, et al. Antemortem detection of colonic alpha-synuclein pathology in a patient with pure autonomic failure. J Neurol. 2014;261(12):2451–2.
59. Donadio V, Cortelli P, Elam M, Di Stasi V, Montagna P, Holmberg B, et al. Autonomic innervation in multiple system atrophy and pure autonomic failure. J Neurol Neurosurg Psychiatry. 2010;81(12):1327–35.
60. Shishido T, Ikemura M, Obi T, Yamazaki K, Terada T, Sugiura A, et al. Alpha-synuclein accumulation in skin nerve fibers revealed by skin biopsy in pure autonomic failure. Neurology. 2010;74(7):608–10.
61. Donadio V, Incensi A, Cortelli P, Giannoccaro MP, Jaber MA, Baruzzi A, et al. Skin sympathetic fiber alpha-synuclein deposits: a potential biomarker for pure autonomic failure. Neurology. 2013;80(8):725–32.
62. Donadio V, Incensi A, El-Agnaf O, Rizzo G, Vaikath N, Del Sorbo F, et al. Skin alpha-synuclein deposits differ in clinical variants of synucleinopathy: an in vivo study. Sci Rep. 2018;8(1):14246.
63. Donadio V, Incensi A, Piccinini C, Cortelli P, Giannoccaro MP, Baruzzi A, et al. Skin nerve misfolded alpha-synuclein in pure autonomic failure and Parkinson disease. Ann Neurol. 2016;79(2):306–16.
64. Klein RL, Baggett JM, Thureson-Klein A, Langford HG. Idiopathic orthostatic hypotension: circulating noradrenaline and ultrastructure of saphenous vein. J Auton Nerv Syst. 1980;2(3):205–22.
65. Guo L, Esler MD, Sari C, Phillips S, Lambert EA, Straznicky NE, et al. Does sympathetic dysfunction occur before denervation in pure autonomic failure? Clin Sci (Lond). 2018;132(1):1–16.
66. Khurana RK. Dysautonomia. In: Schuster MM, Crowell MD, Koch KL, editors. Schuster Atlas of gastrointestinal motility. Hamilton: BC Decker, Inc.; 2002. p. 335–51.
67. Assessment: clinical autonomic testing report of the Therapeutics and Technology Assessment Subcommittee of the American Academy of Neurology. Neurology. 1996;46(3):873–80.
68. Khurana RK, Nicholas EM. Head-up tilt table test: how far and how long? Clin Auton Res. 1996;6(6):335–41.
69. Vogel ER, Sandroni P, Low PA. Blood pressure recovery from Valsalva maneuver in patients with autonomic failure. Neurology. 2005;65(10):1533–7.
70. Denq JC, O'Brien PC, Low PA. Normative data on phases of the Valsalva maneuver. J Clin Neurophysiol. 1998;15(6):535–40.
71. Khurana RK. Valsalva ratio: a noninvasive and quantifiable test of vagal function. Trans Am Neurol Assoc. 1981;106:107–9.
72. Ludbrook J, Vincent A, Walsh JA. Effects of mental arithmetic on arterial pressure and hand blood flow. Clin Exp Pharmacol Physiol. 1975;(Suppl 2):67–70.
73. Khurana RK. Cold face test: adrenergic phase. Clin Auton Res. 2007;17(4):211–6.
74. Khurana RK, Wu R. The cold face test: a non-baroreflex mediated test of cardiac vagal function. Clin Auton Res. 2006;16(3):202–7.
75. Masaoka S, Lev-Ran A, Hill LR, Vakil G, Hon EH. Heart rate variability in diabetes: relationship to age and duration of the disease. Diabetes Care. 1985;8(1):64–8.
76. Fealey RD, Low PA, Thomas JE. Thermoregulatory sweating abnormalities in diabetes mellitus. Mayo Clin Proc. 1989;64(6):617–28.
77. Polinsky RJ, Taylor IL, Chew P, Weise V, Kopin IJ. Pancreatic polypeptide responses to hypoglycemia in chronic autonomic failure. J Clin Endocrinol Metab. 1982;54(1):48–52.
78. Polinsky RJ, Taylor IL, Weise V, Kopin IJ. Gastrin responses in patients with adrenergic insufficiency. J Neurol Neurosurg Psychiatry. 1988;51(1):67–71.
79. Khurana RK, Nelson E, Azzarelli B, Garcia JH. Shy-Drager syndrome: diagnosis and treatment of cholinergic dysfunction. Neurology. 1980;30(8):805–9.
80. Khurana RK. Cholinergic dysfunction in Shy-Drager syndrome: effect of the parasympathomimetic agent, bethanechol. Clin Auton Res. 1994;4(1–2):5–13.
81. Ogata A, Kitano M, Sano H. Cevimeline hydrochloride improved cholinergic dysfunction in a patient with pure autonomic failure. J Neurol. 2006;253(1):119–20.
82. Goldstein DS, Sewell L. Olfactory dysfunction in pure autonomic failure: implications for the pathogenesis of Lewy body diseases. Parkinsonism Relat Disord. 2009;15(7):516–20.
83. Eardley I, Quinn NP, Fowler CJ, Kirby RS, Parkhouse HF, Marsden CD, et al. The value of urethral sphincter electromyography in the differential diagnosis of parkinsonism. Br J Urol. 1989;64(4):360–2.
84. Vodusek DB. Sphincter EMG and differential diagnosis of multiple system atrophy. Mov Disord. 2001;16(4):600–7.
85. Nahm F, Freeman R. Sphincter electromyography and multiple system atrophy. Muscle Nerve. 2003;28(1):18–26.
86. Chelban V, Bocchetta M, Hassanein S, Haridy NA, Houlden H, Rohrer JD. An update on advances in magnetic resonance imaging of multiple system atrophy. J Neurol. 2019;266(4):1036–45.
87. Kondo T, Inoue H, Usui T, Mimori T, Tomimoto H, Vernino S, et al. Autoimmune autonomic ganglionopathy with Sjogren's syndrome: significance of ganglionic acetylcholine receptor antibody and therapeutic approach. Auton Neurosci. 2009;146(1–2):33–5.

88. Pandit A, Gangurde S, Gupta SB. Autonomic failure in primary amyloidosis. J Assoc Physicians India. 2008;56:995–6.
89. Khurana RK. Paraneoplastic autonomic dysfunction. In: Robertson D, Biaggioni I, Burnstock G, Low PA, Paton JFR, editors. Primer on the autonomic Nervous System. London: Academic Press; 2012. p. 593–6.
90. Koike H, Watanabe H, Sobue G. The spectrum of immune-mediated autonomic neuropathies: insights from the clinicopathological features. J Neurol Neurosurg Psychiatry. 2013;84(1):98–106.
91. Goldstein DS, Holmes C, Dendi R, Li ST, Brentzel S, Vernino S. Pandysautonomia associated with impaired ganglionic neurotransmission and circulating antibody to the neuronal nicotinic receptor. Clin Auton Res. 2002;12(4):281–5.
92. Kontos HA, Richardson DW, Norvell JE. Mechanisms of circulatory dysfunction in orthostatic hypotension. Trans Am Clin Climatol Assoc. 1976;87:26–35.
93. Polinsky RJ, Kopin IJ, Ebert MH, Weise V. Pharmacologic distinction of different orthostatic hypotension syndromes. Neurology. 1981;31(1):1–7.
94. Macmillan AL, Spalding JM. Human sweating response to electrophoresed acetylcholine: a test of postganglionic sympathetic function. J Neurol Neurosurg Psychiatry. 1969;32(2):155–60.
95. Low PA, Caskey PE, Tuck RR, Fealey RD, Dyck PJ. Quantitative sudomotor axon reflex test in normal and neuropathic subjects. Ann Neurol. 1983;14(5):573–80.
96. Chung EJ, Kim SJ. (123)I-metaiodobenzylguanidine myocardial scintigraphy in Lewy body-related disorders: a literature review. J Mov Disord. 2015;8(2):55–66.
97. Sakakibara R, Tateno F, Aiba Y, Ogata T, Kishi M, Terada H, et al. MIBG myocardial scintigraphy identifies premotor PD/DLB during a negative DAT scan period: second report. Mov Disord Clin Pract. 2019;6(1):46–50.
98. Kaufmann H, Oribe E, Miller M, Knott P, Wiltshire-Clement M, Yahr MD. Hypotension-induced vasopressin release distinguishes between pure autonomic failure and multiple system atrophy with autonomic failure. Neurology. 1992;42(3 Pt 1):590–3.
99. Williams TD, Lightman SL, Bannister R. Vasopressin secretion in progressive autonomic failure: evidence for defective afferent cardiovascular pathways. J Neurol Neurosurg Psychiatry. 1985;48(3):225–8.
100. Thomaides TN, Chaudhuri KR, Maule S, Watson L, Marsden CD, Mathias CJ. Growth hormone response to clonidine in central and peripheral primary autonomic failure. Lancet. 1992;340(8814):263–6.
101. Kimber JR, Watson L, Mathias CJ. Distinction of idiopathic Parkinson's disease from multiple-system atrophy by stimulation of growth-hormone release with clonidine. Lancet. 1997;349(9069):1877–81.
102. Cohen J, Low P, Fealey R, Sheps S, Jiang NS. Somatic and autonomic function in progressive autonomic failure and multiple system atrophy. Ann Neurol. 1987;22(6):692–9.
103. Meredith IT, Eisenhofer G, Lambert GW, Jennings GL, Thompson J, Esler MD. Plasma norepinephrine responses to head-up tilt are misleading in autonomic failure. Hypertension. 1992;19(6 Pt 2):628–33.
104. Tranchant C, Guiraud-Chaumeil C, Echaniz-Laguna A, Warter JM. Is clonidine growth hormone stimulation a good test to differentiate multiple system atrophy from idiopathic Parkinson's disease? J Neurol. 2000;247(11):853–6.
105. Kaufmann H, Nahm K, Purohit D, Wolfe D. Autonomic failure as the initial presentation of Parkinson disease and dementia with Lewy bodies. Neurology. 2004;63(6):1093–5.
106. Mabuchi N, Hirayama M, Koike Y, Watanabe H, Ito H, Kobayashi R, et al. Progression and prognosis in pure autonomic failure (PAF): comparison iwth multiple system atrophy. J Neurol Neurosurg Psychiatry. 2005;76:947–52.
107. Alves Do Rego C, Namer IJ, Marcel C, Lefebvre F, Lagha-Boukbiza O, Renaud M, et al. Prospective study of relevance of (123)I-MIBG myocardial scintigraphy and clonidine GH test to distinguish Parkinson's disease and multiple system atrophy. J Neurol. 2018;265(9):2033–9.
108. Singer W, Berini SE, Sandroni P, Fealey RD, Coon EA, Suarez MD, et al. Pure autonomic failure: predictors of conversion to clinical CNS involvement. Neurology. 2017;88(12):1129–36.
109. Kaufmann H, Palma JA. Neurogenic orthostatic hypotension: the very basics. Clin Auton Res. 2017;27(Suppl 1):39–43.
110. Bannister R, Ardill L, Fentem P. An assessment of various methods of treatment of idiopathic orthostatic hypotension. Q J Med. 1969;38(152):377–95.
111. Low PA. Neurogenic orthostatic hypotension: pathophysiology and diagnosis. Am J Manag Care. 2015;21(13 Suppl):s248–57.
112. El-Sayed H, Hainsworth R. Salt supplement increases plasma volume and orthostatic tolerance in patients with unexplained syncope. Heart. 1996;75(2):134–40.
113. Jordan J, Shannon JR, Black BK, Ali Y, Farley M, Costa F, et al. The pressor response to water drinking in humans : a sympathetic reflex? Circulation. 2000;101(5):504–9.
114. Mills PB, Fung CK, Travlos A, Krassioukov A. Nonpharmacologic management of orthostatic hypotension: a systematic review. Arch Phys Med Rehabil. 2015;96(2):366–75. e6
115. van Lieshout JJ, ten Harkel AD, Wieling W. Physical manoeuvres for combating orthostatic dizziness in autonomic failure. Lancet. 1992;339(8798):897–8.
116. Harms MP, Wieling W, Colier WN, Lenders JW, Secher NH, van Lieshout JJ. Central and cerebrovascular effects of leg crossing in humans with sympathetic failure. Clin Sci (Lond). 2010;118(9):573–81.
117. Schmid PG, Eckstein JW, Abboud FM. Effect of 9-alpha-fluorohydrocortisone on forearm vascular responses to norepinephrine. Circulation. 1966;34(4):620–6.
118. Chobanian AV, Volicer L, Tifft CP, Gavras H, Liang CS, Faxon D. Mineralocorticoid-induced hypertension in patients with orthostatic hypotension. N Engl J Med. 1979;301(2):68–73.
119. Grijalva CG, Biaggioni I, Griffin MR, Shibao CA. Fludrocortisone is associated with a higher risk of all-cause hospitalizations compared with midodrine in patients with orthostatic hypotension. J Am Heart Assoc. 2017;6(10):e006848.
120. Ten Harkel AD, Van Lieshout JJ, Wieling W. Treatment of orthostatic hypotension with sleeping in the head-up tilt position, alone and in combination with fludrocortisone. J Intern Med. 1992;232(2):139–45.
121. Jankovic J, Gilden JL, Hiner BC, Kaufmann H, Brown DC, Coghlan CH, et al. Neurogenic orthostatic hypotension: a double-blind, placebo-controlled study with midodrine. Am J Med. 1993;95(1):38–48.
122. Low PA, Gilden JL, Freeman R, Sheng KN, McElligott MA. Efficacy of midodrine vs placebo in neurogenic orthostatic hypotension. A randomized, double-blind multicenter study. Midodrine Study Group. JAMA. 1997;277(13):1046–51.
123. Kaufmann H, Norcliffe-Kaufmann L, Palma JA. Droxidopa in neurogenic orthostatic hypotension. Expert Rev Cardiovasc Ther. 2015;13(8):875–91.
124. Kachi T, Iwase S, Mano T, Saito M, Kunimoto M, Sobue I. Effect of L-threo-3,4-dihydroxyphenylserine on muscle sympathetic nerve activities in Shy-Drager syndrome. Neurology. 1988;38(7):1091–4.
125. Perez-Lloret S, Quarracino C, Otero-Losada M, Rascol O. Droxidopa for the treatment of neurogenic orthostatic hypotension in neurodegenerative diseases. Expert Opin Pharmacother. 2019;20(6):635–45.
126. Isaacson S, Vernino S, Ziemann A, Rowse GJ, Kalu U, White WB. Long-term safety of droxidopa in patients with symptom-

atic neurogenic orthostatic hypotension. J Am Soc Hypertens. 2016;10(10):755–62.
127. Lahrmann H, Cortelli P, Hilz M, Mathias CJ, Struhal W, Tassinari M. EFNS guidelines on the diagnosis and management of orthostatic hypotension. Eur J Neurol. 2006;13(9):930–6.
128. Shibao C, Okamoto L, Biaggioni I. Pharmacotherapy of autonomic failure. Pharmacol Ther. 2012;134(3):279–86.
129. Biaggioni I. The pharmacology of autonomic failure: from hypotension to hypertension. Pharmacol Rev. 2017;69(1):53–62.
130. Eschlbock S, Wenning G, Fanciulli A. Evidence-based treatment of neurogenic orthostatic hypotension and related symptoms. J Neural Transm (Vienna). 2017;124(12):1567–605.
131. Young TM, Mathias CJ. Treatment of supine hypertension in autonomic failure with gastrostomy feeding at night. Auton Neurosci. 2008;143(1–2):77–8.
132. Palma JA, Kaufmann H. Treatment of autonomic dysfunction in Parkinson disease and other synucleinopathies. Mov Disord. 2018;33(3):372–90.
133. Goldstein DS, Holmes C, Sato T, Bernson M, Mizrahi N, Imrich R, et al. Central dopamine deficiency in pure autonomic failure. Clin Auton Res. 2008;18(2):58–65.
134. Kaufmann H, Goldstein DS. Pure autonomic failure: a restricted Lewy body synucleinopathy or early Parkinson disease? Neurology. 2010;74(7):536–7.
135. Bousset L, Pieri L, Ruiz-Arlandis G, Gath J, Jensen PH, Habenstein B, et al. Structural and functional characterization of two alpha-synuclein strains. Nat Commun. 2013;4:2575.

Acute Autonomic Neuropathy

25

Walter Struhal

What Is an Acute Autonomic Neuropathy?

An acute autonomic neuropathy is a disease of the peripheral autonomic nervous system developing acutely (e.g., within hours, days, or a few weeks). A number of these diseases are immune-mediated or of paraneoplastic origin. These conditions are in contrast to the pathophysiology of autonomic disorders noted in neurodegenerative diseases. The recognition of autoimmunity in conditions originally termed acute pandysautonomia directed our attention to the diagnostic and therapeutic approach in patients with acute autonomic neuropathies. In the last 20 years, an understanding of these conditions has progressed considerably and is still evolving. As an example, the novel autoimmune encephalitides like dipeptidyl-peptidase-like protein-6 (DPPX), which may also point to the fact that the diseases discussed in that chapter did not entirely exclude the central nervous system involvement. This chapter will focus on the clinically most significant diseases (Box 25.1).

Box 25.1 Acute autonomic neuropathy: the clinically most important diseases

Acute autonomic and sensory neuropathy
Guillain–Barré syndrome
Lambert–Eaton myasthenic syndrome
Limited autonomic neuropathy
Paraneoplastic autonomic neuropathy
Sjögren syndrome
Voltage-gated potassium channel

When to Think of an Acute Autonomic Neuropathy

An important clue is the speed of development of the condition. Severe autonomic failure develops within hours (e.g., Guillain–Barré syndrome [GBS]), days, or weeks (paraneoplastic autonomic neuropathy and autoimmune autonomic ganglionopathy [AAG]). In GBS or AAG, a triggering event is commonly present like a respiratory or gastrointestinal tract infection. Autonomic failure may be cholinergic (e.g., AAG) or noradrenergic (seronegative autonomic ganglionopathy). Most of these diseases may also present with a limited presentation (e.g., only gastrointestinal or other focal manifestation).

The age at onset does not necessarily help; acute autonomic neuropathies may develop in younger or older subjects. Since other autonomic disorders including pure autonomic failure may be clinically similar to acute autonomic neuropathies, the differential diagnosis of an acute autonomic neuropathy should always be kept in mind until excluded (see below).

How to Diagnose Acute Autonomic Neuropathies

A concise history is crucial to evaluate the time course of onset and the clinical presentation. History as obtained from the patient should be followed by a structured autonomic evaluation, for example, COMPASS-31 [1]. A number of scales are available, including a scale for diabetic neuropathy [2]. The Movement Disorder Task Force summary paper may help to introduce several of the tests [3].

The primary goal is to get an idea on the organs involved in the pathologic process. This may be helpful as seropositive AAG has prominent cholinergic (e.g., pupillary involvement) whereas seronegative patients more likely will develop

W. Struhal (✉)
Abteilung für Neurologie, Universitätsklinikum Tulln, Karl Landsteiner Privatuniversität für Gesundheitswissenschaften, Tulln, Austria
e-mail: walter.struhal@tulln.lknoe.at

S. Chokroverty, P. Cortelli (eds.), *Autonomic Nervous System and Sleep*, https://doi.org/10.1007/978-3-030-62263-3_25

orthostatic hypotension [4] (OH), there are, however, contrary reports opposing those differences [5]. Red flags for an autoimmune cause include a personal or family history of an autoimmune disorder (autoimmune thyroiditis, type 1 diabetes mellitus, rheumatoid arthritis, or myasthenia gravis) or cancer [4].

The history will in addition try to highlight symptoms for:

- Orthostatic hypotension (sympathetic dysfunction)
- Heat intolerance (sympathetic sudomotor dysfunction)
- Intolerance of bright light (impaired pupillary light reflex—parasympathetic dysfunction)
- Dry eyes or dry mouth (parasympathetic dysfunction)
- Sexual dysfunction, urinary retention (urogenital dysfunction)
- Abdominal pain, diarrhea, constipation, or nausea (gastrointestinal dysfunction)

A number of patients may only show limited presentations of autonomic failure [6], rather than the full clinical picture of pronounced autonomic dysfunction.

Neurologic examination may give valuable clues: the presence of sensory symptoms is unusual in seropositive AAG apart from eventual mild paresthesia but may be present in seronegative patients [7] and in acute autonomic sensory neuropathy (AASN) [8]. Paraneoplastic patients may have a history of smoking or cancer. Coexisting features including sensory ganglionopathy, neuromuscular features, or symptoms pointing to limbic encephalitis, or paraneoplastic cerebellar degeneration need to be searched for. Eventually, paraneoplastic patients may only show an enteric neuropathy with weight loss, dysphagia, vomiting, early satiety, or constipation [9].

In addition, other diseases including rheumatologic disorders may cause acute autonomic neuropathy. An important example is the primary Sjögren syndrome with a large female predominance (female: male ratio of 9:1), and is estimated to have a prevalence of up to 1% in the adult US population. Autonomic involvement may be quite divergent including orthostatic intolerance, gastrointestinal, sudomotor, and genitourinary symptoms [10]. In fact, autonomic testing in Sjögren patients may resemble POTS.

Additional Tests

History taking, clinical examination and an assessment of autonomic failure using the autonomic function, and antibody testing should be the initial approach to acute and subacute autonomic failure [11].

Cardiovascular reflex and sudomotor testing have been standardized to evaluate the sympathetic and parasympathetic cardiovascular autonomic innervation, as well as the sympathetic sudomotor function [12]. (See also Chap. 9 for details).

Antibody Testing

Identification of an immunological disturbance in some cases of acute autonomic neuropathies is an important development in designing a specific therapy. In 2000, Vernino et al. first described the occurrence of a ganglionic receptor binding antibody in idiopathic autonomic neuropathy and paraneoplastic autonomic neuropathy [13]. This antibody is directed against the alpha3 (ganglionic) subunit of nicotinic acetylcholine receptors (gAChR-AB). The nicotinic acetylcholine receptor is a fast-synaptic transmitter in all autonomic ganglia. Within the ganglion, two alpha-3 subunits and usually three beta-4 subunits are found. Typical patterns of acetylcholine receptors are:

- $(\alpha1)2\beta1\delta\varepsilon$ and $(\alpha1)2\beta1\delta\gamma$ motoric unit
- $(\alpha3)2(\beta4)3$ autonomic ganglion
- $(\alpha4)2(\beta2)3$ brain
- $(\alpha3)2(\beta4)3$ brain

In a number of experimental models, this antibody was proven to be pathogenetic in *Autoimmune Autonomic Ganglionopathy* as well as other syndromes (see below). An active immunization of rabbits caused a syndrome similar to AAG in humans including gastrointestinal hypomotility, urinary retention, impaired light reflex, and even premature pupillary redilation [14, 15].

However, if conditions other than paraneoplastic cause are suspected, gAChR-AB should not be the only antibody to be tested (Table 25.1) [7]. Paraneoplastic autonomic neuropathy most often is associated with gAChR, anti-Hu, and anti-CRMP5 [9]. Anti-Hu and anti-CRMP5 are specific antibodies against intracellular antigens, are associated with a tumor. The immune process is T-cell mediated and the response to immunomodulatory treatment is frequently mild. These patients are generally older [16].

How to Differentiate Among a Variety of Acute Autonomic Neuropathies?

Autoimmune Autonomic Ganglionopathy (AAG)

Acute Phenotype Patients are typically middle-aged and predominantly women [17]. Patients had been typically healthy prior to the acute onset of AAG. An antecedent event (e.g., respiratory infection) is often the trigger for the clinical presentation. The onset evolves during days to weeks.

Table 25.1 Paraneoplastic antibody testing in autonomic neuropathy. (From Golden and Vernino [9], with permission from Springer Nature)

Antibody	Autonomic manifestations	Other manifestations	Cancer frequency (%)	Cancer type	Antigen location
Anti-Hu (ANNA-1)	Diffuse autonomic failure, enteric neuropathy	Sensory ganglionopathy, sensorimotor neuropathy, cerebellar ataxia, limbic encephalitis	88	SCLC	Intracellular
Anit-CRMP5(CV-2)	Diffuse autonomic failure, enteric neuropathy	Somatic neuropathy, cerebellar ataxia, dementia, chorea, cranial neuropathy	91	SCLC, thymoma	Intracellular
Anti-gAChR	Diffuse autonomic failure, enteric neuropathy	None	15	SCLC, thymoma, adenocarcinomas	Cell surface
Anti-P/Q VGCC	Cholinergic impairment (dry mouth, constipation, and erectile dysfunction)	Proximal leg weakness with areflexia, mild oculobulbar weakness	60	SCLC	Cell surface
Anti-VGKC complex	Hyperhidrosis, tachycardia, urinary symptoms, blood pressure abnormalities, and postganglionic sudomotor deficits	Peripheral nerve hyperexcitability, encephalopathy, and limbic encephalitis	13–44	Thymoma, SCLC	Cell surface

gAChR Ganglionic nicotinic acetylcholine receptor, *SCLC* Small-cell lung carcinoma, *VGC* Voltage-gated calcium channel, *VGKC* Voltage-gated potassium channel

Chronic Phenotype After identification of the gAChR-AB as pathologic agent, it became clear that some patients have a chronic course of disease that mimics pure autonomic failure. If the clinical nadir of autonomic failure is reached after 3 months only, the AAG patients are classified as chronic phenotype. In fact, up to 50% account for this chronic phenotype [9]. The clinical presentation may be related to the level of antibody titer found. Prominent cholinergic impairment in this group was linked to 127-fold higher antibody titers than in the group lacking cholinergic impairment [17].

In both phenotypes, patients typically develop diffuse sympathetic, parasympathetic, and enteric dysfunction. Among the sympathetic syndrome patients often present with symptoms of orthostatic hypotension. Parasympathetic and enteric neuropathic symptoms are sicca-symptoms (dry mouth and dry eyes), light and temperature intolerance, sexual dysfunction, and urinary bladder symptoms (neurogenic bladder). Severe gastrointestinal symptoms may occur and have to be addressed to prevent chronic damage (Fig. 25.1) [18]. Some degree of extra-autonomic manifestation is quite common, including sensory disturbances (46%), as well as other comorbid autoimmune diseases (e.g., Sjögren syndrome) [19]. However, there is considerable variation in manifestation. Eventually, only a focal autonomic dysfunction (e.g., dry eyes, dry mouth, OH, or gastrointestinal symptoms) may be present [20]. It is notable that pure autonomic failure may mimic AAG, but may not typically include gastrointestinal dysmotility, and impaired pupillary light reflexes [8, 17].

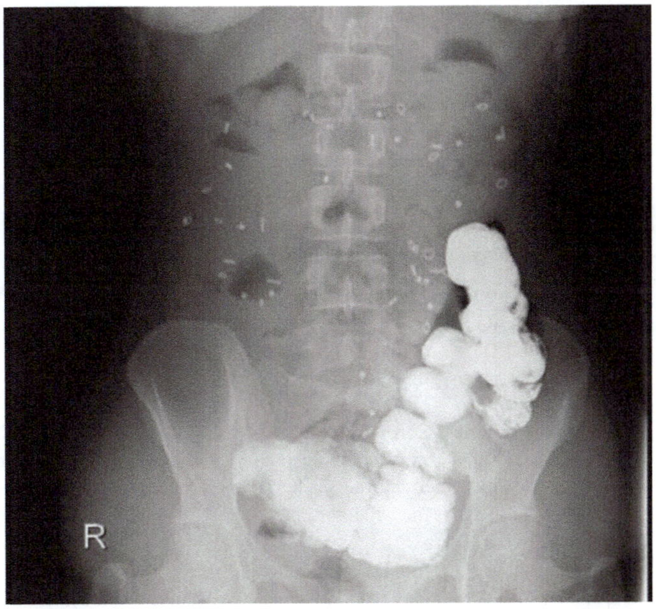

Fig. 25.1 A 24-year-old woman with autoimmune autonomic ganglionopathy—unclear gAChR-AB status. Abdominal X-ray for colon transit time investigation: radiopaque pellets show slow transit obstipation; lower left: remains of X-ray contrast medium 14 days after irrigoscopic application. (From Struhal et al. [18] with permission from Springer Nature)

Autonomic function testing is necessary to confirm the diagnosis of autonomic dysfunction, as well as its extent and severity. Cardiovascular autonomic testing should be performed including supine and standing heart rates and blood pressures. Pupillometry may be especially valuable to diagnose AAG. *Antibody Testing* (see above) is a crucial part in these patients. One has to keep in mind that half of the patients are seronegative. *Paraneoplastic Autonomic Neuropathy* (see below) may clinically resemble AAG.

The patient and caregiver should be advised about supportive care (Box 25.2). Specific management includes intravenous immunoglobulin (IVIG) and plasma exchange as first-line therapies (Table 25.2) [7–9, 21–23]. However, in some cases, rituximab has shown beneficial results [22, 24, 25].

Box 25.2 Supportive care for acute autonomic neuropathy

Orthostatic hypotension
Nonpharmacologic means
Compression stockings, sufficient fluid intake, abdominal binder, enough salt intake
Pharmacologic means
Midodrine, L-DOPS (L-threo-3,4-dihydroxyphenylserine), fludrocortisone
Sicca syndromes
Artificial tears, artificial saliva
Bowel regimen for constipation
Urologic management for neurogenic bladder

Seronegative Autoimmune Autonomic Ganglionopathy

Currently, there is a controversy as to whether this is a distinct entity [7] or not [5]. This condition is most likely an autoimmune disorder. Its length-dependent pattern suggests the pathology to be in the peripheral autonomic nerves rather than in the ganglia. Furthermore, prominent sensory deficits and severe neuropathic pain do occur in seronegative AAG in contrast to seropositive AAG. It is hoped that this controversy will be settled soon.

Management is similar to that in seropositive autoimmune autonomic ganglionopathy with one important difference, in these patients, cortisone treatment may be successful [7]. That cortisone is more effective than other immune therapies as noted in Table 25.2 suggests that this condition is a T-Cell mediated rather than an antibody-mediated disease.

Acute Autonomic and Sensory Neuropathy

In AASN, an autoimmune cause is likely, but until now, there has been no specific antibody identified. Two-thirds of the cases suffer an antecedent event (e.g., upper respiratory tract infection with cough or sore throat) [8]. Initial symptoms consist of sen-

Table 25.2 Current therapeutic options for acute autonomic neuropathy syndromes

Syndrome (Study)	Corticosteroids	IVIG	Plasma exchange	Rituximab	Other
Seropositive AAG (Bouxin et al. [21]; Golden and Vernino [9]	Eventually in combination with first-line therapy	First-line therapy	First-line therapy	Multiple case reports positive	Mycophenolate mofetil azathioprine combination therapy
Seronegative AAG (Bouxin et al. [21]; Golden et al. [7])	Some show tremendous response to high-dose steroids	Same as seropositive AAG	Same as seropositive AAG	Some case reports positive	Same as seropositive AAG
AANS (Koike et al. [8]	First-line therapy	First-line therapy	First-line therapy	–	—
Limited autonomic neuropathy (Golden and Vernino [9])	Idiopathic anhidrosis may respond	Gastrointestinal dysmotility may respond	Gastrointestinal dysmotility may respond	—	—
Paraneoplastic autonomic neuropathy	For cellular autoimmunity	May be helpful in the presence of gAChR ab	May be helpful in the presence of gAChR ab	—	Treat underlying malignancy
LEMS (Titulaer et al. [22])	—	—	—	—	3,4-diaminopyridine screen and treat underlying malignancy in case of P-LEMS
VGKC	May be helpful	May be helpful	May be helpful	–	Treat underlying malignancy
GBS (Willison et al. [23])	—	First-line therapy	First-line therapy	—	Symptomatic treatment for blood pressure and heart rate fluctuations and anti-arrhythmics—may exacerbate symptoms
Sjögren syndrome	–	May be helpful	–	–	

AAG Autoimmune autonomic ganglionopathy, *gAChR* Ganglionic nicotinic acetylcholine receptor, *GBS* Guillain-Barré syndrome, *IVIG* Intravenous immunoglobulin, *P-LEMS* Paraneoplastic Lambert–Eaton myasthenic syndrome, *VGKC* Voltage-gated potassium channel sory features (impaired superficial or deep sensation including vibration or joint position) and gastrointestinal manifestation (vomiting, abdominal distention, and diarrhea). Subsequently, severe and diffuse autonomic dysfunction develops (sympathetic [OH and anhidrosis], parasympathetic [mydriasis and flaccid bladder], and enteric [vomiting, distension, diarrhea, and ileus]), as well as small fiber involvement with neuropathic pain. In half of the patients a sensory ataxia develops. Of note, sensory loss tends to be asymmetrical and segmental, eventually interrupted by patchy areas with minor or no sensory deficit.

Autonomic function testing reveals severe autonomic dysfunction. Nerve conduction studies may reveal a reduction of sensory nerve action potential amplitude. The MRI of the spinal cord may show a high signal intensity in the posterior column in patients with sensory ataxia [4]. The autonomic dysfunction may improve to some extent during the course of the disease, but there may not be an improvement in sensory symptoms.

Treatment consists of i.v. methylprednisolone, IVIG, and plasma exchange as well as supportive care including lifestyle modification to improve the quality of life (see Box 25.2).

Limited Autonomic Neuropathy

This syndrome overlaps with AAG and other autonomic diseases. It has been associated with very low levels of gAChR antibody titers [9]. It was earlier proposed as the cause in some cases of postural orthostatic tachycardia syndrome [26]. This entity may present with pure autonomic failure or isolated pure cholinergic neuropathy including anhidrosis [27] or enteropathy (e.g., gastroparesis). In terms of treatment, anhidrosis responds better to methylprednisolone [28], whereas gastroparesis responds better to IVIG and plasmapheresis (Fig. 25.2).

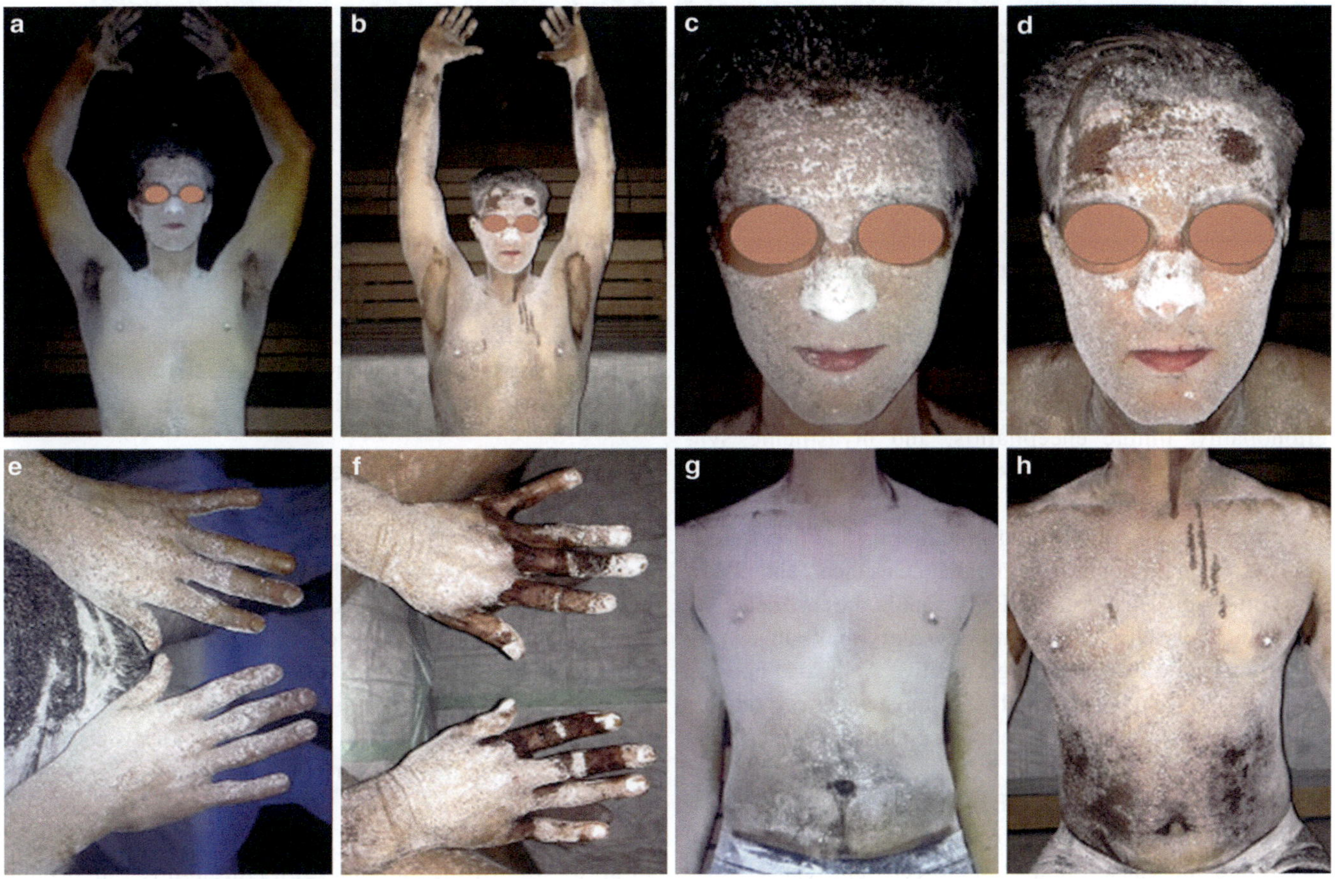

Fig. 25.2 A 30-year-old patient with acquired idiopathic generalized anhidrosis, gAChR-AB negative, severely impaired thermoregulatory sweat test: A, C, E, G, no cooling on thermography: I, and missing QSART response: K; after three cycles of high dose methylprednisolone (1 g on each of 3 consecutive days) improvement: B, D, F, H, cooling on thermography: J, QSART response regained on the left forearm. (From Pargfrieder et al. [28], with permission from Elsevier)

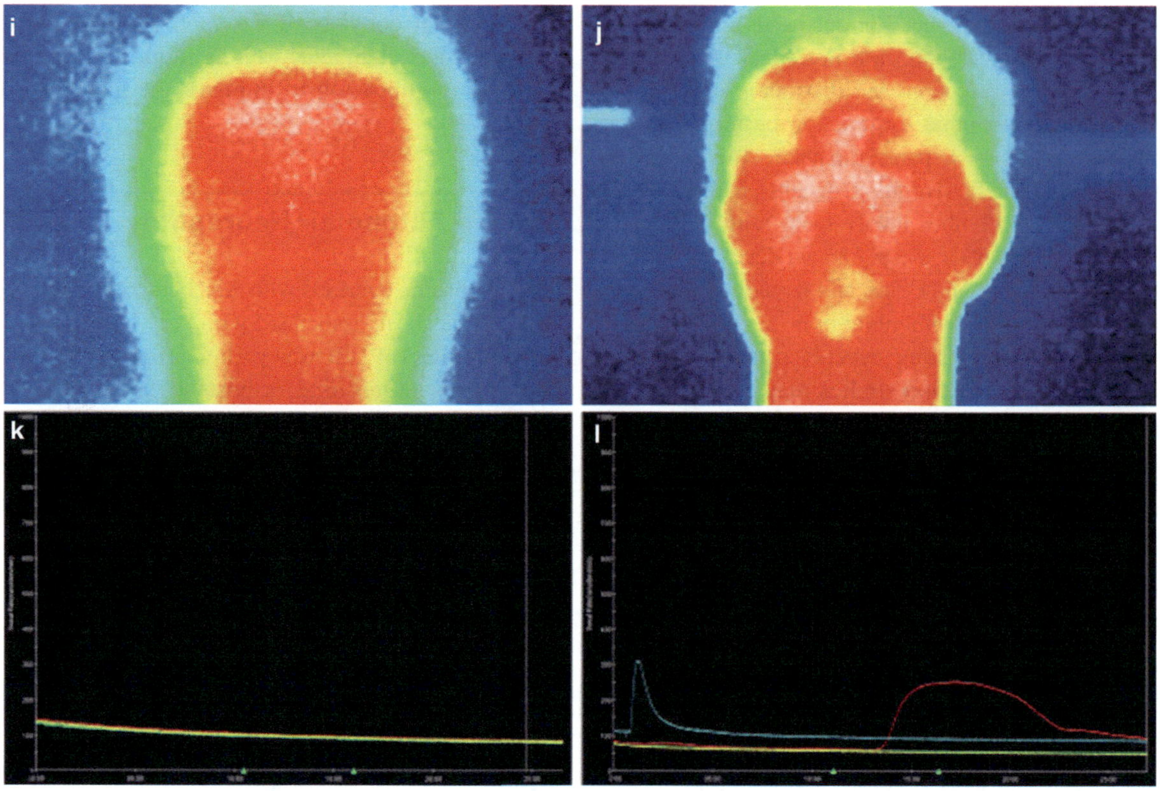

Fig. 25.2 (continued)

Paraneoplastic Autonomic Neuropathy

The presentation of paraneoplastic autonomic neuropathy (PAN) may be similar to AAG. The presence of additional symptoms, such as those noted in ataxia and sensory ganglionopathy, limbic encephalitis, and myasthenic syndrome should raise the suspicion of a paraneoplastic syndrome [29].

Autonomic function testing in addition to antibody testing is essential in confirming the diagnosis (see Table 25.1). Most often anti-Hu and anti-CRMP5 antibodies are detected. Screening for determining antibody titers may suggest an underlying type of cancer (e.g., positive ANNA-1: anti-Hu antibodies may suggest a small-cell lung cancer responsible for such positive titers). Sometimes, patients present with a focal enteric neuropathy only.

Eventually, the gAChR-AB is the paraneoplastic antibody. In that case, the clinical picture is identical with typical AAG, and the cause often is small-cell lung cancer, thymoma, among others [30, 31].

Management includes supportive and immune-modulatory therapy; however, the utmost important endeavor is to search for the underlying neoplastic cause. Therefore, an intensive effort should be made by ordering a computerized tomographic (CT) scan of the thorax and abdomen, and if needed additional tumor markers as well as positron emission tomographic (PET) scan should be obtained.

Other Important Conditions Causing Autonomic Neuropathies

Lambert–Eaton Myasthenic Syndrome (LEMS)

In LEMS, patients report weakness that improves with exercise, dry eyes, and dry mouth. The onset is often insidious and the condition slowly progresses. Typical motor symptoms include proximal muscle weakness (legs often precede arms) and areflexia with the reappearance of reflexes after muscle contraction [32]. While ocular and bulbar symptoms (ptosis, diplopia, dysphagia, and dysarthria) are less common compared to myasthenia gravis, these may be present as well.

Dysautonomia in LEMS is very common and reported in up to 96% of the patients [22]. Autonomic impairment is predominantly cholinergic (dry mouth, dry eyes, erectile dysfunction, and constipation). In addition, orthostatic dizziness with OH and altered sweating may occur less commonly.

More than half of the patients suffer from a paraneoplastic form (P-LEMS), usually caused by a small-cell lung carcinoma (SCLC). The autoimmune LEMS is less common and often overlaps with other autoimmune diseases.

When LEMS is suspected, it is important not to miss autonomic signs and if needed autonomic function testing should be performed to confirm the diagnosis. However, the clinical examination and the distinctive electrophysiological pattern seen with repetitive nerve stimulation are to be tested prior to ordering other tests.

Antibody testing plays a major role in the diagnosis of LEMS. Two antibody types of the voltage-gated calcium channel (VGCC) are to be screened (e.g., P/Q-type VGCC and the N-type VGCC). The P/Q-type percentage is higher in patients with SCLC and also occurs sporadically in SCLC patients without LEMS or even in healthy individuals. Antibody testing was regarded as highly specific in LEMS, but recent data challenged this view. VGCC antibody positivity is therefore only to be interpreted in the clinical context of LEMS [33].

Immune Encephalitides

Voltage-Gated Potassium Channels (VGKC) Encephalitis Autonomic manifestations are also observed in VGKC encephalitides, particularly those with the leucine-rich glioma inactivated protein 1 (LGI1) and the contactin-associated protein-like 2 (Caspr2).

Disorders associated with these antibodies again do not represent a distinct clinical entity [34]:

LGI1 Sixty to seventy percent of this entity occurs in men who suffer from limbic encephalitis.

Caspr2 Again, men constitute 80–90% of such cases and suffer from hyperexcitability of peripheral nerves, Morvan syndrome, and Limbic encephalitis.

Morvan syndrome is associated with Caspr-2 antibodies, but seronegative patients were also reported [35, 36]. This rare disease shows a complex clinical presentation with neuromyotonia, hyperhidrosis, and limbic encephalitis. Neuromyotonia may resemble cramp fasciculation syndrome with muscle cramps in all muscles to some extent as well as myalgias. In neuromyotonia, walking is complicated because of cramps [37, 38]. Muscle relaxation is prolonged resembling pseudomyotonia. In addition, patients suffer from insomnia, hallucinations, memory loss, disorientation as well as constipation, and incontinence [39]. There is a strong male predominance and thymoma is present frequently.

Gadoth et al. described an expanded phenotypic spectrum and long-term outcomes in 196 LGII-IgG O positive, 51 CASPR2-IgG positive, and 9 with double positivity patients identified through neural autoantibody evaluation [40]. Clinical manifestations included pain, peripheral neuropathy, paroxysmal dizzy spells, OH, postganglionic sudomotor deficits, cognitive decline, chronic fatigue, psychiatric symptoms, T2 hyperintensity in *mesiotemporal region* (more common in LGII-IgG than in CASPR2-IgG positive patients), faciobrachial dystonic seizures and an underlying cancer (one-third had thymoma) in varying combination. Age was found to be the only strongest predictor for central neuron system involvement. Most of the patients responded to an initial immunotherapy but some required long-term immunotherapy and antiepileptic medication.

In Morvan syndrome, Na-channel blocking agents including carbamazepine, phenytoin, lamotrigine, and valproate may be helpful.

Anti-NMDA Receptor Encephalitis

This, in fact, is the most common autoimmune encephalitis, more than 80% are noted in women, often below the age of 50 years [41]. A prodromal stage with fever, headache, other signs of infection and eventually mild meningeal sign is followed by psychiatric and amnestic dysfunction. A typical sign consists of bizarre hyperkinetic movement disorder or orofacial dyskinesias eventually followed by mutism and catatonic syndromes.

Patients may show severe autonomic symptoms including episodes of mydriasis, tachycardia, or bradycardia eventually leading to asystole, alternating hypertension and hypotension. Transient sleep dysfunction may occur while recovering. Anti-NMDA-R encephalitis may develop several weeks after recovering from herpes simplex encephalitis [42]. Tumors associated with the anti-NMDA-R antibody are most commonly teratomas, followed by carcinomas.

Dipeptidyl-Peptidase-Like Protein-6 (DPPX)

DPPX is a potassium channel complex antibody. Cognitive disorder and brainstem or spinal cord dysfunction are prominent manifestations [43, 44]. Sleep disorders including insomnia, periodic limb movements, sleep apnea, or hypersomnia are common. Around half of the patients suffer from autonomic dysfunction causing cardiac dysrhythmias, diaphoresis, and temperature dysregulation. Treatment includes corticosteroids, IV immunoglobulin, plasmapheresis, rituximab, and cyclophosphamide.

Guillain–Barré Syndrome (GBS)

GBS is caused by an autoimmune response to peripheral nerves. In the western hemisphere, 40% are preceded by a *Campylobacter jejuni* infection. GBS is characterized by ascending symmetrical weakness, sensory symptoms, and absent deep tendon reflexes. Acute autonomic dysfunction in GBS is common and may increase the mortality. In some patients, autonomic dysfunction precedes the onset of motor dysfunction [45]. During the acute phase, sympathetic hyperactivity dominates and patients are prone to have hypertension, hyperhidrosis, and tachycardia. In patients with baroreflex failure, blood pressure fluctuations with swift alterations are observed [46]. Gastrointestinal dysfunction is regularly seen and 15% of the cases may progress to ileus [47].

Autonomic function (arrhythmia, sweating, blood pressure instability, and ileus) evaluation plays a crucial role in investigating the severity of autonomic nervous system involvement and in deciding whether to transfer the patient to an ICU [23]. Bradyarrhythmia may occur occasionally in GBS patients without the need for artificial ventilation and may need a transient pacemaker [46]. The 24-h heart rate power spectrum analysis may be a valuable surrogate marker to identify those patients who may develop clinically significant arrhythmias [48]. A clinically valuable method to investigate GBS patients at risk for Dysautonomia was reported by Pfeiffer et al. (more than 85 mmHg blood pressure variation daily is a sensitive indicator for autonomic dysfunction) [49].

During recovery, parasympathetic failure is common. Autonomic neuropathy may improve in concert with motor improvement; however, some patients suffer from dysautonomia for quite a long time. First-line therapy for GBS patents is IVIG or plasma exchange.

Sjögren Syndrome

Sjögren syndrome is a common rheumatic disease in the adult population with a female predominance (female: male ratio of 9:1) and a common cause of autonomic neuropathy. It is characterized by sicca symptoms and lymphocytic infiltration in exocrine glands. Autonomic dysfunction is present in more than half of the patients [50]. Structured autonomic testing reveals decreased cardiovagal function, tachycardic response to head-up tilt, and impaired sympathetic vasomotor function. Results may resemble postural tachycardia syndrome [10]. Management for Sjögren syndrome: those presenting with isolated symptoms do not always need therapy, but in the more pronounced disease, steroid treatment is necessary.

Summary

Acute autonomic neuropathies are extremely burdensome to patients and especially autonomic involvement of the heart may be life threatening. Although diagnosis may be a challenge, it is important to consider those entities (described above) presenting with an acute onset of autonomic dysfunction.

Antibody testing is in many of the above–mentioned syndromes a diagnostic hallmark; however, antibody testing is only a piece in the complex puzzle. In addition, antibody test results may take days or even weeks which should not deter initiation of treatment. Figure 25.3 outlines a decision tree for an early diagnosis.

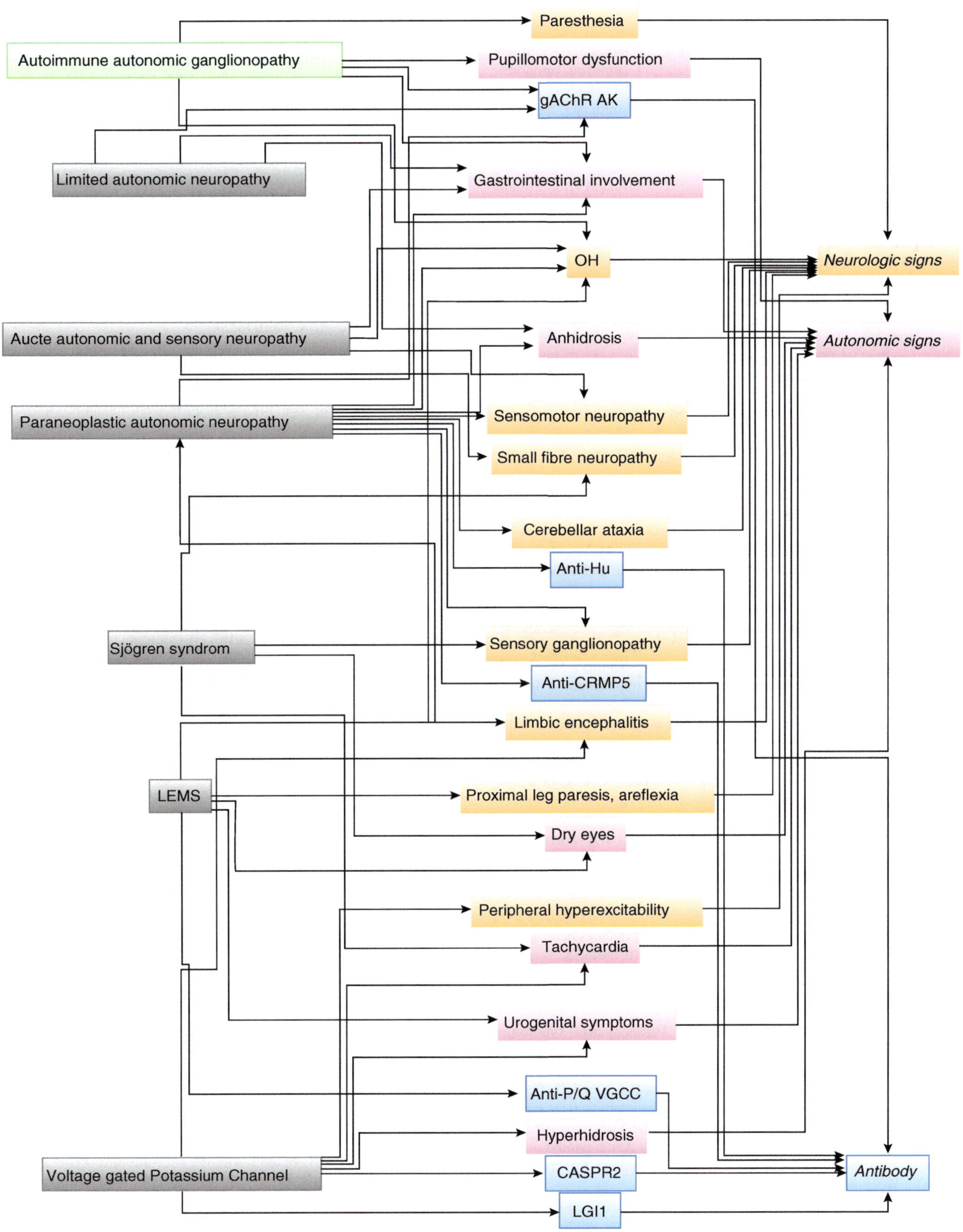

Fig. 25.3 Acute autonomic neuropathy syndromes disease finder—close interconnection of autonomic symptoms, neurologic symptoms, and antibodies

References

1. Sletten DM, Suarez GA, Low PA, Mandrekar J, Singer W. COMPASS 31: a refined and abbreviated Composite Autonomic Symptom Score. Mayo Clin Proc. 2012;87(12):1196–201.
2. Zilliox L, Peltier AC, Wren PA, Anderson A, Smith AG, Singleton JR, et al. Assessing autonomic dysfunction in early diabetic neuropathy: the Survey of Autonomic Symptoms. Neurology. 2011;76(12):1099–105.
3. Pavy-Le Traon A, Amarenco G, Duerr S, Kaufmann H, Lahrmann H, Shaftman SR, et al. The Movement Disorders task force review of dysautonomia rating scales in Parkinson's disease with regard to symptoms of orthostatic hypotension. Mov Disord. 2011;26(11):1985–92.
4. McKeon AB, Benarroch EE. Autoimmune autonomic disorders. In: Pittock SJ, Vincent A, editors. Autoimmune neurology. Handbook of clinical neurology, vol. 133. Philadelphia: Elsevier; 2006. p. 405–16.
5. Tijero B, Del Pino R, Pérez-Concha T, Acera MA, Gabilondo I, Berganzo K, et al. Seronegative and seropositive autoimmune autonomic ganglionopathy (AAG): same clinical picture, same response to immunotherapy. J Neuroimmunol. 2018;319:68–70.
6. Vernino S, Sandroni P, Singer W, Low PA. Invited article: autonomic ganglia: target and novel therapeutic tool. Neurology. 2008;70(20):1926–32.
7. Golden EP, Bryarly MA, Vernino S. Seronegative autoimmune autonomic neuropathy: a distinct clinical entity. Clin Auton Res. 2018;28(1):115–23.
8. Koike H, Atsuta N, Adachi H, Iijima M, Katsuno M, Yasuda T, et al. Clinicopathological features of acute autonomic and sensory neuropathy. Brain. 2010;133(10):2881–96.
9. Golden EP, Vernino S. Autoimmune autonomic neuropathies and ganglionopathies: epidemiology, pathophysiology, and therapeutic advances. Clin Auton Res. 2019;29(3):277–88.
10. Goodman BP, Crepeau A, Dhawan PS, Khoury JA, Harris LA. Spectrum of autonomic nervous system impairment in Sjögren syndrome. Neurologist. 2017;22(4):127–30.
11. Benarroch EE. The clinical approach to autonomic failure in neurological disorders. Nat Rev Neurol. 2014;10(7):396–407.
12. Struhal W, Russell JW. Autonomic nervous system. In: Feldman EL, Grisold W, Russell JW, Löscher WN, editors. Atlas of neuromuscular diseases: a practical guideline. 2nd ed. Vienna: Springer-Verlag Wien; 2014. p. 291–7.
13. Vernino S, Low PA, Fealey RD, Stewart JD, Farrugia G, Lennon VA. Autoantibodies to ganglionic acetylcholine receptors in autoimmune autonomic neuropathies. N Engl J Med. 2000;343(12):847–55.
14. Lennon VA, Ermilov LG, Szurszewski JH, Vernino S. Immunization with neuronal nicotinic acetylcholine receptor induces neurological autoimmune disease. J Clin Invest. 2003;111(6):907–13.
15. Mukherjee S, Vernino S. Dysfunction of the pupillary light reflex in experimental autoimmune autonomic ganglionopathy. Auton Neurosci. 2007;137(1–2):19–26.
16. Rosenfeld MR, Titulaer MJ, Dalmau J. Paraneoplastic syndromes and autoimmune encephalitis: five new things. Neurol Clin Pract. 2012;2(3):215–23.
17. Klein CM, Vernino S, Lennon VA, Sandroni P, Fealey RD, Benrud-Larson L, et al. The spectrum of autoimmune autonomic neuropathies. Ann Neurol. 2003;53(6):752–8. https://doi.org/10.1002/ana.10556.
18. Struhal W, Hödl S, Mazhar S, Ransmayr G. Acute pandysautonomia--restitutio ad integrum by high prednisolone therapy. Wien Klin Wochenschr. 2011;123(15–16):508–11.
19. Nakane S, Mukaino A, Maeda Y, Higuchi O, Matsuo H, Ando Y. Extra-autonomic manifestations in autoimmune autonomic ganglionopathy: a Japanese survey. J Neurol Neurosurg Psychiatry. 2017;88(4):367–8.
20. Dhamija R, Tan KM, Pittock SJ, Foxx-Orenstein A, Benarroch E, Lennon VA. Serologic profiles aiding the diagnosis of autoimmune gastrointestinal dysmotility. Clin Gastroenterol Hepatol. 2008;6(9):988–92.
21. Bouxin M, Schvartz B, Mestrallet S, Debrumetz A, Hentzien M, Tabary T, et al. Rituximab treatment in seronegative autoimmune autonomic neuropathy and autoimmune autonomic ganglionopathy: case-report and literature review. J Neuroimmunol. 2019;326:28–32.
22. Titulaer MJ, Lang B, Verschuuren JJ. Lambert-Eaton myasthenic syndrome: from clinical characteristics to therapeutic strategies. Lancet Neurol. 2011;10(12):1098–107.
23. Willison HJ, Jacobs BC, van Doorn PA. Guillain-Barré syndrome. Lancet. 2016;388(10045):717–27.
24. Gupta A, Harris S, Vernino S, Naina HV. Rituximab-based therapy and long-term control of autoimmune autonomic ganglionopathy. Clin Auton Res. 2015;25(4):255–8.
25. Iodice V, Kimpinski K, Vernino S, Sandroni P, Low PA. Immunotherapy for autoimmune autonomic ganglionopathy. Auton Neurosci. 2009;146(1–2):22–5.
26. Schondorf R, Low PA. Idiopathic postural orthostatic tachycardia syndrome: an attenuated form of acute pandysautonomia? Neurology. 1993;43(1):132–7.
27. Munetsugu T, Fujimoto T, Oshima Y, Sano K, Murota H, Satoh T, et al. Revised guideline for the diagnosis and treatment of acquired idiopathic generalized anhidrosis in Japan. J Dermatol. 2017;44(4):394–400.
28. Pargfrieder C, Struhal W, Sega W, Klein G, Sepp N, Exler G. Acquired idiopathic generalized anhidrosis in a young Austrian patient. JAAD Case Rep. 2018;4(3):222–5.
29. Koike H, Sobue G. Paraneoplastic neuropathy. In: Said G, Krarup C, Vincent A, editors. Peripheral nerve disorders. Handbook of clinical neurology, vol. 115. Philadelphia: Elsevier; 2013. p. 713–26.
30. Lucchinetti CF, Kimmel DW, Lennon VA. Paraneoplastic and oncologic profiles of patients seropositive for type 1 antineuronal nuclear autoantibodies. Neurology. 1998;50(3):652–7.
31. Sharp L, Vernino S. Paraneoplastic neuromuscular disorders. Muscle Nerve. 2012;46(6):841–50.
32. Ivanovski T, Miralles F. Lambert-Eaton Myasthenic syndrome: early diagnosis is key. Degener Neurol Neuromuscul Dis. 2019;9:27–37.
33. Zalewski NL, Lennon VA, Lachance DH, Klein CJ, Pittock SJ, Mckeon A. P/Q- and N-type calcium-channel antibodies: oncological, neurological, and serological accompaniments. Muscle Nerve. 2016;54(2):220–7.
34. van Sonderen A, Schreurs MW, Wirtz PW, Sillevis Smitt PA, Titulaer MJ. From VGKC to LGI1 and Caspr2 encephalitis: the evolution of a disease entity over time. Autoimmun Rev. 2016;15(10):970–4.
35. Irani SR, Pettingill P, Kleopa KA, Schiza N, Waters P, Mazia C, et al. Morvan syndrome: clinical and serological observations in 29 cases. Ann Neurol. 2012;72(2):241–55.
36. Löscher WN, Wanschitz J, Reiners K, Quasthoff S. Morvan's syndrome: clinical, laboratory, and in vitro electrophysiological studies. Muscle Nerve. 2004;30(2):157–63.
37. Maddison P. Neuromyotonia. Clin Neurophysiol. 2006;117(10):2118–27.
38. Hart IK, Maddison P, Newsom-Davis J, Vincent A, Mills KR. Phenotypic variants of autoimmune peripheral nerve hyperexcitability. Brain. 2002;125(Pt 8):1887–95.
39. Löscher W, Cetin H, Schulte-Mattler W, Wanschitz JV. Periphere Nervenübererregbarkeit – Krampf-Faszikulationssyndrom. Neuromyotonie und Morvan Syndrom Klin Neurophysiol. 2014;45(04):201–6.

40. Gadoth A, Pittock SJ, Dubey D, McKeon A, Britton JW, Schmeling JE, et al. Expanded phenotypes and outcomes among 256 LGI1/CASPR2-IgG-positive patients. Ann Neurol. 2017;82(1):79–92.
41. Dalmau J, Tüzün E, Wu HY, Masjuan J, Rossi JE, Voloschin A, et al. Paraneoplastic anti-N-methyl-D-aspartate receptor encephalitis associated with ovarian teratoma. Ann Neurol. 2007;61(1):25–36.
42. Armangue T, Leypoldt F, Málaga I, Raspall-Chaure M, Marti I, Nichter C, et al. Herpes simplex virus encephalitis is a trigger of brain autoimmunity. Ann Neurol. 2014;75(2):317–23.
43. Graus F, Titulaer MJ, Balu R, Benseler S, Bien CG, Cellucci T, et al. A clinical approach to diagnosis of autoimmune encephalitis. Lancet Neurol. 2016;15(4):391–404.
44. Tobin WO, Lennon VA, Komorowski L, Probst C, Clardy SL, Aksamit AJ, et al. DPPX potassium channel antibody: frequency, clinical accompaniments, and outcomes in 20 patients. Neurology. 2014;83(20):1797–803. 1.
45. Koike H, Watanabe H, Sobue G. The spectrum of immune-mediated autonomic neuropathies: insights from the clinicopathological features. J Neurol Neurosurg Psychiatry. 2013;84(1):98–106.
46. Zaeem Z, Siddiqi ZA, Zochodne DW. Autonomic involvement in Guillain-Barré syndrome: an update. Clin Auton Res. 2019;29(3):289–99.
47. Burns TM, Lawn ND, Low PA, Camilleri M, Wijdicks EF. Adynamic ileus in severe Guillain-Barré syndrome. Muscle Nerve. 2001;24(7):963–5.
48. Flachenecker P, Lem K, Müllges W, Reiners K. Detection of serious bradyarrhythmias in Guillain-Barré syndrome: sensitivity and specificity of the 24-hour heart rate power spectrum. Clin Auton Res. 2000;10(4):185–91.
49. Pfeiffer G, Schiller B, Kruse J, Netzer J. Indicators of dysautonomia in severe Guillain-Barré syndrome. J Neurol. 1999;246(11):1015–22.
50. Newton JL, Frith J, Powell D, Hackett K, Wilton K, Bowman S, et al. UK primary Sjögren's syndrome registry. Autonomic symptoms are common and are associated with overall symptom burden and disease activity in primary Sjogren's syndrome. Ann Rheum Dis. 2012;71(12):1973–9.

Familial Dysautonomia

26

Jose-Alberto Palma and Horacio Kaufmann

Introduction

Familial dysautonomia (FD, also known as Riley–Day syndrome, hereditary sensory and autonomic neuropathy type III) is a rare autosomal recessive disease. It was first described in 1949 in children with Jewish Ashkenazi ancestry [1, 2]. The disease is caused by a founder mutation in the IkB kinase-associated protein gene (*IKBKAP* or *ELP1*) resulting in increased levels of mutant, defective, ELP-1 (IKAP) protein, mostly in central and peripheral nervous systems. Lack of functional ELP-1 causes impaired development of primary sensory and autonomic neurons [3–6] resulting in a severe neurological phenotype, which includes arterial baroreflex and chemoreflex failure with high frequency of sleep-disordered breathing and sudden death during sleep [7–12]. FD represents a unique template to study the interactions between sleep-disordered breathing and abnormal chemo- and baroreflex function. We summarize in this chapter recent developments in the understanding of sleep-disordered breathing in patients with FD, the risk factors for sudden death during sleep, and the specific interventions that could prevent it.

Phenotype of Familial Dysautonomia

ELP-1 deficiency in FD affects the development of primary sensory (afferent) neurons, resulting in a complex neurological phenotype. Impaired development of primary sensory nerves results in reduced pain and temperature sensation, absent deep tendon reflexes and gait ataxia [13], as well as optic neuropathy [14], and neurogenic dysphagia contributing to chronic lung disease [15, 16]. In addition, abnormal development of mechano- and chemosensory neurons results in baro- and chemoreflex failure with orthostatic hypotension, paroxysmal hypertension, and abnormal control of heart rate and ventilatory responses to hypoxia and hypercapnia [17, 18]. These contribute to early-onset target organ damage [2, 19, 20] and chronic respiratory disease.

Chemoreflex Failure

Physiology of Respiration and the Chemoreflex The chemoreceptor reflex is a negative feedback mechanism that regulates ventilatory drive to maintain arterial pressures of oxygen (PaO_2) and carbon dioxide ($PaCO_2$) and pH within a narrow range. The *afferent* part of the chemoreflex includes *peripheral* multimodal chemoreceptor cells in the carotid body and *central* CO_2-H^+-sensing chemoreceptor neurons in the brainstem. Peripheral chemoreceptor cells in the carotid bodies, which derive from the neural crest, monitor the partial pressure of oxygen (pO_2), pCO_2, and pH in arterial blood. They synapse with nerve terminals of chemoreceptor neurons, with cell bodies in the petrosal ganglia of the glossopharyngeal nerve, which transmit chemosensory information to neurons in the nucleus of the solitary tract (NTS) in the medulla. These NTS neurons project to the pre-Bötzinger complex, a group of neurons that generates the rhythmic signals underlying the periodic drive for inspiration [21]. Neurons in the pre-Bötzinger complex project to neurons of the dorsal and ventral respiratory groups in the medulla, which control spinal motoneurons innervating respiratory muscles (diaphragm, intercostal and abdominal), as well as pre-motoneurons projecting to vagal (cranial nerve X) and hypoglossal (cranial nerve XII) motor neurons that control the upper airway muscles and tongue [22, 23].

Central breathing networks are also modulated by input from *mechanoreceptors* sensing the stretch of the respiratory muscles (e.g., diaphragm) and lungs. Stretch receptors (mechano-sensors) in smooth muscle of bronchi and bron-

J.-A. Palma (✉) · H. Kaufmann
Dysautonomia Center, Department of Neurology, New York University School of Medicine, New York, NY, USA
e-mail: JoseAlberto.PalmaCarazo@nyulangone.org

S. Chokroverty, P. Cortelli (eds.), *Autonomic Nervous System and Sleep*, https://doi.org/10.1007/978-3-030-62263-3_26

chioles send information via the vagus nerve to the pre-Bötzinger complex and other areas in the brainstem. Lung stretch-receptor afferents conveying signals to brainstem interneurons rhythmically inhibit the pre-Bötzinger complex and activate the lateral parafacial nucleus when lungs are inflated (inspiratory termination reflex) and conversely excite the pre-Bötzinger complex and inhibit the lateral parafacial nucleus when lungs are deflated. This feedback underlies the Hering-Breuer reflexes, essential in controlling inflation and deflation of the lungs.

In normal individuals, most of the respiratory control is exerted by brainstem neurons—*central* chemosensory neurons and glia located in the ventral parafacial nucleus and other regions respond to changes in partial pressure of CO_2 (pCO_2) and pH in the cerebrospinal fluid. These neurons project to the pre-Bötzinger complex – the primary neurons generating the essential periodic drive for inspiration – and other sites to coordinate the breathing cycle [21].

Breathing in humans is extremely sensitive to changes in the levels of pCO_2 in arterial blood, as they directly affect acid-base balance. For instance, in healthy subjects, an increase in arterial pCO_2 from 40 to 41 mmHg (~2.5%) stimulates central and peripheral chemoreceptors and increase minute ventilation from 5 to 7 liters (~40%). In contrast, under normal conditions, breathing is relatively insensitive to changes in levels of pO_2 in arterial blood. However, when oxygen levels decrease and arterial pO_2 is less than ~60 mmHg (e.g., high altitude or intense exercise), hypoxia becomes a powerful stimulus increasing ventilation at any given pCO_2 level [24]. Decreases in pH (i.e., increases in H^+ concentration) stimulate central and peripheral chemoreceptors resulting in hyperventilation. In healthy subjects, reductions in pO_2 cause tachycardia and moderate increases in blood pressure, and both hypoxia and hypercapnia increase ventilatory drive and central sympathetic outflow. Baroreflex activation normally abolishes the increase in sympathetic activity induced by hypoxia, but not by hypercapnia [25–27].

Cardiorespiratory Consequences of Chemo- and Baroreflex Failure Neurological disorders affecting central or peripheral chemoreceptor neurons can manifest with hypoxia and hypercapnia due to hypoventilation and most disturbingly episodes of apnea. In patients with FD, ventilatory responses to hypercapnia are reduced and to hypoxia are almost absent. In response to hypoxia, thee patients develop paradoxical hypoventilation, hypotension, bradycardia, and, potentially, death [7–11]. Impaired ventilatory control due to chemoreflex failure achieves special relevance during sleep when conscious control of respiration withdraws. Virtually all patients with FD have some degree of sleep-disordered breathing [9, 28–30], which is a risk factor for sudden unexpected death during sleep [12].

In patients with FD, cardiorespiratory responses to hypoxia and hypercapnia are markedly abnormal, likely due to impaired afferent chemo- and baroreflex neurons. Several investigations have consistently reported these responses [7–11]. Specifically, in patients with FD (Table 26.1):

(a) Hypercapnia decreases the ventilatory response, instead of increasing it, as it occurs in normal subjects.
(b) Hypoxia results in little or no increase in ventilatory response, rather than the marked increase seen in normal subjects.
(c) During hypoxia and hypercapnia, patients with FD experience bradycardia and hypotension, with some patients experiencing convulsive syncope (frequently misdiagnosed as "grand mal seizures"), instead of tachycardia and a moderate increase in blood pressure as in normal subjects.

Studying six subjects with FD, Edelman and colleagues [8] described that sudden relief of hypoxemia (e.g., with the administration of intranasal 100% O_2) was followed by complete apnea of variable duration (10–56 seconds) in four subjects, instead of only a mild decrease in ventilation (−40% in tidal volume) as in normal subjects. The apnea following the abrupt relief of hypoxia in some subjects with FD might be a consequence of cessation of the hypoxic drive from the peripheral chemoreceptors, suggesting that, at least in some patients, residual peripheral chemoreceptor function might remain.

One dramatic clinical consequence of these cardiorespiratory abnormalities is breath-holding episodes. These are relatively frequent in children with FD after crying or laughing and can result in severe hypotension, hypoxia, and decerebrate posturing before breathing resumes [31]. In addition, during respiratory infections, patients with FD have no compensatory tachypnea and can suffer hypotension and syncope in low-oxygen environments, such as high altitude, airplane travel (although modern airplane cabins are pressurized, partial pressure of O_2 may be low), and underwater swimming [15].

Table 26.1 Cardiorespiratory responses to different setups of hypoxia and hypercapnia in patients with familial dysautonomia compared to healthy controls

	Healthy subjects	Familial dysautonomia
Isocapnic hypoxia [11]	V ↑↑ HR ↑↑	V NC HR NC/↓
Hyperoxic hypercapnia [8, 11]	V ↑↑ HR ↑	V ↑ HR ↑
Hypoxic hypercapnia [8]	V ↑↑↑ HR ↑↑	V NC/↑ HR. NC

V Ventilation, *HR* Heart rate, ↑ Increase, ↓ Decrease, *NC* no change

Sleep-Disordered Breathing

Several studies, some performed decades ago, suggested high prevalence of sleep-disordered breathing in patients with FD [9, 10, 28, 29]. All studies had important limitations, including small sample size, inclusion of subjects before genetic confirmation of the disease was available, lack of end-tidal CO_2 ($EtCO_2$) measurements, selection bias due to inclusion of only symptomatic patients, and inclusion of either adult or pediatric patients only. To overcome these limitations we conducted a large comprehensive study reporting the results of in-hospital polysomnography from 75 consecutive adult and pediatric patients (with genetically confirmed *IKBKAP* mutation) performed regardless of the presence of sleep-related symptoms [30].

Overall, almost all adult (85%) and pediatric (95%) patients had some degree of sleep-disordered breathing [30]. Obstructive apnea events were more frequent in adults, whereas central apnea events were more severe and frequent in children. While the number of central events decreased with advancing age, the severity of hypoventilation (average and maximum $EtCO_2$ levels) progressively worsened with age, suggesting that the mechanisms driving central events tended to have less influence as the brain matured.

The amygdala and hippocampus are specifically involved in breathing control and the pathophysiology of central apneas [32]. Because ELP-1 is required for the normal CNS development and is highly expressed in amygdala and hippocampus [33], it is possible that abnormal development and maturation of these regions may underlie the high frequency of central events during the pediatric years in FD. As these regions mature with age, central events become less frequent.

Not surprisingly, a higher apnea hypopnea index was associated with increased severity of hypoxia and hypoventilation. Notably, in 46% of patients hypoventilation and hypercapnia occurred with no accompanying apnea [30]. This finding has key clinical implications: episodes of hypercapnia not associated with apneas might be missed in polysomnography studies that do not include $EtCO_2$ monitoring. Expert consensus guidelines now recommend $EtCO_2$ monitoring in all sleep studies performed in patients with FD [15].

In addition to chemoreflex failure, additional factors contribute to sleep apnea and the rapid development of hypoxemia in patients with FD. Patients have craniofacial abnormalities with large tonsils and adenoids that predispose to upper airway obstruction, and a smaller thorax and vital capacity due to a physically smaller body habitus and limited chest wall expansion caused by kyphoscoliosis. Additionally, if anemia is present, oxygen-carrying capacity is decreased. Finally, gastroesophageal reflux, frequently present in FD, can cause reflex laryngeal closure resulting in apnea. This laryngeal closure reflex has been implicated in the pathogenesis of sudden-infant death syndrome [34, 35] and could potentially play a role in sleep-disordered breathing in FD. These factors may contribute to prolonged apnea, as well as poor tolerance of environments with low partial pressure of oxygen, such as pressurized airplane cabins and high altitude [15].

Sudden Unexpected Death During Sleep (SUDS)

The two most common causes of death in FD are sudden unexpected death during sleep (SUDS) and respiratory disorders. SUDS is defined as a sudden, unexpected, witnessed or unwitnessed, nontraumatic, and non-drowning death occurring during sleep, with or without evidence of a seizure. Until recently, the risk factors for SUDS in FD remained unidentified. In a recent study, we hypothesized that the high incidence of SUDS in patients with FD was linked to the presence of respiratory abnormalities during sleep. To test this hypothesis, we analyzed the clinical features and polysomnography findings of patients with FD who died suddenly during sleep and compared them to age- and sex-matched patients with FD who remained alive at the time of the study.

This study was based on the New York University (NYU) FD Patient Registry, an ongoing, prospective study of the natural history of patients with FD. The study began in 1970 and contains clinical and diagnostic data, including cause of death, on 670 patients at the time of the study. Of these, 327 (49%) remained alive at the time of the study. All patients have genetic confirmation of FD; more than 99% are homozygous for the same founder mutation (6T>C change) in the *IKBKAP* gene. The majority of patients included in the Registry (above 50%) are from the United States. Patients are followed closely and seen at least once a year [2].

We found that the annual incidence rate of SUDS in patients with FD is 3.4 per 1000 person-year, compared to 0.5–1 per 1000 person-year of sudden unexpected death in epilepsy (SUDEP) [36]. The Registry search specifically identified 32 (14 women) patients with FD and SUDS who had undergone polysomnography in the 18-month period before death. SUDS occurred most frequently during the second and third decades of life (mean age at death was 29.3 ± 12.4 years old). Autopsy was available in six cases. All of them showed brainstem, spinal cord, and dorsal root ganglia atrophy, which are neuropathological hallmarks of FD [37, 38]. These six cases showed no structural cardiac pathology and no acute brain lesions that could otherwise explain their death. Most of them had nonspecific pulmonary congestion or focal hemorrhage, typically seen as a consequence, rather than a cause, of asphyxia.

Multivariable analysis disclosed that treatment with fludrocortisone, plasma potassium levels below 4 mEq/L, and untreated sleep apnea were factors independently associated with increased risk of SUDS in patients with FD. Conversely, treatment with nocturnal noninvasive ventilation was associated with a reduced risk of SUDS.

Taken together, these findings indicate that in patients with FD, sleep-disordered breathing with chemoreflex failure results in episodes of severe hypoxia, hypercapnia, hypotension, and bradycardia. In some patients, hypokalemia is an added factor, potentially contributing to fatal cardiac arrhythmias.

Therapeutic Implications

Noninvasive Ventilation

The finding that untreated sleep apnea and fludrocortisone are independent risk factors for SUDS in patients with FD has important therapeutic implications. Early identification of sleep abnormalities with polysomnography and implementation of noninvasive ventilation with CPAP or BiPAP when required are now encouraged in expert consensus guidelines for the diagnosis and management of respiratory disorders in FD [15].

Treatment with noninvasive ventilation not only decreases the risk of apneas, hypopneas, and sudden death during sleep but also improves daytime ventilatory responses, as recently described [39]. Indeed, treatment with nocturnal noninvasive ventilation in patients with FD results in a marked reduction in daytime arterial pCO_2 suggesting that nocturnal noninvasive ventilation contributes to maintain arterial pCO_2 levels during wakefulness by, perhaps, resetting the chemoreceptor to lower pCO_2 levels.

Role of Potassium

The finding that potassium levels in the low range of normality and treatment with fludrocortisone were associated with SUDS was somewhat unexpected. Fludrocortisone (9α-fluorocortisol) is a synthetic mineralocorticoid that increases renal sodium and water reabsorption, expands intravascular volume, and increases blood pressure. Fludrocortisone for the treatment of orthostatic hypotension in patients with FD became widespread in the 1990s, sometimes at very high dosages (up to 0.6 mg/day). Hypokalemia is a very frequent side effect of fludrocortisone therapy [40]. Thus, it is likely that lower serum potassium levels in cases with SUDS were the result of fludrocortisone treatment. In the general population, hypokalemia and plasma potassium levels in the lower range of normality are independent risk factors for life-threatening arrhythmias and sudden cardiac death [41]. Of note, all drugs proven to reduce mortality and morbidity rates in patients with cardiovascular disease increase plasma potassium concentration [41]. Because specific potassium (TASK-1) channels are key components of the arterial chemoreceptors [42, 43], it is tempting to hypothesize that in patients with FD, lower potassium levels may worsen chemoreceptor failure. Indeed, dysfunction of the TASK-1 receptor in mice results in attenuated cardiorespiratory responses to hypoxia [42], a similar phenotype to that described in patients with FD.

Therefore, reduction or, when possible, discontinuation of fludrocortisone treatment is now recommended. Alternatives to fludrocortisone for the treatment of orthostatic hypotension include non-pharmacological measures and midodrine. Frequent monitoring of plasma potassium concentration during the first 2 weeks following discontinuation is recommended as some patients may develop hyperkalemia. Fludrocortisone discontinuation has other benefits, as long-term treatment with fludrocortisone is associated with target organ damage, including left ventricular hypertrophy and renal failure [44].

Conclusions

The interactions between sleep disorders and autonomic nervous system abnormalities inducing potentially fatal cardiovascular consequences are increasingly recognized in a variety of neurological disorders [45–48]. In FD, discoveries in the last decade have defined the phenotype of the disease, characterized by deafferentation resulting in baroreflex and chemoreflex failure with a high frequency of sleep disordered breathing and SUDS [2, 12, 30]. The recent identification of specific risk factors for SUDS has resulted in the widespread implementation of noninvasive ventilation and reduction or discontinuation of fludrocortisone therapy [12]. Noninvasive ventilation in FD may also have the potential of reversing daytime hypercapnia [39].

A number of questions regarding the pathophysiology of sleep-disordered breathing in FD remain. Chemoreceptor failure should result in central sleep apnea, which is the phenotype in children, but not in adults with FD who have predominantly obstructive sleep apnea. Other factors, such as upper airway abnormalities or interactions between the chemoreceptor signals and upper airway regulation might be responsible and need to be studied. Airway stretch mechanosensing neurons are important for maintaining normal breathing in adults. Functional ablation of mechanosensing neurons in mice abolishes Hering-Breuer reflexes and causes apnea, respiratory failure, and death [49, 50], not unlike the phenotype of FD. It is likely that mechanical signals from airway-innervating sensory neurons are also impaired in FD, but this has not been specifically studied neither in patients nor in animal models of FD [51, 52]. Further investigation of the ventilatory responses during sleep in patients with FD and elucidation of the role of potassium in chemoreceptor function may prove valuable to identify novel therapeutic approaches.

Conflict of Interests The authors report no conflict of interests related to this chapter.

References

1. Riley CM, Day RL, Greeley DM, Langford WS. Central autonomic dysfunction with defective lacrimation; report of five cases. Pediatrics. 1949;3(4):468–78.
2. Norcliffe-Kaufmann L, Slaugenhaupt SA, Kaufmann H. Familial dysautonomia: history, genotype, phenotype and translational research. Prog Neurobiol. 2017;152:131–48.
3. Blumenfeld A, Slaugenhaupt SA, Axelrod FB, Lucente DE, Maayan C, Liebert CB, et al. Localization of the gene for familial dysautonomia on chromosome 9 and definition of DNA markers for genetic diagnosis. Nat Genet. 1993;4(2):160–4.
4. Slaugenhaupt SA, Blumenfeld A, Gill SP, Leyne M, Mull J, Cuajungco MP, et al. Tissue-specific expression of a splicing mutation in the IKBKAP gene causes familial dysautonomia. Am J Hum Genet. 2001;68(3):598–605.
5. Mezey E, Parmalee A, Szalayova I, Gill SP, Cuajungco MP, Leyne M, et al. Of splice and men: what does the distribution of IKAP mRNA in the rat tell us about the pathogenesis of familial dysautonomia? Brain Res. 2003;983(1–2):209–14.
6. Hunnicutt BJ, Chaverra M, George L, Lefcort F. IKAP/Elp1 is required in vivo for neurogenesis and neuronal survival, but not for neural crest migration. PLoS One. 2012;7(2):e32050.
7. Filler J, Smith AA, Stone S, Dancis J. Respiratory control in familial dysautonomia. J Pediatr. 1965;66:509–16.
8. Edelman NH, Cherniack NS, Lahiri S, Richards E, Fishman AP. The effects of abnormal sympathetic nervous function upon the ventilatory response to hypoxia. J Clin Invest. 1970;49(6):1153–65.
9. McNicholas WT, Rutherford R, Grossman R, Moldofsky H, Zamel N, Phillipson EA. Abnormal respiratory pattern generation during sleep in patients with autonomic dysfunction. Am Rev Respir Dis. 1983;128(3):429–33.
10. Guilleminault C, Mondini S, Greenfield M. Abnormal respiratory pattern generation during sleep in patients with autonomic dysfunction. Am Rev Respir Dis. 1984;129(3):512–3.
11. Bernardi L, Hilz M, Stemper B, Passino C, Welsch G, Axelrod FB. Respiratory and cerebrovascular responses to hypoxia and hypercapnia in familial dysautonomia. Am J Respir Crit Care Med. 2003;167(2):141–9.
12. Palma JA, Norcliffe-Kaufmann L, Perez MA, Spalink CL, Kaufmann H. Sudden unexpected death during sleep in familial dysautonomia: a case-control study. Sleep. 2017;40(8):zsx083.
13. Macefield VG, Norcliffe-Kaufmann L, Gutierrez J, Axelrod FB, Kaufmann H. Can loss of muscle spindle afferents explain the ataxic gait in Riley-Day syndrome? Brain. 2011;134(Pt 11):3198–208.
14. Mendoza-Santiesteban CE, Palma JA, Hedges TR 3rd, Laver NV, Farhat N, Norcliffe-Kaufmann L, et al. Pathological confirmation of optic neuropathy in familial dysautonomia. J Neuropathol Exp Neurol. 2017;76(3):238–44.
15. Kazachkov M, Palma JA, Norcliffe-Kaufmann L, Bar-Aluma BE, Spalink CL, Barnes EP, et al. Respiratory care in familial dysautonomia: systematic review and expert consensus recommendations. Respir Med. 2018;141:37–46.
16. Palma JA, Spalink C, Barnes EP, Norcliffe-Kaufmann L, Kaufmann H. Neurogenic dysphagia with undigested macaroni and megaesophagus in familial dysautonomia. Clin Auton Res. 2018;28(1):125–6.
17. Norcliffe-Kaufmann L, Axelrod F, Kaufmann H. Afferent baroreflex failure in familial dysautonomia. Neurology. 2010;75(21):1904–11.
18. Norcliffe-Kaufmann L, Palma JA, Kaufmann H. Mother-induced hypertension in familial dysautonomia. Clin Auton Res. 2016;26(1):79–81.
19. Palma JA, Norcliffe-Kaufmann L, Fuente-Mora C, Percival L, Mendoza-Santiesteban C, Kaufmann H. Current treatments in familial dysautonomia. Expert Opin Pharmacother. 2014;15(18):2653–71.
20. Goldberg L, Bar-Aluma BE, Krauthammer A, Efrati O, Sharabi Y. Ambulatory blood pressure profiles in familial dysautonomia. Clin Autonom Res. 2018;28(4):385–90.
21. Del Negro CA, Funk GD, Feldman JL. Breathing matters. Nat Rev Neurosci. 2018;19(6):351–67.
22. Yang CF, Feldman JL. Efferent projections of excitatory and inhibitory preBotzinger Complex neurons. J Comp Neurol. 2018;526(8):1389–402.
23. Revill AL, Vann NC, Akins VT, Kottick A, Gray PA, Del Negro CA, et al. Dbx1 precursor cells are a source of inspiratory XII premotoneurons. elife. 2015;4 https://doi.org/10.7554/eLife.12301.
24. Hoiland RL, Howe CA, Coombs GB, Ainslie PN. Ventilatory and cerebrovascular regulation and integration at high-altitude. Clin Auton Res. 2018;28(4):423–35.
25. Somers VK, Mark AL, Zavala DC, Abboud FM. Contrasting effects of hypoxia and hypercapnia on ventilation and sympathetic activity in humans. J Appl Physiol. 1989;67(5):2101–6.
26. Somers VK, Mark AL, Zavala DC, Abboud FM. Influence of ventilation and hypocapnia on sympathetic nerve responses to hypoxia in normal humans. J Appl Physiol (1985). 1989;67(5):2095–100.
27. Somers VK, Mark AL, Abboud FM. Interaction of baroreceptor and chemoreceptor reflex control of sympathetic nerve activity in normal humans. J Clin Invest. 1991;87(6):1953–7.
28. Gadoth N, Sokol J, Lavie P. Sleep structure and nocturnal disordered breathing in familial dysautonomia. J Neurol Sci. 1983;60(1):117–25.
29. Weese-Mayer DE, Kenny AS, Bennett HL, Ramirez JM, Leurgans SE. Familial dysautonomia: frequent, prolonged and severe hypoxemia during wakefulness and sleep. Pediatr Pulmonol. 2008;43(3):251–60.
30. Singh K, Palma JA, Kaufmann H, Tkachenko N, Norcliffe-Kaufmann L, Spalink C, et al. Prevalence and characteristics of sleep-disordered breathing in familial dysautonomia. Sleep Med. 2018;45:33–8.
31. Maayan C, Katz E, Begin M, Yuvchev I, Kharasch VS. Laughter is not always funny: breath-holding spells in familial dysautonomia. Clin Pediatr (Phila). 2015;54(2):174–8.
32. Lacuey N, Zonjy B, Londono L, Lhatoo SD. Amygdala and hippocampus are symptomatogenic zones for central apneic seizures. Neurology. 2017;88(7):701–5.
33. Chaverra M, George L, Mergy M, Waller H, Kujawa K, Murnion C, et al. The familial dysautonomia disease gene IKBKAP is required in the developing and adult mouse central nervous system. Dis Model Mech. 2017;10(5):605–18.
34. Cummings KJ. Aspiring to inspire - serotonin, the laryngeal chemoreflex and the sudden infant death syndrome. Exp Physiol. 2016;101(7):790.
35. Horne RSC. Cardiovascular autonomic dysfunction in sudden infant death syndrome. Clin Auton Res. 2018;28(6):535–43.
36. Tomson T, Nashef L, Ryvlin P. Sudden unexpected death in epilepsy: current knowledge and future directions. Lancet Neurol. 2008;7(11):1021–31.
37. Pearson J, Pytel BA, Grover-Johnson N, Axelrod F, Dancis J. Quantitative studies of dorsal root ganglia and neuropathologic

observations on spinal cords in familial dysautonomia. J Neurol Sci. 1978;35(1):77–92.
38. Cohen P, Solomon NH. Familial dysautonomia; case report with autopsy. J Pediatr. 1955;46(6):663–70.
39. Kaufmann H, Norcliffe-Kaufmann L, Palma JA. Improvement of daytime hypercapnia with nocturnal non-invasive ventilation in familial dysautonomia. Clin Auton Res. 2019;29(2):255–6.
40. Chobanian AV, Volicer L, Tifft CP, Gavras H, Liang CS, Faxon D. Mineralocorticoid-induced hypertension in patients with orthostatic hypotension. N Engl J Med. 1979;301(2):68–73.
41. Kjeldsen K. Hypokalemia and sudden cardiac death. Exp Clin Cardiol. 2010;15(4):e96–9.
42. Trapp S, Aller MI, Wisden W, Gourine AV. A role for TASK-1 (KCNK3) channels in the chemosensory control of breathing. J Neurosci. 2008;28(35):8844–50.
43. Buckler KJ. TASK channels in arterial chemoreceptors and their role in oxygen and acid sensing. Pflugers Arch. 2015;467(5):1013–25.
44. Norcliffe-Kaufmann L, Axelrod FB, Kaufmann H. Developmental abnormalities, blood pressure variability and renal disease in Riley Day syndrome. J Hum Hypertens. 2013;27(1):51–5.
45. Fink AM, Bronas UG, Calik MW. Autonomic regulation during sleep and wakefulness: a review with implications for defining the pathophysiology of neurological disorders. Clin Auton Res. 2018;28(6):509–18.
46. Chiaro G, Calandra-Buonaura G, Cecere A, Mignani F, Sambati L, Loddo G, et al. REM sleep behavior disorder, autonomic dysfunction and synuclein-related neurodegeneration: where do we stand? Clin Auton Res. 2018;28(6):519–33.
47. Silvani A. The link between narcolepsy and autonomic cardiovascular dysfunction: a translational perspective. Clin Auton Res. 2018;28(6):545–55.
48. Palma JA. Autonomic dysfunction in sleep disorders: introduction to the series. Clin Auton Res. 2018;28(6):507–8.
49. Physiology GC. Mechanosensor of lung inflation identified. Nature. 2017;541(7636):165–6.
50. Nonomura K, Woo SH, Chang RB, Gillich A, Qiu Z, Francisco AG, et al. Piezo2 senses airway stretch and mediates lung inflation-induced apnoea. Nature. 2017;541(7636):176–81.
51. Lefcort F, Mergy M, Ohlen SB, Ueki Y, George L. Animal and cellular models of familial dysautonomia. Clin Auton Res. 2017;27(4):235–43.
52. Heras-Garvin A. Basic research and model systems in familial dysautonomia: what do we know and what's next? Clin Auton Res. 2017;27(4):211–2.

Diabetic Autonomic Neuropathy

27

Anastasios Tentolouris and Nikolaos Tentolouris

Diabetic Autonomic Neuropathy

Diabetic autonomic neuropathy (DAN) is among the most common but least recognized microvascular complications of diabetes mellitus (DM). DAN often coexists with peripheral neuropathy and other diabetic complications or is isolated, causing increased morbidity, mortality as well as impaired quality of life in subjects with DM [1]. The main clinical manifestations of DAN result from involvement of cardiovascular (CV), gastrointestinal, and urogenital system; sudomotor dysfunction (SD) is also common [2]. In addition, cardiac autonomic neuropathy (CAN) is associated with "hypoglycemia unawareness," and the American Diabetes Association (ADA) recommends that patients with hypoglycemia unawareness should be screened for the presence of CAN [3, 4].

The established pathophysiology mechanisms that lead to the development of DAN are common among all microvascular complications of DM and involve mainly longstanding hyperglycemia [5]. First, the activation of the polyol pathway leads to increased production of polyols and particularly sorbitol [1, 6]. The resultant accumulation of sorbitol causes an increase in intracellular osmotic pressure with consequent cell expansion and lysis [1, 6]. In addition, oxidative stress is increased since glutathione, which is an important intracellular antioxidant, decreases [1, 6]. The activation of the polyol pathway may cause a reduction of neuronal blood flow in addition to a direct cellular injury [1, 6]. Second, hyperglycemia reinforces the production of advanced glycation end products (AGEs) [5]. Every part of nerve tissue can be glycated in diabetic nerves including the axoplasms of nerve fibers and the endoneurial vessels [7]. Intracellular increase of AGEs affects gene transcription, while the interaction of AGEs with their receptor leads to severe structural neuronal changes [7]. Furthermore, AGEs are involved in the damage of the microvasculature [7]. Increased blood glucose levels also activate protein kinase C (PKC) and the hexosamine pathway, leading to vasoconstriction, reduced neuronal blood flow, and neuronal injury [1, 5]. Apart from these four pathways, oxidative stress is another underlying mechanism that causes direct neuronal damage [1, 5]. Hyperglycemia results in increased oxidative stress with generation of free radicals, leading eventually to vascular endothelium damage and decreased bioavailability of nitric oxide [1, 7, 8].

Other factors that may be involved in alteration of nerve function and neuronal damage include immune mechanisms, inflammation, neurovascular insufficiency, reduction of neurotrophic growth factors, activation of genes, and deficiency of fatty acids [1, 7, 9–13]. Moreover, it is known that the ability of neuronal regeneration is impaired in people with DM [14].

A. Tentolouris · N. Tentolouris (✉)
First Department of Propaedeutic Internal Medicine, School of Medicine, Laiko General Hospital, National and Kapodistrian University of Athens, Athens, Greece
e-mail: ntentol@med.uoa.gr

Cardiac Autonomic Neuropathy

According to the ADA and the Toronto Consensus Panel on diabetic neuropathy, CAN is defined as "the impairment of autonomic control of the CV system in the setting of DM after exclusion of other causes" and is the most common, and studied manifestation of DAN [2–4].

The prevalence of CAN was found to vary between 16.6 and 20% in two studies that recruited subjects with type 1 and type 2 DM [15, 16]. The Diabetes Control and Complications Trial (DCCT) demonstrated that among people with newly diagnosed type 1 DM, the prevalence of CAN was low at baseline (3.9% in the intensive and 5.3% in the conventional treatment group); however, the prevalence rate

S. Chokroverty, P. Cortelli (eds.), *Autonomic Nervous System and Sleep*, https://doi.org/10.1007/978-3-030-62263-3_27

increased to 30% after 20 years of DM duration in the DCCT/Epidemiology of Diabetes Interventions and Complications (EDIC) study [17–19]. Similarly, among subjects with long-standing type 2 DM, CAN was found in up to 60% of the population [4]. Prospective studies have shown that the prevalence of CAN increases approximately 6% per year in type 2 and 2% per year in type 1 DM patients [3, 18]. CAN is also diagnosed in subjects with prediabetes, metabolic syndrome, and insulin resistance [20, 21]. The discrepancy between the prevalence rates of CAN may be attributed to the different tests used for the diagnosis of CAN, the different diagnostic criteria, the use of age-related normative values, and the populations studied (differences mainly in patients' age and duration of DM) [2, 3].

The EURODIAB prospective study showed that over a mean period of 7.3 years, baseline age, glycemic control, systolic blood pressure (BP), and presence of peripheral neuropathy as well as retinopathy were the main predictors for the development of CAN in patients with type 1 DM [22]. In type 2 DM, prospective and cross-sectional studies have demonstrated that CAN is associated with age, disease duration, degree of glycemic control, presence of other microvascular complications (retinopathy, nephropathy, and peripheral neuropathy), hypertension, and dyslipidemia. In addition, several other factors such as female gender, CV disease, smoking, obesity, hyperinsulinemia, and waist circumference have been associated with the presence of CAN [3, 23, 24].

In the earliest stages, CAN is asymptomatic and can be detected only by decreased heart rate variability (HRV) during deep breathing [2, 4]. HRV (see further on) is a function of the autonomic nervous system that modulates the response of cardiac rhythm to body's activity [13]. In more advanced stages, CAN causes resting sinus tachycardia and exercise intolerance [2, 4]. Heart rates of approximately 100 beats per minute reflect the damage of the parasympathetic and compensatory increase of the sympathetic activity [13]. Exercise intolerance in people with CAN who are free from CV disease results from the inability of the CV system to increase heart rate and BP in order to increase cardiac output during situations where the body has high energy needs, such as exercise (Table 27.1).

Other common symptoms of CAN include weakness, faintness, visual impairment, light headedness, dizziness, or syncope as a result of orthostatic hypotension (a fall in systolic BP by >20 mmHg or diastolic BP by >10 mmHg within 2 minutes of standing without an appropriate increase in heart rate [3, 4]. Moreover, subjects with CAN have more often a blunted or no physiological fall in the nocturnal arterial BP (nondipper) or even a rise of nocturnal BP (reverse dipper) as compared with subjects without CAN, in whom a normal nocturnal BP drop of more than 10% of the diurnal BP values occurs [13, 25].

All people with DM should be questioned about the presence of CAN symptoms while taking medical history and signs of CAN should be carefully evaluated. Nevertheless, the association between clinical manifestations and autonomic dysfunction is weak [4]. The ADA recommends (with low level of evidence) that symptoms and signs of CAN should be assessed in subjects with microvascular complications [4].

Table 27.1 Symptoms and signs of diabetic autonomic neuropathy

Cardiac autonomic neuropathy	Gastrointestinal neuropathy	Urogenital neuropathy	Sudomotor dysfunction	Ocular manifestations	Metabolic manifestations
Anhidrosis Dry skin Resting tachycardia Exercise intolerance	Esophageal dysfunction Heartburn Dysphagia	Neurogenic bladder: Frequency Urgency Weak stream Dribbling Urinary incontinence	Anhidrosis Dry skin Gustatory sweating Heat intolerance	Pupillomotor function impairment Argyll-Robertson-like pupil	Hypoglycemia unawareness
Abnormal blood pressure regulation	Gastroparesis: Nausea Bloating Loss of appetite Early satiety Vomiting	Male sexual dysfunction: Erectile dysfunction Decreased libido Retrograde ejaculation			
Orthostatic hypotension: Lightheadedness Weakness Faintness Visual impairment Syncope Silent myocardial ischemia Arrhythmias	Diabetic enteropathy: Watery diarrhea Fecal incontinence Constipation	Female sexual dysfunction: Decreased sexual desire Increased pain during intercourse Decreased sexual arousal Inadequate lubrication			

An electrocardiogram (ECG) or commercially available software programs can be used for the assessment of CV autonomic function. Ewing et al. proposed five simple non-invasive tests: heart rate response to deep breathing, heart rate response to standing up, BP response to standing up, Valsalva maneuver, and BP response to sustained handgrip [26, 27]. The first test is the heart rate response to deep breathing and reflects the parasympathetic activity. The person lies quietly and breathes deeply with a frequency of six breaths per minute while a heart monitor records the difference between the maximum and minimum heart rates [1]. The second (30:15 ratio) and the third test examine the heart rate response and the BP response to standing. Normally, on standing a rapid increase in heart rate followed by a reflex bradycardia is recorded, while BP changes slightly. In people with CAN only a progressive increase of heart rate is recorded. An ECG is used to determine the 30:15 ratio, which is the ratio of the longest R-R interval (found at about beat 30) to the shortest R-R interval (found at about beat 15) [1]. Regarding BP, the test is abnormal when the systolic BP falls more than 20 mmHg within 2 minutes after standing [26]. The fourth test is the CV response to the Valsalva maneuver. Under normal circumstances, the response to the Valsalva maneuver is tachycardia and peripheral vasoconstriction followed by reflex bradycardia. In people with CAN, this response is altered and a blunted heart rate response or a lower than normal decline in BP is recorded [1]. The patient is sitting in a supine position and exhales forcibly for 15 seconds against a standard resistance of 40 mmHg [1]. The Valsalva ratio is calculated by measuring the longest R-R interval after the maneuver to the shortest R-R interval during or shortly after the maneuver (Valsalva ratio) [1]. The final test is the diastolic BP response to sustained handgrip. Herein, the patient holds a handgrip dynamometer causing sustained muscle contraction. In healthy people systolic and diastolic BP increase, while individuals with CAN may present a small diastolic BP rise [1].

The tests proposed by Ewing are easy to perform by a general practitioner. They are valid if potential factors such as concomitant illness, drug use (antidepressants, diuretics, b-adrenergic blockers, etc.), and end-organ failure have been excluded [1]. In addition, exercise, smoking, and caffeine intake may alter the CV autonomic function. Normal values that are affected predominantly by age have been recommended for these tests [26].

Apart from Ewing tests, time and frequency domains (power spectral analysis) can be used for the assessment of CAN [1, 13]. Spectral analysis has the advantage that less patients' participation is required, since the subject is lying for several minutes or a 24-hour ECG recording can be performed. The spectrum of heart rate is divided into high-frequency domain that reflects parasympathetic activity and the low-frequency domain that assesses both sympathetic and parasympathetic activity [28]. In addition, baroreflex sensitivity (BRS) examines the capability to increase vagal activity and decrease sympathetic activity when BP increases [13]. QT prolongation has also been proposed as a marker of cardiac autonomic dysfunction [24]. In terms of imaging techniques, quantitative scintigraphy of sympathetic innervation of the human heart with positron emission tomography can be used for the assessment of CAN [13] (for autonomic function laboratory tests.

The presence of CAN is associated with increased mortality due to cardiac arrhythmias and sudden death [13, 29, 30]. In the EURODIAB prospective study after 7 years of follow-up, CAN was the strongest predictor of mortality, exceeding that of traditional CV risk factors in people with type 1 DM [31]. A meta-analysis of 15 studies with 2900 individuals with DM showed that the relative risk of mortality of patients with CAN is 3.45, and increases with the number of abnormal CAN function tests [32]. In addition, another meta-analysis demonstrated that CAN is associated strongly with silent myocardial ischemia [1]. Similarly, CAN predicted silent ischemia and CV events in subjects with type 2 DM [33].

Several potential mechanisms have been proposed for the increased mortality rate in people with DM. First, people with CAN have hypoglycemia unawareness and are not able to recognize and recover from hypoglycemic events [1]. Second, CAN damages respiratory responses to hypoxemia and drugs affecting the respiration that should be avoided [1]. In addition, the concomitant presence of other microvascular complications such as nephropathy and end-stage renal disease increases the risk of CV events. Other potential risks include sudden death due to asymptomatic ischemia and fatal arrhythmias [1]. QT prolongation that is a marker of CAN predisposes to cardiac arrhythmias [1].

The first treatment approach is optimization of glycemic control to prevent or delay the development of CAN [4]. The DCCT trial demonstrated that in subjects with type 1 DM, intensive treatment reduced the incidence of CAN by 53% when compared with conventional management [17]. In addition, in the EDIC trial, the prevalence of CAN increased in both treatment groups; however, CAN remained lower in the intensive treatment arm [18]. In people with type 2 DM, the impact of glycemic control on CAN is not well established. The Steno-2 trial demonstrated that a multifunctional approach involving glycemia and other CV risk factors reduced the prevalence of CAN in people with type 2 DM and microalbuminuria [34]. On the other hand, another study showed that there was no difference in the prevalence of CAN in subjects with type 2 DM after tight glycemic control in comparison with subjects without tight control [35].

Symptomatic treatment includes management of orthostatic hypotension. Patients with CAN should be advised to avoid sudden changes in body posture and medications that enhance hypotension such as tricyclic antidepressants. In addition, physical maneuvers such as leg crossing, muscle pumping, and squatting are encouraged to maintain BP during intense physical activity [13]. Volume repletion, salt, and low dose of fludrocortisone can be used with caution [4].

Regarding pharmacological treatments, midodrine, which is a peripheral selective alpha-1 adrenoreceptor agonist, is the only medication approved by the FDA in doses of 2.5–10 mg three times per day with a gradual titration [4, 13]. Recently, droxidopa was approved by the FDA for the management of neurogenic orthostatic hypotension but not specifically for people with DM [4]. In addition, erythropoietin, nonselective beta-blockers, clonidine, somatostatin analogs, and pyridostigmine bromide have been used for the management of orthostatic hypotension with controversial results and limited use [4, 13].

Gastrointestinal Neuropathy

Gastrointestinal neuropathy (GIN) may affect any part of the gastrointestinal tract such as the esophagus, the stomach, the intestine, and abdominal organs [4, 36]. The main clinical manifestations of GIN are esophageal dysfunction, gastroparesis, diabetic enteropathies including small bowel dysmobility syndromes (e.g., diabetic diarrhea and fecal incontinence) as well as gallbladder atony and enlargement [1, 4, 37].

Epidemiological data regarding the prevalence of GIN are conflicting probably due to studies with small amount of population, difference in methodology, and inconsistency of gastrointestinal symptoms [37–39]. Notably, symptoms are more common when asked by a gastroenterologist than by a diabetologist [38]. In the only community-based study, the cumulative incidence rates for the development of gastroparesis over a 10-year time period were 5.2% in type 1 DM, 1% in type 2 DM, and 0.2% in controls [40]. On the other hand, one-third of subjects with gastroparesis have DM and 26.7% of people hospitalized for gastroparesis have also DM as a comorbidity [37, 39, 41]. Older reports from tertiary care centers reported that up to 60% of people with a long duration of type 1 DM and gastrointestinal symptoms were diagnosed with diabetic gastroparesis [39, 42]. In addition, delayed gastric emptying was found in 27–65% of subjects with type 1 DM and in up to 30% of people with type 2 DM [37]. Disorders of esophageal motility affect up to 50% of the diabetic population [38]. Overall data suggest that gastrointestinal symptoms related to GIN are common among people with DM, and the risk of diabetic gastroparesis and enteropathy is higher in type 1 than in type 2 DM [39, 43]. In terms of gender, most studies have shown a predominance of female sex in diabetic gastroparesis; however, data are not unanimous [37].

In the DCCT-EDIC study, diabetic gastroparesis was associated with the presence of microvascular complications such as severe retinopathy, nephropathy as well as with poor glycemic control [37, 44]. Data are conflicting about the association between DAN and diabetic gastroparesis since one study showed a strong association, while another did not [45, 46].

Esophageal dysfunction is clinically presented with heartburn and dysphagia for solids [1]. The main clinical manifestations of diabetic gastroparesis are nonspecific and include nausea, bloating, loss of appetite, abdominal pain, postprandial fullness, or vomiting [4, 38]. Nevertheless, often gastroparesis is asymptomatic, while the presence of symptoms does not show the extent of gastroparesis [4]. Gastroparesis may cause increased blood glucose variability due to disruption of food absorption, a situation described as "brittle diabetes." Subjects treated with insulin may experience postprandial hypoglycemia, widely known as gastric hypoglycemia, due to delayed food absorption [38]. Hence, people with unexplained poor glycemic control and hypoglycemic events should be tested for diabetic gastroparesis [38]. Complications of gastroparesis include esophagitis, Mallory-Weiss syndrome (gastroesophageal laceration or tear), malnutrition, electrolyte disturbances, volume depletion, and acute renal injury [37].

Exclusion of gastric obstruction or peptic ulcer is needed before testing for gastroparesis [4]. Moreover, other causes that affect gastric emptying such as acute changes in blood glucose levels and medications including opioids or glucagon-like peptide 1 receptor agonists should be evaluated before the diagnosis of diabetic gastroparesis is established [4]. The American College of Gastroenterology (ACG) recommends that a combination of symptoms, signs, and delayed gastric emptying is needed in the absence of gastric outlet obstruction or ulceration to establish the diagnosis of diabetic gastroparesis [47].

Diabetic enteropathy is presented with profuse watery diarrhea, constipation, and fecal incontinence [43]. Diarrhea occurs commonly at night in patients with uncontrolled DM who also have peripheral neuropathy [43]. Even though constipation may affect up to 60% of the diabetic population, complications such as perforation and overflow diarrhea are rare [43]. Fecal incontinence is also predominantly nocturnal and is linked with internal and external anal sphincter dysfunction [43]. The symptoms of diabetic enteropathy have a great impact on the quality of life and people may experience relationship difficulties or social isolation; hence, often psychological support may be needed [43]. However, since antidiabetic medication such as metformin, alpha-glucosidase inhibitors, incretin-based therapies or anticholinergic agents, and psychotropic drugs may cause similar symptoms, titration of dose or discontinuation may be required before testing for diabetic enteropathy [43].

The diagnosis of GIN is based on medical history, physical examination, and imaging techniques. Questions that examine the presence of symptoms related to GIN should be asked to every patient with DM. Physical examination should be focused on the presence of gastrointestinal signs such as abdominal distention and findings of other forms of DAN [37]. Two clinical scoring systems are commonly used for the diagnosis of GIN: the Gastroparesis Cardinal Symptom Index (GCSI) and another multidisciplinary scoring system that is qualitative [37, 48]. Moreover, obstruction caused by a mass or ulcer should be excluded using diagnostic imaging or upper gastrointestinal endoscopy [37]. Antral hypomotility or pylorospasm can be detected with manometry [1].

The gold standard method for the diagnosis of gastroparesis is radiolabeled scintigraphy to quantify the emptying of a physiologic meal and examine stomach's motor function [37]. Acute changes in blood glucose affect gastric emptying and thereby, blood glucose levels should be within normal range before and during the procedure. Alternatively, the ^{13}C-octanoic acid breath test can be used for the assessment of gastric emptying [4]. It is a simple, noninvasive technique without radiation exposure that measures the rate of gastric emptying of the ^{13}C-octanoic acid in a solid meal that is reflected by breath excretion of $^{3}CO_2$ [37]. This technique can be used in circumstances when radiation cannot be performed, such as in pregnant women, women who are breastfeeding or children [37].

In addition, transabdominal ultrasound has been used to measure emptying of a liquid meal by assessing sectional changes in the volume remaining in the gastric antrum over time [37]. Magnetic resonance imaging (MRI) with gadolinium is able to measure with high accuracy semisolid emptying of stomach using sequential transaxial scans [37]. Furthermore, measurement of regional gastric volumes in real time can be examined using single-photon emission computed tomography with 99-Tc administered intravenously [37]. Other methods such as the wireless motility capsule or electrogastrography can be also used [37].

For the diagnosis of constipation methods such as anorectal manometry, assessment of colonic segmental transit time, pelvic examination can be used [1]. Regarding diarrhea, history and specific examination should be performed to exclude several other causes [1].

Dietary management is essential for this disorder and instructions should be given by an experienced dietician who is able to identify patient's tolerance to solids and liquids. Foods with high-fiber or fats should be minimized, since they inhibit gastric emptying, while small-portion multiple meals should be encouraged [49]. People with gastroparesis are advised to take fluids during the meal and to sit or walk for 1–2 hours after meals [37]. If these methods are not effective, the meals should be transformed to liquid, since liquid emptying is not affected. In parallel, behavioral modification and particularly a humanistic approach should be used from health professionals with sympathy for patients' needs [37].

Moreover, glycemic control should be optimized and glycemic variability minimized to avoid acute symptoms of diabetic gastroparesis [37]. Regarding antidiabetic medication, sulfonylureas should be used with caution given the risk of hypoglycemia, whereas glucagon peptide 1-receptor agonists may worsen symptoms [37]. Prandial insulin can be administered after meals to minimize the risk of postprandial hypoglycemia in these patients. In addition, continuous glucose monitoring and insulin pump therapy can be used to optimize glycemic control and minimize glucose variability [37].

The only pharmacological agent that is approved by the FDA for the management of diabetic gastroparesis is metoclopramide [4]. Nevertheless, the level of evidence about the benefits of this drug is weak and the adverse events are common, and hence, its use should not extend beyond 5 days [4]. It is recommended that metoclopramide should be prescribed in severe cases that do not respond to other strategies. Other pharmacological interventions that have been used for the treatment of gastroparesis include prokinetic agents (domperidone, erythromycin, and cisapride), antiemetics (phenothiazines), and low dose of tricyclic antidepressants [37]. Alternative therapy options for severe gastroparesis include intrapyloric botulinum injection, pyloroplasty, or gastric electric stimulation [37]. Surgical options are venting gastrostomy or jejunostomy and gastrectomy, while novel therapies include ghrelin agonists and new generation of 5-hydroxytryptamine receptor 4 agonists [50].

In terms of enteropathy, almost half of the people with diabetic diarrhea have bacterial overgrowth and therefore, antibiotics such as rifaximin or metronidazole may be useful [43, 51]. Furthermore, opioid-based drugs and somatostatin can be used in cases of severe refractory diarrhea [43, 52], while laxatives can be administered when constipation is present [43].

Urogenital Autonomic Neuropathy

Urogenital autonomic neuropathy (UAN) is another clinical manifestation of DAN and refers to bladder and sexual dysfunction in both genders [53, 54]. It is estimated that more than 50% of men and women with DM have bladder dysfunction [53]. DM increases the risk of urinary incontinence by 30–100% [54–56], while the prevalence of lower urinary tract symptoms is twofold higher in men with DM in comparison with those without DM [54, 57]. Regarding sexual dysfunction, epidemiological data suggest that the prevalence ranges between 35% and 90% in men with DM [58]. In a prospective epidemiological study, the 10-year incidence for the development of erectile dysfunction (ED) was 25% among people with type 1 DM [59]. In addition, the risk for

ED in males with DM increases when related comorbidities such as CV disease, nephropathy, diabetic foot ulcer, or retinopathy are present [60]. In women, sexual dysfunction is more common in those with DM than those without DM with an estimated prevalence between 18% and 42%; however, epidemiological data are limited [53].

The main clinical manifestation of bladder dysfunction in women is urinary incontinence that leads to limitations in daily functioning and poor quality of life [53, 61]. On the other hand, men experience lower urinary tract symptoms such as straining, intermittent and post-void dribbling of urine, and weak stream, which are often attributed to increased age and benign prostatic hyperplasia [53, 54]. In addition, urgent, frequent, and nocturnal urination may be present. Generally, there is confusion between bladder dysfunction and prostatic hyperplasia since these two morbidities often coexist [53, 54]. Sexual dysfunction in women presents with dyspareunia, inadequate lubrication, obstructed intercourse, vaginal laxity, and decreased sexual desire/libido or orgasm [1, 53, 54]. In men, sexual dysfunction is presented as ED, reduced libido, orgasmic dysfunction, and retrograde ejaculation [1]. ED is defined as the inability to attain and/or maintain penile erection sufficient for sexual activity [54].

The ADA recommends screening for ED in men who have other forms of DAN with simple questions about libido and inability to reach and maintain an erection [4]. In addition, women with DM that have other forms of DAN should be screened for bladder and female sexual dysfunction in the presence of recurrent urinary tract infections using targeted questioning regarding specific symptoms [4]. Nevertheless, before the diagnosis of ED is established, a hormonal evaluation (testosterone and prolactin) should be performed to exclude hypogonadism, as well as organic causes and medications [4].

The assessment of bladder function can be performed using postvoid ultrasound to assess residual volume and upper urinary tract dilation [1]. In addition, cystometry including voiding cystometry can be used to evaluate bladder sensation and pressure changes [1].

Regarding ED, measurement of nocturnal penile tumescence and measurement of penile and brachial BP, and calculation of the penile-brachial pressure index can be performed [1]. Moreover, the sacral outflow, which represents the sacral parasympathetic activity and the response to intracavernosal injection of vasoactive compound may be useful [1]. In women, sexual dysfunction can be examined with vaginal plethysmography to measure lubrication and vaginal flushing; however, this method is not standardized [1].

The management of ED requires a multifactorial approach. First, in people with type 1 DM optimal glycemic control is associated with lower incidence of ED, while evidence is limited for type 2 DM [62, 63]. Apart from glycemic control, the management of other risk factors such as hypertension and dyslipidemia may improve ED [4]. In addition, lifestyle modifications including increased physical activity, reduced calorie intake, and Mediterranean diet may be helpful by improving endothelial function that is the fundamental issue in ED [8, 60, 64].

Phosphodiesterase type 5 inhibitors (PDE5-i) are the first-line treatment option for men with ED. The mode of action of PDE5-i is the delay of cyclic guanosine monophosphate degradation. Sildenafil (25, 50, and 100 mg on demand), tadalafil (10 and 20 mg on demand; 2.5 and 5 mg for daily dosing), vardenafil (5, 10, and 20 mg on demand; 10 mg on demand in the form of orodispersible tablet), and avanafil (50, 100, and 200 mg on demand) are commercially available [60]. These agents differ in the time to onset and their duration, while safety and efficacy are similar [64]. However, it is known that people with DM respond less to PDE5-i when compared with people without DM [64].

The second line of treatment in patients who do not respond to PDE5-i is intracavernosal injections of prostaglandin E1 (alprostadil), papaverine, or phentolamine [60, 64]. However, patients' education and dose titration are needed. Intraurethral or topical alprostadil can be also delivered without the use of injection. Other treatment options are vacuum erection devices that offer a passive penile engorgement rather than a "true" erection and low-intensity wave therapy [60]. In severe cases, penile prosthesis may be recommended.

Regarding female sexual dysfunction, lifestyle modifications, glycemic control, and psychotherapy can be used; however, no specific guidelines exist [64].

Sudomotor Dysfunction

SD can be presented as dry skin, itching, anhidrosis, and gustatory sweating [4, 65]. Subjects with SD may also experience increased sense of sweating during high environmental temperatures or heat intolerance [66]. It is associated with epidermal moisturization, hyperkeratosis, diabetic foot ulcers, and impaired quality of life [67, 68].

Even though ADA recommends that routine screening for SD in every day practice should not be performed, several methods that examine the integrity of the cholinergic segment of sympathetic nervous system have been developed [4, 65, 66]. First, the thermoregulatory sweat testing (TST) is the gold standard method for the assessment of peripheral and central sympathetic sudomotor function [66]. The main limitations of this method are that it is time consuming, cannot differentiate pre- from postganglionic lesions, and TST requires special equipment [66]. Another method to examine SD is the indicator plaster (Neuropad®; Miro Verbandstoffe, Wiehl-Drabenderhöhe, Germany), which is an adhesive patch measuring skin hydration [69, 70]. The patch contains the blue complex salt anhydrous cobalt (II) chloride. When adequate water is present (sweat), each molecule of this salt absorbs six water molecules and its color changes from blue to pink [69]. The main strength of this method is the high degree of reliability and easiness to perform suggesting that it is proper for self-testing [71]. The quantitative sudomotor axon reflex test (QSART) examines the postganglionic sudomotor function [66]. However, it is expensive, not available in every laboratory, and cannot detect preganglionic lesion [65]. Other methods to assess SD include the sympathetic skin response (SSR) that measures electrodermal activity, the Sudoscan that measures electrochemical skin conductance, and silicone impressions [65, 66].

Regarding management of SD, daily application of glycopyrrolate that is a topical antimuscarinic agent has shown efficacy in the treatment of gustatory sweating [72]. There is little evidence that the use of lubricants on the skin of the feet improves the quality of skin and reduces the incidence of diabetic foot ulceration.

Ocular Manifestations

Ocular manifestations of DAN include pupillomotor function impairment (e.g., decreased diameter of dark-adapted pupil), reduced corneal sensation, eye dryness, and Argyll-Robertson-like pupils [1].

References

1. Vinik AI, Maser RE, Mitchell BD, Freeman R. Diabetic autonomic neuropathy. Diabetes Care. 2003;26(5):1553–79.
2. Tesfaye S, Boulton AJ, Dyck PJ, Freeman R, Horowitz M, Kempler P, et al. Diabetic neuropathies: update on definitions, diagnostic criteria, estimation of severity, and treatments. Diabetes Care. 2010;33(10):2285–93.
3. Spallone V, Ziegler D, Freeman R, Bernardi L, Frontoni S, Pop-Busui R, et al. Cardiovascular autonomic neuropathy in diabetes: clinical impact, assessment, diagnosis, and management. Diabetes Metab Res Rev. 2011;27(7):639–53.
4. Pop-Busui R, Boulton AJ, Feldman EL, Bril V, Freeman R, Malik RA, et al. Diabetic neuropathy: a position statement by the American Diabetes Association. Diabetes Care. 2017;40(1):136–54.
5. Brownlee M. The pathobiology of diabetic complications: a unifying mechanism. Diabetes. 2005;54(6):1615–25.
6. Greene DA, Lattimer SA, Sima AA. Sorbitol, phosphoinositides, and sodium-potassium-ATPase in the pathogenesis of diabetic complications. N Engl J Med. 1987;316(10):599–606.
7. Yagihashi S, Mizukami H, Sugimoto K. Mechanism of diabetic neuropathy: where are we now and where to go? J Diabetes Investig. 2011;2(1):18–32.
8. Tentolouris A, Eleftheriadou I, Tzeravini E, Tsilingiris D, Paschou SA, Siasos G, et al. Endothelium as a therapeutic target in diabetes mellitus: from basic mechanisms to clinical practice. Curr Med Chem. 2019. https://doi.org/10.2174/0929867326666190119154152. [Epub ahead of print].
9. Sundkvist G, Lind P, Bergstrom B, Lilja B, Rabinowe SL. Autonomic nerve antibodies and autonomic nerve function in type 1 and type 2 diabetic patients. J Intern Med. 1991;229(6):505–10.
10. Horrobin DF. Essential fatty acids in the management of impaired nerve function in diabetes. Diabetes. 1997;46(Suppl 2):S90–3.
11. Apfel SC, Arezzo JC, Brownlee M, Federoff H, Kessler JA. Nerve growth factor administration protects against experimental diabetic sensory neuropathy. Brain Res. 1994;634(1):7–12.
12. Satoh J, Yagihashi S, Toyota T. The possible role of tumor necrosis factor-alpha in diabetic polyneuropathy. Exp Diabesity Res. 2003;4(2):65–71.
13. Pop-Busui R. Cardiac autonomic neuropathy in diabetes: a clinical perspective. Diabetes Care. 2010;33(2):434–41.
14. Vincent AM, Russell JW, Low P, Feldman EL. Oxidative stress in the pathogenesis of diabetic neuropathy. Endocr Rev. 2004;25(4):612–28.
15. Ziegler D, Gries FA, Muhlen H, Rathmann W, Spuler M, Lessmann F. Prevalence and clinical correlates of cardiovascular autonomic and peripheral diabetic neuropathy in patients attending diabetes centers. The Diacan Multicenter Study Group. Diabete Metab. 1993;19(1 Pt 2):143–51.
16. Valensi P, Paries J, Attali JR, French Group for R, Study of Diabetic N. Cardiac autonomic neuropathy in diabetic patients: influence of diabetes duration, obesity, and microangiopathic complications--the French multicenter study. Metabolism. 2003;52(7):815–20.
17. The effect of intensive diabetes therapy on measures of autonomic nervous system function in the Diabetes Control and Complications Trial (DCCT). Diabetologia. 1998;41(4):416–23.
18. Pop-Busui R, Low PA, Waberski BH, Martin CL, Albers JW, Feldman EL, et al. Effects of prior intensive insulin therapy on cardiac autonomic nervous system function in type 1 diabetes mellitus: the Diabetes Control and Complications Trial/Epidemiology of Diabetes Interventions and Complications study (DCCT/EDIC). Circulation. 2009;119(22):2886–93.
19. Martin CL, Albers JW, Pop-Busui R, Group DER. Neuropathy and related findings in the diabetes control and complications trial/epidemiology of diabetes interventions and complications study. Diabetes Care. 2014;37(1):31–8.
20. Carnethon MR, Prineas RJ, Temprosa M, Zhang ZM, Uwaifo G, Molitch ME, et al. The association among autonomic nervous system function, incident diabetes, and intervention arm in the Diabetes Prevention Program. Diabetes Care. 2006;29(4):914–9.
21. Ziegler D, Voss A, Rathmann W, Strom A, Perz S, Roden M, et al. Increased prevalence of cardiac autonomic dysfunction at different degrees of glucose intolerance in the general population: the KORA S4 survey. Diabetologia. 2015;58(5):1118–28.
22. Witte DR, Tesfaye S, Chaturvedi N, Eaton SE, Kempler P, Fuller JH, et al. Risk factors for cardiac autonomic neuropathy in type 1 diabetes mellitus. Diabetologia. 2005;48(1):164–71.
23. Balcioglu AS, Muderrisoglu H. Diabetes and cardiac autonomic neuropathy: clinical manifestations, cardiovascular consequences, diagnosis and treatment. World J Diabetes. 2015;6(1):80–91.
24. Serhiyenko VA, Serhiyenko AA. Cardiac autonomic neuropathy: risk factors, diagnosis and treatment. World J Diabetes. 2018;9(1):1–24.
25. Spallone V, Bernardi L, Ricordi L, Solda P, Maiello MR, Calciati A, et al. Relationship between the circadian rhythms of blood pressure and sympathovagal balance in diabetic autonomic neuropathy. Diabetes. 1993;42(12):1745–52.
26. Ewing DJ, Campbell IW, Clarke BF. Assessment of cardiovascular effects in diabetic autonomic neuropathy and prognostic implications. Ann Intern Med. 1980;92(2 Pt 2):308–11.
27. Ewing DJ, Martyn CN, Young RJ, Clarke BF. The value of cardiovascular autonomic function tests: 10 years experience in diabetes. Diabetes Care. 1985;8(5):491–8.

28. Heart rate variability: standards of measurement, physiological interpretation and clinical use. Task Force of the European Society of Cardiology and the North American Society of Pacing and Electrophysiology. Circulation. 1996;93(5):1043–1065.
29. Gerritsen J, Dekker JM, TenVoorde BJ, Kostense PJ, Heine RJ, Bouter LM, et al. Impaired autonomic function is associated with increased mortality, especially in subjects with diabetes, hypertension, or a history of cardiovascular disease: the Hoorn study. Diabetes Care. 2001;24(10):1793–8.
30. Pop-Busui R, Evans GW, Gerstein HC, Fonseca V, Fleg JL, Hoogwerf BJ, et al. Effects of cardiac autonomic dysfunction on mortality risk in the Action to Control Cardiovascular Risk in Diabetes (ACCORD) trial. Diabetes Care. 2010;33(7):1578–84.
31. Soedamah-Muthu SS, Chaturvedi N, Witte DR, Stevens LK, Porta M, Fuller JH, et al. Relationship between risk factors and mortality in type 1 diabetic patients in Europe: the EURODIAB Prospective Complications Study (PCS). Diabetes Care. 2008;31(7):1360–6.
32. Maser RE, Mitchell BD, Vinik AI, Freeman R. The association between cardiovascular autonomic neuropathy and mortality in individuals with diabetes: a meta-analysis. Diabetes Care. 2003;26(6):1895–901.
33. Young LH, Wackers FJ, Chyun DA, Davey JA, Barrett EJ, Taillefer R, et al. Cardiac outcomes after screening for asymptomatic coronary artery disease in patients with type 2 diabetes: the DIAD study: a randomized controlled trial. JAMA. 2009;301(15):1547–55.
34. Gaede P, Vedel P, Larsen N, Jensen GV, Parving HH, Pedersen O. Multifactorial intervention and cardiovascular disease in patients with type 2 diabetes. N Engl J Med. 2003;348(5):383–93.
35. Azad N, Emanuele NV, Abraira C, Henderson WG, Colwell J, Levin SR, et al. The effects of intensive glycemic control on neuropathy in the VA cooperative study on type II diabetes mellitus (VA CSDM). J Diabetes Complications. 1999;13(5–6):307–13.
36. Azpiroz F, Malagelada C. Diabetic neuropathy in the gut: pathogenesis and diagnosis. Diabetologia. 2016;59(3):404–8.
37. Krishnasamy S, Abell TL. Diabetic gastroparesis: principles and current trends in management. Diabetes Ther. 2018;9(Suppl 1):1–42.
38. Kempler P, Varkonyi T, Korei AE, Horvath VJ. Gastrointestinal autonomic neuropathy in diabetes: the unattended borderline between diabetology and gastroenterology. Diabetologia. 2016;59(3):401–3.
39. Bharucha AE. Epidemiology and natural history of gastroparesis. Gastroenterol Clin North Am. 2015;44(1):9–19.
40. Choung RS, Locke GR 3rd, Schleck CD, Zinsmeister AR, Melton LJ 3rd, Talley NJ. Risk of gastroparesis in subjects with type 1 and 2 diabetes in the general population. Am J Gastroenterol. 2012;107(1):82–8.
41. Wang YR, Fisher RS, Parkman HP. Gastroparesis-related hospitalizations in the United States: trends, characteristics, and outcomes, 1995–2004. Am J Gastroenterol. 2008;103(2):313–22.
42. Jones KL, Russo A, Stevens JE, Wishart JM, Berry MK, Horowitz M. Predictors of delayed gastric emptying in diabetes. Diabetes Care. 2001;24(7):1264–9.
43. Maisey A. A practical approach to gastrointestinal complications of diabetes. Diabetes Ther. 2016;7(3):379–86.
44. Bharucha AE, Batey-Schaefer B, Cleary PA, Murray JA, Cowie C, Lorenzi G, et al. Delayed gastric emptying is associated with early and long-term hyperglycemia in type 1 diabetes mellitus. Gastroenterology. 2015;149(2):330–9.
45. Darwiche G, Almer LO, Bjorgell O, Cederholm C, Nilsson P. Delayed gastric emptying rate in type 1 diabetics with cardiac autonomic neuropathy. J Diabetes Complications. 2001;15(3):128–34.
46. Lydon A, Murray C, Cooke T, Duggan PF, O'Halloran D, Shorten GD. Evaluation of standard haemodynamic tests of autonomic function and HbA1c as predictors of delayed gastric emptying in patients with type 1 diabetes mellitus. Eur J Anaesthesiol. 2000;17(2):99–104.
47. Camilleri M, Parkman HP, Shafi MA, Abell TL, Gerson L, American College of G. Clinical guideline: management of gastroparesis. Am J Gastroenterol. 2013;108(1):18–37; quiz 8.
48. Revicki DA, Camilleri M, Kuo B, Szarka LA, McCormack J, Parkman HP. Evaluating symptom outcomes in gastroparesis clinical trials: validity and responsiveness of the Gastroparesis Cardinal Symptom Index-Daily Diary (GCSI-DD). Neurogastroenterol Motil. 2012;24(5):456–63, e215–6.
49. Camilleri M. Clinical practice. Diabetic gastroparesis. N Engl J Med. 2007;356(8):820–9.
50. Abell TL, Johnson WD, Kedar A, Runnels JM, Thompson J, Weeks ES, et al. A double-masked, randomized, placebo-controlled trial of temporary endoscopic mucosal gastric electrical stimulation for gastroparesis. Gastrointest Endosc. 2011;74(3):496–503.e3.
51. Pimentel M. Review of rifaximin as treatment for SIBO and IBS. Expert Opin Investig Drugs. 2009;18(3):349–58.
52. Gatopoulou A, Papanas N, Maltezos E. Diabetic gastrointestinal autonomic neuropathy: current status and new achievements for everyday clinical practice. Eur J Intern Med. 2012;23(6):499–505.
53. Brown JS, Wessells H, Chancellor MB, Howards SS, Stamm WE, Stapleton AE, et al. Urologic complications of diabetes. Diabetes Care. 2005;28(1):177–85.
54. Braffett BH, Wessells H, Sarma AV. Urogenital autonomic dysfunction in diabetes. Curr Diab Rep. 2016;16(12):119.
55. Brown JS, Grady D, Ouslander JG, Herzog AR, Varner RE, Posner SF. Prevalence of urinary incontinence and associated risk factors in postmenopausal women. Heart & Estrogen/Progestin Replacement Study (HERS) Research Group. Obstet Gynecol. 1999;94(1):66–70.
56. Sampselle CM, Harlow SD, Skurnick J, Brubaker L, Bondarenko I. Urinary incontinence predictors and life impact in ethnically diverse perimenopausal women. Obstet Gynecol. 2002;100(6):1230–8.
57. Joseph MA, Harlow SD, Wei JT, Sarma AV, Dunn RL, Taylor JM, et al. Risk factors for lower urinary tract symptoms in a population-based sample of African-American men. Am J Epidemiol. 2003;157(10):906–14.
58. Malavige LS, Levy JC. Erectile dysfunction in diabetes mellitus. J Sex Med. 2009;6(5):1232–47.
59. Klein R, Klein BE, Moss SE. Ten-year incidence of self-reported erectile dysfunction in people with long-term type 1 diabetes. J Diabetes Complications. 2005;19(1):35–41.
60. Hatzimouratidis K, Hatzichristou D. How to treat erectile dysfunction in men with diabetes: from pathophysiology to treatment. Curr Diab Rep. 2014;14(11):545.
61. Wetle T, Scherr P, Branch LG, Resnick NM, Harris T, Evans D, et al. Difficulty with holding urine among older persons in a geographically defined community: prevalence and correlates. J Am Geriatr Soc. 1995;43(4):349–55.
62. Van Den Eeden SK, Sarma AV, Rutledge BN, Cleary PA, Kusek JW, Nyberg LM, et al. Effect of intensive glycemic control and diabetes complications on lower urinary tract symptoms in men with type 1 diabetes: Diabetes Control and Complications Trial/Epidemiology of Diabetes Interventions and Complications (DCCT/EDIC) study. Diabetes Care. 2009;32(4):664–70.
63. Wessells H, Penson DF, Cleary P, Rutledge BN, Lachin JM, McVary KT, et al. Effect of intensive glycemic therapy on erectile function in men with type 1 diabetes. J Urol. 2011;185(5):1828–34.
64. Maiorino MI, Bellastella G, Esposito K. Diabetes and sexual dysfunction: current perspectives. Diabetes Metab Syndr Obes. 2014;7:95–105.
65. Kempler P, Amarenco G, Freeman R, Frontoni S, Horowitz M, Stevens M, et al. Management strategies for gastrointestinal,

erectile, bladder, and sudomotor dysfunction in patients with diabetes. Diabetes Metab Res Rev. 2011;27(7):665–77.
66. Buchmann SJ, Penzlin AI, Kubasch ML, Illigens BM, Siepmann T. Assessment of sudomotor function. Clin Auton Res. 2019;29(1):41–53.
67. Tentolouris N, Marinou K, Kokotis P, Karanti A, Diakoumopoulou E, Katsilambros N. Sudomotor dysfunction is associated with foot ulceration in diabetes. Diabet Med. 2009;26(3):302–5.
68. Argiana V, Eleftheriadou I, Tentolouris N. Screening for the high-risk foot of ulceration: tests of somatic and autonomic nerve function. Curr Diab Rep. 2011;11(4):294–301.
69. Papanas N, Boulton AJ, Malik RA, Manes C, Schnell O, Spallone V, et al. A simple new non-invasive sweat indicator test for the diagnosis of diabetic neuropathy. Diabet Med. 2013;30(5):525–34.
70. Liatis S, Marinou K, Tentolouris N, Pagoni S, Katsilambros N. Usefulness of a new indicator test for the diagnosis of peripheral and autonomic neuropathy in patients with diabetes mellitus. Diabet Med. 2007;24(12):1375–80.
71. Tentolouris N, Achtsidis V, Marinou K, Katsilambros N. Evaluation of the self-administered indicator plaster neuropad for the diagnosis of neuropathy in diabetes. Diabetes Care. 2008;31(2):236–7.
72. Shaw JE, Abbott CA, Tindle K, Hollis S, Boulton AJ. A randomised controlled trial of topical glycopyrrolate, the first specific treatment for diabetic gustatory sweating. Diabetologia. 1997;40(3):299–301.

Spinal Cord Lesion and Dysautonomia

28

Valeria Iodice and Christopher J. Mathias

Introduction

Autonomic Features in Patients with Spinal Cord Lesions

Neurogenic Shock There are differences between the autonomic problems affecting recently and chronically injured patients following a spinal lesion.

Soon after transection there is initially a transient state of hypoexcitability of the isolated cord, leading to 'spinal shock' with flaccid paralysis of the muscles, and lack of tendon reflexes. Analogous to spinal shock, spinal autonomic reflexes are also absent after acute cervical myelopathy and patients experience a transient 'neurogenic shock' characterized by failure of the sympathetic nervous system that results in loss of vascular tone in parts of body deprived of autonomic control (Table 28.1) [1, 2].
Blood pressure is low in the supine posture (SBP < 90 mmHg). Severe bradycardia and even asystole may occur in patients with cervical injuries with the majority requiring admission to intensive care due to haemodynamic instability [3–5].

The pathophysiology of neurogenic shock is not fully understood but is likely to be due to the imbalance in autonomic control, with a relative absence of sympathetic activation leading to an overactivity of vagal activity especially if the functional disconnection is relatively acute and complete [1, 6].

Urinary bladder and large bowel are usually atonic, and there is dilatation of blood vessels particularly in the skin. This stage of spinal cord depression may last from a few days to a few weeks, after which isolated activity of the spinal cord usually returns with the emergence of certain groups of reflexes.

The descriptions below largely relate to tetraplegics and high thoracic spinal cord lesions, unless otherwise indicated.

Cardiovascular Dysfunction

Acute Stage The basal supine blood pressure in recently injured tetraplegics in spinal and neurogenic shock is usually lower than normal, and is likely to be secondary to marked diminution in sympathetic nervous activity, confirmed by the low levels of both plasma noradrenaline and adrenaline from the second day after injury [7].

In tetraplegics in neurogenic shock the basal heart rate is usually below 100 beats/min, unlike in patients with low spinal-cord injuries in whom the heart rate is often higher. This is probably due to a reduction in neural and hormonal sympathetic-mediated chronotropic influences in tetraplegics.

The efferent cardiac parasympathetic pathways, however, are intact and the absence of sympathetic activation may predispose susceptible patients to vagal overactivity. This may result in bradycardia and cardiac arrest, as has been noted during tracheal stimulation [8].

Chronic Stage In the chronic stage, the basal level of both systolic and diastolic blood pressure in high lesions is lower

V. Iodice (✉)
Queen Square Institute of Neurology, National Hospital for Neurology & Neurosurgery, University College London, London, UK

Autonomic Unit, National Hospital for Neurology and Neurosurgery, UCLH Trust, London, UK

Autonomic & Neurovascular Medicine Centre, Hospital of St John & St Elizabeth, London, UK
e-mail: v.iodice@ucl.ac.uk

C. J. Mathias
Queen Square Institute of Neurology, National Hospital for Neurology & Neurosurgery, University College London, London, UK

S. Chokroverty, P. Cortelli (eds.), *Autonomic Nervous System and Sleep*, https://doi.org/10.1007/978-3-030-62263-3_28

Table 28.1 Clinical features of spinal and neurogenic shock

	Spinal shock	Neurogenic shock
Definition	Marked reduction or complete loss of motor and reflex function below the injury level and due to a transient inexcitability (or hypoexcitability) of the lower motor neuron in spinal cord segments disconnected from corticospinal pathway	Failure of sympathetic nervous system resulting in loss of vascular tone in part of body deprived from autonomic control
Onset	Within hours of the injury	Within hours of the injury
Level of injury	Any	Above T6
Duration	4–6 weeks post-injury	Into chronic injury
Symptoms and sign		
	Flaccid paralysis	Hypotension: SBP < 90 mmHg in supine posture in absence of low intravascular volume (blood loss and dehydration)
	Loss of deep tendon and superficial reflex	Bradycardia: HR < 60 bpm
		Vagal hypersensitivity usually lasting for 2–3 weeks. In some cases, implantation of a temporary or permanent pacemaker is required
		Risk of AV conduction block and cardiac arrest, as has been noted during tracheal stimulation
		Orthostatic hypotension risk with mobilization
		Autonomic dysreflexia in minority of patients
		Atonic bladder and large bowel
		Flushed warm skin due to dilatation of blood vessels
		Anhidrosis of cutaneous areas below the lesion

than in normal subjects. A number of secondary mechanisms, particularly hormonal, attempt to compensate for and help maintain blood pressure, including the renin–angiotensin–aldosterone system [7].

In chronic high lesions, the basal heart rate may be marginally lower, or no different, from that of normal subjects. Power spectral analytical techniques in tetraplegics indicate a diminished low-frequency (presumed sympathetic) component with preservation of the high frequency (presumed parasympathetic) component. There are changes in heart rate and RR intervals (heart periods) in response to a rise or a fall in blood pressure suggesting preservation of cardiac vagal function.

Orthostatic Hypotension Patients with high spinal-cord lesions are prone to hypotension, which commonly occurs during postural change from the horizontal to the upright position (Fig. 28.1). This occurs in both recently injured patients in neurogenic shock and in chronically injured patients, especially in the early stages during rehabilitation [9, 10]. Their mobility, even in a wheelchair, can be considerably impeded and patients can experience frequent symptomatic falls in BP with mobilization [11].

The fall in blood pressure is accompanied by symptoms mainly related to diminished cerebral perfusion (Box 28.1). The symptoms can vary in nature and intensity and are not necessarily related to the degree of hypotension [9, 10].

Orthostatic hypotension in individuals with SCI is due to the interruption of efferent pathways from the brainstem projections to the autonomic centres in the intermediolateral cell columns of the Tl to L2 or L3 cord segments involved in vasoconstriction causing failure of short-term blood pressure regulation [9].

As a result of interruption of efferent sympathetic pathways, resting catecholamine levels are lower in acute and chronic phases of SCI and do not significantly increase in tetraplegics undergoing head-up tilt [7, 12].

During head-up postural change the fall in blood pressure is accompanied by a reduction in central venous pressure, stroke volume and cardiac output, which is probably the result of venous pooling, diminished venous return, and the inability to increase sympathetic cardiac inotropic activity. Venous pooling often causes cyanotic discoloration of the legs and may account for ankle oedema, as observed in those with high lesions and in wheelchairs. Urine volume when upright can be reduced to low levels, probably due to a combination of causes that include a fall in blood pressure, thus reducing renal plasma flow and glomerular filtration rate, and an elevation in levels of the antidiuretic hormone, vasopressin [12].

Clinical observations indicate that the symptoms of postural hypotension are often diminished with frequent postural change in the head-up position, along with elevation of the head end of the bed at night. The activation of the renin–angiotensin–aldosterone axis, with both early and longer-acting effects resulting from vasoconstriction and plasma volume expansion, probably helps buffer the fall in blood pressure during head-up postural change. Another possibility is an improved ability to autoregulate cerebral blood flow, which such patients often can do at lower perfusion pres-

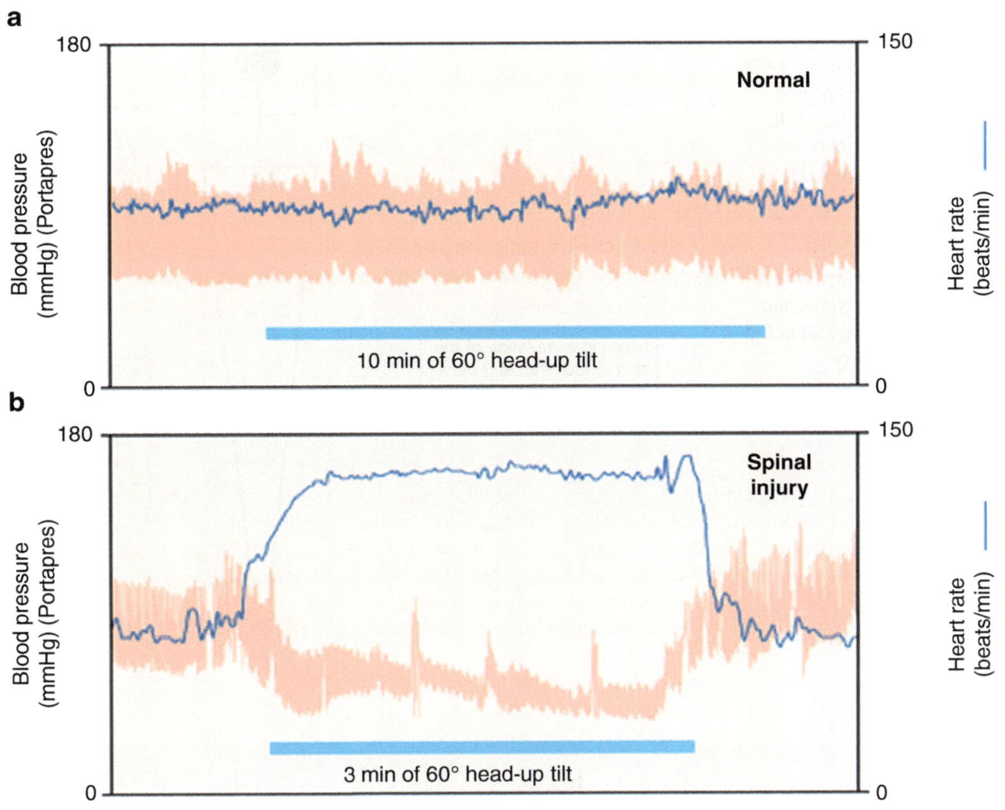

Fig. 28.1 (**a**, **b**) Blood pressure and heart rate measured continuously with the Finometer (Finapres, Enschede, the Netherlands) in a patient with a high cervical spinal cord lesion. There is a fall in blood pressure because of impairment of the sympathetic outflow disrupted in the cervical spine. Heart rate rises because of withdrawal of vagal activity in response to the rise in pressure. (From Mathias [10], with permission of Elsevier)

Box 28.1 Clinical manifestations of postural hypotension

Symptoms of orthostatic hypotension
Giddiness, buzzing and ringing in ears
Blurring, greying out and loss of vision
Facial pallor
Syncope
Clinical signs of orthostatic hypotension
Hypotension and elevation in heart rate
Venous pooling and cyanotic discoloration of lower limbs
Reduced urine secretion

sures than normal subjects [13]. Whether changes in other circulating and locally produced hormones acting on the cerebral vasculature also contribute is not known [9].

Management of OH in SCI A multi-pronged approach, combining non-pharmacological and pharmacological measures, is usually needed in the acute and chronic phase. A variety of physical methods have been used to prevent postural hypotension; these include abdominal binders and thigh cuffs that prevent pooling [14, 15]. Activation of spinal sympathetic reflexes, by induction of muscle spasms or tapping of the anterior abdominal wall suprapubically to activate the urinary bladder, may be of value in some by causing autonomic dysreflexia and thus elevating blood pressure.

Although a range of drugs, as used in patients with autonomic failure, may alleviate postural hypotension in high spinal-cord lesions, spinal patients are prone to paroxysms of hypertension, which may be severe and exacerbated by such drugs. Usually the need for drugs is for limited periods, when postural hypotension is a particular problem, as in the early stages of rehabilitation and after prolonged recumbency.

Ephedrine, in a dose of 15 mg half an hour before postural change, is often of value. Its ability to act directly on adrenoceptors and indirectly by releasing noradrenaline is probably the basis of its efficacy. Dihydroergotamine and other α-adrenoceptor agonists may have a role, especially if they have short-lived effects. Indomethacin, a prostaglandin synthetase inhibitor, also elevates basal blood pressure and reduces the blood pressure fall during postural change but has potential side effects. In the majority of patients, however, drugs are not needed.

Autonomic Dysreflexia Patients with SCI, in addition to orthostatic hypotension, are prone to develop transient exaggerated rise in BP associated with a constellation of symptoms (Fig. 28.2) and triggered by afferent noxious or non-noxious stimuli below the neurological level of injury [6, 16–19].

Autonomic dysreflexia (AD) is frequently associated with complete traumatic spinal cord injury, but has been described in inflammatory disorders, spinal cord tumours

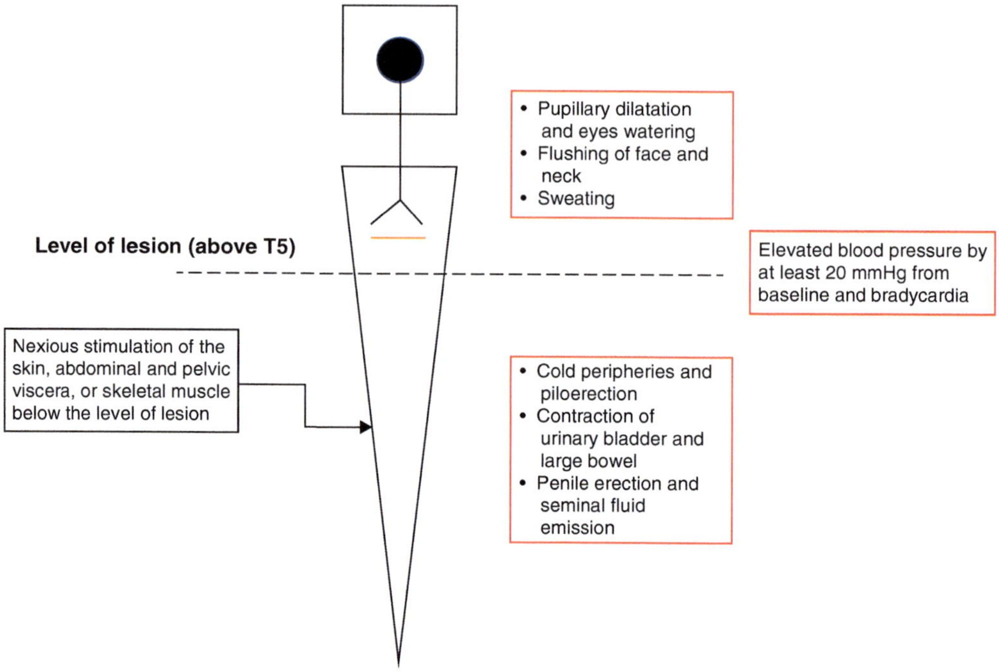

Fig. 28.2 Schematic of clinical manifestation of autonomic dysreflexia (AD). Afferent noxious or non-noxious stimuli below the neurological level of injury lead to paroxysmal rise in blood pressure, which usually is accompanied by a fall in heart rate because of increased vagal activity. A constellation of signs and symptoms above and below the level of injury

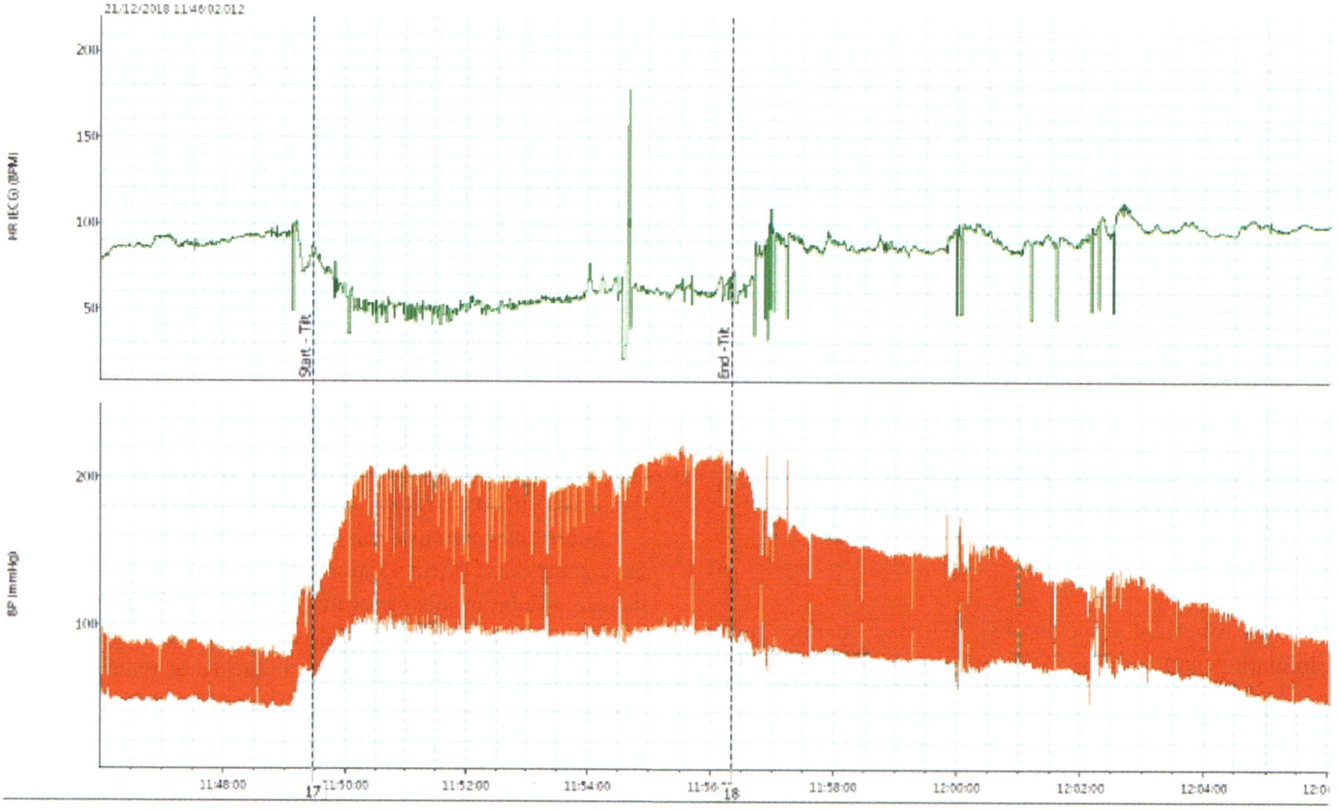

Fig. 28.3 Changes in blood pressure (BP) and heart rate (HR) of a chronic tetraplegic patient undergoing passive postural change from supine to sitting. Sustained increase in BP (episode of autonomic dysreflexia, AD) was documented and associated with reduction in HR. Patient reported recurrent episodes of AD while home, induced by changes in posture

or neurosurgical interventions [20]. AD mainly occurs in the chronic phase of SCI but it has also been documented in a minority (5.7% with SCI above T6) in the acute phase of the injury [16].

Stimulation of the skin, abdominal and pelvic viscera or skeletal muscles, can cause a paroxysmal rise in blood pressure (Fig. 28.3), which usually is accompanied by a fall in heart rate because of increased vagal activity [1].

There is an elevation in both stroke volume and cardiac output, suggestive of activation of spinal cardiac reflexes. These changes occur soon after stimulation, the rapidity indicating that they are of neurogenic origin and likely to be due to reflex sympathetic activity through the isolated spinal cord.

There is a marked reduction in peripheral blood flow which may result in cold limbs, thus accounting for poikilothermia spinalis, in addition to occluded venous pressure, indicating contraction of capacitance vessels.

Increased pressor responses to stimuli do not occur in patients with lesions below the fifth thoracic segment, indicating that the sympathetic neural outflow above that level is of major importance in blood pressure homeostasis. It is likely that in the lesions below T5 there is sparing of the neural control of the large splanchnic circulatory bed [2, 21].

Complication and Management of Autonomic Dysreflexia

Autonomic dysreflexia can be of major clinical importance. Mild episodes probably occur intermittently through the day, often are not noticed, and may be of little consequence (silent autonomic dysreflexia) [6, 17] (Fig. 28.4).

When autonomic dysreflexia is prolonged there may be considerable morbidity, as a result of excessive sweating over the head and neck, and a throbbing headache. Other complications include myocardial failure and neurological deficits such as epileptic seizures, visual defects and cerebral haemorrhage [18, 21]. These may result in extensive and permanent neurological deficits or death.

The key factor in the management of AD is prevention. It is necessary to determine the provoking cause and to rectify it (Fig. 28.5) [10, 17].

In some patients, autonomic dysreflexia may be a major and recurring problem because of difficulty in either defining or resolving the precipitating cause. A more common example, which may easily be missed, is an anal fissure. Despite recognizing the cause, it may be extremely difficult to resolve problems which include severe skeletal muscle spasms or recurrent urinary bladder infection. Autonomic dysreflexia can be a particular problem during surgery, especially if the urinary bladder or the large bowel is involved. In these patients either spinal anaesthesia or a general anaesthetic, such as halothane, along with an increase in positive pressure ventilation, is often successful in controlling the hypertension. Short-acting ganglionic blockers, such as trimethaphan, have been used successfully during surgery.

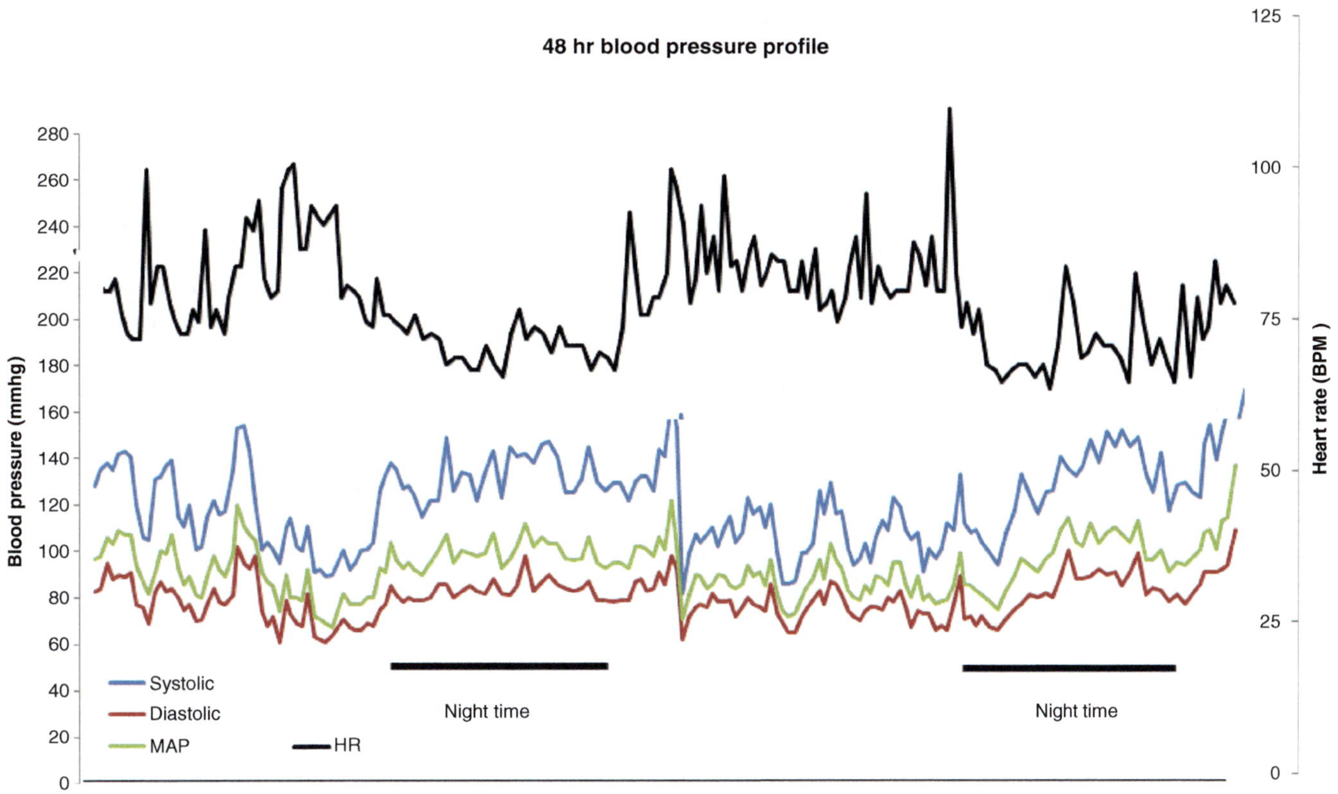

Fig. 28.4 48-hour ambulatory blood pressure and heart rate measurements demonstrating an absent physiological fall in blood pressure at night (loss of the circadian regulation of blood pressure, reversed profile) and multiple episodes of a raised blood pressure due to autonomic dysreflexia in a complete tetraplegic

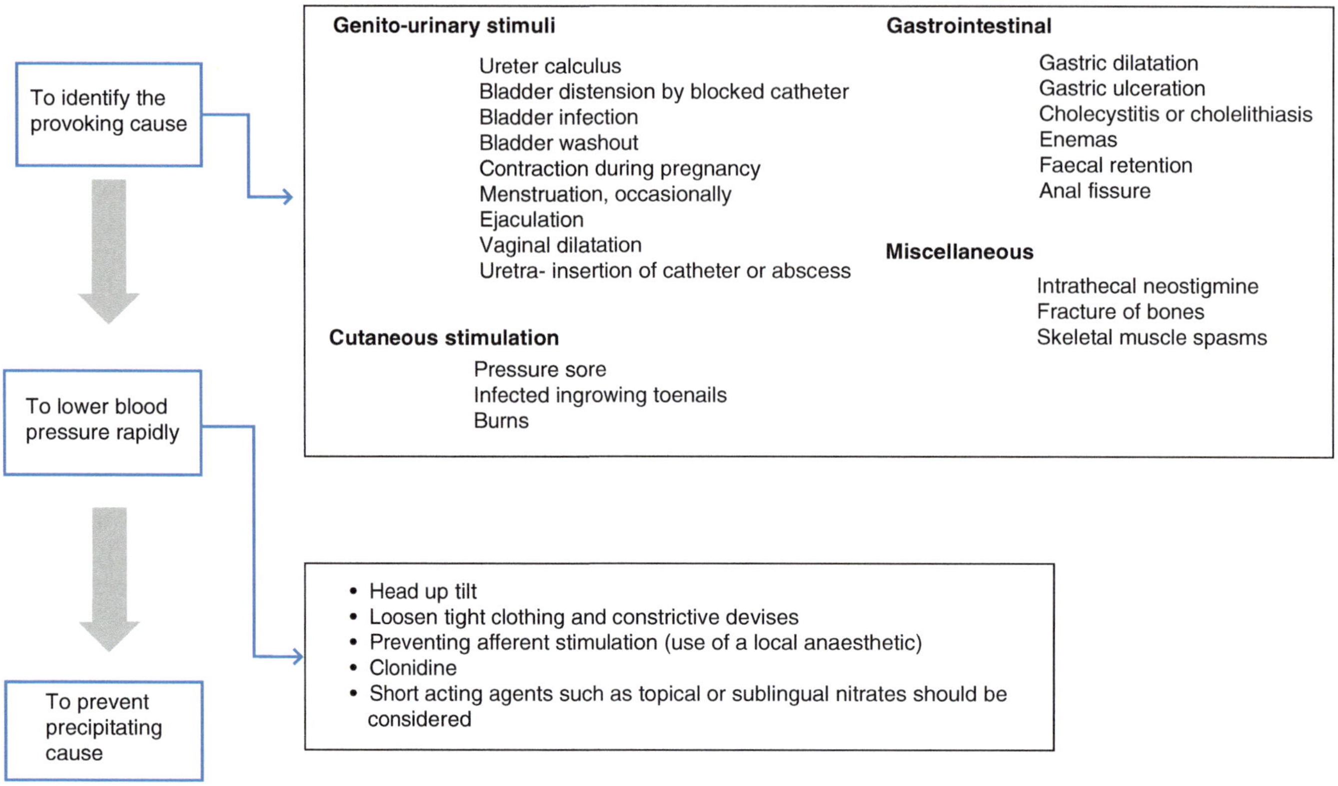

Fig. 28.5 Management of acute autonomic dysreflexia: identify the provoking cause and rectify it. Head-up tilt (which causes venous pooling) may be used initially. Various drugs are helpful: preventing afferent stimulation, for instance by the use of a local anaesthetic such as lignocaine in the urinary bladder, can be effective

Thermodysregulation

Hypothermia, hyperthermia and poikilothermia may be observed in tetraplegics [6].

Hypothermia in tetraplegia is mainly due to lack of activation of skeletal muscles and shivering as a major proportion of skeletal muscle mass is not directly under voluntary control. Tetraplegics maintain the ability to shiver in innervated areas as the body temperature falls, but this often results only in a small increase in metabolism which may be inadequate for body temperature homeostasis. In recently injured tetraplegics in neurogenic shock, cutaneous vasodilatation, and the inability to appropriately vasoconstrict, enhances heat loss and lowers body temperature further [22, 23].

Hyperthermia may occur particularly in tetraplegics and high spinal-cord lesions when environmental temperature is elevated, or in response to infection. Heat loss is dependent on two major mechanisms, vasodilatation and sweating, both of which are impaired in spinal lesions [24].

The maintenance of a suitable environmental temperature is of importance in the prevention of hyperthermia in high spinal lesions. When hyperthermia occurs, cooling with the aid of tepid sponging and increased air flow with a fan accelerates heat loss by a combination of evaporation, conduction and convection. In severe cases, ice-cooled saline by intravenous infusion or urinary bladder irrigation and in extreme cases immersion of the whole body in an ice bath may be necessary. In hyperpyrexia associated with infection, drugs such as aspirin and paracetamol appear to be effective in lowering body temperature. The mechanisms by which they do this are unclear. Chlorpromazine is also effective but has the potential to induce hypotension.

Gastrointestinal Dysfunction

The autonomic nervous system richly innervates the gastrointestinal tract which is often affected especially in the early stages, after spinal-cord lesions.

In recently injured patients increased vagal activity may cause hyperacidity, along with high gastrin levels which also may contribute to gastric hypersecretion and ulceration and gastrointestinal bleeding (Box 28.1).

Paralytic ileus can occur in spinal shock and may be accompanied by gastric dilatation. It may cause meteorism interfering with the movement of the diaphragm, often the only major functional muscle of respiration in these patients.

Paralysis of the sacral parasympathetic results in atony of the colon and rectum with risk of faecal retention. Digital evacuation is often necessary in the early stages.

In the chronic stage, tetraplegics are still prone to paralytic ileus especially after undergoing general anaesthesia and abdominal surgery.

After the initial stage of neurogenic shock, autonomous function of the lower bowel returns is regulated at a spinal level and bowel activity is mainly stimulated by increased volume and distension [25]. The diet should therefore include high residue foods together with mild laxatives and stool softeners, to ensure regular bowel evacuation.

Genito-urinary Dysfunction

Function of the urinary bladder is dependent upon higher centres in the brain and function of sympathetic and parasympathetic nerves and is therefore affected to varying degrees in patients with spinal-cord lesions [14, 26].

In spinal shock there is usually complete paralysis of bladder function with retention of urine followed by distension and urinary overflow after excessive intravesical pressure has developed [25]. With return of parasympathetic activity within the isolated sacral cord there is detrusor muscle contraction, which occurs in response to filling of the urinary bladder or following stimuli such as tapping of the anterior abdominal wall suprapubically. This is the automatic reflex bladder, or neurogenic bladder (Table 28.2). During detrusor contraction there is a need for simultaneous relaxation of the sphincters and pelvic floor to allow the free passage of urine. Retained urine often results in infection, which can involve the kidneys, especially when there is retrograde pressure in the urinary tract. In such patients an indwelling catheter, or various forms of urological and neurological surgery, may be needed to relieve the functional obstruction and prevent autonomic dysreflexia. There are emerging treatments for neurogenic detrusor overactivity which may also reduce the risk of AD in this patient group.

Penile erection is dependent largely upon the sacral parasympathetic nerves with ejaculation dependent upon the sympathetic nerves. In spinal shock there is an absence of both erectile and ejaculatory function. In some patients, however, passive penile enlargement and priapism may occur, probably due to paralytic dilatation resulting in engorgement of the corpora cavernosa. Following the return of isolated spinal-cord reflex activity, penile erection may occur if the glans penis is stimulated, or as part of autonomic dysreflexia. Ejaculation is usually retrograde, as the associated contraction of muscles at the bladder neck which prevents seminal fluid flowing back into the bladder does not usually occur. In spinal-cord injuries, therefore, procreation in the male is largely dependent on the collection of seminal fluid for artificial insemination.

Table 28.2 Gastrointestinal and genito-urinary dysfunction in spinal cord injury

In recently injured	Chronic injured
Gastrointestinal dysfunction	
Upper gastrointestinal bleeding with gastric hypersecretion and ulceration Greater risk in those with higher lesions	Tetraplegics and high thoracic lesions are at risk of paralytic ileus
Risk of perforation	Return of autonomous function of the lower bowel regulated at a spinal level
Paralytic ileus and gastric dilatation	Increased volume and distension stimulate bowel activity
Atony of the colon and rectum with faecal retention	
Genito-urinary dysfunction	
Complete paralysis of bladder function with retention of urine	Neurogenic bladder with risk of retention, infection and autonomic dysreflexia
Absence of both erectile and ejaculatory function	Penile erection with glans penis stimulation and retrograde ejaculation
Priapism	Transient disruption of the menstrual cycle
	Pregnancies carry the risk of severe autonomic dysreflexia and paroxysmal hypertension

In women transient disruption of the menstrual cycle is often observed after spinal lesions, as may occur during other traumatic conditions or illnesses. There is usually a return to normal menstrual periods within a year. Successful pregnancies have been reported in both tetraplegics and paraplegics. In those with high lesions a particular problem is severe autonomic dysreflexia and paroxysmal hypertension which may be accompanied by cardiac dysrhythmias, especially during uterine contractions. Such patients are particularly prone to epileptic seizures and cerebral haemorrhage, and it is essential to lower their blood pressure.

Sleep Disorders in SCI

Sleep problems are common in spinal cord injury (SCI) and contribute to poor quality of life and to increased cardiovascular risk [27, 28].

Patients often present with poor or decreased sleep, mainly related to increased risk for sleep-disordered breathing (SDB), including intermittent hypoxemia and sleep fragmentation and contributing to nocturnal hypertension [29].

SDB is also frequent in non-traumatic spinal cord disorders such as spinal muscular atrophy, myelomeningocele, multiple sclerosis, rheumatoid arthritis, tumours or infections [30, 31].

The pathogenesis of sleep dysfunction is not fully understood and likely to be multifactorial, including the level and completeness of injury. Low concentrations of melatonin in serum, plasma and saliva have been documented in combination with lack of diurnal rhythm in cervical complete SCI patients [32–34].

Impaired core body temperature rhythmicity might also play a role in sleep onset and maintenance [35, 36].

Bladder dysfunction with urinary retention and increased risk of autonomic dysreflexia may contribute to sleep fragmentation.

Pain and secondary complications have been correlated with poor sleep after paediatric-onset SCI [37].

Increasing interest in systematic assessment of sleep in patients with SCI might shed some light on pathophysiology, diagnosis and management of sleep disorders in this population.

Assessing Cardiovascular Autonomic Function in Patients with Spinal Cord Lesion

Autonomic Screening Tests

Autonomic screening tests, in addition to head-up tilt testing, help determine the extent of the cardiovascular autonomic abnormality [6].

Pressor stimuli dependent on sympathetic activation that either originate in, or are modulated by, the brain do not raise blood pressure in patients with complete cervical cord transaction. Stimuli such as mental arithmetic, a loud noise and cutaneous stimulation by either pain or cold in areas above the lesion have no effect in tetraplegics, unlike in normal subjects in whom they elevate blood pressure. The lack of response to these stimuli provides evidence of severance of sympathetic pathways descending within the cervical spinal cord.

Orthostatic hypotension is a common manifestation in both the acute and chronic phase of spinal injury. Patients may have a fall of ≥20 mmHg of systolic or a decrease in diastolic blood pressure of ≥10 mmHg when moved from the supine to the upright position. In the laboratory head-up tilt to 60° often is used as the postural stimulus, and blood pressure and heart rate can be accurately measured using automated non-invasive and continuous techniques.

During head-up postural change, as on a tilt table, there usually is an immediate fall in both systolic and diastolic blood pressure in high lesions. The pressure may fall to extremely low levels that may cause loss of consciousness in recently injured tetraplegics or in chronic tetraplegics following prolonged recumbency. Tolerance to a low cerebral perfusion pressure often occurs in patients with chronic autonomic failure, who are also able to autoregulate their cerebral circulation despite an extremely low perfusion blood pressure [13].

Following an initial fall in blood pressure when upright, subsequent responses vary including a further fall in BP in the early stage of the disease, (Fig. 28.1), or a partly recovery in blood pressure in chronically injured patients. In some, especially in the early stages, blood pressure continues to fall (Fig. 28.1). There is no rise in levels of plasma noradrenaline in the early phases following head-up postural change, consistent with their inability to reflexively increase sympathetic nervous activity in response to postural change, as should occur normally. In many chronically injured patients, however, if tilt is prolonged, the blood pressure tends to partly recover, often with oscillations. This recovery may be related to activation of the renin–angiotensin–aldosterone system [12]. A further mechanism contributing to blood pressure recovery during tilt is the activation of spinal reflexes either from stimulation of the skin, the skeletal muscles or the viscera. This is more likely to account for the reduction in peripheral blood flow and rise in occluded venous pressure observed during head-up tilt in tetraplegics than the spinal postural reflexes that were previously proposed. Local sympathetic reflexes (veno-arteriolar reflexes) may operate in high lesions during postural change.

During head-up postural change there often is a rapid rise in heart rate, which is inversely related to the fall in blood pressure [1, 26]. This is likely to be due to withdrawal of vagal tone in response to unloading of baroreceptor afferents, as it is markedly attenuated, although not abolished, by atropine. Propranolol also reduces the heart rate rise during tilt, suggesting that beta-adrenoceptor stimulation may partially contribute. In the majority heart rate does not usually rise above 100 beats/min when upright, even when there is a marked fall in blood pressure. This therefore is different from patients with an intact sympathetic nervous system who are in 'shock' with a similarly low level of blood pressure.

Valsalva Manoeuvre In high spinal lesions the responses to the Valsalva manoeuvre are abnormal because the baroreceptor reflex is impaired due to the disruption of sympathetic efferent pathways through the cervical and thoracic spinal cord. When intrathoracic pressure is elevated there is a fall in blood pressure, despite a fairly modest increase in intrathoracic pressure that is often difficult to achieve and maintain because of the inability to activate intercostal muscles. There is no recovery in blood pressure while the intrathoracic pressure is elevated. Heart rate rises with the fall in blood pressure because the cardiac vagi respond to the fall in blood pressure. On reducing the elevated intrathoracic pressure, there is a gradual recovery of blood pressure with a reduction in heart rate that does not fall below the basal level.

This ability to lower blood pressure has also been used to the benefit of patients, to prevent hypertension during urological surgery by increasing positive pressure during assisted ventilation.

Additional investigations may be needed to determine factors causing or contributing to orthostatic hypotension. These include the responses to food ingestion and exercise.

Liquid Meal Challenge Tests

In tetraplegics, unlike patients with chronic primary autonomic failure, ingestion of food does not result in a substantial fall in supine blood pressure. The modest fall in blood pressure is accompanied by an elevation in heart rate [38]. Levels of forearm venous plasma noradrenaline do not change, excluding a generalized increase in sympathetic nerve activity. The mechanisms responsible for preventing a substantial fall in blood pressure in tetraplegics are unclear; these could include the stimulation of reflexes from the gastrointestinal tract and mesentery.

Exercise Testing

This is not possible in patients with complete lesions but possible in those with incomplete lesions.

Responses are obtained during graded incremental supine exercise using a bicycle ergometer with measurement of postural responses before and after exercise.

Ambulatory 24 BP and HR Monitoring

Intermittent ambulatory blood pressure and heart rate recordings over a 24- or 48-hour period using small computerized lightweight devices are of particular value, especially at home, in determining the effects of various stimuli in daily life and assessing the occurrence of BP and HR abnormalities of circadian rhythm. It is essential that an accurate diary of events is maintained to determine the effects of postural change, food and exercise.

Non-invasive ambulatory 24-hour recordings indicate loss of the nocturnal circadian fall in blood pressure, as should occur normally.

Plasma Catecholamines

Plasma catecholamine measurements are available in specialized laboratories and may be of value in acute and chronic phase to evaluate severity of autonomic impairment.

Plasma noradrenaline (norepinephrine) provides a measure of sympathetic neural activity and plasma adrenaline (epinephrine) of adrenal medullary activity [7].

Conclusion

This chapter has focused on patients with cervical and high thoracic spinal cord injuries, as these patients often have major clinical problems resulting from autonomic dysfunction. The level of the last functioning cord segment is important in autonomic cardiovascular problem, with lesions at or above T5 causing the most disabling orthostatic hypotension, and severity of autonomic dysreflexia. Clinicians should be aware of the most common noxious and non-noxious stimuli below the level of injury capable of triggering an exaggerated sympathetic response and hypertension which may result in potentially fatal complications.

Loss of supraspinal control over sympathetic preganglionic neurons and reflex sympathetic activity through the isolated spinal cord are the primary cause of disordered blood pressure regulation and AD after spinal cord injury

References

1. Mathias CJ, Christensen NJ, Frankel HL, Spalding JM. Cardiovascular control in recently injured tetraplegics in spinal shock. Q J Med. 1979;48(190):273–87.
2. Krassioukov A, Claydon VE. The clinical problems in cardiovascular control following spinal cord injury: an overview. Prog Brain Res. 2006;152:223–9.
3. Frankel HL, Mathias CJ, Spalding JM. Mechanisms of reflex cardiac arrest in tetraplegic patients. Lancet. 1975;2(7946):1183–5.
4. Hadley MN, Walters BC, Grabb PA, Oyesiku NM, Przybylski GJ, Resnick DK, et al. Blood pressure management after acute spinal cord injury. Neurosurgery. 2002;50(3 Suppl):S58–62.
5. Hadley MN, Walters BC, Grabb PA, Oyesiku NM, Przybylski GJ, Resnick DK, et al. Guidelines for the management of acute cervical spine and spinal cord injuries. Clin Neurosurg. 2002;49:407–98.
6. Curt A, Nitsche B, Rodic B, Schurch B, Dietz V. Assessment of autonomic dysreflexia in patients with spinal cord injury. J Neurol Neurosurg Psychiatry. 1997;62(5):473–7.
7. Mathias CJ, Christensen NJ, Corbett JL, Frankel HL, Goodwin TJ, Peart WS. Plasma catecholamines, plasma renin activity and plasma aldosterone in tetraplegic man, horizontal and tilted. Clin Sci Mol Med. 1975;49(4):291–9.
8. Mathias CJ. Bradycardia and cardiac arrest during tracheal suction--mechanisms in tetraplegic patients. Eur J Intensive Care Med. 1976;2(4):147–56.
9. Claydon VE, Steeves JD, Krassioukov A. Orthostatic hypotension following spinal cord injury: understanding clinical pathophysiology. Spinal Cord. 2006;44(6):341–51.
10. Mathias CJ. Orthostatic hypotension and paroxysmal hypertension in humans with high spinal cord injury. Prog Brain Res. 2006;152:231–43.
11. Illman A, Stiller K, Williams M. The prevalence of orthostatic hypotension during physiotherapy treatment in patients with an acute spinal cord injury. Spinal Cord. 2000;38(12):741–7.
12. Mathias CJ, Christensen NJ, Frankel HL, Peart WS. Renin release during head-up tilt occurs independently of sympathetic nervous activity in tetraplegic man. Clin Sci (Lond). 1980;59(4):251–6.
13. Gonzalez F, Chang JY, Banovac K, Messina D, Martinez-Arizala A, Kelley RE. Autoregulation of cerebral blood flow in patients

with orthostatic hypotension after spinal cord injury. Paraplegia. 1991;29(1):1–7.

14. Alexander MS, Biering-Sorensen F, Bodner D, Brackett NL, Cardenas D, Charlifue S, et al. International standards to document remaining autonomic function after spinal cord injury. Spinal Cord. 2009;47(1):36–43.
15. Mathias CJ, Luckitt J, Desai P, Baker H, el Masri W, Frankel HL. Pharmacodynamics and pharmacokinetics of the oral antispastic agent tizanidine in patients with spinal cord injury. J Rehabil Res Dev. 1989;26(4):9–16.
16. Krassioukov AV, Furlan JC, Fehlings MG. Autonomic dysreflexia in acute spinal cord injury: an under-recognized clinical entity. J Neurotrauma. 2003;20(8):707–16.
17. Consortium for Spinal Cord M. Acute management of autonomic dysreflexia: individuals with spinal cord injury presenting to health-care facilities. J Spinal Cord Med. 2002;25 Suppl 1:S67–88.
18. Fausel RA, Paski SC. Autonomic dysreflexia resulting in seizure after colonoscopy in a patient with spinal cord injury. ACG Case Rep J. 2014;1(4):187–8.
19. Sharif H, Hou S. Autonomic dysreflexia: a cardiovascular disorder following spinal cord injury. Neural Regen Res. 2017;12(9):1390–400.
20. Furlan JC, Fehlings MG, Halliday W, Krassioukov AV. Autonomic dysreflexia associated with intramedullary astrocytoma of the spinal cord. Lancet Oncol. 2003;4(9):574–5.
21. Lee ES, Joo MC. Prevalence of autonomic dysreflexia in patients with spinal cord injury above T6. Biomed Res Int. 2017;2017:2027594.
22. Nicotra A, Asahina M, Mathias CJ. Skin vasodilator response to local heating in human chronic spinal cord injury. Eur J Neurol. 2004;11(12):835–7.
23. Nicotra A, Asahina M, Young TM, Mathias CJ. Heat-provoked skin vasodilatation in innervated and denervated trunk dermatomes in human spinal cord injury. Spinal Cord. 2006;44(4):222–6.
24. Handrakis JP, Trbovich M, Hagen EM, Price M. Thermodysregulation in persons with spinal cord injury: case series on use of the autonomic standards. Spinal Cord Ser Cases. 2017;3:17086.
25. Ditunno JF, Little JW, Tessler A, Burns AS. Spinal shock revisited: a four-phase model. Spinal Cord. 2004;42(7):383–95.
26. Krassioukov AV, Karlsson AK, Wecht JM, Wuermser LA, Mathias CJ, Marino RJ, et al. Assessment of autonomic dysfunction following spinal cord injury: rationale for additions to International Standards for Neurological Assessment. J Rehabil Res Dev. 2007;44(1):103–12.
27. Fogelberg DJ, Hughes AJ, Vitiello MV, Hoffman JM, Amtmann D. Comparison of sleep problems in individuals with spinal cord injury and multiple sclerosis. J Clin Sleep Med. 2016;12(5):695–701.
28. Giannoccaro MP, Moghadam KK, Pizza F, Boriani S, Maraldi NM, Avoni P, et al. Sleep disorders in patients with spinal cord injury. Sleep Med Rev. 2013;17(6):399–409.
29. Chiodo AE, Sitrin RG, Bauman KA. Sleep disordered breathing in spinal cord injury: a systematic review. J Spinal Cord Med. 2016;39(4):374–82.
30. Mellies U, Dohna-Schwake C, Stehling F, Voit T. Sleep disordered breathing in spinal muscular atrophy. Neuromuscul Disord. 2004;14(12):797–803.
31. Waters KA, Forbes P, Morielli A, Hum C, O'Gorman AM, Vernet O, et al. Sleep-disordered breathing in children with myelomeningocele. J Pediatr. 1998;132(4):672–81.
32. Golder FJ, Reier PJ, Davenport PW, Bolser DC. Cervical spinal cord injury alters the pattern of breathing in anesthetized rats. J Appl Physiol (1985). 2001;91(6):2451–8.
33. Sankari A, Bascom AT, Badr MS. Upper airway mechanics in chronic spinal cord injury during sleep. J Appl Physiol (1985). 2014;116(11):1390–5.
34. White LH, Bradley TD. Role of nocturnal rostral fluid shift in the pathogenesis of obstructive and central sleep apnoea. J Physiol. 2013;591(5):1179–93.
35. Rizwan A, Sankari A, Bascom AT, Vaughan S, Badr MS. Nocturnal swallowing and arousal threshold in individuals with chronic spinal cord injury. J Appl Physiol (1985). 2018;125(2):445–52.
36. Sankari A, Martin JL, Badr M. A retrospective review of sleep-disordered breathing, hypertension and cardiovascular diseases in spinal cord injury patients. Spinal Cord. 2015;53(6):496–7.
37. January AM, Zebracki K, Chlan KM, Vogel LC. Poor sleep in adults with pediatric-onset spinal cord injury: associations with pain, health, and activity. J Spinal Cord Med. 2017;40(5):560–6.
38. Baliga RR, Catz AB, Watson LD, Short DJ, Frankel HL, Mathias CJ. Cardiovascular and hormonal responses to food ingestion in humans with spinal cord transection. Clin Auton Res. 1997;7(3):137–41.

Dysautonomia and Sleep Dysfunction in Pediatric Practice

29

Suresh Kotagal

Introduction

The control of heart rate and breathing is intimately related to sleep. The continuous neuromaturation that is characteristic of infancy and childhood brings with it the need for adaptation to the internal and external milieu. There are several conditions with sleep-related autonomic dysfunction that are unique to infants and children. They form the substance of this overview.

Physiological Changes in Cardiorespiratory Control

Rapid eye movement (REM) (active) sleep constitutes about 80% of total sleep in preterm infants at 32–34 weeks postconceptional age. By full term or 40 weeks postconceptional age, REM sleep has decreased to about 50% of total sleep, and by the age of around 3 years to 20–25% of total sleep time [1]. The preponderance of REM sleep in infancy confers a mortality and morbidity risk to patients of this age. For instance, upper airway collapsibility is increased during REM sleep and at the same time, the central nervous response to hypercarbia remains blunted during this stage of sleep [2]. In other words, while there is increased risk of sleep-related upper airway obstruction, the ability of the central nervous system to compensate for hypoxia and hypercarbia is limited.

S. Kotagal (✉)
Center for Sleep Medicine and Department of Neurology, Mayo Clinic, Rochester, Minnesota, USA
e-mail: kotagal.suresh@mayo.edu

Sudden Infant Death Syndrome (SIDS)

SIDS is defined as the sudden death of an infant below 1 year of age which remains unexplained despite thorough case investigation, including a complete autopsy, examination of the death scene, and review of the clinical history [3]. The prevalence is about 0.6/1000 live births. Sixty percent of the deaths occur by the age of 3 months and 85% by age 6 months. Infants are generally between 1 and 6 months of age. The infant is usually found cold, limp, unresponsive, not breathing, and lifeless in the crib by the parent or guardian. Risk factors include premature birth, maternal cigarette smoking, overheating and prone sleeping position, and bed sharing with the parent [4]. Soft bedding may increase the risk of compression of the face against the mattress and predispose to hypercarbia and consequent respiratory depression. There is increased risk of rebreathing and hypercarbia in the prone position. The Back to Sleep program that was initiated by the Centers for Disease Control in 1992 is credited for significantly reducing the incidence of SIDS. While for the most part infants are now placed to sleep in the supine position, occasional instances of infants being placed in the prone position still do occur.

The triple risk model hypothesis for SIDS consists of the vulnerable infant, environmental factors, and critical neurodevelopmental stage of the infant (Fig. 29.1) [5]. Neuropathological examination of the brain stem may reveal lesions in the ventral medullary surface, especially involving the arcuate nucleus that has a role in the automatic control of breathing and is part of the medullary serotonergic network. Other components of the medullary serotonergic network that have been implicated in SIDS are the raphe nucleus, the gigantocellular nucleus, the lateral paragigantocellular nucleus, and the intermediate reticular zone (Fig. 29.2) [5, 6]. The medullary serotonergic network contains pH sensitive K+ channels, and is involved in chemosensitivity, and in the regulation of blood pressure and temperature. It also projects to the hypoglossal and phrenic nuclei. The hypocretin

S. Chokroverty, P. Cortelli (eds.), *Autonomic Nervous System and Sleep*, https://doi.org/10.1007/978-3-030-62263-3_29

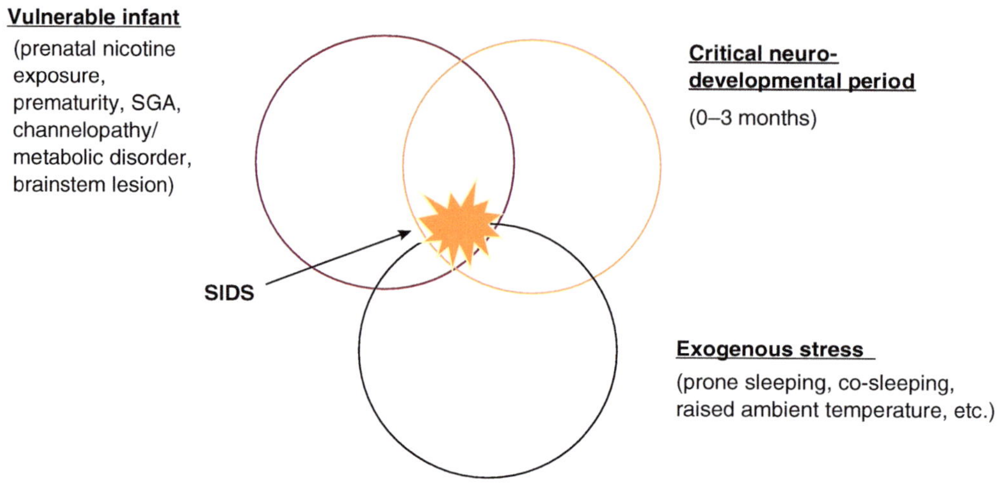

Fig. 29.1 Venn diagram, depicting the interaction among host, environment, and vulnerability at a critical neurodevelopmental stage that is associated with sudden infant death syndrome (SIDS). (Adapted from Kinney et al. [5], with permission of Oxford University Press on behalf of the American Association of Neuropathologists)

	Medulla	Serotonergic Cell Bodies	Raphe Terminals	Rhombic lip-derived	Autonomicl Respiratory Function
N. Raphé Obscurus	+	+	+	+	+
Arcuate Nucleus	+	+	+	+	Post-ulated
Principal Inferior Olive	+	–	+	+	+
N. Gigantocellularis	+	+	+	Unknown	+
N. Paragigantocellularis lateralis	+	+	+	+	+
Intermediate Reticular Zone	+	+	+	Unknown	+

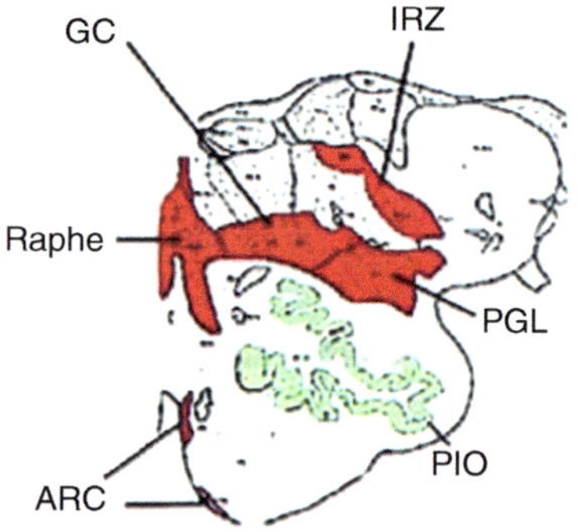

Fig. 29.2 Cross section of the medulla, depicting components of the medullary serotonergic network that are implicated in sudden infant death syndrome (SIDS). Key areas are shaded in dark. (From Kinney et al. [5], with permission of Oxford University Press on behalf of the American Association of Neuropathologists)

system might also be implicated in SIDS as it projects from the hypothalamus to the nucleus tractus solitarius, and mediates central arousal responses, the failure of which may be a key agonal process in SIDS [7]. Incidentally, the highest levels of CSF hypocretin are in infants, with a gradual decline thereafter [8]. Cardiac rhythm disturbances such as long QT interval may also contribute to SIDS in about 12% of cases [9]. Mutations implicated are known to involve seven different genes—*KCNQ1*, *KCNH2/HERG*, *SCN5A*, *KCNE2*, *CAV3*, *SCN4B*, and *SCNTA1* that predispose to long QT interval [9]. A small percentage of cases may have inborn errors of metabolism, such as fatty acid oxidation disorders that can now be detected on newborn screening panels, for example, medium chain acetyl coenzyme A dehydrogenase deficiency. A targeted assay utilizing a combination of direct injection mass spectrometry and reverse phase mass spectrometry recently found seven acyl carnitines (involved in fatty acid metabolism) to significantly differ in concentration in brains from SIDS patients as compared to controls [10].

Management strategies are essentially preventative in nature and include avoidance of smoking by the mother during pregnancy, teaching adult caretakers to always place infants in the crib in the supine position, and avoidance of pillows and soft mattresses that can pose a suffocation hazard. Newborn screening methods on dried blood spots and urine are able to identify disorders of acylcarnitine and amino acid metabolism that have been implicated in SIDS [11].

Brief Resolved Unexplained Events (BRUE)

BRUE occurs in infants less than 1 year. The observer reports a sudden, brief, and now resolved episode of cyanosis or pallor/absent, decreased or irregular breathing/marked change in muscle tone (decreased or increased), and altered responsiveness [12]. The previous diagnosis term was apparent life-threatening episodes but it has now been dropped due to the fact that the episodes are not always "life threatening." The prior clinical course during pregnancy and the perinatal period is normal. Development overall up to the point of occurrence of the event is also normal. An event qualifies for the diagnosis of BRUE only if no clear etiology has been identified. Consequently, an episode of choking or gagging due to gastroesophageal reflux does not qualify for the BRUE diagnosis. There is no increased risk of SIDS in BRUE patients, but child maltreatment may be a concern in this category.

Risk stratification is important [13]. High-risk BRUE patients are those of less than age 2 months, those born prematurely with gestational age <32 weeks, suspected child abuse, need for cardiopulmonary resuscitation, and a history of more than one event. They need hospitalization for further observation and work up for cardiopulmonary, gastrointestinal, neurological, metabolic, and traumatic etiologies. Low-risk BRUE patients are those who are older than age 60 days, gestational age is >32 weeks, first episode, duration <1 minute, no need for cardiopulmonary resuscitation, and no concerning features on history or examination. Low-risk BRUE patients may not require hospitalization or extensive diagnostic work up, though screening overnight oximetry is still appropriate to conduct. Chest radiographs are not usually indicated in the low-risk BRUE category, and the same applies to blood gas analysis.

Congenital Central Hypoventilation Syndrome (CCHS)

CCHS is characterized by failure of the automatic control of the breathing. Onset of symptoms is generally in the newborn period. Patients show hypoxemia and hypercarbia in the absence of any significant cardiopulmonary disease. Those requiring ventilators for initial apnea, hypercarbia or oxygen desaturation experiences difficulty in weaned off the ventilator despite otherwise healthy lungs. Respiratory function is normal initially during wakefulness but impaired in quiet (NREM) sleep and less impaired during active (REM) sleep. Autonomic dysfunction can be widespread, with associated pupillary abnormalities, prolonged sinus pauses, constipation, Hirschsprung disease, and neural crest tumors like neuroblastoma and ganglioneuroma [14].

Nocturnal polysomnography shows decreased respiratory rate and elevated levels of transcutaneous CO_2 or end tidal CO_2. A ventilatory challenge with a mixture of 5% CO_2 and 95% oxygen during NREM sleep is not accompanied by the physiologic three- to fivefold increase in minute volume. Capillary blood gas analysis may reveal hypercarbia and respiratory acidosis. Respiratory function is generally normal during wakefulness till the late stages when it gets affected. Cognitive and language development remains normal to mildly impaired.

Dysfunction in the automatic control of breathing is due to lesions affecting the brain stem ventilatory control apparatus, which includes the arcuate nucleus, nucleus tractus solitarius, the nucleus ambiguous, and the chemosensitive ventral medullary surface. CCHS occurs as a consequence of disruption in function of the PHOX2B gene that localized to chromosome 4 [15]. The PHOX2B gene is a transcription factor. It modulates differentiation of the neural crest cells that ultimately form the mature autonomic nervous system. This gene has three exons. Mutations in the PHOX2B gene are present in over 90% of cases of CCHS, with increased number of polyalanine repeats in exon 3. Normally, each of the two alleles of third exon of PHOX2B has 20 polyalanine repeats in the tail. CCHS is associated with a heterozygous polyalanine expansion mutation in one of the alleles, with the end result of a genotype that is 20/25 or 20/24–20/33. Larger polyalanine expansions are associated with more severe disease [15]. Some patients do not have expansion of the polyalanine tail but show nonpolyalanine repeat expansion mutations (NPARM). Disease severity is more in those with NPARMS. These mutations can be missense, nonsense, or frame shift in type. Hirschsprung disease is likely to occur in close to 90% of patients with NPARM. Neuroblastoma is also more likely to occur in NPARMS [16]. Those with PARMs are predisposed to develop ganglioneuroma or ganglioneuroblastoma.

Testing for the PHOX2B gene abnormalities in CCHS is recommended in a step-wise manner. The first step is to analyze for the polyalanine expansions. If this test is noninformative, the next step is to proceed to gene sequence testing for nonsense, missense, and frame shift mutations. If this step is also not informative, one obtains multiplex ligation dependent probe amplification to look for large deletions of exon 3 [14].

Management consists of supportive care. Families are informed of the life-long nature of the disorder. Infants may require tracheostomy combined with home ventilators. Monitoring of oxygen saturation and end tidal CO_2/transcutaneous CO_2 in the home environment is needed on a routine basis. Older children may be able to tolerate noninvasive home ventilation. Diaphragmatic pacing can help older children. Autonomic dysfunction may involve the cardiovascular system also, hence periodic monitoring of heart rhythm using Holter studies is indicated. A cardiac pacemaker may be needed if there are recurrent sinus pauses of 3 seconds or longer [14]. Periodic surveillance for neural crest tumors may require 24-hour urinary catecholamine measurements, chest radiographs, and magnetic resonance imaging of the posterior mediastinum and retroperitoneal region. Comprehensive management also requires a skilled multidisciplinary team of experts that is familiar with the disorder [14, 15]. Ideally, the patient is admitted to the hospital annually for 3–5 days for the purpose of undergoing this multidisciplinary assessment and for making periodic changes to the management plan.

Central Hypoventilation Secondary to Other Brainstem Lesions

Patients with brainstem cavernomas [17], brainstem tumors [18], paraneoplastic encephalitis [19], bulbar poliomyelitis [20], and less frequently, patients with Chiari malformations [21] may be vulnerable to developing sleep-related hypoventilation. Patients generally present with symptoms of fatigue, and early morning headache. Nocturnal polysomnography shows sleep-related hypoventilation levels of end tidal CO_2 or transcutaneous CO_2 are above 50 mm for 25% or more of the total sleep time. Morning capillary blood gas analysis may also confirm hypercarbia. Those with Chiari type 1 malformation may require suboccipital decompression with the help of neurosurgical colleagues. Management is otherwise supportive, with use of noninvasive home ventilation or tracheostomy plus home respirator. There is insufficient experience with modalities like diaphragmatic pacing.

Rapid-Onset Obesity with Hypoventilation, Hypothalamic, Autonomic Dysregulation (ROHHAD)

ROHHAD is a recently established pediatric multisystem entity. Onset is in the first decade, with the child being previously well. It is slightly more common in girls than boys. The median age of onset in a recent meta-analysis was around 4 years [22]. There is abrupt onset of obesity which is associated with fatigue, hypersomnia, behavioral dysregulation, and a variety of neuroendocrine abnormalities. Besides sleep-related hypoventilation, the patients may exhibit endocrine abnormalities such as hyperprolactinemia, hyponatremia, hypernatremia, diabetes insipidus, or growth hormone deficiency [23]. Autonomic dysfunction generally manifests itself as impaired gastrointestinal motility, cold intolerance, excessive sweating, urinary incontinence, and altered perception to pain. Nocturnal polysomnography consistently shows obstructive or central sleep apnea in association with hypoventilation. About half the patients have associated neuroendocrine tumors (NET), hence the label ROHHAD-NET. Most commonly associated neuroendocrine tumors were ganglioneuromas and ganglioneuroblastomas. The tumors are generally located in the posterior mediastinum or the retroperitoneal space. No specific genetic mutation has been identified. The condition is progressive, and in some instances may be fatal. Management is essentially symptomatic. It requires monitoring of serum sodium levels, and sleep-related breathing. Respiration may need to be supported by noninvasive ventilation or in rare cases, using tracheostomy and home ventilators.

Autonomic Dysfunction in Pediatric Primary Hypersomnia Syndromes

Primary hypersomnia syndromes include narcolepsy types 1 and 2, idiopathic hypersomnia, and the Kleine Levin syndrome. There is a well-defined physiological basis for alterations in autonomic function in narcolepsy because neurons of the orexin system influence autonomic function via descending projections to the intermediate reticular zone of the medulla, the nucleus tractus solitarius, and the intermediolateral column in the spinal cord [24]. In rats, the orexin system has also been found to influence sympathetic activity and cardiovascular activity [25].

Orthostatic intolerance (OI) is the most common clinical manifestation of the autonomic nervous system dysfunction. It is defined as impaired ability to tolerate the upright position due to symptoms that subside when the supine position is assumed [26]. The most common manifestations of OI are lightheadedness, fatigue, nausea, heat intolerance, headache, and memory and attention impairment [26]. More severe cases of OI can be associated with postural orthostatic tachycardia syndrome (POTS), a condition that can be comorbid with narcolepsy type 2 and lesions in the thalamus and amygdala [27].

Autonomic dysfunction in pediatric primary hypersomnia syndromes has not been investigated. In a retrospective study (unpublished observation) at our institution, the author reviewed the medical records of patients with primary hypersomnia syndromes, age less than 18 years, who had been seen between 2000 and 2017 at our sleep disorder center. Inclusion criteria were diagnosis of narcolepsy type 1, narcolepsy 2, or idiopathic hypersomnia. The age at initial presentation was less than 18 years. Subjects with comorbidities, like obstructive sleep apnea, depression, or other sleep disorders were excluded. The medical records were reviewed for symptoms of orthostatic intolerance (see above). If orthostatic symptoms were present, the medical chart was reviewed in more detail to determine whether an autonomic reflex screening (ARS) battery had been conducted. The ARS is a composite of the tilt table test, heart rate response to the Valsalva maneuver and deep breathing, the quantitative sudomotor axon reflex test, and sweat test [28]. The autonomic studies were reviewed and reported independently of knowledge of the diagnosis of the primary hypersomnia syndrome by a specialist in autonomic neurology. Medication history at the time of autonomic reflex screen testing was also extracted from the chart.

There were 89 patients with primary hypersomnia disorders. The diagnoses had been established on the basis of history, polysomnogram and multiple sleep latency test (46 patients with narcolepsy type 1; 17 patients with narcolepsy type 2; 18 with idiopathic hypersomnia; 1 with Klein Levin syndrome; and 7 with medical disorders). Symptoms of OI were not associated with any one specific hypersomnia disorder. Thirty-three of 89 subjects (37%) had symptoms of OI, hence had undergone the autonomic reflex test battery. The mean age at hypersomnia diagnosis for the 33 subjects with autonomic testing was 13.6 ± 2.9 years; 25/33 were not on medications at the time of autonomic testing. The male:female ratio in the OI subgroup was 1:2 ($n = 33$), whereas in the subgroup without OI, it was reversed (2.1:1[$n = 56$; $p = 0.0015$]). Symptoms of OI included fatigue in 25/33, headache in 15/33, palpitations in 6/33, nausea and vomiting in 4/33, and constipation in 3/33. OI symptoms were reproducible during the tilt table test in 17/33 subjects. In 5 of these 17, they were severe enough to qualify for the diagnosis of postural orthostatic tachycardia syndrome (POTS). Overall, around the time of initial hypersomnia syndrome diagnosis, one-third of the group of 89 children had OI, with female predominance. One-half of this subgroup exhibited heart rate perturbations that were detectable on the autonomic reflex screening battery.

A limitation of our findings is that they are retrospective in nature. Nevertheless, we feel that autonomic dysfunction is common in children with primary hypersomnia disorders. It frequently goes unrecognized and can masquerade as fatigue. Once the patients get started on stimulants, wake promoting agents, sodium oxybate, or tricyclic agents for the treatment of the hypersomnia syndrome, proper testing for autonomic dysfunction is no longer feasible. Nevertheless, the importance of enquiring about orthostatic intolerance at the time of primary hypersomnia syndrome diagnosis and when appropriate, obtaining a comprehensive evaluation of the autonomic nervous system is emphasized. Prospective studies are also needed in this area. The pathophysiology of OI is unclear, but it may simply be a manifestation of hypersomnia patients spending excessive time in the recumbent or sitting positions.

Conclusion

Autonomic dysfunction with cardiorespiratory disturbance may be the sole initial manifestation of pediatric sleep–wake disorders (e.g., CCHS) or may constitute a significant comorbidity (e.g., narcolepsy). History and assessment of the autonomic system utilizing a comprehensive test battery and molecular genetic studies are needed for diagnosis. A team management approach is required.

References

1. Sheldon SH. The function, phylogeny and ontogeny of sleep. In: Sheldon SH, Ferber R, Kryger MH, Gozal D, editors. Principles and practice of pediatric sleep medicine. Philadelphia: Elsevier Saunders; 2014. p. 3–11.
2. Home RS, Parslow PM, Harding R. Respiratory control and arousals in sleeping infants. Pediatr Resp Rev. 2004;5(3):190–8.
3. Willinger M, James LS, Catz C, et al. Defining the sudden infant death syndrome (SIDS): deliberations of an expert panel convened by the National Institute of Child Health and Human Development. Pediatr Pathol. 1991;11(5):677–84.
4. Moon RY, Fu L. Sudden infant death syndrome: an update. Pediatr Rev. 2012;33(7):314–20.
5. Kinney HC, Filiano JJ, White WF. Medullary serotonergic deficiency in the sudden infant death syndrome: review of a 15-year study of a single data set. J Neuropathol Exp Neurol. 2001;60(3):228–47.
6. Rubens D, Sarnat HB. Sudden infant death syndrome: an update and new perspectives of etiology. Handb Clin Neurol. 2013;112:867–74.
7. Kotagal S. The emerging role of hypocretin (orexin A) in the developing central nervous system. Sleep. 2012;35(2):171–2.
8. Aran A, Shors I, Lin L, et al. CSF levels of hypocretin-1 (orexin-A) peak during early infancy in humans. Sleep. 2012;35(2):187–91.
9. Ioakeimidis NS, Papamitsou T, Meditskou S, Iakovdou-Krist Z. Sudden infant death due to long QT syndrome: a brief review of the genetic substrate and prevalence. J Biol Res (Thessalon). 2017;24:6.
10. Graham SF, Turkoglu O, Kumar P, Yilmaz A, Bjorndahl TC, Han B, et al. Targeted metabolic profiling of post-mortem brain from infants who died of sudden infant death syndrome. J Proteome Res. 2017;16(7):2587–96.
11. van Rijt WJ, Koolhaas GD, Bekhof J, Heiner Fokkema MR, de Koning TJ, et al. Inborn errors of metabolism that cause sudden infant death: a systematic review with implications for population neonatal screening programmes. Neonatology. 2016;109(4):297–302.
12. Tieder JS, Bonkowsky JL, Etzel RA, Franklin WH, Gremse DA, Herman B, Subcommittee on Apparent Life-Threatening Events, et al. Brief resolved unexplained events (formerly apparent life-threatening events) and evaluation of lower risk infants: executive summary. Pediatrics. 2016;137(5). https://doi.org/10.1542/peds.2016-0591.
13. Zwemer E, Claudius I, Tieder J. Update on the evaluation and management of brief resolved unexplained events (previously apparent life-threatening events). Rev Recent Clin Trials. 2017;12(4):233–9.
14. Patwari PP. Congenital central hypoventilation syndrome. In: Sheldon SH, Ferber R, Kryger MH, Gozal D, editors. Principles and practice of pediatric sleep medicine. Philadelphia: Elsevier Saunders; 2014. p. 301–5.
15. Weese-Mayer DE, Berry-Kravis EM, Ceccherini I, Keens TG, Loghmanee DA, Trang H, ATS Congenital Central Hypoventilation Syndrome Subcommittee. An official ATS clinical policy statement: congenital central hypoventilation syndrome: genetic basis, diagnosis and management. Am J Respir Crit Care Med. 2010;181(6):626–44.
16. Berry-Kravis EM, Zhou L, Rand CM, Weese-Mayer DE. Congenital central hypoventilation syndrome: PHOX2B mutations and phenotype. Am J Respir Crit Care Med. 2006;174(10):1139–44.
17. Rao GS, Ramesh VJ, Lalla RK. Ventilatory management and weaning in a patient with central hypoventilation caused by a brainstem cavernoma. Acta Anesthesiol Scand. 2005;49(8):1214–7.
18. Hui SH, Wing YK, Poon W, Chan YL, Buckley TA. Alveolar hypoventilation in brainstem glioma with improvement after surgical resection. Chest. 2000;118(1):266–8.
19. Najjar M, Taylor A, Agrawal S, Fojo T, Merkler AE, Rosenblum MK, et al. Anti-Hu paraneoplastic brainstem encephalitis caused by a pancreatic neuroendocrine tumor presenting with central hypoventilation. J Clin Neurosci. 2017;40:72–3.
20. Solliday NH, Gaensler EA, Schwaber JR, Parker TF. Impaired central chemoreceptor function following and chronic hypoventilation many years following poliomyelitis. Case report. Respiration. 1974;31(2):177–92.
21. Ferré Á, Poca MA, de la Calzada MD, Moncho D, Romero O, Sampol G, Sahuquillo J. Sleep disordered breathing in Chiari

malformation type 1: a prospective study of 90 patients. Sleep. 2017;40(6). https://doi.org/10.1093/sleep/zsx069.
22. Lee JM, Shin J, Kim S, Gee HY, Lee JS, Cha DH, et al. Rapid-onset obesity with hypoventilation, hypothalamic, autonomic dysregulation, and neuroendocrine tumors (ROHHADNET) syndrome: a systematic review. Biomed Res Int. 2018;2018:1250721.
23. Patwari PP, Rand CM. Rapid onset obesity with hypothalamic dysfunction, hypoventilation, and autonomic dysregulation (ROHHAD). In: Sheldon SH, Ferber R, Kryger MH, Gozal D, editors. Principles and practice of pediatric sleep medicine. Philadelphia: Elsevier Saunders; 2014. p. 307–10.
24. Miglis MG. Autonomic dysfunction in primary sleep disorders. Sleep Med. 2016;19:40–9.
25. Shirasaka T, Nakazato M, Matsukura S, Takasaki M, Kannan H. Sympathetic and cardiovascular actions of orexins in conscious rats. Am J Physiol. 1999;277(6):R1780–5.
26. Stewart JM, Boris JR, Chelimsky G, Fischer PR, Fortunato JE, Grubb BP, Pediatric Writing Group of the American Autonomic Society, et al. Pediatric disorders of orthostatic intolerance. Pediatrics. 2018;141(1):e20171673. Review.
27. Kim P, During E, Miglis M. A case of narcolepsy type 2 and postural tachycardia syndrome secondary to lesions of the thalamus and amygdala. J Clin Sleep Med. 2018;14(3):479–81.
28. Low PA. Evaluation of autonomic function. Curr Opin Neurol Neurosurg. 1992;5(4):461–3.

Autonomic Regulation of Sleep-Related Gastrointestinal Function

30

William C. Orr and Samih Raad

Introduction

Alterations in gastrointestinal (GI) function during sleep have been shown via an avalanche of recent research to be an integral part of normal function and an important element in the pathogenesis of GI disease [1]. Since the autonomic nervous system (ANS) is integrally involved in the control of GI function, it is essential to understand the role of the ANS to allow a more complete understanding of the pathogenesis and optimal treatment of GI disease. A cogent example of the role of ANS in sleep-related alterations of GI function relates to the pathogenesis of duodenal ulcer disease (DUD). Gastric acid secretion plays an important part, along with the presence of *Helicobacter pylori*, in the pathogenesis of DUD. Among the early successful treatments for DUD was a vagotomy which markedly diminished gastric acid secretion and promoted the healing of duodenal ulcers. Gastric acid secretion reaches a peak during sleep, and the inhibition of sleep-related acid secretion is an essential element for the healing of duodenal ulcers. In the development of H2 blockers such as ranitidine, the inhibition of nocturnal acid secretion was considered important and the 24-hour measurement of gastric pH became an important variable in the assessment of acid inhibition, particularly during the sleeping interval [2]. Two of the most common GI diseases are those with considerable involvement of autonomic function and sleep alterations associated with the clinical presentation, and pathogenesis of the diseases: gastroesophageal reflux disease (GERD) and irritable bowel disease (IBS). Disturbed sleep has also been shown to be involved with other less common disorders such as inflammatory bowel disease (IBD) and nonalcoholic fatty liver disease, but this review will focus on GERD and IBS.

Esophageal function is largely regulated by the vagus nerve. Swallowing induces a relaxation of both the upper esophageal sphincter (UES) and the lower esophageal sphincter (LES). These responses allow the transit of a bolus of food into the cervical esophagus and this initiates a peristaltic wave which transits the entire esophagus moving the bolus into the stomach via the relaxation of the LES. The main mechanism which allows this is the transient relaxation of the LES (TLESR) which is a spontaneous decrease in the resting LES pressure to near the intragastric baseline. These functions are initiated and perpetuated by the autonomic nervous system, predominately via afferent and efferent branches of the vagus nerve. This neural innervation allows the relaxation of the skeletal cricopharyngeal muscle and smooth muscle of the lower esophageal sphincter which is initiated by a swallow. Esophageal transit is also largely mediated via the vagal innervation of the esophagus, but also involved in this process are the glossopharyngeal, hypoglossal, and trigeminal cranial verves. LES relaxation is mediated by the afferent sensory branch of the vagus nerve. This stimulates the nucleus of the tractus solitarius which in turn activates the efferent branch of the vagus through the dorsal motor nucleus of the vagus which then initiates relaxation of the LES. Together, this innervation allows the coordinated contraction of the esophagus and transit of a swallowed bolus from the pharynx to the stomach. These autonomic functions mediating swallowing and esophageal peristalsis are essential in the normal functioning of the esophagus. These mechanisms are substantially altered during sleep [2]. Since swallowing is a volitional act, it is markedly diminished during sleep.

The main stimulus for the induction of a TLESR is gastric distention which occurs predominately subsequent to food ingestion. Since food ingestion does not occur during sleep, TLESRs are rare during sleep and it is well established that

W. C. Orr (✉)
University of Oklahoma Health Sciences Center, Oklahoma City, OK, USA

OU Medical Center, Gastroenterology, Oklahoma City, OK, USA
e-mail: worr@lhsi.net

S. Raad
Department of Pulmonary, Critical Care & Sleep Medicine, University of Oklahoma Health Sciences Center, Oklahoma City, OK, USA

S. Chokroverty, P. Cortelli (eds.), *Autonomic Nervous System and Sleep*, https://doi.org/10.1007/978-3-030-62263-3_30

reflux events are relatively fewer during sleep in GERD patients, and in fact rarely occur in normal individuals. Thus, patients and normal individuals do often observe belching and occasionally, heartburn, after a meal, but sleep-related reflux, and heartburn are relatively rare. It has been demonstrated that, although TLESRs are essentially absent during sleep, they do occur during transient arousals from sleep [3]. Along with the marked reduction in salivation and swallowing during sleep, esophageal clearance of refluxed gastric contents during sleep is substantially prolonged. The prolonged acid contact resulting from sleep-related gastroesophageal reflux (GER) is now accepted as a major factor in the pathogenesis of esophagitis [4]. Furthermore, sleep-related GER and its consequences have been suggested to constitute a distinct clinical entity that deserves special consideration and altered approach to treatment [5].

Gastroesophageal Reflux Disease (GERD)

A rational hypothesis regarding the pathogenesis of GERD would be altered vagal function. This hypothesis was tested by Chakraborty and colleagues in a study in which they assessed a variety of cardiovascular autonomic functions in addition to pupil cycle time which is a nonvagal function [6]. The study revealed that 40% of the GERD patients had significant abnormalities in vagally mediated autonomic function. Only a few patients showed any abnormal pupillary response suggesting that the autonomic abnormalities are part of a generalized vagal dysfunction. This study was published in 1989 and since then other studies have been done using somewhat more sophisticated methods of autonomic function assessment. A subsequent study in 2001 was conducted by Campo and colleagues in which they measured not only several standard cardiovascular tests of autonomic function, but they also did a spectral analysis of heart rate variability (HRV) in GERD patients and controls [7]. Spectral analysis of HRV is a more sophisticated technique of autonomic assessment which calculates heart rate functioning in the frequency domain rather than in the time domain. The power spectral analysis reveals relative activity in the high and low-frequency bands of heart rate functioning. The high-frequency (HF) band reflects vagal tone, the low-frequency (LF) band reflects sympathetic tone, and the LF/HF ratio reflects the sympathovagal balance. Figure 30.1 depicts normal autonomic function during sleep. It can be seen that there are two peaks in this analysis reflecting vagal and sympathetic tone. Twenty-four-hour esophageal pH monitoring was also measured. Results showed no significant heart rate variability changes associated with a reflux event (defined as a decrease in the esophageal pH below 4 for at least 5 minutes). A decrease in sympathetic tone was noted in the GERD group with only one of the cardiovascular measures.

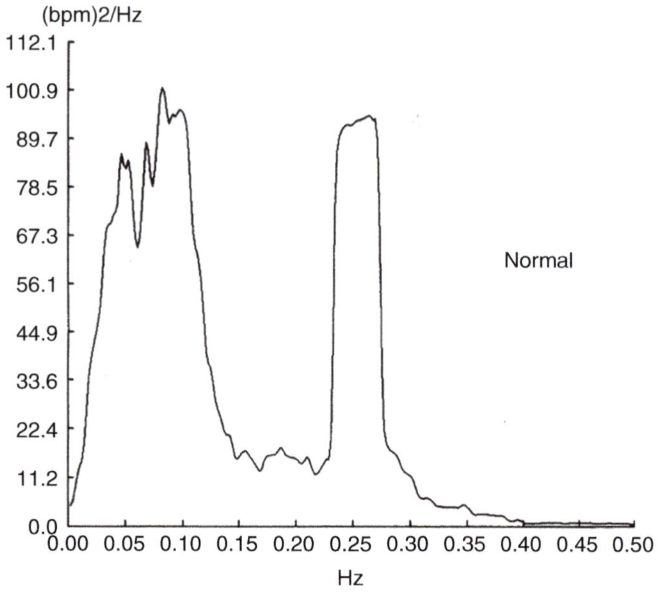

Fig. 30.1 Heart rate variability spectral analysis showing normal vagal and sympathetic responses to resting heart rate. Vagal tone is the peak in the high-frequency range and sympathetic tone is depicted in the low-frequency peak

However, total reflux time did show an inverse correlation with sympathetic tone in the GERD group. Thus, there appears to be some evidence for decreased sympathetic activity in the GERD group. The authors speculate that these changes could result in a decrease in intrinsic inhibitory control and thereby facilitate an increase in spontaneous relaxations of the LES.

It is of note that sleep disturbances in GERD patients have been shown to induce an alteration of visceral perception and pain thresholds [8]. This investigation showed that in GERD patients with sleep disturbance documented via actigraphy chest pain induced by acid infusion was clearly exacerbated after three nights of poor sleep. These functions are modulated by the afferent branch of the vagus nerve. This observation prompted study by Chen and Orr to test the hypothesis that altered autonomic function may be playing a role in the pathogenesis of GERD [9]. This was accomplished via the use of the spectral analysis of heart rate variability during the esophageal infusion of 0.1 N hydrochloric acid. In this study, water and acid infusion produced decreased vagal tone in GERD patients compared to normal controls. There was enhanced sympathetic dominance during acid infusion in GERD patients which was not noted in controls. This is most likely due to the decreased vagal tone noted in GERD patients. This provides support for the notion of altered autonomic function via the combined effects of enhanced sympathetic tone and decreased vagal input in GERD patients in response to acid mucosal contact. This is in contrast to the study noted by Campo et al. [7], which did show evidence of decreased sympathetic tone correlating with the percent acid contact time. The different measures of autonomic function are difficult to compare, but there does seem to be some agreement that sympathetic tone, as reflected in the overall sympathovagal balance may be associated with the pathogenesis of or a consequence of GERD.

In a subsequent study, Dobrek and colleagues examined autonomic functioning in GERD patients with and without esophagitis [10]. They examined the question of whether autonomic functioning would differentiate patients with esophagitis (i.e., mucosal inflammation) from those with heartburn symptoms but without esophagitis. If autonomic functioning was more altered in the esophagitis, it would suggest that the mucosal inflammation per se resulted in the autonomic changes since both groups have similar symptom manifestations. If autonomic functioning is not significantly different, it would suggest that any autonomic changes would be more generic and not related to the inflammation noted in the esophagitis group. In this study, spectral analysis was again used to assess autonomic functioning in three groups: patients with erosive esophagitis (EE); patients with nonerosive reflux disease (NERD) and normal controls. Autonomic functioning was assessed via HRV. Vagal tone was also decreased, but significantly more in the esophagitis patients. Thus, overall both patient groups showed a decrease in sympathetic tone while the EE group also had a more pronounced decrease in vagal tone. Both groups did show decreased vagal tone compared to controls suggesting that inflammatory changes alone do not account for these findings. Since the authors did not present any data on the LF/HF ratio, these results remain somewhat difficult to interpret definitively.

A similar subsequent study was conducted by Chen and colleagues in which they also examined autonomic functioning in patients with erosive and nonerosive esophagitis [11] Again, the primary measure of autonomic function was the spectral analysis of heart rate variability. This study demonstrated that the high-frequency power (vagal tone) was lower in patients with EE compared to NERD patients and controls, while the LF and LF/HF ratio was significantly lower in the NERD patients compared to the EE patients and controls. No relationship was noted between symptom severity score in either patient group. The authors concluded that autonomic changes do distinguish EE from NERD patients in that the EE patients tended to show decreased vagal tone while diminished sympathetic modulation distinguishes the NERD group. This study demonstrates that, in contrast to the results noted by Dobrek et al. [10], autonomic function does vary in terms of mucosal involvement. As noted above, Chen and Orr addressed this issue directly by assessing autonomic responses to acid mucosal contact via esophageal acid infusion [9]. The patient group experienced a greater degree of heartburn as would be expected. There were no changes in sympathetic tone as measured by HRV; however, there was a significant decrease in vagal tone and a corresponding increase in sympathovagal balance (LF/HR ratio). This would suggest that mucosal inflammation does have some effect on autonomic function, but it remains to be determined as to whether these changes represent a cause or an effect of the inflammatory process. These data are somewhat in agreement with the Campo study noted above which showed decreased sympathetic tone in GERD patients although no information was provided as to whether or not these patients had esophagitis.

In conclusion, autonomic changes have been clearly documented in GERD patients. These relate largely to a *diminished sympathetic tone* and an *enhanced sympathetic dominance* which appears to be related to decreased vagal tone. None of these investigations involved sleep or circadian rhythm assessments. It is, however, of interest to note that in a study of diabetic patients with autonomic neuropathy showed impairment of the circadian cycle of both the LF and HF components compared to diabetics without neuropathy [12]. This suggests that there may be some sleep-related alterations in the autonomic functioning of GERD patients which may further distinguish GERD patients with and without inflammatory changes in the esophageal mucosa.

Irritable Bowel Syndrome

Irritable bowel syndrome (IBS) is an enigmatic but extremely prevalent GI disorder [13]. The prevalence in the general population is noted between 10% and 25% [13]. In addition, it is thought to be the most commonly encountered functional GI disorder encountered in primary care [14]. IBS is vaguely defined as a disorder which is characterized by abdominal pain with relief with defecation, altered bowel habits (diarrhea, constipation or alternating constipation and diarrhea), and abdominal bloating [15, 16]. Although numerous pathophysiological mechanisms have been proposed there is no definitive biomarker for IBS. Among the proposed pathophysiological mechanisms associated with IBS is autonomic dysfunction. The autonomic nervous system is critical in the modulation and transformation of environmental and psychological variables into physiological function or dysfunction during sleep. Thus, alterations in autonomic function will affect physiological functioning during sleep and conversely autonomic dysfunction can alter physiological function in sleep. Sleep is largely a parasympathetic state with periodic bursts of sympathetic activity noted with arousals from sleep and during phasic REM sleep as noted with episodes of gastroesophageal reflux or upper airway obstruction in sleep apnea. The transient relaxation of the LES (TLESRs) is largely modulated by vagal function, and it is well known that these relaxations are inhibited during sleep resulting in a marked decrease in reflux events. Furthermore, a disruption in the brain–gut axis via altered sleep was suggested in a study which showed an increase in REM sleep and disruption in gastric electrical rhythms in IBS patients [16]. In addition, visceral pain sensitivity, a vagally mediated function, has been shown to be enhanced as a result of sleep disturbance [8]. In addition, a study by Jarrett and colleagues has shown a link between sleep disturbance and GI symptoms [17]. In this study, they demonstrated a significant relationship between daytime GI symptoms and poor sleep on the subsequent night. This was maintained when stress and other psychological variables were controlled. This relationship is likely mediated via the ANS. There is, therefore, a clear and important integration of sleep, autonomic function, and gastrointestinal disorders.

The most commonly used technique to assess autonomic dysfunction is HRV. Studies utilizing HRV in IBS have been reviewed by Mazurak and colleagues [18]. This review points out the variability of results and the many variables that can affect results such as BMI, age, and respiratory rate that need to be routinely controlled. They also note that there are many issues which impair the comparability of results such as use of a small number of validated parameters in many studies and the inherent variability of the measures making comparability of results difficult. In addition, HRV analysis and autonomic activity are very sensitive to many modulators such as BMI, respiratory rate, age, menstrual cycle, and medications use. Furthermore, the computation of Fourier transforms is complicated and dependent on many physiological characteristics such as how closely the measured cycle simulates a perfect sine wave. These factors all mitigate comparability of results.

Relevant studies on autonomic functioning in IBS involve both waking and sleep studies. The ANS plays an integral role in symptom manifestation in IBS due to the pervasive role of the ANS, particularly the vagus nerve, in GI functioning. IBS symptoms involve alterations in both sensory and motor functioning. It has been suggested, for example, that IBS patients have a visceral hyperalgesia which makes them more susceptible to pain from stimuli that would be considered part of normal GI functioning; these pain symptoms are modulated by the ANS. A seminal study addressing these issues was conducted by Iovino and colleagues [19]. In this study, they assessed the effects of sympathetic activation via enhanced lower body negative pressure. Autonomic reflexes were measured by duodenal and gastric barostat measures. Visceral but not somatic pain responses were enhanced by increased sympathetic activation. These results offer an explanation as to how symptoms of abdominal pain and bloating can occur to normal intestinal distention in patients with IBS. Abnormal responses to normal levels of intestinal gas may be a common culprit in generating abdominal pain and bloating which are classic symptoms of IBS. Further emphasizing these symptoms is the relief of abdominal pain after a bowel movement which constitutes one of the cornerstones of the diagnosis of IBS.

Sleep and Irritable Bowel Syndrome

Also important in the pathogenesis of IBS symptoms are the very prevalent comorbid symptoms of anxiety and depression, and disturbed sleep [20]. Of particular importance is the coincidental symptom of insomnia commonly noted with complaints of anxiety and depression, and the very common occurrence of sleep complaints in IBS patients [18, 21]. It is well established that depression has a negative impact on sleep and that IBS patients have significant symptoms of clinical depression [21, 22]. There is a bidirectional relationship: IBS is 33% more common in patients with sleep disturbance, and the risk of having IBS is 1.6 times greater in individuals with sleep disturbance compared to those without sleep disturbance [20]. These data are of particular interest since, as noted above, sleep disturbance can exacerbate visceral pain responses. For example, Chen and colleagues have shown that patients with subjective sleep disturbance as assessed by the Pittsburg Sleep Quality Index (PSQI) revealed enhanced sensitivity to rectal distention [23]. Thus, it has been suggested that this may result in a vicious cycle of enhanced pain that creates and causes an enhanced sleep disturbance as noted in the study by Maneerattanaporn and Chey (Fig. 30.2) [24]. This brain–gut connection is modulated through the ANS. It is relevant that insomnia has been noted to be associated with autonomic abnormalities. For example, Bonnet and Arand showed a significant sympathetic dominance in insomnia patients using HRV analysis [25]. In a study from our laboratory, Elsenbruch et al. noted that subjective sleep abnormalities were noted in IBS patients compared to controls, but objective PSG measures were not significantly different [26]. It was pointed out that this pattern is commonly noted in insomnia patients and is described as sleep state misperception (paradoxical insomnia). Similar results have been noted by Heitkemper et al., which showed only a very weak relationship between the objective and subjective sleep measures [27]. However, their study related PSG measures to subjective sleep quality the following morning while the Elsenburch study utilized the Pittsburg Sleep Quality Index to assess sleep quality over the previous month. Insomnia complaints have also been associated with high-frequency EEG activity and Maes et al. have correlated this subjective complaint with K complexes and alpha intrusion, and an ANS pattern of reduced parasympathetic activity and increased sympathetic dominance [28]. Thus, the presence of difficulty sleeping, associated ANS changes, and poor sleep-related visceral hyperalgesia coalesce to help explain the symptoms commonly noted in IBS patients. An understanding of the pathogenesis of IBS, its sleep, and autonomic correlates requires an assessment of the sleep and autonomic consequences resulting from comorbidities such as anxiety and depression [20, 22].

Among the first studies to utilize HRV analysis in long-term recordings with IBS patients was accomplished by

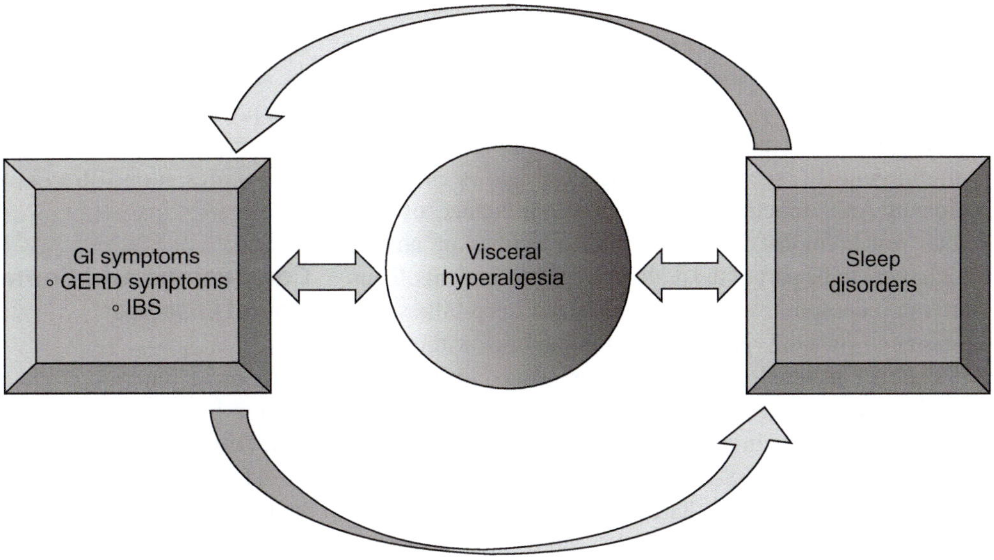

Fig. 30.2 Proposed relationship between sleep disorders and gastrointestinal symptoms. (From Maneerattanaporn and Chey [24], with permission John Wiley & Sons)

Heitkemper et al., and our group [29, 30]. Our study utilized HRV analysis during PSG-monitored sleep. The results revealed an increase in the low-frequency HRV band during waking in IBS patients corresponding to increased sympathetic dominance. No differences were noted in the high-frequency band corresponding to vagal tone during any state. However, the LF/HR ratio was significantly greater in IBS patients during REM sleep. These results are consistent with increased sympathetic activity in IBS patients and this is particularly noted during REM sleep. It was observed by the authors that these data could support the hypothesis of an enhanced sympathetic activity contributing to increased waking susceptibility to pain. The Heitkemper study did not specifically note sleep-related changes in autonomic functioning, but rather employed ANS functioning utilizing EKG data from a 24-hour Holter monitoring system. Vagal tone was significantly decreased and the LR/HF ratio was increased in the constipation (IBS-C) predominant group. These differences were most notable in patients with more severe symptoms. Thus, sleep state, symptom severity, and IBS subgroup are all important variables in understanding autonomic functioning during sleep.

As stated above, visceral sensitivity is modulated largely by the ANS and subtle abnormalities in autonomic functioning may contribute to the clinical presentation of patients in IBS symptom subgroups. It is well established that autonomic function is altered during sleep and particularly during REM sleep. Alterations in sleep patterns have not shown consistent differences in IBS patients, but it seems clear that changes in sleep functioning are an important element in the pathogenesis of IBS [21]. Results of various studies and the suggestion that ANS functioning may be different during sleep in IBS subgroups demonstrate the complexity of the pathogenesis of IBS and that the presenting bowel habit pattern (constipation, diarrhea or alternating) may constitute phenotypical presentations of this complicated disease entity.

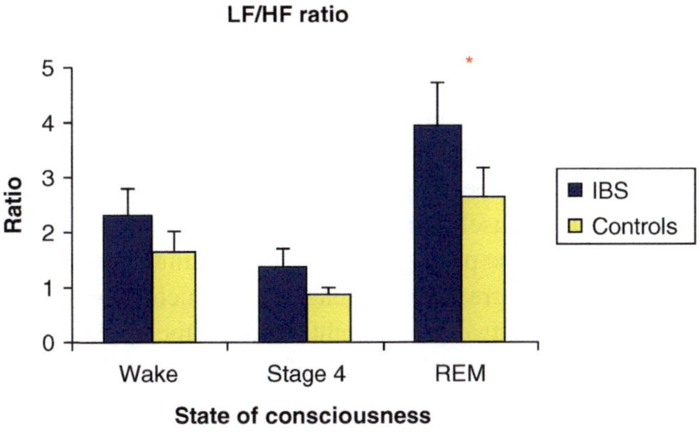

Fig. 30.3 Heart rate variability data during different stages of sleep in IBS patients. Sympathetic balance is depicted in terms of the ration of sympathetic and vagal tone. Note that sympathetic dominance is significantly greater during REM sleep in the IBS patients. (Data from Thompson et al. [31])

Differences in autonomic function likely play an important role in the expression of the clinical symptoms in these IBS subgroups. In the Heitkemper study [27], the overall 24-hour assessment of HRV noted differences in ANS function in IBS symptom subgroups. Subsequent studies have looked more closely at this issue. Two studies from our laboratory have addressed the issue of ANS functioning during sleep in different IBS symptom subgroups. Shortly after the publication of the study by Heitkemper et al., we embarked on a more detailed study in which HRV was assessed during different sleep stages and compared across different IBS symptom groups (dyspeptic vs. nondyspeptic) [31]. In the IBS patients without dyspeptic symptoms, a substantial vagal withdrawal was noted during REM sleep and the LF/HF ratio was greater indicating enhanced sympathetic tone (Fig. 30.3). Although this study did not incorporate typical IBS symptom subgroups such as IBS-C or IBS-D, it does illustrate that autonomic involvement in symptom generation may be different when other GI organs are involved. It was noted that IBS patients had an increase in REM sleep which did appear to manifest itself in altered basic gastric electrical rhythm [16].

The ability to study autonomic functioning in patients with different IBS subgroups during sleep allows an examination of ANS functioning without the influence of conscious psychological influences such as stress or anxiety which seem to be part of the daily lives of IBS patients. Thus, studying autonomic functioning during sleep allows an assessment of pure physiologic functioning without the influence of psychological state. Our group attempted to describe autonomic functioning during sleep [32] by using the HRV techniques in three typical IBS subgroups: constipation predominant (IBS-C), diarrhea predominant (IBS-D), and IBS with alternating diarrhea and constipation symptoms (IBS-A). It was found in this study that the IBS-D group experienced significant vagal withdrawal during REM and non-REM sleep compared to the IBS-A group. This resulted in a greater degree of sympathetic dominance noted primarily during non-REM sleep in the IBS-D group. The IBS-D patients were physiologically distinct from the IBS-A patients, but not from the IBS-C group. Although not definitive, this study does suggest that these investigative techniques can be useful in a more complete and revealing explanation of the pathogenesis of IBS. A similar study was conducted by Jarrett and colleagues in which they had an advantage of a two-study night PSG protocol [33]. This study did not confirm the results of the Robert et al.'s study, and in fact the results of the study by Jarrett et al. were notably different. In the study by Jarrett et al. [33], the vagal was enhanced and the sympathovagal balance was diminished in the IBS-D compared to both IBS-C and IBS-A during both REM and non-REM sleep. These discrepancies bring into focus the complexity of IBS diagnosis and the likelihood that these IBS subgroups are not clear-cut phenotypes.

IBS patients frequently have comorbid symptoms of sleep disturbance and psychological issues such as anxiety and depression. In order to assess the role of depression in sleep quality and autonomic function in IBS patients, our laboratory undertook a study in which we compared a group of IBS patients with depressive symptoms as assessed by the Beck Depression Inventory compared to a group of IBS patients without depressive symptoms [34]. HRV analysis was assessed during PSG-monitored sleep and subjective sleep quality was determined via the PSQI. The IBS depression group revealed more disturbed sleep as measured by the PSQI compared to the nondepressed group. The IBS-depressed group revealed a more prolonged REM onset latency than normal controls, but this was not significantly different in the nondepressed group. The depressed group also showed a significant increase in GI symptom severity. HRV analysis did not reveal significant differences between the study groups either during waking or sleep stages. These data provide additional support for the importance of comorbid conditions such as depression and sleep disturbance in the manifestation IBS symptoms.

Conclusions and Comments on Inflammatory Bowel Disease

Autonomic function is the critical link to the intimate connection between brain and gut. Autonomic function affects both GI function and sleep, and the link to these phenomena would seem to provide a clearer and more in-depth understanding of GI function and associated sleep disorders. It is well established that autonomic function is critical to the modulation of visceral sensation and visceral pain. Autonomic function is also modulated substantially by state of consciousness such as sleep and psychological states (e.g., anxiety, depression, and stress). It has been demonstrated that all of these variables affect sleep and that sleep plays an important role in the pathogenesis of commonly encountered diseases such as GERD and IBS. Although no definitive conclusions can made given the current state of research in this area of sleep-related autonomic functioning in GI disease, the studies have provided an important impetus to further research. The cited studies differ in many variables such as sample size, age, male, female composition, and effects of the menstrual cycle. Since the majority of IBS patients are women, this is an important variable (e.g., menstrual cycle) in any study on IBS patients. More recently, sleep has been shown to affect symptom manifestation and disease progression in IBD [35]. The ANS is heavily involved in the perception of visceral pain, and inflammation of the gut wall can clearly influence the perception of visceral pain. Thus, any stimulus that alters visceral perception can affect the manifestation and progression of IBD. It has been noted in this review that sleep disturbance can induce visceral hyperalgesia. Thus, sleep disturbances noted in IBD patients can enhance the perception of visceral pain and therefore enhance disease symptom manifestation in IBD patients.

Autonomic functioning in IBD has been reviewed by Taylor et al., but there are no references specifically to autonomic functioning during sleep [36]. This review has focused on the commonly noted sleep disturbances with IBD patients. Autonomic disturbances have been extrapolated from existing data on autonomic disturbances during waking noted in IBD patients. However, the dearth of studies related to autonomic function specifically during sleep is notable and emphasizes this as a fruitful area for future investigation.

References

1. Johnson DA, Orr WC, Ware JC, editors. Sleep effect on gastrointestinal health and disease: translational opportunities for promoting health and optimizing disease management. New York: Nova Biomedical; 2018.
2. Chokroverty S, Ferini-Strambi L, editors. Oxford textbook of sleep disorders. Oxford: Oxford University Press; 2017.
3. Freidin N, Fisher MJ, Taylor W, Boyd D, Surratt P, Mccallum RW, et al. Sleep and nocturnal acid reflux in normal subjects and patients with reflux oesophagitis. Gut. 1991;32(11):1275–9.
4. Orr W. Sleep and gastroesophageal reflux disease: a wake-up call. Rev Gastroenterol Disord. 2004;4(Suppl 4):S25–32.
5. Orr WC. Review article: sleep-related gastro-oesophageal reflux as a distinct clinical entity. Aliment Pharmacol Ther. 2010;31(1):47–56.
6. Chakraborty TK, Ogilvie AL, Heading RC, Ewing DJ. Abnormal cardiovascular reflexes in patients with gastro-oesophageal reflux. Gut. 1989;30(1):46–9.
7. Campo SMA, Capria A, Antonucci F, Martino G, Ciamei A, Rossini PM, et al. Decreased sympathetic inhibition in gastroesophageal reflux disease. Clin Auton Res. 2001;11(1):45–51.
8. Schey R, Dickman R, Parthasarathy S, Quan SF, Wendel C, Merchant J, et al. Sleep deprivation is hyperalgesic in patients with gastroesophageal reflux disease. Gastroenterology. 2007;133(6):1787–95.
9. Chen C-L, Orr WC. Autonomic responses to heartburn induced by esophageal acid infusion. J Gastroenterol Hepatol. 2004;19(8):922–6.
10. Dobrek L, Nowakowski M, Mazur M, Thor PJ. Disturbances of the parasympathetic branch of the autonomic nervous system in patients with gastroesophageal reflux disease (GERD) estimated by short-term heart rate variability recordings. J Physiol Pharmacol. 2004;55(Suppl 2):77–90.
11. Chen C-L, Orr WC, Yang CC, Kuo TB. Cardiac autonomic regulation differentiates reflux disease with and without erosive esophagitis. Scand J Gastroenterol. 2006;41(9):1001–6.
12. Yamamoto M, Yamasaki Y, Kodama M, Matsuhisa M, Kishimoto M, Ozaki H, et al. Impaired diurnal cardiac autonomic function in subjects with type 2 diabetes. Diabetes Care. 1999;22(12):2072–7.
13. Saito Y. The epidemiology of irritable bowel syndrome in North America: a systematic review. Am J Gastroenterol. 2002;97(8):1910–5.
14. Bellini M, Tosetti C, Costa F, Biagi S, Stasi C, Punta AD, et al. The general practitioners approach to irritable bowel syndrome: from intention to practice. Dig Liver Dis. 2005;37(12):934–9.
15. Drossman D, Whitehead W, Camilleri M. Irritable bowel syndrome: a technical review for practice guideline development. Gastroenterology. 1997;112(6):2120–37.
16. Orr WC, Crowell MD, Lin B, Harnish MJ, Chen JDZ. Sleep and gastric function in irritable bowel syndrome: derailing the brain-gut axis. Gut. 1997;41(3):390–3.
17. Jarrett M, Heitkemper M, Cain KC, Burr RL, Hertig V. Sleep disturbance influences gastrointestinal symptoms in women with irritable bowel syndrome. Dig Dis Sci. 2000;45(5):952–9.
18. Mazurak N, Seredyuk N, Sauer H, Teufel M, Enck P. Heart rate variability in the irritable bowel syndrome: a review of the literature. Neurogastroenterol Motil. 2012;24(3):206–16.
19. Iovino P, Azpiroz F, Domingo E, Malagelada JR. The sympathetic nervous system modulates perception and reflex responses to gut distention in humans. Gastroenterology. 1995;108(3):680–6.
20. Vege SS, Locke GR, Weaver AL, Farmer SA, Melton LJ, Talley NJ. Functional gastrointestinal disorders among people with sleep disturbances: a population-based study. Mayo Clin Proc. 2004;79(12):1501–6.
21. Tu Q, Heitkemper MM, Jarrett ME, Buchanan DT. Sleep disturbances in irritable bowel syndrome: a systematic review. Neurogastroenterol Motil. 2016;29(3):e12946.
22. Spiller R. Clinical update: irritable bowel syndrome. Lancet. 2007;369(9573):1586–8.
23. Chen CL, Liu TT, Yi CH, Orr WC. Evidence for altered anorectal function in irritable bowel syndrome patients with sleep disturbance. Digestion. 2011;84(3):247–51.
24. Maneerattanaporn M, Chey WD. Sleep disorders and gastrointestinal symptoms: chicken, egg or vicious cycle? Neurogastroenterol Motil. 2009;21(2):97–9.
25. Bonnet MH, Arand DL. Heart rate variability in insomniacs and matched normal sleepers. Psychosom Med. 1998;60(5):610–5.
26. Elsenbruch S, Harnish MJ, Orr W. Subjective and objective sleep quality in irritable bowel syndrome. Am J Gastroenterol. 1999;94(9):2447–52.
27. Heitkemper M, Burr R, Jarrett M, Hertig V, Lustyk M, Bond E. Evidence for autonomic nervous system imbalance in patients with irritable bowel syndrome. Dig Dis Sci. 1998;43(9):2093–9.
28. Maes J, Verbraecken J, Willemen M, Volder ID, Gastel AV, Michiels N, et al. Sleep misperception, EEG characteristics and autonomic nervous system activity in primary insomnia: a retrospective study on polysomnographic data. Int J Psychophysiol. 2014;91(3):163–71.
29. Orr W. Autonomic regulation of cardiac function during sleep in patients with irritable bowel syndrome. Am J Gastroenterol. 2000;95(10):2865–71.
30. Heitkemper M, Jarrett M, Cain KC, Burr R, Levy RL, Feld A, et al. Autonomic nervous system function in women with irritable bowel syndrome. Dig Dis Sci. 2001;46(6):1276–84.
31. Thompson JJ, Elsenbruch S, Harnish MJ, Orr W. Autonomic functioning during REM sleep differentiates IBS symptom subgroups. Am J Gastroenterol. 2002;97(12):3147–53.
32. Robert JJT, Elsenbruch S, Orr WC. Sleep-related autonomic disturbances in symptom subgroups of women with irritable bowel syndrome. Dig Dis Sci. 2006;51(12):2121–7.
33. Jarrett ME, Burr RL, Cain KC, Rothermel JD, Landis CA, Heitkemper MM. Autonomic nervous system function during sleep among women with irritable bowel syndrome. Dig Dis Sci. 2008;53(3):694–703.
34. Robert JJ, Orr WC, Elsenbruch S. Modulation of sleep quality and autonomic functioning by symptoms of depression in women with irritable bowel syndrome. Dig Dis Sci. 2004;49(7/8):1250–8.
35. Ranjbaran Z, Keefer L, Farhadi A, Stepanski E, Sedghi S, Keshavarzian A. Impact of sleep disturbances in inflammatory bowel disease. J Gastroenterol Hepatol. 2007;22:1748–53.
36. Taylor CT, Keely SJ. The autonomic nervous system and inflammatory bowel disease. Auton Neurosci. 2007;133(1):104–14.

Index

S. Chokroverty, P. Cortelli (eds.), *Autonomic Nervous System and Sleep*, https://doi.org/10.1007/978-3-030-62263-3

Q

R

GPSR Compliance

The European Union's (EU) General Product Safety Regulation (GPSR) is a set of rules that requires consumer products to be safe and our obligations to ensure this.

If you have any concerns about our products, you can contact us on ProductSafety@springernature.com

In case Publisher is established outside the EU, the EU authorized representative is:

Springer Nature Customer Service Center GmbH
Europaplatz 3
69115 Heidelberg, Germany

Batch number: 10731667

Printed by Printforce, the Netherlands